WITHDRAWN

CHRONIC ILLNESS

IMPACT AND INTERVENTION

EIGHTH EDITION

EDITED BY

ILENE MOROF LUBKIN, MS, RN, CGNP
Professor Emeritus
California State University
Hayward, California

PAMALA D. LARSEN, PHD, RN, CRRN, FNGNA
Associate Dean for Academic Affairs and Professor
Fay W. Whitney School of Nursing
University of Wyoming
Laramie, Wyoming

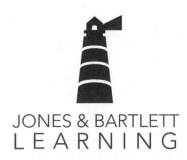

JONES & BARTLETT
LEARNING

World Headquarters
Jones & Bartlett Learning
5 Wall Street
Burlington, MA 01803
978-443-5000
info@jblearning.com
www.jblearning.com

Jones & Bartlett Learning books and products are available through most bookstores and online booksellers. To contact Jones & Bartlett Learning directly, call 800-832-0034, fax 978-443-8000, or visit our website, www.jblearning.com.

Substantial discounts on bulk quantities of Jones & Bartlett Learning publications are available to corporations, professional associations, and other qualified organizations. For details and specific discount information, contact the special sales department at Jones & Bartlett Learning via the above contact information or send an email to specialsales@jblearning.com.

Production Credits

Publisher: Kevin Sullivan
Acquisitions Editor: Amanda Harvey
Editorial Assistant: Sara Bempkins
Production Editor: Amanda Clerkin
Marketing Manager: Elena McAnespie
V.P., Manufacturing and Inventory Control: Therese Connell

Composition: Laserwords Private Limited, Chennai, India
Cover Design: Kristin E. Parker
Cover Image: © Jeffery Clathenburg/Dreamstime.com
Printing and Binding: Malloy, Inc.
Cover Printing: Malloy, Inc.

To order this product, use ISBN: 978-1-4496-4905-0

Library of Congress Cataloging-in-Publication Data
Chronic illness : impact and intervention / [edited by] Ilene M. Lubkin and Pamala D. Larsen.—8th ed.
    p. ; cm.
  Includes bibliographical references and index.
  ISBN-13: 978-0-7637-9966-3
  ISBN-10: 0-7637-9966-1
  I. Lubkin, Ilene Morof, 1928-2005. II. Larsen, Pamala D., 1947-
  [DNLM: 1. Chronic Disease—psychology. 2. Professional-Family Relations. 3. Professional-Patient Relations. WT 500]
  LC classification not assigned
  616'.044—dc23

                                                                              2011029659

6048

Printed in the United States of America
16 15 14 13 12   9 8 7 6 5 4 3 2

To Randy, as we continue the chronic illness journey together

This text was developed by and originated with Ilene Morof Lubkin in 1986 and was the first work of its kind to address the psychosocial concepts of chronic illness. Pamala Larsen joined the project in its fourth edition in 1998. It remains a landmark work in the healthcare field.

Contents

Part IV Impact of the System   511

Preface

A VIEW FROM THAT OTHER PLACE

The first draft of the preface for this edition covered the usual topics—our expensive healthcare system providing limited access to some Americans, falling behind in life expectancy in the world and also in infant mortality, and a plea that we can't keep putting our head in the sand merely hoping that something will change, along with my usual plea that everyone with chronic illness needs a nurse as a case manager. Yes, it was very preachy, but how I feel.

However, during this past year my husband of 42 years was diagnosed with esophageal cancer. As Susan Sontag (1988) notes, "illness is the night-side of life, there is a kingdom of the well and a kingdom of the sick, and that eventually everyone is obligated, at least for a spell, to identify ourselves as citizens of that other place" (p. 3). My husband and I are now in "that other place"—the land of chronic illness. One would think that being a registered nurse for 42 years and caring for those with chronic illness in many settings would have made me an expert in this land. This is my area; I teach about it, know about it, and edit this textbook. This is "me." However, I didn't realize how little I knew about the kingdom of the sick. In the past I was confident that I knew what my patients/clients and families were going through. I was supportive. I was empathetic. I was working with them for optimal wellness. But I didn't *know*.

From the day of diagnosis, the day before Thanksgiving 2010 (funny, I don't even remember the date, just the relationship with Thanksgiving), you think your loved one's tests have been mixed up with someone else's, that it must be a mistake. These things happen to other people. You just had Christmas family pictures taken the prior weekend with all 11 grandchildren......you are happy, healthy, alive. This diagnosis isn't real. But it soon becomes your reality.

I think of the chapters in this book and how my husband and I can now relate to most of them. I've added a few quotes of my own in some of the chapters, but in reality, I could have added a thousand quotes about our experience. Luckily my husband's hospitalizations, surgeries, chemotherapy, radiation, and care have been in two Magnet hospitals. The nursing and medical care have been fantastic. We've been actively involved in care decisions and have never felt like outsiders. But that care doesn't touch "that other place."

As nurses we advocate that one's illness shouldn't take over an individual's life, that illness is just part of who the person is. A lofty goal, but the reality is that your life is often your illness. They are one and the same. Your life revolves around how many times you've vomited today; endless doctor appointments; electrolytes are off, need a bag of IV fluids and some potassium as an out-patient; titrating nocturnal jejunostomy feedings with oral intake; IV antibiotics for an infection of some kind; fatigue and weakness; and iatrogenic effects of treatment, to name just a few of the new additions to daily life. Hospitalizations become a blur as to what happened when. Some things, however, are permanently recorded in my brain, such as the night my husband had a cardiac arrest in ICU. Then the thought surfaces that none of this treatment will make any difference, and you talk, again, about advance directives, wills, and so on.

That other place. I didn't know until now.

Pamala D. Larsen

REFERENCES

Sontag, S. (1988). *Illness as metaphor*. Toronto, Canada: Collins Publishers.

Contributors

Susan J. Barnes, PhD, RN, CNE
Associate Professor and Chair
Transformative and Global Education
Kramer School of Nursing
Oklahoma City University
Oklahoma City, Oklahoma

Jill Berg, PhD, RN
Associate Professor
Program in Nursing Science
University of California, Irvine
Irvine, California

Diana Luskin Biordi, PhD, RN, FAAN
Associate Dean
Nursing Research and Scholarship
College of Nursing
The University of Akron
Akron, Ohio

Donna Carruthers, PhD, RN
Assistant Professor
School of Nursing
University of Pittsburgh
Pittsburgh, Pennsylvania

Anne Deutsch, PhD, RN, CRRN
Clinical Research Scientist
Rehabilitation Institute of Chicago *and*
Research Assistant Professor
Department of Physical Medicine and Rehabilitation &
Institute for Healthcare Studies
Northwestern University Feinberg School of Medicine
Chicago, Illinois

Jacqueline M. Dunbar-Jacob, PhD, RN, FAAN
Dean, School of Nursing
Professor, Nursing, Psychology, Epidemiology and Occupational Therapy
Director, Center for Research in Chronic Disorders
University of Pittsburgh
Pittsburgh, Pennsylvania

Lorraine S. Evangelista, PhD, RN
Associate Professor
Program in Nursing Science
University of California, Irvine
Irvine, California

Patricia McCann Galon, PhD, CNS
Associate Professor
College of Nursing
The University of Akron
Akron, Ohio

Sonya R. Hardin, PhD, RN, CCRN, NP-C
Professor
School of Nursing
University of North Carolina, Charlotte
Charlotte, North Carolina

Ann Marie Hart, PhD, APRN-BC, FNP
Associate Professor
Fay W. Whitney School of Nursing
University of Wyoming
Laramie, Wyoming

Judith E. Hertz, PhD, RN, FNGNA
Associate Professor
School of Nursing and Health Studies
Northern Illinois University
DeKalb, Illinois

Alicia Huckstadt, PhD, RN, APRN, FNP-BC, GNP-BC
Professor and Director, DNP Program
School of Nursing
Wichita State University
Wichita, Kansas

Faye I. Hummel, PhD, RN, CTN
Professor
School of Nursing
University of Northern Colorado
Greeley, Colorado

Cynthia S. Jacelon, PhD, RN-BC, CRRN, FAAN
Associate Professor
Director of Departmental Honors
School of Nursing
University of Massachusetts, Amherst
Amherst, Massachusetts

Pamala D. Larsen, PhD, CRRN, FNGNA
Associate Dean for Academic Affairs, Professor
Fay W. Whitney School of Nursing
University of Wyoming
Laramie, Wyoming

Barbara J. Lutz, PhD, RN, CRRN, FAHA
Associate Professor
College of Nursing
University of Florida
Gainesville, Florida

Kristin L. Mauk, PhD, DNP, RN, CRRN, GCNS-BC, GNP-BC, FAAN
Professor of Nursing
Kreft Endowed Chair
Valparaiso University
Valparaiso, Indiana

Elaine T. Miller, PhD, RN, CRRN, FAAN, FAHA
Professor of Nursing
Coordinator, Center for Aging with Dignity
College of Nursing
University of Cincinnati
Cincinnati, Ohio

Nicholas R. Nicholson, Jr., PhD, MPH, RN, PHCNS-BC
Postdoctoral Fellow
Geriatric Clinical Epidemiology and Aging-Related Research
Yale University School of Medicine
New Haven, Connecticut

Linda L. Pierce, PhD, RN, CNS, CRRN, FAHA, FAAN
Professor
College of Nursing
University of Toledo
Toledo, Ohio

Barbara M. Raudonis, PhD, RN, FNGNA, FPCN
Associate Professor
College of Nursing
University of Texas, Arlington
Arlington, Texas

Victoria Schirm, PhD, RN
Director of Nursing Research
Penn State Milton S. Hershey Medical Center
Hershey, Pennsylvania

Betty Smith-Campbell, PhD, RN
Professor
School of Nursing
Wichita State University
Wichita, Kansas

Diane L. Stuenkel, EdD, RN
Professor
The Valley Foundation School of Nursing
San Jose State University
San Jose, California

Margaret Chamberlain Wilmoth, PhD, RN, MSS, FAAN
Professor
School of Nursing
University of North Carolina, Charlotte
Charlotte, North Carolina

Vivian K. Wong, PhD, RN
Associate Professor
The Valley Foundation School of Nursing
San Jose State University
San Jose, California

PART I

Impact of the Disease

CHAPTER 1

Chronicity

Pamala D. Larsen

The prevalence of chronic disease worldwide is similar if not greater than it is in the United States. Chronic diseases are the leading cause of death in the world, accounting for 60% of all deaths worldwide (World Health Organization [WHO], 2011). Twenty percent of chronic disease deaths occur in high-income countries, whereas the remaining 80% occur in low- and middle-income countries, where most of the world's population resides (WHO, 2011).

There is a wide variety of conditions that are considered chronic, and each condition needs a diverse array of services to care for affected individuals. For example, consider clients with Alzheimer's disease, cerebral palsy, heart disease, acquired immunodeficiency syndrome (AIDS), or spinal cord injury; each of these clients has unique physical needs, and each needs different services from a healthcare system that is attuned to delivering acute care.

The first baby boomers turned 65 in 2011, and this event has focused increased attention on the capabilities of the healthcare system. The baby boomer generation, in particular, has been vocal about the inability of the healthcare system to meet current needs, let alone future needs.

INTRODUCTION

In 2005 it was estimated that there were 133 million individuals living with at least one chronic disease (Centers for Disease Control and Prevention [CDC], 2010a), and that 7 of every 10 Americans who die each year—or more than 1.7 million people—die of a chronic disease. Chronic disease accounts for one-third of the years of potential life lost before age 65. The data that have quantified the costs from chronic disease are quite sobering as well:

- The direct and indirect costs of diabetes were $174 billion in 2007 (American Diabetes Association, 2011).
- In 2010, the cost of heart disease and stroke was $316.4 billion (CDC, 2010b).
- The direct cost of cancer care in 2010 was $124 billion (National Cancer Institute, 2011).
- The medical costs of people with chronic disease account for more than 75% of the nation's $2 trillion medical care costs each year (CDC, 2008).

These facts indicate that chronic disease is the nation's greatest healthcare problem and the number one driver of health care today. With the aging population and the advanced technologies that assist clients in living longer lives, the costs will only increase.

The influx of baby boomers into organizations such as AARP has distinctly flavored the activities of that and other similar types of organizations. In addition, this new group of seniors is the most ethnically and racially diverse of any previous generation. This well educated, consumer-driven generation wants to be knowledgeable about their conditions and all treatment options. They question their healthcare providers and do not necessarily accept their healthcare advice and treatment options.

In 2000, minorities represented 16% of older American adults. By 2020 that percentage will increase to 24% (Administration on Aging [AOA], 2010). Unfortunately, the healthcare disparities that we have seen in the past regarding ethnic and racial groups are not decreasing, but rather increasing. Three key themes emerged from the 2009 National Health Disparities Report: 1) disparities are common and lack of health insurance is an important contributor; 2) many disparities are not decreasing; and 3) some disparities merit particular attention, especially care for cancer, heart failure, and pneumonia (Agency for Healthcare Research and Quality [AHRQ], 2010a). How will the current system or a future system cope with this diverse group of seniors and their accompanying chronic conditions?

Multiple factors have produced the increasing number of individuals with chronic disease. Developments in the fields of public health, genetics, immunology, technology, and pharmacology have led to a significant decrease in mortality from acute disease. Medical success has contributed, in part, to the unprecedented growth of chronic illness by extending life expectancy

and by earlier detection of disease in general. Living longer, however, leads to greater vulnerability to the occurrence of accidents and disease events that can become chronic in nature. The client who may have died from a myocardial infarction in earlier years now needs continuing health care for heart failure. The cancer survivor has healthcare needs related to the iatrogenic results of life-saving treatment. The adolescent, who is a quadriplegic because of an accident, may live a relatively long life with our current rehabilitation efforts, but needs continuous preventive and maintenance care from the healthcare system. Children with cystic fibrosis have benefited from lung transplantation, but need care for the rest of their lives. Therefore, many previously fatal conditions, injuries, and diseases have become chronic in nature.

Disease versus Illness

Although the terms, *disease* and *illness*, are often used interchangeably, there is a distinct difference between them. Disease refers to the pathophysiology of the condition, such as an alteration in structure and function. Illness, on the other hand, is the human experience of symptoms and suffering, and refers to how the disease is perceived, lived with, and responded to by individuals, their families, and their healthcare providers. Although it is important to recognize the pathophysiological process of a chronic disease, understanding the illness experience is essential to providing holistic care.

> I put my elbows on my knees and let my forehead sink into my palms. I'm tired. Not just tired…weary. My husband's catheter went AWOL at one in the morning, and we've spent the rest of the night in the ER (How many nights does that make now?

How many hours?) Noise and cold and too-bright lights and too-bright student doctors. Repeating Bruce's history, over and over. (Harleman, 2008, p. 74)

Today is the 19th day in a row that my husband has seen a healthcare provider, and actually a few of those times, he's seen two different ones on the same day. It's either radiation therapy, receiving IV fluids and/or replacement potassium, an IV antibiotic for a resistant infection, receiving blood as an out-patient, a mishap with the jejunostomy tube . . . something every day. Will this ever stop? Will we ever have a normal life again? Right now I don't even remember what normal is.

—*Jenny, wife of a 63-year-old cancer patient*

These patient stories chronicle part of the illness experience. The illness experience is nursing's domain. Thus, the focus of this book is on the illness experience of individuals and families, and not specific disease processes. While nursing cannot cure chronic disease, nursing can make a difference in the illness experience.

Acute Conditions versus Chronic Conditions

When an individual develops an acute disease, there is typically a sudden onset, with signs and symptoms related to the disease process itself. Acute diseases end in a relatively short time, either with recovery and resumption of prior activities, or with death.

Chronic illness, on the other hand, continues indefinitely. Although a welcome alternative to death in most, but not all cases, the illness is often seen as a mixed blessing to the individual and to society at large. In addition, the illness

often becomes the person's identity. For example, an individual having any kind of cancer, even in remission, acquires the label of "that person with cancer" (see Stigma, Chapter 3). Chronic conditions take many forms, and there is no single onset pattern. A chronic disease can appear suddenly or through an insidious process, have episodic flare-ups or exacerbations, or remain in remission with an absence of symptoms for long periods. Maintaining wellness or keeping symptoms in remission is a juggling act of balancing treatment regimens while focusing on quality of life.

Defining Chronicity

Defining chronicity is complex. Many individuals have attempted to present an all encompassing definition of chronic illness. Initially, the characteristics of chronic diseases were identified by the Commission on Chronic Illness as all impairments or deviations from normal that included one or more of the following: permanency; residual disability; nonpathologic alteration; required rehabilitation; or a long period of supervision, observation, and care (Mayo, 1956). The extent of a chronic disease further complicates attempts in defining the term. Disability may depend not only on the kind of condition and its severity, but also on the implications it holds for the person. The degree of disability and altered lifestyle, part of traditional definitions, may relate more to the client's *perceptions and beliefs* about the disease than to the disease itself.

Long-term and iatrogenic effects of some treatment may constitute chronic conditions in their own right, making them eligible to be defined as a chronic illness. Take, for example, the changes in lifestyle required of clients receiving hemodialysis for end-stage renal disease (ESRD). Life-saving procedures can create other problems. For instance, abdominal radiation that arrested metastatic colon cancer when an individual was 30 years of age contributes to a malabsorption problem years later. Chemotherapy or radiation given to a client for an initial bout with cancer may be an influencing factor in the development of leukemia years later.

Chronic illness, by its very nature, is never completely cured. Biologically the human body wears out unevenly. Medical advances cause older adults to need a progressively wider variety of specialized services for increasingly complicated conditions. In the words of Emanuel (1982): "Life is the accumulation of chronic illness beneath the load of which we eventually succumb" (p. 502).

Although definitions of chronic disease are important, from a nursing perspective we are far more interested in how the illness is affecting the client and family. What is the illness experience of the client and family? Price (1996) suggests that the onus of defining chronic illness, and similarly, quality of life and comfort, should be that of the client's, as only the client truly understands the illness. However, that aside, the following definition of chronic illness is offered: "Chronic illness is the irreversible presence, accumulation, or latency of disease states or impairments that involve the total human environment for supportive care and self-care, maintenance of function, and prevention of further disability" (Curtin & Lubkin, 1995, pp. 6–7).

IMPACT OF CHRONIC ILLNESS

This section addresses the influence of chronic illnesses and impact on society in general.

The Older Adult

Although chronic diseases and conditions exist in children, adolescents, and young and middle-aged adults, the bulk of these conditions occur in adults age 65 years and older. Julie Gerberding, former Director of the CDC, stated: "The aging of the U.S. population is one of the major public health challenges we face in the 21st century" (CDC & the Merck Company Foundation, 2007). In 2009 persons older than 65 years of age numbered 39.6 million and represented 12.9% of Americans (AOA, 2010). Since 1900, the percentage of older Americans has tripled. By 2030 there will be 72.1 million adults in the United States who are older than age 65 years, nearly double the current number and roughly 19% of the U.S. population (AOA, 2010). Increased life expectancy and medical advances have contributed to these demographic changes.

With age comes chronic disease. Six of the seven leading causes of death among older Americans are chronic diseases (Federal Interagency Forum on Aging-Related Statistics, 2010). Medicare data document that 83% of all of its beneficiaries have at least one chronic condition (Anderson, 2005). However, 23% of Medicare beneficiaries with five or more conditions account for 68% of the program's funding (Anderson, 2005, p. 305).

A compounding factor in the physical health of older adults is the presence of depression, the occurrence of which is increasing in the older population. Himelhoch, Weller, Wu, Anderson, and Cooper (2004) analyzed data in a randomized sample of 1,238,895 Medicare recipients, with 60,382 of those clients meeting the criteria for a depressive syndrome. For each of eight chronic medical conditions, Medicare beneficiaries with a depressive syndrome were at least twice as likely to use emergency department services and medical inpatient hospital services as those without depression (Himelhoch et al., 2004, p. 512).

As people age, it is clear they will have more chronic conditions and will access, if their socioeconomic status permits, an acute care system. How will the needs of these aging adults affect our healthcare delivery system? As mentioned previously, there is evidence of growing inequities in healthcare services that racial and ethnic minorities receive. Combine those inequities with being an older adult, and there is a significant population that will be without quality health care or perhaps any health care at all.

The Healthcare Delivery System

The current healthcare system was largely designed and shaped in the 2 decades following World War II (Lynn & Adamson, 2003). In 1946 Congress passed Public Law 79-725, the Hospital Survey and Construction Act, sponsored by Senators Lister Hill and Harold Burton. The Hill-Burton Act was designed to provide federal grants to modernize hospitals that had become obsolete, owing to lack of capital investment throughout the Great Depression and World War II (1929–1945). The healthcare system was designed to provide acute, episodic, and curative care, and it was never intended to address the needs of individuals with chronic conditions. At the time, little, if any, thought was given to what "future patients" would look like. Generally, our present healthcare delivery system provides acute care effectively and efficiently. However, it is based on a component style of care in which each component or care setting of the system is reimbursed separately, that is, hospital, home care, physician visit.

Each component of the healthcare system views the client through its narrow window of care. No one entity, practice, institution, or agency is managing the entire disease, and certainly none is managing the illness experience of the client and family. No one entity is responsible for the overall care of the individual, only their own independent component of care. Typically this approach produces higher costs for the client.

The current healthcare delivery system is disease oriented. Clients fit within the "standards of care," or the algorithm of a specific disease. With diagnosis-related groups (DRGs), payment is predetermined according to diagnosis as opposed to how many services are used. Think about an older adult in this system: Mr. Jones, with several comorbidities, enters the acute care institution. His admitting diagnosis is pneumonia, but now his diabetes is flaring up along with his hypertension, and his kidneys are not working as well as they should. A specialty physician is treating each of his conditions, but there is no coordinator of his care. He is taking multiple medications, and soon he becomes confused and incontinent. In addition, the focus of the acute care facility is the disease processes of this individual and not the illness experience of the patient and his elderly wife. What does our acute care system do with this older adult with multiple chronic health problems? How does our healthcare delivery system care for Mr. Jones and the multitude of others like him on the horizon?

Healthy People 2020

Healthy People 2020 provides science-based, 10-year national objectives for improving the health of all Americans (http://www.healthypeople.gov). For the 2020 document, there is a renewed focus on identifying, measuring, tracking, and reducing health disparities through a determinants-of-health approach. The mission of *Healthy People 2020* is to:

1) Identify nationwide health-improvement priorities.
2) Increase public awareness and understanding of the determinants of health, disease, and disability and the opportunities for progress.
3) Provide measurable objectives and goals that are applicable at the national, state, and local levels.
4) Engage multiple sectors to take actions to strengthen policies and improve practices that are driven by the best available evidence and knowledge.
5) Identify critical research, evaluation, and data-collection needs.

The topic areas and objectives of *Healthy People 2020* are based on four overarching goals: 1) attain high-quality, longer lives free of preventable disease, disability, injury, and premature death; 2) achieve health equity, eliminate disparities, and improve the health of all groups; 3) create social and physical environments that promote good health for all; and 4) promote quality of life, healthy development, and healthy behaviors across all life stages. Topic areas of *Healthy People 2020* are listed in **Table 1-1**. Many of the topics relate to chronic disease and/or prevention of chronic disease.

Quality of Care

In 1996 the Institute of Medicine (IOM) initiated a focus on assessing and improving the quality of care in the United States. A number of documents and books have evolved from that initiative. Perhaps the most known of those include *Crossing the Quality Chasm* (IOM, 2001)

and *To Err is Human* (IOM, 1999). The intent of these books and other documents was to increase awareness of quality and improve the health outcomes of individuals in the nation.

The quest for quality continues. Chassin and Loeb (2011) chronicle the quality improvement journey from Semmelweis, the Hungarian physician who discovered that childbed fever could be drastically cut by the use of hand washing standards in obstetric clinics, to the present day. These authors characterize healthcare quality and safety as "showing pockets of excellence on specific measures or in particular services at individual healthcare facilities" (p. 562). One example provided is that hospitals, on average, provide life-prolonging beta-blockers to heart attack patients 98% of the time (as cited in Chassin & Loeb, 2011). However, they contend that what is missing is *maintenance* of high levels of safety over time and across all healthcare services and settings.

> Moreover, the available evidence suggests that the harmful error in health care may be increasing. As new devices, equipment, procedures, and drugs are added to our therapeutic arsenal, the complexity of delivering effective care increases. Complexity greatly increases the likelihood of error, especially in systems that perform at low levels of reliability. (Chassin & Loeb, 2011, p. 563)

This complex care causes medical errors. It has been documented that surgical procedures performed either on the wrong patient or at the wrong site on a patient still occur (Stahel et al., 2010). Medicare has termed these events as "never events"—serious, costly errors in patient care that should never happen (Centers for Medicare and Medicaid, 2008). Van Den Bos and colleagues (2011) estimate that the annual

Table 1-1	**Topics of** *Healthy People 2020*
Access to health services	HIV
Adolescent health*	Immunization and infectious diseases
Arthritis, osteoporosis, and chronic back conditions	Injury and violence prevention
Blood disorders and blood safety*	Lesbian, gay, bisexual, and transgender health*
Cancer	Maternal, infant, and child health
Chronic kidney disease	Medical product safety
Dementias, including Alzheimer's disease*	Mental health and mental disorders
Diabetes	Nutrition and weight status
Disability and health	Occupational safety and health
Early and middle childhood*	Older adults*
Educational and community-based programs	Oral health
Environmental health	Physical activity
Family planning	Preparedness*
Food safety	Public health infrastructure
Genomics*	Respiratory diseases
Global health*	Sexually transmitted diseases
Health communication and health information technology	Sleep health*
Healthcare-associated infections*	Social determinants of health*
Health-related quality of life and well-being*	Substance abuse
Hearing and other sensory or communication disorders	Tobacco use
Heart disease and stroke	Vision

Source: Healthy People 2020. Topics and objectives index. Retrieved July 24, 2011, from: http://healthypeople.gov/2020/topicsobjectives2020/default.aspx

*New Topic Area

cost of medical errors that harm patients was $17.1 billion in 2008 (p. 596).

Since 2003 the AHRQ with the Department of Health and Human Services (DHHS) has reported on quality measures. In the past, reports were based on 250 measures across 6 dimensions: effectiveness, patient safety, timeliness, patient centeredness, efficiency, and access to care. For 2010 the AHRQ produced the National Healthcare Quality Report (NHQR) and the National Healthcare Disparities Report (NHDR), combining their summary of findings into one document in an effort to reinforce the need to consider simultaneously the quality of health care and disparities across populations when assessing the healthcare system. Four themes from the 2010 NHQR and the 2010 NHDR emphasize the need to accelerate progress if the United States wants to achieve higher quality and more equitable health care in the near future:

- Healthcare quality and access are suboptimal, especially for minority and low-income groups.
- While quality is improving, access and disparities are not improving.
- Urgent attention is warranted to ensure improvements in quality and progress on reducing disparities with respect to certain services, geographic areas, and populations, including:
  - Cancer screening and management of diabetes
  - States in the central part of the country
  - Residents of inner city and rural areas
  - Disparities in preventive services and access to care
- Progress is uneven with respect to eight national priority areas:
  - Two are improving in quality: 1) palliative and end-of-life care, and 2) patient and family engagement
  - Three are lagging: 3) population health, 4) safety, and 5) access
  - Three require more data to assess: 6) care coordination, 7) overuse, and 8) health system infrastructure
  - All eight priority areas showed disparities related to race, ethnicity, and socioeconomic status. (AHRQ, 2010b)

Data across the country are contradictory. Although progress has been made in some areas, other areas have not seen any improvement. Data involving quality of care include the following:

- On average, patients received chronic disease management services three-quarters

of the time. Receipt of chronic disease management services varied widely, from 17% of dialysis patients being registered on a kidney transplant waiting list to 95% of hospice patients receiving the right amount of pain medication.
- On average, patients received preventive services two-thirds of the time, but there was a wide variation in receipt of those services. For instance, only 20% of high-risk adults ages 18–64 years received the pneumococcal vaccination, but 94% of children ages 19–35 months received 3 doses of polio vaccine.
- Access to care is limited. On average, Americans report barriers to care one-fifth of the time, ranging from 3% of people saying they were unable to get or had to delay getting prescription medications to 60% of people saying their usual provider did not have office hours on weekends or nights. (AHRQ, 2011).

Certainly, these data demonstrate that as a nation we have much work to do to improve the quality of care that our clients receive. More information is available in the AHRQ's annual reports, including a data breakdown by individual states. In addition, AHRQ includes *State Snapshots* on their website (http://statesnapshots. ahrq.gov/). This website documents the quality measures of each individual state.

Health Disparities

The first National Healthcare Disparities Report (NHDR) sponsored by AHRQ was released in 2003. In 2011, the ninth report was issued. As mentioned in the section on quality, this year AHRQ integrated the findings from the 2010 NHDR and the 2010 NHQR to produce one summary document. Disparities continue. The following are some examples from the summary (AHRQ, 2011):

- Blacks, American Indians, and Alaska Natives received worse care than whites for about 40% of the core measures.
- Hispanics/Latinos received worse care than non-Hispanic/Latino whites for about 60% of the core measures.
- Poor people received worse care than high-income people for about 80% of the core measures.
- Hispanics/Latinos had worse access to care than non-Hispanic/Latino whites for five of six core measures.
- Poor people had worse access to care than high-income people for all six core measures.
- Measures of acute treatment are improving; measures of preventive care and chronic disease management are lagging.

Culture

Illness belief systems form a cultural milieu that defines one's attitudes about illness, both acute and chronic. Conceptions or misconceptions about the source of the disease, potential treatment, and possible outcomes are all influenced by these belief systems, and one's belief system is influenced by one's culture. Providing culturally competent care may be a daunting task; however, health care is not "one size fits all," and healthcare professionals must take the extra steps to ensure culturally competent care (see Culture and Cultural Components, Chapter 13).

Another way to view culture is to consider chronic illness as a culture. Although we often believe that each disease is different, there are multiple tasks that are similar, and illness experiences may look alike across diseases.

Strauss (1975) was among the first researchers to recognize the similar issues and tasks within the culture of chronic illness. Generally, the culture of chronic illness includes preventing and managing medical crises; managing a treatment regimen; controlling symptoms; the reordering of time; and social isolation. In 1984 Strauss and colleagues suggested that the basic strategy to cope with these issues was to normalize, not just to stay alive or keep symptoms under control, but to live as normally as possible (p. 79). Essentially, for a number of clients with chronic illness, a "new normal" must be created.

A number of years ago when teaching a chronic illness practicum to graduate students, this author developed a mini-ethnography project of the individuals who the students were caring for that semester. Students were caring for clients with a variety of diseases—HIV, liver disease, heart failure, rheumatoid arthritis, and breast cancer. Using grand tour questions that had been developed as a class, students interviewed their clients over the course of the semester. During the final weeks of seminar after the practicum was completed, students compiled the data from all of the clients and looked at the themes that emerged. The class was able to develop a clear concept of the culture of what it is like to have a chronic illness and to understand the vast number of similarities between individuals with a variety of chronic conditions.

Social Influences

As a society we often stereotype individuals according to the color of their skin, their culture, and their ethnicity. Unfortunately, we behave in a similar fashion with individuals with chronic conditions and disabilities (see Stigma, Chapter 3). To this day there are some individuals who avoid others who may be in a wheelchair, have visible signs of disease (burns, paralysis, amputations, etc.), have a diagnosis of AIDS, and so forth. While some efforts such as department store advertisements depicting individuals in wheelchairs may positively influence some behavior, as a nation, there is much progress to be made.

Publicly recognized individuals have stepped forward with stories about their own chronic conditions. The courage of these individuals to share their experiences and speak out for more comprehensive legislation to support those with chronic disease and increase research funding is admirable. Examples include Michael J. Fox and Muhammed Ali, with diagnoses of Parkinson's disease; Magic Johnson, with his diagnosis of HIV; and the late Christopher and Dana Reeve, as advocates for spinal cord injury research.

Financial Impact

Healthcare spending in the United States grew only 4% in 2009—the lowest rate of increase in the 50-year history of the National Health Expenditure Accounts—to $2.5 trillion, or $8,086 per person (Martin, Lassman, Whittle, Catlin, & the National Health Expenditure Accounts Team, 2011). Researchers attribute several factors to this low rate of increase: "deceleration in private health insurance spending, a decline in spending on structures and equipment in the healthcare system, and slower growth in out-of-pocket spending" (p. 11).

Despite the slower growth, healthcare spending accounted for 17.6% of the gross domestic product (GDP) in 2009, up from 16.6% in 2008. This is the largest 1-year increase in the history of the national health accounts

(Martin et al., 2011). Martin and colleagues (2011) note several important findings:

- The growth rate of health spending outpaced the growth of the overall economy, which experienced its largest drop since 1938.
- The recession contributed to slower growth in private health insurance spending and out-of-pocket spending by consumers.
- Declining federal revenues and strong growth in federal health spending increased the health spending share of total federal revenue from 37.6% in 2008 to 54.2% in 2009.
- Faster growth in Medicaid spending, from 4.9% in 2008 to 9% in 2009, was driven by the addition of 3.5 million new enrollees.
- The number of uninsured people increased by 3.8 million, from 42.7 million in 2008 to 46.5 million in 2009.

Using Medical Expenditure Panel Survey (MEPS) data, five conditions have been identified as the most costly conditions in the noninstitutionalized population, and four of them are chronic conditions. The five conditions—heart disease, cancer, trauma-related disorders, mental disorders, and asthma—ranked highest in terms of direct medical spending in 1996 and again in 2006 (Soni, 2009). These data are based on expenditures (what is paid for healthcare services), and do not include any indirect costs. Heart disease had the largest medical expenditures in 2006 with $78 billion, followed by trauma-related disorders at $68.1 billion, cancer and mental disorders tied at $57.5 billion, and asthma at $51.3 billion (Soni, 2009). The largest increases in expenditures from 1996 to 2006 were for mental disorders and trauma-related disorders. The biggest increase in number of people accounting for expenditures was for mental disorders, which nearly doubled in the 10-year period, while in terms of mean expenditures per person, costs were highest for cancer and heart disease in both 1996 and 2006 (Soni, 2009).

Compounding chronic disease is the issue of the uninsured. The long-term uninsured, versus those uninsured for short periods, is a significant population. MEPS data for 2002 to 2005 (the most current available) demonstrate the following in the population younger than 65 years of age: 17.4 million U.S. residents were uninsured for the entire 4-year period, and those reporting fair/poor health (11.2%) were the most likely to be uninsured for the entire 4-year period (Rhoades & Cohen, 2007). During the first half of 2009, 18.5% of the U.S. civilian noninstitutionalized population, numbering 55.6 million people, was uninsured. Among those under age 65, 55.3 million were uninsured. Young adults aged 19 to 24 and 25 to 29 were at the greatest risk of being uninsured. For the uninsured, 42.4% lived in the South, while 12.8% lived in the Northeast, 18.7% lived in the Midwest, and 26.2% lived in the West (Roberts & Rhoades, 2010). Among people under age 65, Hispanics/Latinos accounted for 29% of the uninsured U.S. civilian noninstitutionalized population even though they represented only 17% of the overall population of this age group (Roberts & Rhoades, 2010).

The Organization for Economic Cooperation and Development (OECD) annually tracks and reports on more than 1,200 health system measures across 30 industrialized countries. Since 1998, the Commonwealth Fund has sponsored an analysis of cross-national health systems based on OECD health data. According to data from 2006, the United States continues to differ markedly from other countries (Anderson & Squires, 2010). The United States continues to outspend other countries in healthcare spending per capita at more than twice the median per capita expenditure of the 30 countries tracked by OECD. Compared with other countries, the United States has a low number of hospital beds and physicians per capita, and patients in the Unites States have fewer hospital and physician visits than most other countries. However, spending per hospital visit is the highest in the United States. Also, the United States ranks in the bottom quartile in life expectancy among these 30 countries and has seen the smallest improvement in this statistic over the past 20 years (Anderson & Squires, 2010). Life expectancy at birth in the United States was 77.8 years in 2006; however, ten countries had life expectancies at birth of more than 80 years. The United States' investment in technology has surely influenced health expenditure costs; however, Anderson and Squires contend that there is a gap between the investment in technically advanced equipment and procedures and what services are delivered in return. Either these health services are less effectively implemented or come at a higher price.

INTERVENTIONS

Chronic disease is an issue that is all encompassing, such that interventions from many sources will be needed to make a difference. What follows are examples of ways to decrease the impact of chronic disease.

Professional Education

One of the challenges in chronic disease care and management is educating healthcare professionals about providing care tailored to those with chronic disease. The differences are vast between caring for a person with an acute illness on a short-term basis, and caring for those over the long haul with a chronic condition. The WHO developed a document outlining the steps to prepare a healthcare workforce for the 21st century that can appropriately care for individuals with chronic conditions. The WHO document calls for a transformation of healthcare training to better meet the needs of those individuals with chronic conditions. The document, *Preparing a Healthcare Workforce for the 21st Century: The Challenge of Chronic Conditions* (WHO, 2005), has the support of the World Medical Association, the International Council of Nurses, the International Pharmaceutical Federation, the European Respiratory Society, and the International Alliance of Patients' Organizations.

The competencies delineated by the WHO (2005) were identified with a process that included an extensive document/literature review and international expert agreement (p. 14). All competencies were based on addressing the needs of patients with chronic conditions and their family members from a longitudinal perspective, and focused on two types of "prevention" strategies: initial prevention of the chronic disease; and secondly, prevention of complications from the condition (p. 18). The five competencies include: patient-centered care; partnering; quality improvement; information and communication technology; and public health perspective (see **Table 1-2**). At first glance, the competencies might not seem unique. However, in an acute care–oriented healthcare delivery system, these concepts are not as prominent. Clients are in and out of the care system quickly, and there is less need for implementation of these concepts.

Table 1-2   WHO Core Competencies

Patient-centered care
   Interviewing and communicating effectively
   Assisting changes in health-related behaviors
   Supporting self-management
   Using a proactive approach

Partnering
   Partnering with patients
   Partnering with other providers
   Partnering with communities

Quality improvement
   Measuring care delivery and outcomes
   Learning and adapting to change
   Translating evidence into practice

Information and communication technology
   Designing and using patient registries
   Using computer technologies
   Communicating with partners

Public health perspective
   Providing population-based care
   Systems thinking
   Working across the care continuum
   Working in primary healthcare–led systems

Source: World Health Organization. (2005b). *Preparing a health care workforce for the 21st century: The challenge of chronic conditions* (p. 20). Geneva, Switzerland: WHO.

In 2007, the IOM charged an ad hoc committee with the task of determining the healthcare needs of an aging America, and, more importantly, developing recommendations to address those needs. On April 14, 2008, the IOM report, *Retooling for an Aging America: Building the Health Care Workforce*, was released to the public. This report suggests a three-pronged approach that includes the following: 1) enhance the geriatric competence of the entire workforce; 2) increase the recruitment and retention of geriatric specialists and caregivers; and 3) improve the way care is delivered (IOM, 2008).

The report states a well known fact: Little attention is paid to educating healthcare professionals about caring for older adults. The committee recommends that healthcare professionals be required to demonstrate their competence in caring for older adults as a criterion for licensure and certification. More stringent training standards would be implemented for direct-care providers by increasing existing federal training requirements and establishing state-based standards. And finally, because informal caregivers continue to play important roles in the care of older adults (with and without chronic illness), training opportunities should also be available for them (IOM, 2008).

Currently only a small percentage of the healthcare workforce specializes in caring for older adults. The IOM report recommends that financial incentives be provided to increase the number of geriatric specialists in every health profession. Incentives would include an increase in payments for clinical services, development of awards to increase the number of faculty in geriatrics, and the establishment of programs that would provide loan forgiveness, scholarships, and direct financial incentives for individuals to become specialists in geriatrics. For the direct-care workers in long-term care facilities that typically have high levels of turnover and job dissatisfaction, the recommendation is to improve job desirability, improve supervisory relationships, and provide opportunities for career growth. In addition, the report recommends that state Medicaid programs increase pay for direct-care workers and provide access to fringe benefits (IOM, 2008).

Lastly, models of care for older adults need to improve. The report envisions three key principles in improving care: 1) the healthcare needs of older adults must be addressed comprehensively, 2) services need to be provided efficiently, and 3) older adults need to be encouraged to be active partners in their own care. Because no one model of care will be appropriate for all persons, the IOM recommends that Congress and public and private foundations significantly increase support for research and programs that promote development of new models of care (IOM, 2008).

Chronic Disease Practitioner Competencies

From another point of view, the National Association of Chronic Disease Directors (NACDD) developed the document "Competencies for Chronic Disease Practice." The organization was founded in 1988 to link the directors of chronic disease programs in each state and U.S. territory. It created these competencies to assist state and local healthcare programs with developing competent workforces and effective programs. The NACDD document is based on domains, with individual competencies within each domain. Several of the domains address the WHO competencies (i.e., partnering, evidence-based interventions). Furthermore, the NACDD has developed an assessment tool for practitioners to gauge their level of proficiency in each of the seven domains. **Table 1-3** lists the competencies for chronic disease practitioners.

Resources

Centers for Disease Control and Prevention Programs

The CDC has provided both leadership and funding in developing state-based programs

Table 1-3   National Association of Chronic Disease Directors: Competencies for Chronic Disease Practice

Domain 1—Build Support	Chronic disease practitioners establish strong working relationships with stakeholders, including other programs, government agencies, and nongovernmental lay and professional groups, to build support for chronic disease prevention and control.
Domain 2—Design and Evaluate Programs	Chronic disease practitioners develop and implement evidence-based interventions and conduct evaluations to ensure ongoing feedback and program effectiveness.
Domain 3—Influence Policies and Systems Change	Chronic disease practitioners implement strategies to change the health-related policies of private organizations or governmental entities capable of affecting the health of targeted populations.
Domain 4—Lead Strategically	Chronic disease practitioners articulate health needs and strategic vision, serve as catalysts for change, and demonstrate program accomplishments to ensure continued funding and support within their scope of practice.
Domain 5—Manage People	Chronic disease practitioners oversee and support the optimal performance and growth of program staff as well as themselves.
Domain 6—Manage Programs and Resources	Chronic disease practitioners ensure the consistent administrative, financial, and staff support necessary to sustain successful implementation of planned activities and to build opportunities.
Domain 7—Use Public Health Science	Chronic disease practitioners gather, analyze, interpret, and disseminate data and research findings to define needs, identify priorities, and measure change.

Source: National Association of Chronic Disease Directors. *Competencies for chronic disease.* Retrieved July 24, 2011, from: http://www.chronicdisease.org/professional-development/documents/workforce-dev/CompetenciesforChronicDiseasePractice.pdf

nationwide. Programs have been developed to look at risk factors and prevention of disease and to examine ways to prevent complications and delay death resulting from chronic disease.

One example of the CDC's preventive work is with diabetes. The CDC's programs with diabetes encompass several components and include: promoting effective state programs, monitoring the burden and translating science, providing education and sharing expertise, supporting primary prevention, and targeting populations at

risk. What follows is a brief description of what each of these components provides.

- *Promoting effective state programs.* In 2007 the CDC provided funding for capacity building to 22 states, 8 current or former U.S. territories, and the District of Columbia for diabetes prevention and control programs. In addition, the CDC provided funding for basic implementation of programs in the other 28 states. The state programs identify the disease burden in each state, develop and evaluate new prevention strategies, establish partnerships, increase awareness of prevention and control opportunities, and improve access to quality care. These projects continue in 2011 (CDC, 2011a).

- *Monitoring the burden and translating science.* The CDC analyzes data from several national sources, including the Behavioral Risk Factor Surveillance System. The translating of these data into quality practice is implemented with the assistance of other research partners, managed care organizations, and community health centers.

- *Providing education and sharing expertise.* Another component of the CDC's work is providing education. The National Diabetes Education Program (NDEP) is sponsored by both the CDC and the National Institutes of Health (NIH). The NDEP was launched in 1997 to improve diabetes management and reduce the morbidity and mortality from diabetes and its complications. The NDEP comprises more than 200 public and private partners. NDEP's major campaigns are based on landmark scientific studies on diabetes prevention and control, including the following:

  - Diabetes Control and Complications Trial
  - Epidemiology of Diabetes Interventions and Complications Study
  - United Kingdom Prospective Diabetes Study
  - Action to Control Cardiovascular Risk in Diabetes
  - Veterans Affairs Diabetes Trial
  - Diabetes Prevention Program

  - Diabetes Prevention Program Outcomes Study
  - Action for Health in Diabetes
  - SEARCH for Diabetes in Youth (CDC, 2011b)

REACH US

The Racial and Ethnic Approaches to Community Health Across the United States (REACH US) is a national, multilevel program that serves as the cornerstone of the CDC's efforts to eliminate racial and ethnic disparities in health. Through REACH US, the CDC supports 40 grantee partners that establish community-based programs and culturally appropriate interventions to eliminate health disparities among African Americans, American Indians, Hispanics/Latinos, Asian Americans, Alaska Natives, and Pacific Islanders (CDC, 2011c). REACH US communities empower residents to 1) seek better health; 2) help change local healthcare practices; and 3) mobilize communities to implement evidence-based public health programs that address their unique social, historical, economic, and cultural circumstances.

Agency for Healthcare Research and Quality

AHRQ sponsors a number of programs that are working to reduce or eliminate health disparities. These programs are described here because, as previously noted, 80% of U.S. healthcare dollars are spent on chronic disease. Therefore, healthcare inequities largely involve chronic care.

AHRQ's goal of reducing/eliminating disparities is met through continued commitment to:

- Improving the quality of health care and healthcare services for patients and their families, regardless of their race/ethnicity, socioeconomic status, and literacy level

- Continuing to improve the quality of data collected to address disparities among priority populations and subpopulations
- Promoting representation and inclusion of racial/ethnic minority populations in all health services research activities
- Monitoring and tracking changes in disparities by priority populations, subpopulations, and conditions
- Identifying and implementing effective strategies to reduce/eliminate disparities
- Partnering with communities to ensure that research activities are relevant to their populations and that the research findings are adopted and implemented effectively (AHRQ, 2009)

World Health Organization

The WHO has updated its 2000 plan for the prevention and control of noncommunicable disease. Working with partners/agencies across the world, the 2008–2013 plan focuses on cardiovascular diseases, diabetes, cancer, and chronic respiratory disease, as well as the four shared risk factors of tobacco use, physical inactivity, unhealthy diet, and the harmful use of alcohol. The six objectives of the action plan are:

- To raise the priority accorded to noncommunicable disease in development work at global and national levels, and to integrate prevention and control of such diseases into policies across all government departments
- To establish and strengthen national policies and plans for the prevention and control of noncommunicable diseases

- To promote interventions to reduce the main shared modifiable risk factors for noncommunicable diseases—tobacco use, unhealthy diet, physical inactivity, and harmful use of alcohol
- To promote research for the prevention and control of noncommunicable diseases
- To promote partnerships for the prevention and control of noncommunicable diseases
- To monitor noncommunicable diseases and their determinants and evaluate progress at the regional, national, and global levels (WHO, 2008)

Evidence-Based Practice

The evidence-based practice movement had its beginnings in the 1970s with Dr. Archie Cochrane, a British epidemiologist. In 1971 Cochrane published a book that criticized physicians for not conducting rigorous reviews of evidence in making appropriate treatment decisions. Cochrane was a proponent of randomized clinical trials, and in his exemplar case noted that thousands of low birthweight premature infants died needlessly. At the same time there were several randomized clinical trials (RCTs) that had been conducted on the use of corticosteroid therapy to halt premature labor in pregnant women, but the data had never been reviewed or analyzed. After review, these studies demonstrated that this therapy was effective in halting premature labor and thus reducing infant deaths due to prematurity. Cochrane died in 1988, but as a result of his influence and call for systematic review of the literature, the Cochrane Collaboration was launched in Oxford, England, in 1993. It also hosts the Cochrane Library, which is a sophisticated collection of databases containing current, high-quality research that supports practice.

However, evidence-based practice does not rely on RCTs alone. A number of definitions have been brought forth, but Porter-O'Grady (2006) offers a clear and succinct definition: "Evidence-based practice is simply the integration of the best possible research to evidence with clinical expertise and with patient needs. Patient needs in this case refer specifically to the expectations, concerns, and requirements that patients bring to their clinical experience" (p. 1).

As healthcare professionals examine the evidence to improve the care of their clients, there are a number of sources for reference. The following agencies and organizations are a sample of the resources available:

- Agency for Healthcare Research and Quality (AHRQ) (www.ahrq.gov)
- *Clinical Evidence* (www.clinicalevidence.com)
- Cochrane Library (www.thecochranelibrary.com)
- The Joanna Briggs Institute (www.joannabriggs.edu.au)
- National Guideline Clearinghouse (www.guideline.gov)
- Task Force on Community Preventive Services (www.thecommunityguide.org)
- U.S. Preventive Services Task Force (www.ahrq.gov/clinic/uspstfab.htm)
- Veterans Evidence-Based Research Dissemination Implementation Center (VERDICT): (www.verdict.research.va.gov)

Legislation

On March 21, 2010, President Barack Obama signed legislation to reform the healthcare delivery system: the Patient Protection and Affordable Care Act and the Health Care and Education Reconciliation Act expand, health insurance coverage to individuals who were not previously covered by any health plan through the implementation of individual and employer mandates as well as through expansion of federal and state programs such as Medicare and Medicaid. According to the Congressional Budget Office (CBO), an estimated 32 million additional individuals will be covered by 2019 (Albright et al., 2010). Some components of the law address individuals with chronic illness:

- It established a Patient's Bill of Rights.
- High-risk insurance pools were created to make insurance available to individuals with pre-existing health conditions until healthcare coverage exchanges are operational in 2014.
- Insurers are no longer able to exclude children with pre-existing conditions from being covered under their parents' insurance.
- Insurers are not able to rescind policies to avoid paying medical bills when a person becomes ill.
- Lifetime limits on coverage are prohibited.
- Children are able to stay covered under their parents' insurance plan until age 26.
- Funding for scholarships and loan repayments for primary care practitioners working with underserved populations was expanded.
- Insurers will no longer be able to refuse to sell or renew policies because of an individual's health status, and will no longer be able to exclude coverage for an individual of any age because of a pre-existing condition (effective 2014).

- Insurers can no longer charge higher rates because of an individual's health status or gender (effective 2014).
- Health plans will be prohibited from imposing any annual limits on coverage (effective 2014).
- Health plans will no longer be able to charge copays and deductibles for recommended preventive care (effective 2014).
- Health insurance exchanges will open in each state, allowing individuals and small employers to shop for health insurance policies (effective 2014).
- Tax credits will be available to those whose income is above Medicaid eligibility and below 400% of the poverty level and do not receive acceptable coverage. Additionally, Medicaid eligibility will increase to 133% of the poverty level for all non-elderly individuals. (The Affordable Care Act: One Year Later, 2011; The White House, 2011)

SUMMARY

The United States touts the most sophisticated and technologically advanced health care in the world. Such health care should produce optimal patient outcomes rivaled by none. With healthcare expenditures amounting to 17.6% of the GDP, apparently sophisticated health care comes at a price. Currently the United States spends $8,086 per capita to provide this care. However, even with all of the money that the nation has allocated to health care, outcomes are not optimal. When compared with the countries in the OECD, the United States ranks below the median on most core measures while having the most expensive health care in the world. Life expectancy of U.S. citizens now ranks in the bottom quartile of the 30 countries in the OECD. How can we explain that? What can be done to improve care?

STUDY QUESTIONS

Summarize the state of chronic disease in the United States and globally today.

What factors and influences have led to the increased incidence of chronic disease in the United States?

What factors should be considered in defining chronicity?

How can we better educate healthcare professionals to care for those with chronic disease? To care for older adults with chronic disease?

What changes does the healthcare delivery system need to embrace to better care for those with chronic disease?

Compare and contrast chronic disease and chronic illness.

What action should the United States take to decrease healthcare disparities?

For a full suite of assignments and additional learning activities, use the access code located in the front of your book and visit this exclusive website: **http://go.jblearning.com/larsen**. If you do not have an access code, you can obtain one at the site.

REFERENCES

Administration on Aging. (2010). *A profile of older Americans: 2009*. Washington, DC: U.S. Department of Health and Human Services.

The Affordable Care Act: One Year Later (2011). Retrieved July 24, 2011, from: http://www.healthcare.gov/law/introduction/index.html

Agency for Healthcare Research and Quality. (2009). *AHRQ activities to reduce racial and ethnic disparities in health care* (AHRQ Publication No. 09(10)-P008). Rockville, MD: AHRQ.

Agency for Healthcare Research and Quality. (2010a). *National healthcare disparities report 2009* (AHRQ 10-0004). Rockville, MD: U.S. Department of Health and Human Services.

Agency of Healthcare Research and Quality (2010b). *Highlights from the National Healthcare Quality and Disparities Reports.* Retrieved July 24, 2011, from: http://www.ahrq.gov/qual/nhqr10/Key.htm.

Agency for Healthcare Research and Quality. (2011). *Disparities in healthcare quality among racial and ethnic minority groups: Selected findings from the 2010 national healthcare quality and disparities reports* (Fact Sheet, AHRQ Publication # 11-0005-3-EF). Rockville, MD: Author. Retrieved July 24, 2011, from: http://www.ahrq.gov/qual/nhqrdr10/nhqrdrminority10.htm

Albright, H. W., Moreno, M., Feeley, T. W., Walters, R., Samuels, M., Pereira, A., & Burke, T. W. (2010). The implications of the 2010 Patient Protection and Affordable Care Act and the Health Care and Education Reconciliation Act on Cancer Care Delivery. *Cancer, 117*(8), 1564–1174.

American Diabetes Association. (2011). *Diabetes statistics.* Retrieved July 24, 2011, from: http://www.diabetes.org/diabetes-basics.

Anderson, G. F. (2005). Medicare and chronic conditions [Electronic version]. *New England Journal of Medicine, 343*(3), 305–309.

Anderson, G. F., & Squires, D. A. (2010). *Measuring the U.S. Health Care System: A cross-national comparison. The Commonwealth Fund.* Retrieved July 24, 2011, from: http://www.commonwealthfund.org/~/media/Files/Publications/Issue%20Brief/2010/Jun/1412_Anderson_measuring_US_hlt_care_sys_intl_ib.pdf

Centers for Disease Control and Prevention & the Merck Company Foundation. (2007). *The state of aging and health in America 2007.* Whitehouse Station, NJ: The Merck Company Foundation.

Centers for Disease Control and Prevention. (2008). *Chronic disease prevention and health promotion: Press room.* Retrieved July 24, 2011, from: http://www.cdc.gov/nccdphp/press/index.htm

Centers for Disease Control and Prevention. (2010a). *Chronic diseases and health promotion.* Retrieved July 24, 2011, from: http://www.cdc.gov/chronicdisease/overview/index.htm

Centers for Disease Control and Prevention. (2010b). *Heart disease facts.* Retrieved July 24, 2011, from: http://www.cdc.gov/heartdisease/facts.htm

Centers for Disease Control and Prevention. (2011a). *Diabetes public health resource. State-based diabetes prevention and control programs.* Retrieved July 24, 2011, from: http://www.cdc.gov/diabetes/states/Index.htm

Centers for Disease Control and Prevention. (2011b). *Diabetes public health resource. National Diabetes Education Program (NDEP).* Retrieved July 24, 2011, from: http://www.cdc.gov/diabetes/ndep/index.htm

Centers for Disease Control and Prevention. (2011c). *Racial and ethnic approaches to community health: REACH US.* Retrieved July 24, 2011, from: http://www.cdc.gov/reach/

Centers for Medicare and Medicaid. (2008). *Fiscal year 2009 quality measure reporting for 2010 payment update.* Retrieved July 24, 2011, from: http://www.cms.gov/HospitalQualityInits/downloads/HospitalRHQDAPU200808.pdf

Chassin, M. R., & Loeb, J. M. (2011). The ongoing quality improvement journey: Next stop, high reliability. *Health Affairs, 30*(4), 559–568.

Cochrane, A. L. (1971). *Effectiveness and efficiency: Random reflections on health services.* London: Nuffield Provincial Hospitals Trust.

Curtin, M., & Lubkin, I. (1995). What is chronicity? In I. Lubkin (Ed.) *Chronic illness: Impact and interventions* (3rd ed.). Sudbury, MA: Jones & Bartlett.

Emanuel, E. (1982). We are all chronic patients. *Journal of Chronic Diseases, 35*, 501–502.

Federal Interagency Forum on Aging-Related Statistics. (2010). *Older Americans 2010: Key Indicators of Well-Being.* Washington, DC: U.S. Government Printing Office.

Harleman, A. (2008, January & February). My other husband. *AARP Magazine*, pp. 74–78.

Healthy People 2020. (2011). Topics and objectives. Retrieved July 24, 2011, from: http://healthypeople.gov/2020/topicsobjectives2020/default.aspx

Himelhoch, S., Weller, W. E., Wu, A. W., Anderson, G. F., & Cooper, L. A. (2004). Chronic medical illness, depression and use of acute medical services among Medicare beneficiaries [Electronic version]. *Medical Care, 42*, 512–521.

Institute of Medicine. (1999). *To err is human: Building a safer health system.* Washington, DC: National Academies Press.

Institute of Medicine. (2001). *Crossing the quality chasm.* Washington, DC: National Academies Press.

Institute of Medicine. (2008). *Retooling for an aging America: Building the health care workforce.* Washington, DC: National Academies Press.

Lynn, J. & Adamson, D. M. (2003). *Living well at the end of life: Adapting healthcare to serious chronic illness in old age.* Santa Monica, CA: RAND.

Martin, A., Lassman, D., Whittle, L., Catlin, A., & the National Health Expenditure Accounts Team (2011). Recession contributes to slowest annual rate of increase in health spending in five decades. *Health Affairs, 30*(1), 11–21.

Mayo, L. (Ed.). (1956). *Guides to action on chronic illness.* Commission on Chronic Illness. New York: National Health Council.

National Association of Chronic Disease Directors. *Competencies for chronic disease practice.* Retrieved July 24, 2011, from: http://www.chronicdisease.org/professional-development/documents/workforce-dev/CompetenciesforChronicDiseasePractice.pdf/

National Cancer Institute. (2011). *The cost of cancer.* Retrieved July 24, 2011, from: http://www.cancer.gov/aboutnci/servingpeople/cancer-statistics/costofcancer/

Porter-O'Grady, T. (2006). A new age for practice: Creating the framework for evidence. In K. Malloch & T. Porter-O'Grady (Eds.), *Introduction to evidence-based practice in nursing and health care.* Sudbury, MA: Jones & Bartlett.

Price, B. (1996). Illness careers: The chronic illness experience. *Journal of Advanced Nursing, 24,* 275–279.

Rhoades, J. A., & Cohen, S. B. (2007). *The long-term uninsured in America, 2002–2005: Estimates for the U.S. population under age 65* (Statistical Brief #183). Rockville, MD: Agency for Healthcare Research and Quality. Retrieved July 24, 2011, from: http://www.meps.ahrq.gov/mepsweb/data_files/publications/st183/stat183.shtml

Roberts, M., & Rhoades, J. A., (2010). *The uninsured in America, first half of 2009: Estimates for the U.S. civilian noninstitutionalized population under age 65* (Statistical Brief #291). Rockville, MD: AHRQ. Retrieved July 24, 2011, from: http://www.meps.ahrq.gov/mepsweb/data_files/publications/st291/stat291.pdf

Soni, A. (2009). *The five most costly conditions, 1996 and 2006: Estimates for the U.S. civilian noninstitutionalized population* (Statistical Brief #248). Rockville, MD: Agency for Healthcare Research and Quality. Retrieved July 24, 2011, from: http://www.meps.ahrq.gov/mepsweb/data_files/publications/st248/stat248.pdf

Stahel, P. F., et al. (2010). Wrong-site and wrong-patient procedures in the universal protocol era: Analysis of a prospective database of physician self-reported occurrences. *Archives of Surgery, 145*(1), 978–984.

Strauss, A. (1975). *Chronic illness and the quality of life.* St. Louis: Mosby.

Strauss, A., Corbin, J., Fagerhaugh, S., Glaser, B., Maines, D., Suczek, B., et al. (1984). *Chronic illness and the quality of life* (2nd ed.). St. Louis: Mosby.

Van Den Bos, J., Rustagi, K., Gray, T., Halford, M. Ziemkiewicz, E., & Shreve, J. (2011). The $17.1 billion problem: The annual cost of measurable medical errors. *Health Affairs, 30*(4), 596–602.

The White House. (2011). *Health reform in action.* Retrieved July 24, 2011, from: http://www.whitehouse.gov/healthreform

World Health Organization (2008). *2008–2013 action plan for the global strategy for the prevention and control of noncommunicable diseases.* Geneva. Switzerland: Author.

World Health Organization. (2011). *Chronic diseases and health promotion.* Retrieved July 24, 2011, from: http://www.who.int/chp/en/index.html

World Health Organization. (2005). *Preparing a health care workforce for the 21st century: The challenge of chronic conditions.* Geneva, Switzerland: Author.

CHAPTER 2

The Illness Experience

Illness is the night-side of life, a more onerous citizenship. Everyone who is born holds dual citizen-ship, in the kingdom of the well and in the kingdom of the sick. Although we all prefer to use only the good passport, sooner or later each of us is obligated, at least for a spell, to identify ourselves as citizens of that other place.

—Susan Sontag, *Illness as Metaphor,* 1988, p. 3

Pamala D. Larsen

INTRODUCTION

Commonly, healthcare providers are educated in the medical model and understand its applicability and use in practice. Clients enter a healthcare system with symptoms, which are then diagnosed based on pathological findings, and as such are treated and/or cured with medical treatment. For acute disease, this is the pattern. One isn't concerned about the client's illness behavior associated with appendicitis, tonsillitis, or a fractured leg. An individual may be concerned that the tonsillitis will return, the fractured leg may not heal normally, or there may be an adverse event associated with the appendectomy, but by and large, these concerns pass quickly because of the acuteness of the event. The United States' acute care–focused healthcare system acts upon the pathology that is present, with the goal that an individual will fully recover from the condition and return to prior behaviors and roles.

What happens however, when the recovery is incomplete or the illness continues or becomes chronic in nature? The individual and family have to modify or adapt previous behavior and roles to accommodate the chronicity of the condition. Societal expectations, their own expectations, and their health status all influence illness behavior. This chapter provides an overview of the illness experience and corresponding behavior demonstrated by those with chronic illness—it presents a sociological view of illness rather than a medical view of illness. It is not meant to be a comprehensive review of the entire body of knowledge, which is vast.

Historical Perspectives

Chronic disease involves not only the physical body, but it also affects one's relationships, self-image, and behavior. The social aspects of disease may be related to the pathophysiologic changes that are occurring, but may be independent of them as well. The very act of diagnosing a condition as an illness has consequences far beyond the pathology involved (Conrad, 2005). Freidson (1970) discussed this more than 40 years ago in his writings about the meaning that is ascribed to a diagnosis by an individual and family (p. 223). It is not merely pathology or a diagnosis anymore, and the individual and family develop their own meanings and perceptions of the condition, and ultimately their own, unique illness behaviors. The earliest concept of illness behavior was described in a 1929 essay by Henry Sigerist. His essay described the "special position of the sick" (as cited in Young, 2004). Talcott Parsons developed this concept further and described the "sick role" in his 1951 work, *The Social System.* A brief examination of the sick role provides context to the illness experience, perceptions, and behavior.

Sick Role

Talcott Parsons, a proponent of structural–functionalist principles, viewed health as a functional prerequisite of society. From Parsons's point of view, sickness was dysfunctional and was a form of social deviance (Williams, 2005). From this functionalist viewpoint, social systems are linked to systems of personality and culture to form a basis for social order (Cockerham, 2001, p. 160). Parsons viewed sickness as a response to social pressure that permitted the avoidance of social responsibilities. Anyone could take on the role he identified, as the role was achieved through failure to keep well.

The four major components of the sick role include:

- The person is exempt from normal social roles.
- The person is not responsible for his/her condition.
- The person has the obligation to want to become well.
- The person has the obligation to seek and cooperate with technically competent help. (Williams, 2005, p. 124)

Although the sick role may have been accepted when developed by Parsons in the 1950s, it is no longer considered relevant today. American culture for the most part has embraced a role of self-care and self-management of disease and participation with care providers to obtain optimal health. Parsons's sick role was based on assumptions about the nature of society and the nature of illness during a previous period of time (Weitz, 2007).

Using Parsons's work as a basis, Mechanic (1962) proposed the concept of illness behavior as symptoms being perceived, evaluated, and acted (or not acted) upon differently by different persons (p. 189). He believed it was essential to understand the influence of norms, values, fears, and expected rewards and punishments on how an individual with illness acts. Mechanic (1995) defines illness behavior as the "varying ways individuals respond to bodily indications, how they monitor internal states, define and interpret symptoms, make attributions, take remedial actions and utilize various sources of formal and informal care" (p. 1208).

Around the time of Mechanic's earlier work, Kasl and Cobb (1966) identified three types of health-related behavior:

1. *Health behavior* is any activity undertaken by a person believing himself to be healthy, for the purpose of preventing disease or detecting it in an asymptomatic stage.
2. *Illness behavior* is any activity, undertaken by a person who feels ill, to define the state of his health and to discover a suitable remedy.
3. *Sick-role behavior* is the activity undertaken, for the purpose of getting well, by those who consider themselves ill.

McHugh and Vallis (1986) suggest that perhaps instead of categorizing behavior as health-related, illness-related, or sick-role–related that it makes more sense to look at illness behavior on a continuum. By doing this, the term *illness behavior* can be broadly defined, and this characterization is more helpful, because the distinction between health and illness behaviors is arbitrary at times (p. 8).

A more current definition of illness behavior suggests that illness behavior "includes all of the individual's life which stems from the experience of illness, including changes in functioning and activity, and uptake of health services and other welfare benefits" (Wainwright, 2008, p. 76). Simply put, when an individual defines him/herself as ill, different behaviors may be displayed. A behavior could be as simple as seeking medical treatment or as complex as the individual's emotional response to the diagnosis. As more acute conditions become chronic in nature, there is more interest in how individuals behave in these circumstances. Individuals with chronic illness are living longer and are creating new norms of illness behavior.

Illness Perceptions

According to Rudell, Bhui, and Priebe (2009), two theories have dominated illness perception research: 1) the explanatory model (EM) from Kleinmann (1985); and 2) illness representations (IR) as a part of the self-regulatory theory (Leventhal, Leventhal, & Cameron, 2001). Explanatory models are associated with mental illness as Kleinmann is a cross-cultural psychiatrist and anthropologist. Leventhal and colleagues, on the other hand, based their research on psychological theory. They argue that there is both a cognitive and an emotional representation

of illness (Rudell et al., 2009). Although both models hold credence for individuals and families with chronic illness, this text uses the work of Leventhal and colleagues as a basis for the discussion of illness perceptions and behaviors.

Prior to focusing on behaviors, a discussion of illness perceptions is needed, as they are the basis for the behaviors exhibited by individuals and families. The literature uses two terms, *illness representations* and *illness perceptions*. Both refer to how the client (and family) view the illness. Illness representations belong to clients and are interpreted by clients and may not conform to scientific beliefs (as cited in Lee, Chaboyer, & Wallis, 2010; Diefenbach, Leventhal, Leventhal, & Patrick-Miller, 1996). In a majority of studies, illness representations are measured by the Illness Perception Questionnaire, the Illness Perception Questionnaire-Revised, or the Brief Illness Perception Questionnaire. Each of these questionnaires assesses the cognitive and emotional responses to illness (www.uib.no.ipq). For purposes of this chapter, the words will be used interchangeably, although medical sociologists might question that decision.

Why are illness perceptions of interest to healthcare providers? The primary reason is that these perceptions directly influence the emotional response that clients and families have to the illness (Petrie & Weinman, 2006). How one behaves due to the illness, implements coping strategies, and generally responds to the illness is based on one's perceptions. Clients and their families do not simply develop their own illness beliefs and perceptions within a vacuum, but they are molded by their everyday social interactions (Marks et al., 2005), their past experiences, and their culture.

Clients and families build mental models to make sense of an event (Petrie & Weinman, 2006). Thus, when a client and family face a health threat, a model of that event is developed. The idea behind a model is that clients can then visualize the threat and become active problem solvers. Within those models are their perceptions of the diagnosis, the illness experience, the treatment, and the consequences, which in turn, forecast how they will behave and/or respond to the crisis. Often these models may not make sense to an outsider, and often they may be built on faulty information. The model is dynamic, changing as new data from healthcare providers, their own experiences, and other sources are presented to the client and family and become incorporated into the model.

Leventhal and colleagues (2001) identified five dimensions that represent a client's view of their illness: 1) identity of the illness—connecting the symptoms with the illness and having an understanding of the illness; 2) timeline—duration and progression of the illness; 3) causes—perceived reason for the illness; 4) consequences—what will be the physical, psychosocial, and economic impact of the illness; and lastly 5) controllability—can this disease be controlled or cured? After identification of these dimensions, Leventhal and colleagues. believe that coping and appraisal follow.

However, is it that simple? Leventhal and colleagues' explanation leads one to believe that everything fits into a neat little box and there is a natural, linear progression from identity to control/curability. Imagine that a chronic illness has either entered your life or affected someone in your family. You may have had some sort of identity of it prior to diagnosis, but now that the condition is "yours," that perception changes. Plus, you have the Internet to provide you with more information than you can absorb. You begin with the idea that this condition is controllable, and perhaps curable, but you find a plethora of websites and data that tell you

otherwise. Thus, your beliefs and perceptions of the situation can be changed overnight, and in turn, your attitudes and behaviors do so as well.

Clients and families with chronic illness need to make sense of their illness. They construct models of the illness in an attempt to be logical and inject sense into their lives. Often the diagnosis of a chronic condition doesn't make sense to clients. The model is created to make the situation rational to the individual and family. The model is dynamic and fluid throughout the illness or threat; it's what clients and families with chronic illness "hang their hat on"—it helps them cope.

The literature about the effects of illness perceptions and beliefs on behavior and treatment is vast. What follows are some representative research studies that demonstrate current and continuing work in this area. Although there is work with clients who have a number of different chronic illnesses or injuries such as spinal cord injury (deRoon-Cassini, de St. Aubin, Valvano, Hastings, & Horn, 2009), the majority of studies have focused on heart disease.

Heart Disease

Several studies have explored the relationships among quality of life, adherence to and choice of treatment, and illness beliefs/perceptions. Juergens, Seekatz, Moosdorf, Petrie, and Rief (2010) studied 56 patients undergoing coronary artery bypass grafting (CABG). Participants were assessed using the Illness Perception Questionnaire-Revised (IPQ-R) prior to and 3 months post-surgery. The researchers concluded that patients' beliefs before surgery strongly influenced their recovery from surgery. They added that perhaps patients could benefit from some pre-surgery cognitive interventions to change maladaptive beliefs (p. 553). Similarly, Alsen, Brink, Persson, Brandstrom, and Karlson (2010) found that patients' illness perceptions influenced health outcomes after myocardial infarction. Broadbent, Ellis, Thomas, Gamble, and Petrie (2009) indicate that a brief in-hospital illness perception intervention changed perceptions and improved rates of return to work in patients with myocardial infarction.

In a sample of clients with atrial fibrillation, patients' perceptions about their symptoms and medication at diagnosis affected their health-related quality of life (Lane, Langman, Lip, & Nouwen, 2009). Negative illness beliefs were significantly predictive of higher levels of depressive symptomology at 3 and 9 months in clients with coronary artery disease (Stafford, Berk, & Jackson, 2009). Illness beliefs were also significantly associated with depressive symptomology and health-related quality of life in clients with coronary artery disease. In a study examining adherence to secondary prevention regimens, illness beliefs contributed to adherence to those behaviors (Stafford, Jackson, & Berk, 2008).

Two representative studies in hypertension have included the relationships between treatment and illness perceptions. Chen, Tsai, and Chou (2010) tested a hypothetical model of illness perception and adherence to prescribed medications. Using a sample of 355 hypertensive patients, findings suggested that adherence could be enhanced by improving the patient's perception of controllability. Other researchers have argued that illness perceptions/beliefs about hypertension have played a role in the choice of medication for treatment of hypertension (Figueiras et al., 2010).

Work Participation

Hoving, van der Meer, Volkova, and Frings-Dresen (2010) completed a systematic review of illness perceptions and participating in work (however, only three studies met the authors' criteria for review). They found that nonworking clients perceived more serious consequences, expected their illness to last a long period of time, and reported more symptoms and emotional responses. The working clients had a strong belief in the controllability of their condition and a better understanding of the disease (its identity).

Influences on Illness Behavior

Illness behavior is shaped by sociocultural and social-psychological factors (Mechanic, 1986). What follows in this section are examples of these factors.

Culture of Poverty

The culture of poverty (see Chapter 13) influences the development of social and psychological traits among those experiencing it. These traits include dependence, fatalism, inability to delay gratification, and a lower value placed on health (Cockerham, 2001, p. 123). The poor, who have to work to survive, often deny sickness unless it brings functional incapacity (Helman, 2007). Different cultures may define and interpret health and illness in a variety of ways (see Chapter 13). Individuals with chronic illness in the culture of poverty will have different looking illness perceptions and behaviors depending on their unique ethnic origins.

Demographic Status

Marital status may influence illness behavior as well. In general, married individuals require fewer services because they are healthier, but utilize other services because they are more attuned to preventive care (Thomas, 2003). Searle, Norman, Thompson, and Vedhara (2007) examined the influence of the illness perceptions of clients' significant others and their impact on client outcomes and illness perceptions. Differences in illness representations of significant others and clients have been shown to influence psychological adaptation in chronic fatigue syndrome and Addison's disease (cited in Searle et al., 2007). Searle and colleagues sought to understand illness representations in clients with type II diabetes and their partners. However, in this study, almost without exception, there was agreement between the illness representations of patients and their partners. Another aim of the study was to determine the influence of the partner or significant other on the clients' illness representation. There was some evidence to suggest that partners' representations partially mediated clients' representations on exercise and dietary behaviors (Searle et al., 2007).

Gender may influence illness behavior and "help-seeking" behavior in chronic conditions. Sociologic analysis has suggested that women are more likely than men to seek medical help for nonfatal and chronic illness (Bury, 2005). Morbidity rates demonstrate that women are more likely to be sick than men and thus seek more professional medical help (Bury, 2005, p. 55). Lorber (2000) states that women are not more fragile than men, but are just more self-protective of their health status.

Increasing age often brings chronic conditions and disability. However, older individuals in poor health (as measured by medicine's standard measures) often do not see themselves in this way. What may influence older adults' perceptions of their illness and subsequent behavior may not even be considered by healthcare professionals as "relevant." Kelley-Moore, Schumacher, Kahana, and Kahana (2006) identified that cessation of driving and receiving home health care influenced older adults' illness perceptions, causing them to self-identify as disabled.

Past Experience

One's education and learning, socialization, and past experience, as defined by one's social and cultural background, mediate illness behavior. Past experiences of observing one's parents being stoic, going to work when they were ill, avoiding medical help, all influence their children's future responses. If children see that "hard work" and not giving in to illness pays off with rewards, they will assimilate those experiences and mirror them in their own lives. Elfant, Gall, and Perlmuter (1999) evaluated the effects of avoidant illness behavior of parents on their adult children's adjustment to arthritis. Even after several decades, children's early observations of their parents' illness behaviors appear to affect their own adjustment to arthritis. Those clients whose parents avoided work and other activities when ill with a minor condition reported greater severity of arthritis and its limitations, depression, and helplessness when compared to clients whose parents did not respond to minor illness with avoidance (Elfant et al., 1999, p. 415).

What if parents and adolescents have differing views on illness perceptions? The illness perceptions of 30 adolescents and their parents were compared to see the effects on the adolescents' outcomes (Salewski, 2003). Parents' illness representations had little impact on their children's outcomes. In families with high similarity between the parents' perceptions and the adolescents' perceptions, the adolescents reported more well-being (Salewski, 2003, p. 587).

In another vein, how parents respond to their children's health complaints may later influence how the children, as adults, cope with illness. Whitehead and colleagues (1994) studied the influence of childhood social learning on the adult illness behavior of 383 women aged 20 to 40 years of age. Illness behavior was measured by frequency of symptoms, disability days, and physician visits for menstrual, bowel, and upper respiratory symptoms. Findings included that childhood reinforcement of menstrual illness behavior significantly predicted adult menstrual symptoms and disability days, and childhood reinforcement of cold illness behavior predicted adult cold symptoms and disability days. The study's data supported the hypothesis that specific patterns of illness behavior are learned during childhood through parental reinforcement and modeling, and that these behaviors continued into adulthood (Whitehead et al., 1994, p. 549).

In a small study examining illness perceptions in clients with critical illness in a medical intensive care unit, as well as their surrogates, it was hypothesized that perceptions would vary by demographic, personal, and clinical measures (Ford, Zapka, Gebregziabher, Yang, & Sterba, 2010). Although client/surrogate factors, including race, faith, and pre-critical illness quality of life were significant, clinical measures were not. Researchers concluded that clinicians should recognize the variability in illness perceptions and the possible implications this might have for patient/surrogate and healthcare provider communication.

One cannot minimize the impact of the past experiences of the individual and family on how they deal with their own chronic illnesses, their children's, parents', and/or siblings'. Each of those experiences affects how the individual and family perceive their current health challenge. These experiences could be positive as well as negative. A negative healthcare experience with a relatively minor injury/illness could have a stronger influence than that of a positive experience

with serious illness. As healthcare providers, do not underestimate the client's and family's perception of their illness and its effect on outcomes.

IMPACT AND ISSUES RELATED TO ILLNESS BEHAVIOR

As illness behavior is described, it is important to reiterate the difference between the terms *disease* and *illness*. Disease is the pathophysiology—the change in body structure or function that can be quantified, measured, and defined. Disease is the objective "measurement" of symptoms. As Wainwright (2008) states,

> disease within the medical model is materialist and assumes that the mechanisms of the body can be revealed and understood in the same way that the working of the solar system can be understood through gazing at the night sky. (p. 77)

Illness is what the client and family experience. It is what is experienced and "lived" by the client and family, and includes the "meaning" the client gives to that experience (Helman, 2007). Both the meaning given to the symptoms and the client's response, or behavior, are influenced by the client's background and personality as well as the cultural, social, and economic contexts in which the symptoms appear (p. 126).

The Illness Experience and Subsequent Behavior

The diagnosis of a chronic disease and subsequent management of that disease bring unique experiences and meanings of that process to the client and family. The biomedical world disregards illness and its meaning and focuses instead on disease. Disease can be quantified and measured, and it can be considered a "black-and-white" concept. Disease fits into the medical model's framework.

Illness, and the unique meaning that each of us attaches to it, does not fit into a neat little box; it is not black and white, but consists of many shades of gray and thus defies measurement and categorization. Illness is a subjective label that reflects both personal and social ideas about what is normal as much as the pathology behind it (Weitz, 1991). Kleinmann (1985) expressed concern that researchers have "reduced sickness to something divorced from meaning in order to avoid the hard and still unanswered technical questions concerning how to actually go about measuring meaning and objectivizing and quantifying its effect on health status and illness behavior" (Kleinmann, 1985, p. 149). While realizing the importance of this scientific work, Kleinmann (1985) sees it as "detrimental to the understanding of illness as human experience, because they redefine the problem to subtract that which is mostly innately human, beliefs, feelings" (p. 149).

The common sense self-regulation model (Leventhal et al., 2001) seeks to explain that individual illness perceptions influence coping responses to an illness. This perspective explains that clients construct their own illness representations to help them make sense of their illness experience. It is these representations that form a basis for appropriate or inappropriate coping responses (Leventhal et al., 2001). Stuifbergen Phillips, Voelmeck, & Browder (2006) used a convenience sample of 91 women with fibromyalgia to explore their illness representations. Overall, the women had fairly negative perceptions of their illness. Emotional representations explained 41% of the variance in mental health

scores. Using the model of Levanthal and colleagues (2001), less emotional distress predicted more frequent health behaviors and more positive mental health scores; whereas those women who perceived their fibromyalgia to have more serious consequences and as less controllable were more likely to have higher scores on the Fibromyalgia Impact Questionnaire (p. 359).

Price (1996) describes individuals with a chronic disease as developing an illness career that responds to changes in health, his or her involvement with healthcare professionals, and the psychological changes associated with pathology, grief, and stress management (p. 276). This illness career is dynamic, flexible, and goes through different stages of adaptation as the disease itself may change.

Powerlessness

This construct is a major component of the illness experience. As such, an entire chapter in this book has been devoted to this subject (see Chapter 12).

Loss of Self

Charmaz (1983) coined the phrase "loss of self" with her research in the 1980s, interviewing individuals with chronic illness through a symbolic interactionist perspective. The influences on the loss of self develop from the chronic condition(s) and the illness experience. Charmaz describes clients' illness experience as living a restricted life, experiencing social isolation, being discredited, and burdening others. Slowly the individual with chronic illness feels his or her self-image disappear: a loss of self, without the development of an equally valued new one (p. 168).

In another study of 40 men with chronic illness, Charmaz (1994) describes different identity dilemmas than with women. Charmaz sees these men as "preserving self." As men come to terms with illness and disability, they preserve self by limiting the effect from illness in their lives. They intensify control over their lives. Many assume that they can recapture their past self, and they try to do so. They may devote vast amounts of energy to keeping their illness contained and the disability invisible to maintain their masculinity. At the same time, they often maintain another identity at home—thus they create a public identity and a private identity to preserve self (Charmaz, 1994, p. 282).

Moral Work

Townsend, Wyke, and Hunt (2006) describe the moral dimension of the chronic illness experience in their qualitative study. Their work speaks to the fact that moral work is integral to the illness, similar to the biographical and everyday "work" of Corbin and Strauss (1988). The participants in their study spoke about the need to demonstrate their moral worth as individuals, that it was their moral obligation to manage symptoms alongside their daily life (Townsend et al., 2006, p. 189).

Devalued Self

In a qualitative study of Chinese immigrant women in Canada, Anderson (1991) describes how these women with type I diabetes have a devalued self, not only from the disease but also because of dealing with being marginalized in a foreign country where they do not speak the language. Similar to the "loss of self" described by Charmaz, Anderson discusses women who need to reconstruct a new self. Influencing this devalued self were the interactions with healthcare professionals, which were frequently negative in nature, adding to their stress.

Similarly, eight older women with a chronic disease were asked to describe the meaning of living with a long-term illness. Five themes emerged: loss and uncertainty, learning one's capacity and living accordingly, maintaining fellowship and belonging, having a source of strength, and building anew. However, clearly the guiding premise of each woman was that chronic illness brought about reassessment and formation of a new understanding of self, and a sense of being revalued by the world (Lundman & Jansson, 2007).

Chronic Sorrow

The concept of chronic sorrow was first described by Olshansky in 1962 when he was working with parents of children with learning disabilities. His conclusion was that chronic sorrow was a natural response to a tragedy instead of becoming neurotic (p. 193). Two more recent studies discuss the existence of chronic sorrow in individuals with chronic illness. Sixty-one clients with multiple sclerosis were interviewed about chronic sorrow and also screened for depression. Thirty-eight of the 61 clients met the criteria for chronic sorrow. The participants in the study described feeling sorrow, fear, anger, and anxiety. Frustration and sadness were constantly present, or were periodically overwhelming (Isaksson, Gunnarsson, & Ahlstrom, 2007, p. 318). Seven themes were identified: loss of hope, loss of control over the body, loss of integrity and dignity, loss of a healthy identity, loss of faith that life is just, loss of social relations, and loss of freedom (Isaksson et al., 2007). Implications for healthcare providers included providing psychological support for these individuals. How does one provide the appropriate help when the client perceives such significant losses? What realistic help can healthcare professionals provide?

Similarly, Ahlstrom (2007) interviewed 30 adults of working age with an average disease duration of 18 years. Sixteen of the 30 adults experienced chronic sorrow. The losses in this study are consistent with other studies on chronic sorrow even though the group was heterogeneous regarding diagnosis.

The Legitimization of Chronic Illness

With some illnesses, especially when symptoms are not well defined and diagnostic tests may be ambiguous, receiving legitimization from a physician or other healthcare professional may be difficult and frustrating. Denial of opportunity to move into the sick role leads to "doctor hopping," placing clients in problematic relationships in which they must "work out" solutions alone (Steward & Sullivan, 1982). As a result, symptomatic persons may be left to question the truth of their own illness perceptions. How do you build a mental model of your illness (as a basis for problem solving) if healthcare providers and society in general are skeptical of your symptoms?

As examples, two current chronic conditions often defy diagnosis and are slow to respond to treatment. Chronic fatigue syndrome (CFS) and fibromyalgia are typically seen as diseases of young women. In both diseases there is uncertainty with respect to etiology, treatment, and prognosis. They have been contested illnesses, in that some question their existence (Asbring, 2001). Without legitimatization from physicians or the healthcare system, these clients are labeled as hypochondriacs or malingerers. Some of these clients are referred to psychologists or psychiatrists when a physical diagnosis cannot be made and diagnostic test results are normal.

When a diagnosis is finally made, the client frequently shows a somewhat joyous initial response to having a name for the recurrent and troublesome symptoms. This reaction results from the decrease in stress over the unknown. These clients have an enormous stake in how their illnesses are understood. They seek to achieve the legitimacy necessary to elicit sympathy and avoid stigma, and to protect their own self-concept (Mechanic, 1995).

Asbring (2001) identified two themes from her qualitative study in which women with CFS or fibromyalgia were interviewed. She describes an earlier identity partly lost, and coming to terms with a new identity. Asbring uses the term *identity transformation* with the women she interviewed. However, she also saw illness gains in these women. The illness and its limitations provided the women with time to think and reflect on their lives and perhaps rearrange priorities. Therefore, the illness experience of these women may be seen as a paradox with both losses and gains (Asbring, 2001, p. 318).

Larun and Malterud (2007) examined 20 qualitative studies in a meta-ethnography about the illness experiences of individuals with CFS to summarize the illness experiences of the individuals as well as the physicians' perspectives. Across studies, clients spoke of being "controlled and betrayed by their bodies" (Larun & Malterud, 2007, pp. 22–23). Although physical activities were mostly curtailed, individuals spoke of mental fatigue that affected memory and concentration, they described difficulty with following conversations, and several clients felt that their learning abilities had decreased (p. 24). One of the themes that emerged was telling stories about *bodies that no longer held the capacity for social involvement.* For some individuals the most distressing part of the illness were the negative responses from family members, the workplace, and their physicians, who *questioned the legitimacy of their illness behavior* because of the dynamic symptoms of CFS (p. 25). Thus their physicians' beliefs about CFS influenced the clients' perceptions of the disease and therefore their illness experience. To summarize, the researchers' analysis determined that clients' sense of identity becomes more or less invalid and that a change in identity of the individuals was experienced.

Dickson, Knussen, and Flowers (2008) describe the personal loss and identity crisis in their study of 14 individuals diagnosed with CFS. Participants talked about the illness that is their life and controls every aspect of their daily lives. Self-comparison took place between the participants' former selves and their "ill selves." Skepticism from others brought further crises of self.

Lastly Nettleton (2006) describes interviews with 18 neurology patients in the United Kingdom with MUS—medically unexplained symptoms. Not having a diagnosis limits legitimate access to the sick role and the ability to build a mental model of the illness. One of the biggest hurdles is that society does not grant permission to be ill in the absence of a disease with a name.

Professional Responses to Illness Behavior and Roles

Healthcare professionals generally expect those entering the acute hospital setting to conform to sick role behaviors. Most people entering the hospital for the first time are quickly socialized and expected to cooperate with treatment, to recover, and to return to their normal roles. Provider expectations and client responses are in line with social expectations and fit with the traditional medical model of illness as acute and curable. When clients are compliant and cooperative,

CASE STUDY

Mary Ellen is a 35-year-old woman with unexplained neurological symptoms. She is a relatively new client to the clinic where you work. However, she has been seen by your clinic several times over the last 3 months. Originally her diagnosis was "probable multiple sclerosis." However, that diagnosis has been ruled out. Mary Ellen's clinical symptoms include double vision (at times), transient numbness and tingling down the right side of her body, and general weakness and fatigue. Although she has been employed full time as a staff associate at the county assessor's office, she has been forced to go on short-term disability. In her phone call to the office this morning, she is frustrated. She states, "I feel like no one is believing me—that you people think that I am making this up. I'm going to lose my job if you can't figure this out. I'm not a psych case."

Discussion Questions

1. How do you make sense of this client's illness behavior?
2. What strategies might you use to deal with this client?
3. How could you apply the frameworks for practice mentioned in this chapter to this client situation?

healthcare professionals communicate to them that they are "good patients" (Lorber, 1981). When clients are less cooperative, the staff may consider them problematic or nonadherent.

The percentage of individuals with chronic illness entering hospitals is increasing, and often these admissions are due to superimposed acute illness or exacerbations of the chronic condition. Additionally, older adults in particular may have more than one chronic condition. Many of these individuals have had their chronic illnesses for long periods and have had prior hospital experiences. Multiple contacts with the healthcare system result in loss of the "blind faith" that the individual once had in that system. Individuals with chronic illness seek a different kind of relationship with healthcare professionals, in which there is "give and take" and that can empower the client. The extent to which a client with chronic illness is included in the formulation of his or her treatment plan likely influences the assumption of responsibility for it and, ultimately, its success (Weaver & Wilson, 1994).

Thorne's (1990) study of individuals with chronic illness and their families found that their relationships with healthcare professionals evolved from what was termed "naïve trust" through "disenchantment" to a final stage of "guarded alliance." She proposed that the "rules" that govern these relationships should be entirely different for acute illness and chronic illness. Although assuming sick-role dependency may be adaptive in acute illness, where medical expertise offers hope of a cure, it is not so in chronic illness. Individuals with chronic illness are the "experts" in their illnesses and should have the ultimate authority in managing those illnesses over time.

When individuals with chronic illness are hospitalized, they view the situation quite differently than do the healthcare professionals with whom they interact. Clients with multiple chronic conditions may focus on maintaining stability of their chronic conditions to prevent unnecessary symptoms, whereas their healthcare providers are more likely to focus on managing the current acute disorder. In addition, clients who have had multiple prior admissions are more likely to use their hospital savvy to gain what they want or need from the system. During hospitalization, these individuals may demand certain treatments, specific times for treatment, or routines outside of hospital parameters. They may keep track of times that various routines occur or complain about or report actions of the staff as a means to an end they consider important. In a grounded theory study in the United Kingdom, Wilson, Kendall, and Brooks (2006) explored how client expertise is viewed, interpreted, defined, and experienced by both clients and healthcare professionals. With nursing playing a key role in empowering clients with chronic disease to self-manage their conditions, knowing how that client expertise is viewed (by the care provider) is extremely important. Generally, in this study of 100 healthcare professionals (physicians, nurses, physical therapists), the nurses found the expert patients to be more threatening than other healthcare professionals did. The nurses had issues with accountability, perceived threats to their professional power, and potential litigation. The data from the study demonstrated that the nurses lacked a clear role definition and distinct expertise in working with patients with chronic disease and were unable to work in a flexible partnership with self-managing patients (Wilson et al., 2006, p. 810).

Lack of Role Norms for Individuals with Chronic Illness

Chronic illnesses require a variety of tasks be performed to fulfill the requirements of both the medical regimen and the individual's personal lifestyle. However, there is a lack of norms for those with chronic illness. What is expected of a client recovering from cancer surgery? An exacerbation of rheumatoid arthritis? A flare-up of inflammatory bowel disease? Assume sick-role behaviors are discouraged, or not? These individuals enter and remain in a type of impaired, "at-risk" role. Implicit behaviors for this role are not well defined by society, leading to a situation of role ambiguity. Given this lack of norms, influences on the client include the degree of disability (with different attributes of disability producing different consequences), visibility of the disability (the less the visibility, the more normal the response), self-acceptance of the disability (resulting in others' reciprocating with acceptance), and societal views of the disabled as either economically dependent or productive. Without role definition, whether disability is present or not, individuals are unable to achieve maximum levels of functioning. Individuals must adapt their definitions of themselves to their limitations, and to what the anticipated future imposes on them because of the chronic condition (Watt, 2000). What is normal illness behavior?

INTERVENTIONS

There is no "magic" list of interventions to assist and support clients and their families with the illness experience. The current healthcare system with its acute-care focus, fix-and-cure model, and a prescription for each symptom, does not fit with caring for individuals long term. These clients do not need their illness behavior "fixed" or "cured," but instead they need a healthcare professional who will listen and understand the illness experience and not the disease process. What follows are suggestions that *assist and support* clients and their families.

Frameworks and Models for Practice

A review of the literature since the last edition of this book did not yield any new frameworks for caring for those with chronic illness. With chronic illness increasing, evidence-based frameworks need to be developed. As stated previously, not all healthcare providers have the skills to care for those with long-term illness. Meeting the psychosocial needs of clients with chronic illness, alone, is an ominous task. Caring for a client with chronic illness requires a framework or model for practice that differs from that of caring for those with acute, episodic disease. The frameworks that follow are examples, and are not intended to be all inclusive.

These frameworks and models should not be confused with the disease management models discussed in Chapter 19. Disease management models address the physical symptoms of a condition. Some of those models assign an algorithm to the condition where clients receive certain "care" when their blood work is at an inappropriate level, or their symptoms "measure" a certain degree of seriousness. These models manage the disease, but not the illness. Illness frameworks and models address the illness experience of the individual and family that occurs as a result of changing health status.

Chronic Illness and Quality of Life

In the early 1960s, Anselm Strauss, working with Barney Glaser, a social scientist, and Jeanne Quint Benoliel, a nurse, interviewed dying patients to determine what kind of "care" was needed for these clients (Corbin & Strauss, 1992). As a result of those early interviews, Strauss and colleagues (Strauss & Glaser, 1975; Strauss et al., 1984) published a rudimentary framework that addressed the issues and concerns of individuals with chronic illness. Although the term *trajectory* was coined at that time, it did not become fully developed until 20 years later. Strauss and colleagues' framework was simple, but it was an early attempt to examine the illness experience of the individual and family as opposed to the disease. If healthcare professionals could better understand the illness experience of clients and families, perhaps more appropriate care would be provided. Basic to this care is understanding the key problems of chronic illness, including:

- Prevention of medical crises and their management if they occur
- Controlling symptoms
- Carrying out of prescribed medical regimens
- Prevention of, or living with, social isolation
- Adjustment to changes in the disease
- Attempts to normalize interactions and lifestyle
- Funding—finding the necessary money
- Confronting attendant psychological, marital, and familial problems (Strauss et al., 1984, p. 16)

After identifying the key problems of the individual and family with chronic illness, Strauss and colleagues (1984) suggested basic problem-solving strategies, family and organizational arrangements, and then re-evaluating the consequences of those arrangements.

The Trajectory Framework

From the work of Strauss and colleagues in the 1960s and 1970s, the trajectory framework was further refined in the 1980s. Corbin and Strauss (1992) developed this framework so that nurses could: 1) gain insight into the chronic illness experience of the client; 2) integrate existing literature about chronicity into their practice; and 3) provide direction for building nursing models that guide practice, teaching, research, and policy-making (p. 10).

A trajectory is defined as the course of an illness over time, plus the actions of clients, families, and healthcare professionals to manage that course (Corbin, 1998, p. 3). The illness trajectory is set in motion by pathophysiology and changes in health status, but there are strategies that can be used by clients, families, and healthcare professionals that shape the course of dying and thus the illness trajectory (Corbin & Strauss, 1992). Even if the disease may be the same, each individual's illness trajectory is different and takes into account the uniqueness of each individual (Jablonski, 2004). Shaping does not imply that the ultimate course of the disease will be changed or the disease will be cured, merely that the illness trajectory may be shaped or altered by actions of the individual and family so that the disease course is stable, fewer exacerbations occur, and symptoms are better controlled (Corbin & Strauss, 1992).

Within the model, the term *phase* indicates the different stages of the chronic illness experience for the client. There are nine phases in the trajectory model, and although it could be conceived as a continuum, it is not linear. Clients may move through these phases in a linear fashion, regress to a former phase, or plateau for an extended period. In addition, having more than one chronic disease influences movement along the trajectory. Another term used in the model is *biography*. A client's biography consists of previous hospital experiences and useful ways of dealing with symptoms, illness beliefs, and other life experiences

The initial phase of the trajectory model is the pretrajectory phase, or preventive phase, in which the course of illness has not yet begun; however, there are genetic factors or lifestyle behaviors that place an individual at risk for a chronic condition. An example would be the individual who is overweight, has a family history of cardiac disease and high cholesterol, and does not exercise.

During the trajectory phase, signs and symptoms of the disease appear and a diagnostic workup may begin. The individual begins to cope with implications of a diagnosis. In the stable phase, the illness symptoms are under control and management of the disease occurs primarily at home. A period of inability to keep symptoms under control occurs in the unstable phase. The acute phase brings severe and unrelieved symptoms or disease complications. Critical or life-threatening situations that require emergency treatment occur in the crisis phase. The comeback phase signals a gradual return to an acceptable way of life within the symptoms that the disease imposes. The downward phase is characterized by progressive deterioration and an increase in disability or symptoms. The trajectory model ends with the dying phase, characterized by gradual or rapid shutting down of body processes (Corbin, 2001, pp. 4–5).

Chronic Illness and the Life Cycle

Rolland's (1987) illness trajectory model encompasses three phases: 1) crisis, 2) chronic, and 3) terminal. The crisis phase has two subphases consisting of the symptomatic period prior to diagnosis and the period of initial adjustment just after diagnosis. The chronic phase is the period between the beginning of treatment and the terminal phase. Rolland was one of the first authors to describe chronic illness, and in this case the chronic phase, as the "long haul," the day-to-day living with chronic illness. Lastly, the terminal phase is divided into the preterminal phase, where the client and family acknowledge that death is inevitable, and the period following death (Jablonski, 2004, p. 54).

Shifting Perspectives Model of Chronic Illness

This model resulted from the work of Thorne and Paterson (1998), who analyzed 292 qualitative studies of chronic physical illness that were published from 1980 to 1996. Of these, 158 studies became a part of a metastudy in which client roles in chronic illness were described. The work of Thorne and Paterson reflects the "insider" perspective of chronic illness as opposed to the "outsider" view, the more traditional view. This change in perspective is a shift from the traditional approach of patient-as-client to one of client-as-partner in care (p. 173). Results from the metastudy also demonstrated a shift away from focusing on loss and burden, and an attempt to view health within illness.

Analysis of these studies led to the development of the Shifting Perspectives Model of Chronic Illness (Paterson, 2001). The model depicts chronic illness as an ongoing, continually shifting process where people experience a complex dialectic between the world and themselves (p. 23). Paterson's model considers both the "illness" and the "wellness" of the individual (Paterson, 2003). The illness-in-the-foreground perspective focuses on the sickness, loss, and burden of the chronic illness. This is a common reaction of those recently diagnosed with a chronic disease. The overwhelming consequences of the condition, learning about their illness, considerations of treatment, and long-term effects contribute to putting the illness in the foreground. The disease becomes the individual's identity.

Illness-in-the-foreground could also be a protective response by the individual and be used to conserve energy for other activities. However, it could be used to maintain their identity as a "sick" person, or because it is congruent with their need to have sickness as their social identity and receive secondary gains (Paterson, 2001).

With the wellness-in-the-foreground perspective, the "self" is the source of identity rather than the disease (Paterson, 2001, p. 23). The individual is in control and not the disease. It does not mean, though, that the individual is physically well, cured, or even in remission of the disease symptoms. The shift occurs in the individual's thinking, allowing the individual to focus away from the disease. However, any threat that cannot be controlled will transition the individual back to the illness-in-the-foreground perspective. Threats include disease progression and lack of ability to self-manage the disease, stigma, and interactions with others (Paterson, 2001).

Lastly, neither the illness perspective nor the wellness perspective is right or wrong, but each merely reflects the individual's unique needs, health status, and focus at the time (Paterson, 2001). In Paterson's research published in 2003, one of her study participants was concerned that those reading about the Shifting Perspectives Model might interpret the two perspectives as "either/or"—that one has to have either wellness or illness in the foreground. This individual states:

> I think there is danger when researchers think there is a right way to have a chronic illness. There is only one way . . . the one you choose at the moment . . . generally I live in the orange. If red is illness and yellow represents wellness, then I like to be a blend of both things . . . in the orange . . . It is not a good idea for me to be completely yellow because then I forget that I have MS and I do stupid things that I pay for later. And if I am totally in the red, I am too depressed to do anything. (Paterson, 2003, p. 990)

Dealing with Dependency

Chronic illness is fraught with unpredictable dilemmas. Even when an acute stage is past, the client's energy for recovery may be sapped by the uncertainty about the future course of the illness, the effectiveness of medical regimens, and the disruption of usual patterns of living. Awareness of behavioral responses and when they occur can help the professional avoid premature emphasis on independence until the client can collaborate in working toward a return to normal roles.

Miller (2000) recommends several strategies for decreasing clients' feelings of powerlessness as they work toward independence:

- Modifying the environment to afford clients more means of control
- Helping clients set realistic goals and expectations
- Increasing clients' knowledge about their illness and its management

- Increasing the sensitivity of health professionals and significant others to the powerlessness imposed by chronic illness
- Encouraging verbalization of feelings

Utilizing knowledge of illness roles in planning interventions allows the healthcare professional to maximize time spent with the client. One such intervention that could be improved by integrating knowledge of illness roles is education (see Chapter 15). The client who is still in the highly dependent phase cannot benefit from education. As improvement in physical status occurs, emphasis on the desire to return to normal roles creates motivation to learn about the condition and necessary procedures for maximizing health. As the client moves into the impaired role and becomes aware of the necessity to maximize remaining potential, education provides a highly successful tool both in the hospital and at home.

phenomenological method, four major themes emerged: 1) needing to be normal, 2) dealing with the behaviors of others, 3) enduring the restrictions of illness, and 4) learning from self to care for others. Throughout the students' experiences, they tried to negate their illness or their abnormal behavior and maintain their valued social role as students. Participants felt that their chronic illness created an inner strength and gave them intuitive knowledge about the body and how to better understand the needs of others.

Source: Dailey, M. (2010). Needing to be normal: The lived experience of chronically ill nursing students. *International Journal of Nursing Education Scholarship, 7*(1), Article 15. 10.2202/1548-923X.1798.

Evidence-Based Practice Box

Ten full-time nursing students, all diagnosed with at least one chronic illness, were interviewed to examine their illness experience. Participants looked for ways to be ordinary because they perceived they were different from the norm. Chronic conditions included systemic lupus erythematous, Raynaud's syndrome, rheumatoid arthritis, psoriasis, chronic back pain, irritable bowel syndrome, fibromyalgia, relapsing-remitting multiple sclerosis, type I diabetes mellitus, chronic urinary tract infections, anorexia/bulimia, and adrenal hyperplasia. Using Colaizzi's

Self-Management

The participants in the study by Kralick, Koch, Price, and Howard (2004) identified self-management as a process that they initiated to bring about order in their lives. This is in sharp contrast to how most healthcare professionals describe self-management in a structured patient education program that assists clients in adhering to their medical regimen. The participants saw self-management as creating a sense of order, and a process that included four themes: 1) recognizing and monitoring the boundaries; 2) mobilizing the resources; 3) managing the shift in self-identity; and 4) balancing, pacing, planning, and prioritizing (Kralick et al., 2004, pp. 262–263). Kralick and colleagues suggest that self-management is a combination of a process by clients and families and a structure of patient education.

The Women to Women project has been instrumental in helping women with chronic illness in rural states manage their illnesses. Through a computer intervention model that provides education, support groups, and fosters self-care, women have successfully managed their illness responses (Sullivan, Weinert, & Cudney, 2003).

Clients with chronic illness use multiple techniques to manage symptoms, maintain social roles, be the "good patient," and maintain some degree of normality. Townsend, Wyke, and Hunt (2006) describe the moral obligation of individuals to self-manage their symptoms and manage their selves. Although individuals are trying to manage both symptoms and social roles, the priority is always given to behaviors that typify a "normal" life and identity management over managing the symptoms of the disease (p. 193).

Critical to working with clients and families in self-managing both their disease and their illness is appropriate client–healthcare provider communication. Thorne, Harris, Mahoney, Con, and McGuiness (2004) interviewed clients with end-stage renal disease, type II diabetes, multiple sclerosis, and fibromyalgia to determine what clients perceived as priorities. Across all diseases, the concepts of courtesy, respect, and engagement were important. Certainly courtesy and respect are fairly clear in their meaning. Engagement was described by clients as an extension of courtesy and respect. An example would be a healthcare professional engaged with a client in problem solving and care management, in which they experienced a feeling of teamwork/working together (p. 301).

Such communication enhanced their relationships with clients.

Kaptein, Klok, Moss-Morris, and Brand (2010) reviewed 19 studies that examined how illness perceptions could impact an individual's control of asthma. Using the Common Sense Model of Self-Regulation as a basis, the authors created their own model of how these perceptions affected self-management. The conclusion of the authors was that self-management was determined mainly by behavioral factors and not sociodemographic factors. One of those behavioral factors was illness perceptions. They note that changing a client's illness perceptions is called for to help the client and healthcare provider achieve optimal asthma control (Kaptein et al., 2010, p. 199).

Research

Do we understand and can we place in an appropriate context the meaning of illness for clients? Why do some individuals ignore symptoms and refuse to seek medical advice, while others with the same condition seek immediate care and relief from their "social roles" at the slightest symptom? A relatively minor symptom in one individual causes great distress, whereas more serious health conditions in others cause little concern.

Stuifbergen and colleagues (2006) suggest that it is unclear from the literature how illness perceptions change over time and how specifically these perceptions are influenced. These researchers believe that if illness perceptions can be altered, then interactions with those in a positive manner could be encouraged. Bijsterbosch and colleagues (2009) noted that illness perceptions did change over time and were related to the progression of the disability (p. 1058). Illness perceptions regarding the number of symptoms attributed to osteoarthritis (OA), and the level of perceived control and perceived consequences of OA were predictive of more disability.

Mechanic (1986, 1995) asks a question that is still pertinent today: What are the processes or factors that cause individuals exposed to similar stressors to respond differently and present unique illness behavior? There is such variation in how individuals perceive their health status, seek or not seek medical care, and function in their social and work roles. What causes these differences?

This author poses another question. What can we do as healthcare providers to change illness perceptions of clients? A growing body of evidence shows that more negative views of illness held by clients are associated with poorer outcomes (Petrie & Weinman, 2006). What can we do to effect change in chronic sorrow? How can we give clients a sense of hope? How do we value clients so that they don't feel they have devalued lives? Chronic illness is the condition as the client and family experience it. What can we do to make a difference in the lives of our clients and families?

OUTCOMES

Illness behavior is not deviant and does not need to be fixed. However, we need to support our clients and understand the lived experience of the illness. As healthcare professionals, we are efficient and effective working within the disease model. However, the client lives in the illness model as well. Because nursing is an art and a science, there is a strong "fit" with the illness model. The best outcome for clients with chronic illness would be the healthcare professional supporting and assisting the client through the illness experience.

STUDY QUESTIONS

Using this chapter as a guide, how would you support and work with an individual that has either CFS or fibromyalgia? How do your own past healthcare experiences influence your practice with these clients?

Dealing with "expert" patients can be difficult. Often your own "power" as a healthcare professional is threatened. How do you deal with "expert" patients and make it a collaborative relationship?

There are no norms for individuals with long-term illness. What does this mean and how does it apply to the clients with chronic illness that you care for?

Differentiate between health and illness behavior and give examples of each for someone with end-stage heart failure, endometriosis, or esophageal cancer.

How do healthcare professionals influence the illness behavior of clients and families in positive ways or negative ways?

Apply each of the frameworks for practice described in this chapter to clients with chronic illness that you care for.

Reflect on your own past and present health and illness experiences. What influences your own illness behaviors?

REFERENCES

Ahlstrom, G. (2007). Experiences of loss and chronic sorrow in persons with severe chronic illness. *Journal of Nursing and Healthcare of Chronic Illness* in association with *Journal of Clinical Nursing, 16*(3a), 76–83.

Alsen, P., Brink, E., Persson, L, Brandstrom, Y., & Karlson, B. W. (2010). Illness perceptions after myocardial infarction: Relations to fatigue, emotional distress, and health-related quality of life. *Journal of Cardiovascular Nursing, 25*(2), E1–E10.

Anderson, J. M. (1991). Immigrant women speak of chronic illness: The social construction of the devalued self. *Journal of Advanced Nursing, 16*, 710–717.

Asbring, P. (2001). Chronic illness—a disruption in life: Identity transformation among women with chronic fatigue syndrome and fibromyalgia. *Journal of Advanced Nursing, 34*(3), 312–319.

Bijsterbosch, J., Scharlooo, M., Visser, A. W., Watt, I., Meulenbelt, T. W., Huzinga, J., et al. (2009). Illness perceptions in patients with osteoarthritis: Change over time and association with disability. *Arthritis and Rheumatism, 61*(8), 1054–1061.

Broadbent, E., Ellis, C. J., Thomas, J., Gamble, G., & Petrie, K. J. (2009). Further development of an illness perception intervention for myocardial infarction patients: A randomized controlled trial. *Journal of Psychosomatic Research, 67*, 17–23.

Bury, M. (2005). *Health and illness*. Cambridge, UK: Polity Press.

Charmaz, K. (1983). Loss of self: A fundamental form of suffering in the chronically ill. *Sociology of health and illness, 5*(2), 168–195.

Charmaz, K. (1994). Identity dilemma of chronically ill men. *The Sociological Quarterly, 35*(2), 269–288.

Chen, S. L., Tsai, J. C., & Chou, K. R. (2010). Illness perceptions and adherence to therapeutic regimens among patients with hypertension: A structural modeling approach. *International Journal of Nursing Studies, 8*(2), 235–245.

Cockerham, W. C. (2001). The sick role. In *Medical sociology* (8th ed.; pp. 156–178). Upper Saddle River, NJ: Prentice-Hall.

Conrad, P. (2005). *The sociology of health and illness: Critical perspectives* (7th ed.). New York: Worth Publishers.

Corbin, J. (1998). The Corbin & Strauss chronic illness trajectory model: An update. *Scholarly Inquiry for Nursing Practice, 12*(1), 33–41.

Corbin, J. (2001). Introduction and overview: Chronic illness and nursing. In R. Hyman & J. Corbin (Eds.), *Chronic illness: Research and theory for nursing practice* (pp. 1–15). New York, Springer.

Corbin, J. M., & Strauss, A. (1988). *Unending work and care: Managing chronic illness at home*. San Francisco: Jossey-Bass.

Corbin, J., & Strauss, A. (1992). A nursing model for chronic illness management based upon the trajectory framework. In P. Woog (Ed.), *The chronic illness trajectory framework: The Corbin and Strauss nursing model* (pp. 9–28). New York: Springer.

Dailey, M. (2010). Needing to be normal: The lived experience of chronically ill nursing students. *International Journal of Nursing Education Scholarship, 7*(1), Article 15.10.2202/1548-923X.1798.

deRoon-Cassini, T., de St. Aubin, E., Valvano, A., Hastings, J., & Horn, P. (2009). Psychological well-being after spinal cord injury: Perception of loss and meaning making. *Rehabilitation Psychology, 54*(3), 306–314.

Dickson, A., Knussen, C., & Flowers, P. (2008). 'That was my old life; it's almost like a past-life now': Identify crisis, loss and adjustment among people living with chronic fatigue syndrome. *Psychology and Health, 23*(4), 459–476.

Diefenbach, M. A., Leventhal, E. A., Leventhal, H., & Patrick-Miller, L. (1996). Negative affect relates to cross-sectional but not longitudinal symptom reporting: Data from elderly adults. *Health Psychology, 15*(4), 282–288.

Elfant, E., Gall, E., & Perlmuter, L. C. (1999). Learned illness behavior and adjustment to arthritis. *Arthritis Care and Research, 12*(6), 411–416.

Figueiras, M., Marcelino, D., Claudino, A., Cortes, M., Maroco, J., & Weinman, J. (2010). Patients' illness schemata of hypertension: The role of beliefs for the choice of treatment. *Psychology and Health, 25*(4), 507–517.

Ford, D., Zapka, J., Gebregziabher, M., Yang, C., & Sterba, K. (2010). Factors associated with illness perception among critically ill patients and surrogates. *Chest, 138*, 59–67.

Freidson, E. (1970). *Profession of medicine*. New York: Dodd, Mead.

Helman, C. G. (2007). *Culture, health and illness* (5th ed.). London: Arnold.

Hoving, J. L., van der Meer, M., Volkova, A. Y., & Frings-Dresen, M. H. W. (2010). Illness perceptions and work participation: A systematic review. *International Archives of Occupational & Environmental Health, 83*(6), 595–605.

The Illness Perception Questionnaire. Retrieved August 2, 2011 from http://www.uib.no/ipq

Isaksson, A., Gunnarsson, LO., & Ahlstrom, G. (2007). The presence and meaning of chronic sorrow in patients with multiple sclerosis. *Journal of Nursing and Healthcare of Chronic Illness* in association with *Journal of Clinical Nursing, 16*(11c), 315–324.

Jablonski, A. (2004). The illness trajectory of end-stage renal disease dialysis patients. *Research and Theory for Nursing Practice: An International Journal, 18*(1), 51–72.

Juergens, M. C., Seekatz, B., Moosdorf, R. G., Petrie, K. J., & Rief, W. (2010). Illness beliefs before cardiac surgery predict disability, quality of life and depression 3 months later. *Journal of Psychosomatic Research, 68*, 553–560.

Kaptein, A. A., Klok, T., Moss-Morris, R., & Brand, P. L. P. (2010). Illness perceptions: Impact on self-management and control in asthma. *Current Opinion in Allergy and Clinical Immunology, 10*, 194–199.

Kasl, S. V., & Cobb, S. (1966). Health behavior, illness behavior, and sick-role behavior. *Archives of Environmental Health, 12*, 531–541.

Kelley-Moore, J. A., Schumacher, J. G., Kahana, E., & Kahana, B. (2006). When do older adults become "disabled"? Social and health antecedents of perceived disability in a panel study of the oldest old. *Journal of Health and Social Behavior, 47*, 126–141.

Kleinmann, A. (1985). Illness meanings and illness behavior. In S. McHugh & M. Vallis (Eds.), *Illness behavior: A multidisciplinary model* (pp. 149–160). New York: Plenum.

Kralick, D., Koch, T., Price, K., & Howard, N. (2004). Chronic illness management: Taking action to create order. *Journal of Clinical Nursing, 13*, 259–267.

Lane, D. A., Langman, C. M., Lip, G. Y. H., & Nouwen, A. (2009). Illness perceptions, affective response, and health-related quality of life in patients with atrial fibrillation. *Journal of Psychosomatic Research, 66*, 203–210.

Larun, L., & Malterud, K. (2007). Identity and coping experiences in chronic fatigue syndrome: A synthesis of qualitative studies. *Patient Education and Counseling, 69*, 20–28.

Lee, B., Chaboyer, W., & Wallis, M. (2010). Illness representations in patients with traumatic injury: A longitudinal study. *Journal of Clinical Nursing, 19*, 556–463.

Leventhal, H., Leventhal, E. A., & Cameron, L. (2001). Representations, procedures, and affect in illness self-regulation: A perceptual-cognitive model. In A. Baum, T. A. Revenson, & , J. E. Singer (Eds.), *Handbook of health psychology* (pp. 19–47). Mahwah, NJ: Lawrence Erlbaum Associates.

Lorber, J. (2000). Gender and health. In P. Brown (Ed.), *Perspectives in Medical Sociology* (3rd ed., pp. 40–70). Prospect Heights, IL: Waveland Press.

Lorber, J. (1981). Good patients and problem patients: Conformity and deviance in a general hospital. In P. Conrad & R. Kern (Eds.), *The sociology of health and illness: Critical perspectives*. New York: St. Martin's.

Lundman, B., & Jansson, L. (2007). The meaning of living with a long-term disease: To revalue and be revalued. *Journal of Nursing and Healthcare of Chronic Illness* in association with *Journal of Clinical Nursing 16*, 7b, 109–115.

Marks, D. F., Murray, M., Evans, B., Willig, C., Woodall, C., & Sykes, C. (2005). *Health psychology: Theory, research and practice* (2nd ed.). Thousand Oaks, CA: Sage.

McHugh, S., & Vallis, M. (1986). Illness behavior: Operationalization of the biopsychosocial model. In S. McHugh & M. Vallis (Eds.), *Illness behavior: A multidisciplinary model* (pp. 1–32). New York: Plenum.

Mechanic, D. (1962). The concept of illness behavior. *Journal of Chronic Diseases, 15*, 189–194.

Mechanic, D. (1986). The concept of illness behavior: Culture, situation, and personal predisposition. *Psychological Medicine, 16*, 1–7.

Mechanic, D. (1995). Sociological dimensions of illness behavior. *Social Science and Medicine, 41*(9), 1207–1216.

Miller, J. F. (2000). *Coping with chronic illness: Overcoming powerlessness* (3rd ed.). Philadelphia: F. A. Davis.

Nettleton, S. (2006). 'I just want permission to be ill': Towards a sociology of medically unexplained symptoms. *Social Science and Medicine, 62,* 1167–1178.

Olshanky, S. (1962). Chronic sorrow: A response to having a mentally defective child. *Social Casework, 43,* 190–193.

Parsons, T. (1951). *The social system.* New York: The Free Press.

Paterson, B. (2001). The shifting perspectives model of chronic illness. *Journal of Nursing Scholarship, 33*(1), 21–26.

Paterson, B. (2003). The koala has claws: Applications of the shifting perspectives model in research of chronic illness. *Qualitative Health Research, 13*(7), 987–994.

Petrie, K. J., & Weinman, J. (2006). Why illness perceptions matter. *Clinical Medicine, 6*(6), 536–539.

Price, B. (1996). Illness careers: The chronic illness experience. *Journal of Advanced Nursing, 24,* 275–279.

Rolland, J. S. (1987). Chronic illness and the life cycle: A conceptual framework. *Family Process, 26,* 203–221.

Rudell, K., Bhui, K., & Priebe, S. (2009). Concept, development and application of a new mixed method assessment of cultural variations in illness perceptions: Barts explanatory model inventory. *Journal of Health Psychology, 24,* 336-347.

Salewski, C. (2003). Illness representations in families with a chronically ill adolescent: Differences between family members and impact on patients' outcome variables. *Journal of Health Psychology, 8*(5), 587–598.

Searle, A., Norman, P., Thompson, R., & Vedhara, K. (2007). Illness representations among patients with type 2 diabetes and their partners: Relationships with self-management behaviors [Electronic version]. *Journal of Psychosomatic Research, 63*(2), 175–184.

Sontag, S. (1988). *Illness as metaphor.* Toronto: Collins Publishers.

Stafford, L., Berk, M. & Jackson, H. L. (2009) Are illness perceptions about coronary artery disease predictive of depression and quality of life outcomes? *Journal of Psychosomatic Research, 66,* 211–220.

Stafford, L., Jackson, H. J., & Berk, M. (2008). Illness beliefs about heart disease and adherence to secondary prevention regimens. *Psychosomatic Medicine, 70,* 942–948.

Steward, D. C., & Sullivan, T. J. (1982). Illness behavior and the sick role in chronic disease: The case of multiple sclerosis. *Social Science and Medicine, 16,* 1397–1404.

Stuifbergen, A., Phillips, L., Voelmeck, W., & Browder, R. (2006). Illness perceptions and related - outcomes among women with fibromyalgia syndrome. *Women's Health Issues, 16,* 353–360.

Strauss, A., & Glaser, B. (1975). *Chronic illness and the quality of life.* St. Louis: Mosby.

Strauss, A., Corbin, J., Fagerhaugh, S., Glaser, B., et al. (1984). *Chronic illness and the quality of life* (2nd ed.). St. Louis: Mosby.

Sullivan, T., Weinert, C., & Cudney, S. (2003). Management of chronic illness: Voices of rural women. *Journal of Advanced Nursing, 44*(6), 566–574.

Thomas, R. (2003). *Society and health: Sociology for health professionals.* New York: Kluwer.

Thorne, S. E. (1990). Constructive noncompliance in chronic illness. *Holistic Nursing Practice, 5*(1), 62–69.

Thorne, S. E., Harris, S. R., Mahoney, K., Con, A., & McGuinness, L. (2004). The context of health care communication in chronic illness [Electronic version]. *Patient Education and Counseling, 54*(3), 299–306.

Thorne, S. E., & Paterson, B. (1998). Shifting images of chronic illness. *Image, 30*(2), 173–178.

Townsend, A., Wyke, S., & Hunt, K. (2006). Self-managing and managing self: Practical and moral dilemmas in accounts of living with chronic illness. *Chronic Illness, 2,* 185–194.

Wainwright, D. (2008). Illness behavior and the discourse of health. In D. Wainwright (Ed.), *A sociology of health* (pp. 76–96). London: Sage.

Watt, S. (2000). Clinical decision-making in the context of chronic illness. *Health Expectations, 3,* 6–16.

Weaver, S. K., & Wilson, J .F. (1994). Moving toward patient empowerment. *Nursing and Health Care, 15*(9), 380–483.

Weitz, R. (2007). *The sociology of health, illness, and health care* (4th ed.). Belmont, CA: Thomson Higher Education.

Weitz, R. (1991). *Life with AIDS.* New Brrunswick, NJ: Rutgers University Press.

Whitehead, W. E., Crowell, M. D., Heller, B. R., Robinson, J. C., Schuster, M. M., & Horn, S. (1994). Modeling and reinforcement of the sick role during childhood predicts adult illness behavior. *Psychosomatic Medicine, 56,* 541–550.

Williams, S. J. (2005). Parsons revisited: From the sick role to . . .? *Health, 9*, 123–144.

Wilson, P. M., Kendall, S., & Brooks, F. (2006). Nurses' responses to expert patients: The rhetoric and reality of self-management in long term conditions: A grounded theory study. *International Journal of Nursing Studies, 43*, 803–818.

Young, J. T. (2004). Illness behavior: A selective review and synthesis. *Sociology of Health and Illness, 26*(1), 1–31.

CHAPTER 3

Stigma

My car came to a stop at the intersection. I looked around me at all the people in the other cars, but no one there was like me. They were apart from me, distant, different. If they looked at me, they couldn't see my defect. But if they knew, they would turn away. I am separate and different from everybody that I can see in every direction as far as I can see. And it will never be the same again.
—Client with new diagnosis of cancer

Diane L. Stuenkel and Vivian K. Wong

INTRODUCTION

This chapter demonstrates how the concept of stigma has evolved and is a significant factor in many chronic illnesses and disabilities. It also explores the relationship of stigma to the concepts of prejudice, stereotyping, and labeling. Because stigma is socially constructed, it varies from setting to setting. In addition, individuals and groups react differently to the stigmatizing process. Those reactions must be taken into consideration when planning strategies to improve the quality of life for individuals with chronic illnesses.

Although stigmatizing is common, not all individuals attach a stigma to their disease or disability. This chapter does not assume that all who come in contact with those who are disabled or chronically ill devalue them; rather, it insists that each of us examine our values, beliefs, and actions carefully.

Merriam Webster (2011a) defines stigma as a "mark of shame or discredit, an identifying mark or characteristic," and as a "mark of guilt or disgrace" (2011b). Goffman (1963) traced the historic use of the word stigma to the Greeks, who referred to "bodily signs designed to expose something unusual and bad about the moral status of the signifier" (p. 1). These signs were cut or burned into a person's body as an indication of being a slave, a criminal, or a traitor. Notice the moral and judgmental nature of these stigmas. The disgrace and shame of the stigma became more important than the bodily evidence of it. Labeling, stereotyping, separation, status loss, and discrimination can all occur at the same time and are considered components of the stigma (Link & Phelan, 2001).

THEORETICAL FRAMEWORKS: STIGMA, SOCIAL IDENTITY, AND LABELING THEORY

Society teaches its members to categorize persons by common defining attributes and characteristics (Goffman, 1963). Daily routines establish the usual and the expected. When we meet strangers, certain appearances help us anticipate what Goffman called "social identity." This identity includes personal attributes, such as competence, as well as structural ones, such as occupation. For example, university students usually tolerate some eccentricities in their professors, but stuttering, physical handicaps, or diseases may bestow a social identity of incompetence. Although this identity is not based on actuality, it may be stigmatizing.

One's social identity may include: 1) physical activities, 2) professional roles, and 3) the concept of self. Anything that changes one of these, such as a disability, changes the individual's identity and, therefore, potentially creates a stigma (Markowitz, 1998). Goffman (1963) used the idea of social identity to expand previous work done on stigma. His theory defined stigma as something that disqualifies an individual from full social acceptance. Goffman argued that social identity is a primary force in the development of stigma, because the identity that a person conveys categorizes that person. Social settings and routines tell us which categories to anticipate. Therefore, when individuals fail to meet expectations because of attributes that are different and/or undesirable, they are reduced from accepted people to discounted ones—that is, they are stigmatized.

Goffman recognized that people who had stayed in a psychiatric institute or a prison were labeled. To label a person as different or deviant by powers of the society is applying a stigma (Goffman, 1963). In general, labeling theory is the way that society labels behaviors that do not conform to the norm. For instance, an individual experiencing constant drooling or the leakage of food that requires frequent wiping of the mouth exhibits behaviors different from the norm. The difficulty in swallowing may be labeled by society as deviant behavior, despite the fact that tremor and dyskinesias associated with Parkinson's disease may be the cause (Miller, Noble, Jones, & Burn, 2006). Therefore, the concept of deviance versus normality is a social construct. That is, individuals are devalued because they display attributes that some call deviant (Kurzban & Leary, 2001).

During the 2 decades following Goffman's work in the 1960s, extensive criticism arose concerning the impact and long-term consequences of stigma on social identity. In the area of mental illness, critics resisted the theory that stigma could contribute to the severity and chronicity of mental illness. In a series of studies, Link proposed a modified labeling theory that asserted that labeling, derived from negative social beliefs about behavior, could lead to devaluation and discrimination. Ultimately, these feelings of devaluation and discrimination could lead to negative social consequences (Link, 1987; Link et al., 1989; Link et al., 1997). Those who are labeled with mental illness often are excluded from social activities and discriminated against when they do participate.

In 1987, Link compared the expectations of discrimination and devaluation and the severity of demoralization among clients with newly diagnosed mental illness, repeat clients with mental illness, former clients with mental illness, and community residents (Link, 1987). He found that both new and repeat clients with mental illness scored higher on measures of demoralization and discrimination than community residents and former clients with mental illness. Further, he demonstrated that high scores were related to income loss and unemployment.

In 1989, Link and colleagues tested a modified labeling theory on a similar group of clients with newly diagnosed mental illness, repeat clients with mental illness, former clients, untreated clients, and community residents who were well (Link et al., 1989). They found that all groups expected clients to be devalued and discriminated against. They also found that, among current clients, the expectation of devaluation and discrimination promoted coping mechanisms of secrecy and withdrawal. Such coping mechanisms have a strong effect on social networks, reducing the size of those networks to persons considered to be safe and trustworthy.

In 1997, Link and colleagues tested modified labeling theory in a longitudinal study that compared the effects of stigma on the well-being of clients who had mental illness and a pattern of substance abuse to determine the strength of the long-term negative effects of stigma and whether the effects of treatment have counterbalancing positive effects (Link et al., 1997). They found that perceived devaluation and discrimination, as well as actual reports of discrimination, continued to have negative effects on clients even though clients were improved and had responded well to treatment. They concluded that healthcare professionals attempting to improve quality of life for clients with mental illness must contend initially with the effects of stigma in its own right to be successful.

Fife and Wright (2000) studied stigma using modified labeling theory as a framework in individuals with HIV/AIDS and cancer. They found that stigma had a significant influence on the lives of persons with HIV/AIDS and with cancer. However, they also found that the nature of the illness had few direct effects on self-perception, whereas the effects on self appeared to relate directly to the perception of stigma. Their findings suggested that stigma has

different dimensions, which have different effects on self. Rejection and social isolation lead to diminished self-esteem. Social isolation influences body image. A lack of sense of personal control stems from social isolation and financial insecurity. Social isolation appears to be the only dimension of stigma that affects each component of self.

Camp, Finlay, and Lyons (2002) questioned the inevitability of the effects of stigma on self based on the hypothesis that, in order for stigma to exert a negative influence on self-concept, the individuals must first be aware of and accept the negative self-perceptions, accept that the identity relates to them, and then apply the negative perceptions to themselves. A study of women with long-term mental health problems found that these women did not accept negative social perceptions as relevant to them. Rather, they attributed the negative perceptions to deficiencies among those who stigmatized them. These researchers found no evidence of the passive acceptance of labels and negative identities. These women appeared to avoid social interactions where they anticipated feeling different and excluded, and formed new social networks with groups in which they felt accepted and understood. Whereas they acknowledged the negative consequences of mental illness, there did not appear to be an automatic link between these consequences and negative self-evaluation. Factors that contributed to a positive self-evaluation included membership in a supportive in-group, finding themselves in a more favorable circumstance than others with the same problems, and sharing experiences with others who had knowledge and insight about mental illness.

In summary, stigma, defined as discrediting another, arises from widely held social beliefs about personality, behavior, and illness, and is communicated to individuals through a process of socialization. When individuals display the condition that engenders the mark of discredit, they may experience social devaluation and discrimination. Stigma clearly attaches to individuals with mental illness as well as individuals with infectious and terminal diseases. Stigma may produce changes in perception of body image, social isolation, rejection, loss of status, and perceived lack of personal control. However, there is some evidence to suggest that stigma does not attach universally to individuals with marked behavior or conditions. Some individuals appear resistant to stigma, identifying flaws in the society conveying the negative beliefs. These individuals share experiences with others who have knowledge of and sensitivity to being stigmatized and benefit from the ability to perceive themselves as equal to or better off than others with the same condition.

Unique Aspects of Stigma

There are special circumstances in which stigma can be perceived with enhanced distinction. Individuals who lack a fully developed sense of personal identity and who are reliant upon external sources to reinforce their internal sense of worthiness may be uniquely prone to a sense of stigma. Adolescence can be used as an example. There are aspects of society that tend to be highly valued by individuals, and when that society communicates stigma, the stigmatizing beliefs are uniquely powerful. Religion and culture are examples, as well as issues concerning self-infliction and punishment.

The task of developing a stable, coherent identity is one of the most important tasks of adolescence (Erikson, 1968). To successfully complete this task, the adolescent must be able to utilize formal operational thinking within a context of expanded social experiences to evolve a sense of self that integrates not only the similarities, but also the differences observed between the self and others. Social interactions and messages from the sociocultural environment about what is desirable and what is not desirable guide and direct the adolescent toward an identity that incorporates desired similarities and rejects undesired differences. The influences and preferences of peers become important as the adolescent seeks acceptance of this newly developed sense of identity. The skill of labeling and stigmatizing individuals with intolerable differences is wielded with frightening force and sometimes terrible consequences—the 1999 Columbine High School tragedy is one example.

Intolerance often results in bullying and peer aggressiveness in the adolescent. Wang, Iannotti, Luk, and Nansel (2010) examined subtypes of bullying in a national sample of 7,475 adolescents in the United States. Bullying of all types (verbal, physical, relational, cyber, and cell phone) that occurred among students in grades 6 to 10 was related to depression, physical injuries, and increased medication use to manage nervousness and insomnia. Bullying, including cyberbullying, has also been linked to suicidal thoughts and behaviors in the adolescent (Brunstein Klomek, Sourander, & Gould, 2010; Hinduja & Patchin, 2010).

Normal adolescent maturation may include dealing with sudden growth spurts, changes in body image, and even acne associated with fluctuating hormone levels. Australian researchers (Magin, Adams, Heading, Pond, & Smith, 2006) explored the experience of adolescents living with very visible skin disorders (e.g., severe acne, psoriasis). These youth (aged 11–18 years) were stigmatized and frequently were the targets of teasing and bullying behaviors by peers.

Culture may determine stigma as well. For some conditions, such as traumatic brain injury (Simpson, Mohr, & Redman, 2000), HIV/AIDS (Heckman et al., 2004), and epilepsy (Baker, Brooks, Buck, & Jacoby, 2000), stigma and social isolation cross cultural boundaries. On the other hand, in a study of attitudes about homelessness in 11 European cities, Brandon, Khoo, Maglajlie, and Abuel-Ealeh (2000) found marked differences in attitudes between countries, with high levels of stigma predominating in former Warsaw Pact countries. A determination of racial and/or cultural inferiority of a minority group by a dominant group may result in racism, discrimination, and stigma (Weston, 2003).

Religion may also play a role in stigma. In a study of five large religious groups in London that examined attitudes about depression and schizophrenia, it was found that fear of stigma among nonwhite groups was prevalent, and particularly the fear of being misunderstood by white healthcare professionals not of the same religious group (Cinnirella & Loewenthal, 1999).

The label and associated stigma of a disability or disease excludes individuals from social interaction or alters social relationships whereas their intellectual or physical handicaps alone may not (Link et al., 1997). Vulnerable populations are in jeopardy of forming unhealthy relationships. Results from a South African study (Rohleder, 2010) indicated that the stigma of disability increased participation in risky behaviors. Individuals with a physical or mental disability were more likely to engage in unsafe sexual practices, thereby increasing their risk of contracting HIV/AIDS. The desire to form an attachment and establish a physical relationship with another human being

outweighed the need to protect oneself. The concepts of self-worth and self-esteem are interwoven with stigma.

Most stigmas are perceived as threatening by and to others. Criminals and social deviants are stigmatized because they create a sense of anxiety by threatening society's values and safety. Similarly, encounters with sick and disabled individuals also cause anxiety and apprehension, but in a different way. The encounter destroys the dream that life is fair. Sick people remind us of our mortality and vulnerability; consequently, physically healthy individuals may make negative value judgments about those who are ill or disabled (Kurzban & Leary, 2001). For example, some sighted individuals may regard those who are blind as being dependent or unwilling to take care of themselves, an assumption that is not based on what the blind person is willing or able to do. Individuals with AIDS are often subjected to moral judgment. Those with psychiatric illness have been stigmatized since medieval times (Keltner, Schwecke, & Bostrom, 2003). As a result, these individuals deal with more than their symptomatology; on a daily basis they contend with those who perceive them as less worthy or valuable, because they possess a stigma.

Some individuals are stigmatized because the behavior or difference is considered to be self-inflicted and, therefore, less worthy of help. Alcoholism, drug-related problems, and mental illness are frequently included in this category (Crisp et al., 2000; Ritson, 1999). In fact, alcoholism as a disease is highly stigmatized as compared to other mental illnesses (Schomerus et al., 2010). HIV/AIDS and hepatitis B are examples of infectious diseases in which the mode of infection is considered to be self-inflicted as a result of socially unacceptable behavior; therefore, affected individuals are stigmatized (Halevy, 2000; Heckman et al., 2004).

In the past, the words "shame" and "guilt" were used to describe a concept similar to stigma—a perceived difference between a behavior or an attribute and an ideal standard. From this perspective, guilt is defined as self-criticism, and shame results from the disapproval of others. Guilt is similar to seeing oneself as discreditable. Shame is a painful feeling caused by the scorn or contempt of others. For example, a person with alcoholism may feel guilty about drinking and also feel ashamed that others perceive his or her behavior as less than desirable.

Whenever a stigma is present, the devaluing characteristic is so powerful that it overshadows other traits and becomes the focus of one's personal evaluation (Kurzban & Leary, 2001). This trait, or differentness, is sufficiently powerful to break the claim of all other attributes (Goffman, 1963). As an example, the fact that a nurse has unstable type I diabetes may cancel her/his remaining identity as a competent health professional. The stigma attached to a professor's stutter may overshadow academic competence.

The extent of stigma resulting from any particular condition cannot be predicted. Individuals with a specific disease do not universally feel the same degree of stigma. On the other hand, very different disabilities may possess the same stigma. In writing about individuals with mental illness, Link and colleagues (1997) described variations in symptomology among them; however, individuals without mental illness did not take those variations into account. All individuals who were disabled were seen as sharing the same stigma—mental illness—regardless of their capabilities or severity of their illness. That is, people responded to the mental illness stereotype rather than to the person's actual physical and mental capabilities.

Similarly, Herek, Capitanio, and Widaman (2003) reported on the stigmatizing effects of the label of HIV/AIDS. They found that those individuals who reported a perceived reduction in the level of stigma attached to HIV/AIDS overall still generally expressed negative feelings toward people with AIDS and favored a name-based reporting system such as that used by the public health department for other communicable diseases.

Types of Stigma

Stigma is a universal phenomenon and every society stigmatizes. Goffman (1963) distinguished among three types of stigma. The first is the stigma of physical deformity. The actual stigma is the deficit between the expected norm of perfect physical condition and the actual physical condition. For example, many chronic conditions create changes in physical appearance or function. These changes frequently create a difference in self- or other-perception (see Chapter 6).

Stigma can arise from a normal physiological process—aging. The normal aging process creates a body far different from the television commercial "norm" of youth, physical beauty, and leanness. Younger people tend to differentiate themselves from older people based on the differences in appearances, physique, and mentality. Butler (1975) first termed "the process of systemically stereotyping and discriminating against people because they are old" as ageism (p. 894). Detrimental consequences may follow after labeling a person as elderly, senior citizen, or aged. For example, a person who is hard of hearing may refuse to use a hearing aid to avoid being labeled as "getting old". In fact, hearing loss was considered a perceived stigma in aging and the use of hearing aids was associated with being disabled in one longitudinal qualitative study (Wallhagen, 2010). In another study, adults (n = 103) 60 to 70 years old were found to be more sensitive to stereotyping threats affecting memory performance (Hess, Hinson, & Hodges, 2009). In other words, if the older adult is conscious of how his or her behavior may reflect negatively on the older adult population, he or she may have increased anxiety and reduced memory capacity. Although physical decline, loneliness, and depression in the older adult have been well documented in the literature, interventions must be implemented to enhance "positive aging" (Stephens & Flick, 2010). Health promotion and positive aging attitudes can only be accomplished when the stigma of ageism is abolished.

The second type of stigma is that of character blemishes. This type may occur in individuals with HIV/AIDS, alcoholism, mental illness, or sexually transmitted diseases. For example, individuals infected with HIV face considerable stigma because many believe that the infected person could have controlled the behaviors that resulted in the infection (Halevy, 2000; Heckman et al., 2004; Herek et al., 2003; Weston, 2003). Likewise, individuals with eating disorders such as anorexia nervosa fear being stigmatized (Stewart, Keel, & Schiavo, 2006). The fear of stigma can be a major barrier to seeking treatment.

The third type of stigma is tribal in origin and is known more commonly as prejudice. This type of stigma originates when one group perceives features of race, religion, or nationality of another group as deficient compared with their own socially constructed norm. Most healthcare professionals agree that prejudice has no place in the healthcare delivery system. Although some professionals display both subtle and overt intolerance, others strive to treat persons of every age, race, and nationality with sensitivity. However, prejudice against individuals with chronic illnesses exists as surely as racial or religious prejudice.

The three types of stigma may overlap and reinforce each other (Kurzban & Leary, 2001). Individuals who are already socially isolated because of race, age, or poverty will be additionally hurt by the isolation resulting from another stigma. Heukelbach and Feldmeier (2006) stated that scabies infestations are associated with poverty in undeveloped countries, which contributes to the stigmatization of both diagnosis and treatment. Those who are financially disadvantaged or culturally distinct (that is, stigmatized by the majority of society) will suffer more stigma should they become disabled. Poor women with HIV feared the stigma associated with HIV/AIDS more than dying of the disease (Abel, 2007).

Psychologists and sociologists have built on Goffman's theory to address the concepts of felt stigma and enacted stigma (Jacoby, 1994; Scambler, 2004). Felt stigma is the internalized perception of being devalued or "not as good as" by an individual. It may be related to fears of being treated differently or of being labeled by others, even though the stigmatizing attribute is not known or outwardly apparent. The other component of felt stigma is shame (Scambler, 2004). Individuals view themselves as discreditable. The quote at the beginning of this chapter is an example of a client experiencing felt stigma.

Enacted stigma, on the other hand, refers to behaviors and perceptions by others toward the individual who is perceived as different. Enacted stigma is the situational response of others to a visible, overt stigmatizing attribute of another (Jacoby, 1994; Scambler, 2004). Hesitating or failing to shake hands with a person who has vitiligo, a dermatologic condition characterized by hypopigmentation of the skin, is an example of enacted stigma.

Felt and enacted stigma may overlap. "Smoke-free" regulations are now in effect across the United States and abroad. Whereas these laws have been enacted to protect the public from the carcinogens and toxins present in secondhand smoke, the smoking behavior may be viewed as an unfavorable attribute. By association, the individual who smokes may be seen as "less than" or as less favorable. Thus, the individuals who smoke may experience both felt stigma and enacted stigma. Indeed, some smokers and recent ex-smokers in Scotland described themselves as "lepers" (Ritchie, Amos, & Martin, 2010). The temporary segregation occurring as a result of "smoking sections" led them to stigmatize themselves as well as their behaviors and that of other smokers.

Stigma is prevalent in our society and, once it occurs it endures (Link et al., 1997). If the cause of stigma is removed, the effects are not easily overcome. An individual's social identity has already been influenced by the stigmatizing attribute. A person with a history of alcoholism or mental illness continues to carry a stigma in the same way that a former prison inmate does.

Chronic Disease as Stigma

Individuals with chronic illness present deviations from what many people expect in daily social interchanges. In general, most people do not expect to meet someone with an electronic voice-box following treatment for laryngeal cancer. Both the cancer and the assistive device may not be readily visible, but once the person begins to speak, the individual is at risk of being labeled as "different" by others.

American values contribute to the perception of chronic illness as a stigmatizing condition. That is, the dominant culture emphasizes qualities of youth, attractiveness, and personal accomplishment. The work ethic and heritage of the Western frontier provide heroes who are strong, conventionally productive, and physically healthy. Television and magazines demonstrate, on a daily basis, that physical perfection is the standard against which all are measured, yet these societal values collide with the reality of chronic disease. A discrepancy exists between the realities of a chronic condition, such as arthritis or HIV/AIDS, and the social expectation of physical perfection.

A disease characteristic or one having an unknown etiology may contribute to the stigma of many chronic illnesses. In fact, any disease having an unclear cause or ineffectual treatment is suspect, including Alzheimer's disease (Jolley & Benbow, 2000) and anxiety disorders (Davies, 2000). Clients with Alzheimer's disease also may be stigmatized because of perceptions relating to their level of decision-making competence (Werner, 2006). Diseases that are somewhat mysterious and at the same time feared, such as leprosy, are often felt to be morally contagious.

Stigma can be associated with inequitable treatment, although the relative severity of such inequitable treatment often varies with the degree of severity of the stigmatized condition. For example, public policy about HIV/AIDS has acted both to increase accessibility to treatment and potentially to limit the civil rights of the stigmatized individuals (Herek et al., 2003). In addition, the shame, guilt, and social isolation of some stigmatized individuals may lead to inequitable treatment for their families. Because of the secrecy associated with being HIV-positive, affected clients and family members may not be able to access needed mental health, substance abuse rehabilitation, or infectious disease therapies (Salisbury, 2000).

The stigma associated with HIV/AIDS or the associated high-risk behaviors may impact public health screening efforts (Glasman, Weinhardt, DiFranceisco & Hackl, 2010). Men of Mexican descent were less likely to participate in free HIV-screening events. Findings suggested that participation in HIV testing could stigmatize these men due to the association of HIV infection with high-risk behaviors (men having sex with men, illicit drug use). By avoiding testing, these men were avoiding the possibility of enacted stigma. A study of Irish women of childbearing age found the same reasoning behind avoiding screening for chlamydia (Balfe et al., 2010). Undergoing screening for the disease was associated with risky behaviors and promiscuity, which would result in felt stigma and possibly enacted stigma.

This chapter has defined stigma and presented a framework for understanding stigma as a social construct. All types of stigma share a common tie: In every case, an individual who might have interacted easily in a particular social situation may now be prevented from doing so by the discredited trait. The trait may become the focus of attention and potentially turn others away.

IMPACT OF STIGMA

Stigma has an impact on both the affected individual and those persons who do not share the particular trait. Responses to stigma vary and will be discussed from the perspective of the person living with stigma, the layperson, and the healthcare professional.

The Individual Living with Stigma

Stigmatized individuals respond to the reactions of others in a variety of ways. They are often unsure about the attitudes of others and, therefore, may feel a constant need to make a good impression. Individuals living with stigma each and every day may choose to accept society's or others' view of them, or choose to reject others' discrediting viewpoints. Culture may limit the coping choices that are available, particularly in relation to disclosing a mental illness. In a study of West Indian women coping with depression, Schreiber, Stern, and Wilson (2000) found that "being strong" was the culturally sanctioned behavior for depression, rather than disclosure.

Passing

Passing oneself off as "normal" is one strategy used by individuals living with a stigmatizing condition. Pretending to have no disability or a less stigmatic identity (Dudley, 1983; Goffman, 1963; Joachim & Acorn, 2000) may be an option if the stigmatizing attribute is not readily visible. Passing is a viable option for those with felt stigma associated with conditions such as type II diabetes or a positive AIDS antibody test but no symptoms. The process of passing may include the concealment of any signs of the stigma. Some individuals refuse to use adaptive devices, such as hearing aids, because this tells others of their disability. Another example is the abused client who provides reasonable explanations for bruises, swelling, and injuries. The practice of "passing" may significantly impair the health-seeking behavior of the abused individual, particularly where sociocultural barriers to disclosure exist (Bauer, Rodriguez, Quiroga, & Flores-Ortiz, 2000).

CASE STUDY

Case Study #1

Richard Wilson is a 43-year-old, married, high school science teacher. He is 100 pounds over-weight and smokes cigarettes (1 pack per day for the past 20 years). He is thankful that he is in reasonably good health, although he does state that "my doctor started making me take a blood pressure pill every day when I saw her 2 months ago." Mr. Wilson lives in a state that has recently enacted smoke-free legislation. He rarely travels because he is concerned that he "will not fit in those tiny airplane seats."

Discussion Questions

1. What type of stigma is Mr. Wilson at risk for? How would you assess this client's self-perception of stigma?
2. What strategies can the healthcare provider offer this client to reduce the effects of stigma?
3. At Mr. Wilson's next blood pressure check appointment, how can the nurse evaluate whether the client has made progress in reducing felt and/or enacted stigma?
4. What strategies can the healthcare professional use to help break through the barriers of enacted stigma by members of the healthcare team toward individuals with negatively perceived lifestyle behaviors?
5. One goal stated in the *Healthy People 2020* document is to promote healthy nutrition and weight. How can the healthcare professional assess nutritional status and make recommendations for behavioral change without stigmatizing the individual?

Case Study #2

Dr. Min Pak is a 78-year-old retired nursing professor from Korea. While visiting her son in the United States, she developed nausea, vomiting, diarrhea, and abdominal pain. She went to a nearby urgent care center. The nurse at the urgent care center just finished checking her vital signs.

Dr. Pak: What are my blood pressure and temperature?

Nurse: Blood pressure is a little low and you have a low-grade temperature.

Dr. Pak: Could you please tell me the numbers?

Nurse: Blood pressure is in the 90s and you have a slight fever. Trust me, you don't need to know the exact numbers. By the way, when was the last time you had something to eat or drink, sweetie?

Dr. Pak: [thinking]

Nurse: When did you last have something to eat or drink? [*speaking louder and gesturing eating and drinking with mouth and hand*]

Dr. Pak: I heard you. That was 3 hours ago.

CASE STUDY   (Continued)

Nurse: You marked on the health form that you have chronic pancreatitis. How often and how much do you drink? And, of what kind?

Discussion Questions

1. What type of stigma is Dr. Pak experiencing?
2. Describe the nurse's attitudes and perceptions of stigma.
3. What interventions to reduce stigma would you suggest the client and the healthcare provider implement?
4. What are the implications for professional nursing practice?

Covering

Because of the potential threat and anxiety-provoking nature of disclosing a stigmatizing difference, most people deemphasize their differentness. This response, called covering, is an attempt to make the difference seem smaller or less significant than it really is (Goffman, 1963). Covering involves understanding the difference between visibility and obtrusiveness; that is, the condition is openly acknowledged, but its consequences are minimized. Persons with special dietary requirements may deny the importance of maintaining the restriction in a social situation, even though they follow it. The goal is to divert attention from the defect, create a more comfortable situation for all, and minimize the risk of experiencing enacted stigma.

Humor, used in a skillful and lighthearted manner by the stigmatized individual, may decrease the anxiety of others and avoid an awkward encounter. This form of covering neutralizes the anxiety-producing subject; therefore, it is no longer taboo and can more easily be managed.

Disregard

A person's first response to enacted stigma may be disregard. In other words, they may choose not

to reflect on or discuss the painful incidents. Well adjusted individuals who are comfortable with their identity, have dealt with stigma for a long time, and choose not to respond to the reaction of others, may disregard it (Dudley, 1983).

Other examples are wheelchair athletes. These athletes disregard perceptions that their disabilities prohibit them from participating in strenuous, athletic endeavors. Any person who has observed these well conditioned athletes racing their wheelchairs up hills in competitive meets may find it difficult to consider them discredited.

Going public with a serious medical diagnosis is another example of disregard by acting in the face of negative consequences. One positive aspect of going public is the potential for assertive political action and social change. Celebrities such as Muhammed Ali, Earvin (Magic) Johnson, Michael J. Fox, and the late Christopher and Dana Reeve, among others, have captured public attention and acted positively to reduce enacted stigma by disclosing their personal struggles with a variety of conditions.

Resistance and Rejection

Similar to disregard, resistance and rejection are additional strategies used in response to stigma

(Dudley, 1983). Individuals may speak out and challenge rules and protocol if their needs are not met. More recently, Franks, Henwood, and Bowden (2007) noted that resisting and rejecting were strategies used by maternal mental health clients. These disadvantaged mothers outright rejected or actively resisted the judgments of professionals who held negative opinions. Broader societal misconceptions, such as the belief all teen mothers are on welfare, also were rejected. The use of resistance or rejection can be used to preserve or bolster a more positive self-identity and effect larger societal changes.

Isolation

Human beings have a proclivity for separating themselves into small subgroups because staying with one's own group is easier, requires less effort, and, for some individuals, is more congenial. However, this separation into groups tends to emphasize differences rather than similarities (Link et al., 1989; see Chapter 5).

Closed interaction from within may enhance one's feelings of normality because the individual is surrounded by others who are similar (Camp et al., 2002). The process of isolation can occur any time outsiders are seen as threatening or are reminders that the world is different from the in-group.

Staying with like others may be a source of support, but some individuals with a disability or chronic illness may feel more comfortable when they are surrounded by nondisabled individuals. A young woman, disabled since birth, feels better around nondisabled people because she has always considered herself normal. Her attitude reminds us to use caution when making assumptions about the perceptions of others.

Information Management

In addition to the stigmatized individual, family members often acquire a secondary stigma as a result of association (Goffman, 1963) and must deal with their own responses to situations of enacted stigma. Mothers who are HIV-positive expend significant effort to protect their children from the negative effects of disclosure of their HIV status (Sandelowski & Barroso, 2003). Likewise, family members who care for persons with HIV/AIDS share the stigma and are discredited, resulting in rejection, loss of friends, and harassment (Gewirtz & Gossart-Walker, 2000; Salisbury, 2000).

Information management is used by both the individual and loved ones in dealing with felt and enacted stigma. The world may be divided into a large group of people to whom they tell nothing and a small group of insiders who are aware of the stigmatizing condition. Healthcare professionals may use information management in an attempt to lessen the likelihood of stigma for a client. For example, listing a diagnosis of Hansen's disease or mycobacterial neurodermatitis gives the client the option of revealing the alternate name of leprosy, with its accompanying historical stigma.

The Layperson: Responses to and Effects of Stigma

Responses of an individual to a stigmatized person vary with the particular stigma and the individual's past conditioning. Because society specifies the characteristics that are stigmatized, it also teaches its members how to react to that stigma. Differences between groups based on nationality and culture have been found in attitudes toward those with disabilities (Brandon et al., 2000; Cinnirella &

Loewenthal, 1999). Just as children learn to interact with others who are culturally different by watching and listening to those around them, they also learn how to treat individuals with chronic illness or disabilities by incorporating societal judgments. Sadly, these reactions are often negative.

With the advances in telecommunication and electronic communication, the general public is more aware of chronic physical and mental illnesses. Yet an online survey by the American Psychiatric Association (2010) on the perception of mental illness found that the stigma still persisted. Adults (n = 2,285) who responded to the survey revealed an increased acceptance to mental disorders, especially when they had a personal experience of the disease with family and friends. Other responders kept a more open mind after obtaining accurate information on mental illnesses from the mass media, celebrity figures, and Internet sources.

Devaluing

People may believe that the person with the stigma is less valuable, less human, or less desired. Unfortunately, many of us practice more than one kind of discrimination and, by so doing, effectively reduce the life chances of the stigmatized individual (Goffman, 1963). Devaluing results in enacted stigma as demonstrated by those who categorize individuals as inferior or even dangerous. Use of words such as "cripple" or "moron" also represent a devaluing of individuals.

Stereotyping

Categories simplify our lives. Instead of having to decide what to do in every situation, we can respond to categories of situations. Stereotypes are a negative type of category. They are a social reaction to ambiguous situations and allow us to react to group expectations rather than to individuals. When individuals meet those with physical impairments, expectations are not clear (Katz, 1981). People often are at a loss as to how to react, so placing the individual with chronic illness in a stereotyped category reduces the ambiguousness toward him or her and makes the situation more comfortable for those doing the stereotyping. Much less effort is required to sustain a bias than is required to reconsider or alter it.

Using stereotypes to understand individuals decreases our attention to other positive characteristics (Hynd, 1958). Categorizing tends to make one see the world as a dichotomy. For example, people are categorized as either mentally delayed or not, even though mental capabilities exist on a continuum, with all of us falling somewhere along the line.

Responses such as scapegoating and ostracizing people with HIV/AIDS have increased the impact of this disease and delayed treatment (Distabile, Dubler, Solomon, & Klein, 1999; Rehm & Franck, 2000; Salisbury, 2000). These responses also impede appropriate health education aimed at prevention.

Labeling

The label attached to an individual's condition is crucial and influences the way we think about that individual. The diagnosis of HIV/AIDS is a powerful label, possibly resulting in the loss of relationships and jobs. People with learning disabilities may not mind being called slow learners, but may be startled by being called mentally retarded (Dudley, 1983). Their response indicates that they see this latter term as a negative label.

Professional Responses: Attitudes and Perceptions of Stigma

In the United States, most healthcare professionals share the American dream of achievement, attractiveness, and a cohesive, healthy family. These values influence our perceptions of individuals who are disabled, chronically ill, or otherwise considered "less than normal." Although the factors that contribute to these individual differences vary, the consequences of stigma associated with chronic illnesses are similar in different health conditions and cultures (Van Brakel, 2006).

Attitudes

It is not surprising that society's values and definitions of stigma affect the attitudes of healthcare professionals. Attitudes can be changed by interactions with clients and acquaintances with chronic illness (Sandelowski & Barroso, 2003). Students' confidence in clients' ability to cope with a disease increased with professional experience. In a similar manner, knowing someone with a chronic disease increased positive attitudes. When healthcare professionals (general practitioners, nurses, and counselors) were asked about their perceptions of depression among older adults, they agreed that the older adults displayed embarrassment and shame when disclosing feelings of depression. Older adults were perceived as reluctant to seek mental health services because depression was identified as a stigma. Whether these perceptions of the healthcare professionals are consistent with those of the older adults will require further examination (Murray et al., 2006).

Perceptions

Healthcare professionals' perceptions of stigma affect care outcomes. Liggins and Hatcher (2005) studied the stigma of mental illness in the hospital setting. Labeling a client as mentally ill had a negative impact on both the client and the healthcare professional. Clients believed that they were ignored or treated differently because they had mental illness. They feared how the healthcare professional would respond to them. The healthcare professional showed disbelief toward physical ailments because the client had "mental disease." Healthcare providers also assumed that mental illness was associated with an unpredictable behavior that might affect the healthcare professional–client relationship (Liggins & Hatcher, 2005). Clearly, interventions to reduce perceptions of stigma and episodes of enacted stigma in the hospital setting are needed.

The attitude of the healthcare provider is vital in reducing the stigma associated with chronic illness. Healthcare professionals who are nonjudgmental, empathic, and knowledgeable were observed to reduce the perception of stigma in a specialized HIV/AIDS unit. Stigma was minimized when nurses and other interdisciplinary team members identified themselves with the behaviors of the clients, held a positive view of the disease, and reached consensus in the delivery of appropriate care (Hodgson, 2006).

Another study of medical students' perspectives of illness disclosed a surprising aspect of stigma. Medical students revealed a high level of concern over the perception of social stigma attached to their own personal health problems and the resulting professional jeopardy they might encounter upon disclosure (Roberts, Warner, & Trumpower, 2000).

Healthcare professionals potentially display all the reactions and responses toward discredited individuals that laypersons do.

Therefore, caregivers need a thorough understanding of these responses if we are to overcome the effects of stigmatizing behavior or to eliminate it outright. Understanding the concept of stigma increases one's ability to plan interventions for clients with chronic illnesses (Joachim & Acorn, 2000).

INTERVENTIONS: COPING WITH STIGMA OR REDUCING STIGMA

A chronic illness or disability imposes various constraints on an individual's life. The stigma of a specific disorder adds additional burdens, often far greater than those caused by the disorder itself (Joachim & Acorn, 2000). Individuals with chronic conditions usually receive medical treatment, but few interventions may be directed at reducing the effects of the associated stigma.

Helping others to manage the effects of stigma is not simple and should be approached with care. At best, change will be slow and uneven. However, consistent and knowledgeable interventions aimed specifically at reducing the impact of stigma are as crucial as those that reduce blood pressure or chronic pain. The following section discusses appropriate strategies healthcare providers can employ in their practice to address the issue of stigma.

National Healthcare Reform

Alleviating stigma is more effective in a politically supportive environment. As part of the healthcare reform under the Obama administration, the U.S. Congress passed the Health Reform Act (Healthcare.gov, 2010). This act combined both the Patient Protection and Affordable Care Act and the Healthcare Education and Reconciliation Act of 2010. The Health Reform Act proposed an increase in coverage in the treatment of mental illness and substance abuse. Clients with a pre-existing health condition such as cancer, HIV/AIDS, substance abuse, or mental illness will not be denied treatment. Funding will be provided to develop programs in Medicaid and in the community to improve the coordination and quality of behavioral healthcare services. In addition, grants will be offered for projects and research to increase the public awareness of mental health and substance abuse prevention and management. It is hoped that by increasing awareness of the nature of chronic illnesses and addictions among the general public, and with increased accessibility to health care for all, the issue of stigma attached to the aforementioned problems will be decreased.

Healthcare Professional and Client Interactions

The healthcare professional who is aware of his or her own biases, beliefs, and behaviors has already begun to mitigate the effects of stigma for the client and family members. Being aware of the societal context and implications that a diagnosis of chronic illness carries with it enables the healthcare professional to work with the client to develop strategies to prevent, reduce, or cope with potentially stigmatizing conditions.

Professional Attitudes: Cure versus Care

Traditionally, the goal of health care has been to cure the client. Because chronic illness is now more prevalent than infectious disease or acute illness, this criterion of success may be inappropriate. Cure is neither essential nor necessary in order that the client benefit. Instead, caring, demonstrated by valuing and assisting, should be the criterion. With the increasing number of people with chronic illnesses, professionals must learn to accept those characteristics accompanying chronic illness: an indeterminate course of disease, relapses, and multiple treatment modalities. Cost containment is a central focus in healthcare delivery. Providers must not lose sight, however, of health policy considerations that include ideas of personhood and equitable health care sensitive to the reality of stigmatizing chronic illness (Gewirtz & Gossart-Walker, 2000; Roskes, Feldman, Arrington, & Leisher, 1999; Salisbury, 2000).

The Mutual Participation Model

The manner in which health care is delivered may increase or decrease the effects of stigma. Encouraging a client's participation in healthcare decision making is an outward demonstration of respect and regard for that person. Establishing the client as a partner in setting goals demonstrates one's acceptance and valuing of the individual. On the other hand, when healthcare professionals make decisions regarding treatment or goals without consulting a client, they reinforce the person's feeling of being discredited or discreditable. Therefore, any mode of care delivery that increases client participation enhances that person's perception of self-worth and reduces the effects of stigma. The mutual participation model is the model of choice in managing chronic diseases because it enhances the client's feelings of self-worth. The client is responsible for long-term disease management, and the healthcare professional is responsible for helping the client help him- or herself.

Mutual participation divides power evenly between professional and client and leads to a relationship that can be mutually satisfying. In other words, the client should be as satisfied with the recommendations and decisions as the provider is. In addition, each party depends on the other for information culminating in a satisfactory solution. The client needs the provider's experience and expertise; the provider needs not only the client's history and symptoms but his or her priorities, expectations, and goals. Sometimes a choice between treatments with relatively equal mortality rates is necessary—for example, surgery or radiation for cancer treatment. The professional can offer expert knowledge regarding long-term effects of radiation and changes in body image due to surgery. The client must decide the relative value of side effects of the alternative proposed treatments. Because the "right" decision depends on the individual, input from both client and healthcare provider is necessary to produce a course of action that is mutually acceptable.

When healthcare professionals become more comfortable with allowing clients a greater range of participation and decision making, the relationship decreases some of the stigmatizing effects of the disability. Healthcare professionals must create an atmosphere in which individuals with chronic conditions not only are expected to cooperate, but are encouraged to express their concerns, observations, expectations, and limitations. Together, they explore alternative strategies and decide on one that is agreeable to both. When a client's priorities and goals are valued and incorporated into the regimen, an increased sense of acceptance emerges. Therefore, the respect and regard for clients demonstrated by this model provide effective tools to counteract some stigmatizing effects of illness.

Healthcare professionals who establish a therapeutic relationship with their client are ideally situated to assess their client's perceptions of felt or enacted stigma. Asking open-ended questions to ascertain how the client perceives himself or herself, the meaning of the disease to the client, and types of interactions with others may elicit valuable information. Family members and significant others may be included in the assessment as well.

It is particularly important to distinguish between nonparticipation and nonacceptance when caring for stigmatized individuals. Nonparticipation is an abstinence from social activities that is based on limitations caused by a disability or illness. Nonacceptance, on the other hand, is a negative attitude—a resistance or reluctance on the part of the nondisabled person to admit the disabled person to various kinds and degrees of social relationships (Ladieu-Leviton, Adler, & Dembo, 1977). A person with a disability who chooses not to join a camping trip is a nonparticipant; the physical disability serves as the basis for that person's decision not to participate. Deciding not to invite that person to join the group, whether or not participation is possible, is nonacceptance; it preempts the person's choice and is a form of enacted stigma.

Commonly, individuals without a disability cannot accurately estimate the limits of potential participation for those with a disease or disability—a key point for healthcare professionals to remember. Typically, the physical limitations imposed by a disability are overestimated by others. If nondisabled individuals incorrectly assume that a disabled individual is not able to participate, that is a form of nonacceptance. Such nonacceptance is created by the difference between the degree of participation that is actually possible and the degree assumed possible by those who are not disabled. If the difference can be resolved, nonacceptance ceases to be a problem.

The remedy for this dilemma is simple. Nondisabled individuals can simply indicate that they want the disabled individual to participate, leaving to him or her the decision of whether to become involved. Perhaps the individual with the disability would like to participate, but in a different way. For example, the young adult who has juvenile arthritis may not regret being unable to actually fish if he or she can go along on the trip and spend time socializing with friends. Healthcare professionals can encourage their clients to look for these opportunities to participate as they are able.

Family members or significant others who are involved in the client's care must not be forgotten. An ethnographic study of immediate family members of burn survivors explored the perceptions of stigma (Rossi, Vila Vda, Zago, & Ferreria, 2005). The stigma associated with the burn and the accompanying feelings of loss of control affected both the client and the family. The family had fears of facing the reactions from society, which encompassed feelings of sadness, anger, denial, resignation, and/or anxiety. Some family members expressed feelings of shame when living with someone whose role and appearance changed due to the burn injuries. Thus, it is imperative that the perceptions of both the stigmatized person and the family are assessed.

Client-Centered Interventions

Strategies to Increase Self-Worth

Societal norms and values are a major determinant of an individual's sense of self-esteem and self-worth. The person who does not possess the expected attribute is quite aware of this discredit as an equal and desired individual in society. In addition, individuals with chronic conditions may find their own deformities or failings decrease their self-respect. That is, not only do stigmatized individuals have to deal with the responses of others (enacted stigma), but some experience strong negative feelings about their own self-worth (felt stigma). These internalized perceptions may be more difficult to deal with than the illness or disability itself. Examples of negative feelings were described by 60 study participants with epilepsy. More than half of the participants experienced feelings of shame, fear, worry, and low self-esteem, and one-fourth had the perception of stigma (de Souza & Salgado, 2006).

In another study, obese individuals and their family members noted both stigmatization and discrimination on the basis of weight. They reported being constantly reminded by family members, peers, healthcare providers, and strangers that they were inferior as compared to those who were not obese (Rogge, Greenwald, & Golden, 2004).

In an attempt to change self-perception of stigma, Abel (2007) utilized an intervention of emotional writing disclosure for women with HIV. Women who participated in the intervention had more positive scores on the Stigma Scale tool at the end of the 12-week pilot study than women in the control group. The stigma scale is a 28 item self-report questionnaire developed to measure the stigma felt by clients with psychiatric illness (King, Dinos, Shaw, Watson, Stevens, Passett et al., 2007). This journaling strategy may be one way the healthcare provider can help individuals change their internal perception of stigma.

With these internalized negative perceptions, some people with chronic illness choose to conceal the disease. When 14 people with a diagnosis of multiple sclerosis and their families

were interviewed, it was found that the disease was purposefully concealed or selectively disclosed to shield from social judgment or to enhance social belonging at work (Grytten & Maseide, 2005). In describing studies of clients with cerebral palsy, cancer, facial deformity, arthritis, and multiple sclerosis, Shontz (1977) noted that the personal meaning of the disability to each client was uniformly regarded as crucial. For example, individuals who feel valuable because they are healthy and physically fit usually experience feelings of worthlessness if they contract a chronic condition. But people with diabetes will never be without a regimen and the necessary paraphernalia; visually impaired individuals will never see normally again. Therefore, the individuals' reactions and ability to accommodate these discrepancies determine their attitudes of worth and value.

In contrast, some individuals with chronic conditions can accept deviations from expected norms and feel relatively untouched. They have reordered life's priorities; no longer is the absence of disease or disability their major criterion for self-worth. Rather, an alternative ideology evolves to counter the "standard" ideologies. A strong sense of identity protects them, and they are able to feel acceptable in the face of the stigma (Goffman, 1963).

This identity belief system, also called cognitive belief patterns, refers to a person's perspective. It includes one's perceptions, mental attitudes, beliefs, and interpretations of experiences (Link et al., 1997). Individuals who are stigmatized by the major society may believe and perceive that their groups are actually superior or at least preferable. These belief patterns offer protection from the stigmatized reactions of others. Yet, being in a specific cultural or ethnic group does not always provide protection against stigma in certain diseases. In fact, the stigma of having a mental illness is even more prominent among some ethnic groups. A literature review by Gary (2005) found that African Americans, Asian Americans, Hispanic Americans, and Indian Americans all perceived stigma related to mental illness in addition to the prejudice and discrimination already experienced due to the affiliation with their particular ethnic group.

Cognitive belief patterns help individuals with chronic illnesses achieve identity acceptance and protection in the face of stigmatizing conditions. For example, after extensive cancer surgery, clients may consciously tell themselves that they are full human beings because the missing part was diseased or useless. The body, although disfigured, is now healthy and totally acceptable. Similarly, wheelchair athletes take pride in their superb physical condition and competitiveness. That is, one's perception of self-worth influences one's reactions to disease or disability. An individual's question, "Am I worthwhile?" is answered by determining his or her own values and perspective. Therefore, clients' definitions of themselves are crucial factors in self-satisfaction.

Support Groups

Goffman (1963) used the term *the own* for those who share a stigma. Those who share the same stigma can offer the "tricks of the trade," acceptance, and moral support to a person living with stigma. Self-help or support groups are examples of persons who are the own. Alcoholics Anonymous (AA), for instance, provides a community of the own as well as a way of life for its members. Members speak publicly, demonstrating that people with alcoholism are treatable, not terrible, people.

Groups composed of people with similar conditions can be formal or informal and are enormously helpful. First, peer groups can be used to explore all of the potential response options discussed previously, such as resisting and passing. Second, problem-solving sessions in these groups explore possible solutions to common situations (Dudley, 1983). Finally, others who share the stigma provide a source of acceptance and support for both the individuals with the chronic condition and their families. Maternal mental health clients developed and implemented an ongoing support group in consultation with a healthcare professional (Franks et al., 2007). These women were able to promote and sustain their group for a 12-month period.

O'Sullivan (2006) reported on a unique twist to the self-help group. A Barcelona, Spain radio program was planned and implemented by persons with mental illness. The program sought to inform, educate, and break down the stigma and stereotypes associated with mental illness. Benefits to the participants included an increase in self-esteem and more positive self-perception.

A word of caution is needed. Sometimes stigmatized individuals feel more comfortable with nonstigmatized individuals than with like others as a result of a closer identity with the former. For example, not all women with cancer respond positively to the American Cancer Society's Reach to Recovery support groups; some may feel more discomfort than support.

Reputable online support groups present another option for people with the technologic equipment and skills to access these resources. The ability to control the encounter with like others in a safe haven may be appealing to many clients. The advent of social media sites such as Facebook may alter the way individuals access and develop support networks as well. Social sites may offer another means of establishing both social and supportive relationships with the amount of disclosure controlled by the person. One must be aware of the potential for misuse, misrepresentation, and violations of privacy that could occur. Research in this area is sorely needed. Ultimately, the "best" solution varies from individual to individual.

Other Considerations

Other points for the healthcare professional to consider are issues of "inclusion" and "exclusion," and how they impact stigma. Technology and assistive devices are significant factors because they underline the fact that "quality of life" is not a static entity. Until relatively recently, electric wheelchairs were not readily available. Now such wheelchairs exist, in pediatric to bariatric sizes, as well as electric scooters that allow mobility for clients with a variety of conditions. Formerly, a person with paralyzed arms could only type slowly with a stick fastened to a headband; now there are increasingly accurate voice-activated home computers that type as the person speaks. In the same vein, a person whose speech is unintelligible to most others can press symbols on a display board that produces full sentences spoken in a nonrobotic, smooth human voice. The savvy healthcare professional will attend to technologic advances and assist clients in obtaining necessary aids to promote full functioning of the individual.

To that end, the opportunity to hire personal assistants is also important. Having such assistance allows individuals with severe disabilities to have a far richer life than those without such help. Many disability advocates are pressing for public money that is currently spent on nursing homes and other institutions to be redirected to enable individuals who are disabled or chronically ill to live in their own homes (see Chapter 23). Maintaining function and independence may lessen the impact of both felt and enacted stigma.

Developing Supportive Others

Supportive others are persons (professional and nonprofessional) who do not carry the stigmatizing trait but are knowledgeable and offer sensitive understanding to individuals who do carry it. These people are called *the wise* by Goffman (1963) and are accorded acceptance within the group of stigmatized individuals. Desired behaviors are simply the ones friends or acquaintances would use. The stigmatized person must be seen and treated as a full human being—viewed as more than body changes or orthopedic equipment, seen as a person who is more than a stigmatized condition.

The AIDS epidemic has added to the impetus for the development of groups of supportive others. In many cities, the model of care for those with HIV/AIDS depends on volunteer, community-based groups that supply food, transportation, in-home care, acceptance, and support. This community network is an adjunct to hospital care and provides a vivid example of wise others who are essential to the care of these clients.

Implications for Professional Practice

One way an individual can become wise is by asking straightforward, sensitive questions, such as inquiring about the disabled person's condition. Many individuals with disabilities would welcome the opportunity to disclose as much or as little as they wish, because that would mean that the disability was no longer taboo. For example, the disabled person may prefer that others ask about a cane or a walker rather than ignore it. This opportunity allows the disabled individual to reply with whatever explanation he or she wishes. Therefore, the disability is acknowledged, not ignored. It goes without saying that these questions should be asked after a beginning relationship is established, as opposed to being asked out of idle curiosity.

The process of becoming wise is not simple; it may mean offering oneself and waiting for validation of acceptance. Healthcare professionals who encounter individuals with chronic illness cannot prove themselves as wise immediately. Validation requires consistent behavior by the professional that is sensitive, knowledgeable, and accepting. Being wise is not a new role for nurses or other caring healthcare professionals. Nurses have traditionally worked in medically underserved areas with discredited persons and are accustomed to treating clients as individuals, not as conditions. Nurses often assume the predominant role of gatekeepers to the healthcare delivery system for many devalued individuals. Often, clients with chronic illnesses receive effective and efficient care from these nurses and other healthcare professionals, who have great opportunities to perform the role of the wise.

Evidence-Based Practice Box

This chapter has dealt primarily with adults' perceptions of stigma and interventional strategies that healthcare providers can use to both raise awareness of and to decrease the incidence of stigma. The aging of the population in the United States and the continuing negative perceptions surrounding mental illness are addressed in the *Healthy People 2020*

document. One goal is to improve the health and well-being of our elder members through such methods as screening, diagnosing, and treating mood disorders.

A study by Conner and colleagues (2010) offers some insight into the impact of stigma and race on elders seeking treatment for depression.

Purpose: To explore the impact of stigma (external and internal) on treatment-seeking behaviors of older adults with depression by race (African American, Caucasian).

Sample: A random sample of African American and Caucasian adults (n = 248) aged 60 years and older (mean age = 72) with mild to moderate depressive symptoms as identified by the Patient Health Questionnaire-9.

Method: Participants were surveyed via telephone to assess treatment-seeking attitudes and behavior and related factors. Perceived external (public) stigma was measured using a revised Perceived Devaluation Discrimination Scale. Internalized stigma were measured using the Internalized Stigma of Mental Illness tool. Attitudes toward mental health treatment were measured using a researcher-modified Attitudes Toward Seeking Professional Psychological Help Scale. Intention to seek treatment was measured by one item using a Likert-type scale. Chi squares, *t*-tests, and regression analyses were conducted.

Select Findings: Older adults who were depressed perceived more external stigma and were less likely to seek treatment.

(continues)

There were no statistically significant differences noted by race. A statistically significant difference was found for treatment. African Americans were significantly less likely ($X^2 = 11.1$, df = 1, p < .0001) to have received mental health treatment. African American elders reported more internal stigma ($t = -2.18$, p = .04) and held less favorable attitudes toward seeking treatment than Caucasians. A higher degree of internalized stigma was correlated ($r = .136$, p < .05) with intention to seek treatment. Regression analyses indicated that "internalized stigma partially mediated the relationship between race and attitudes toward treatment" (p. 538).

Conclusions: Perceptions of stigma negatively influenced treatment-seeking behaviors for all older adults with depression. All participants perceived high levels of public stigma. Strategies to reduce internalized stigma for African American older adults should be implemented in order to improve attitudes toward seeking mental health treatment. Although increased internal stigma was positively related to intent to seek treatment, this may be due to the individual's depressive symptoms and perceived need. Implementing interventions to reduce internalized stigma for older adults should be individualized.

Source: Connor, K. O., Copeland, V. C., Grote, N. K., Koeske, G., Rosen, D., Reynolds, C. F., et al. (2010). Mental health treatment seeking among older adults with depression: The impact of stigma and race. *American Journal of Geriatric Psychiatry, 18*(6), 531–543.

Another strategy healthcare professionals can use to acquire real-life knowledge about individuals with a particular illness is to increase their interaction with people who have the disorder (Heijenders & Van Der Meij, 2006). In addition to increasing exposure to and interaction with people who have a particular stigmatizing condition, Corrigan and Penn (1999) suggest that it is important for healthcare professionals to be exposed to people who are successfully coping with a condition; those who have recovered from mental illness, who are in remission, or who have been successfully rehabilitated. This knowledge can enable them to offer not only sensitive understanding and practical suggestions to individuals with chronic illness, but also hope. Nurses who work with HIV/AIDS clients, for instance, have the opportunity to find out which behavior is really effective and can learn about outcomes and clients' reactions. This information is extremely valuable as providers advocate for similar clients and their families.

Implications for Professional Education

Healthcare professionals' attitudes are representative of general societal views and so can be expected to include prejudices. Because healthcare professionals have prolonged relationships with chronically ill individuals, the impact of these prejudices can be great. Programs to teach professional staff to identify and correct preconceived and often subconscious notions of categories and stereotypes deserve high priority (Dudley, 1983).

Providing intensive staff education for the purpose of reducing stigma perception by all employees in any particular agency is beneficial. In addition, professional staff are then in a position to role model desired behaviors and to share information to help nonprofessional staff treat clients in an accepting manner.

One study of stigma-promoting behaviors provides ideas for healthcare professionals who wish to change their attitudes (Dudley, 1983). In Dudley's study, the most frequent stigma-promoting behaviors included the following: staring, denial of opportunities for clients to present views, inappropriate language in referring to clients, inappropriate restrictions of activities, violation of confidentiality, physical abuse, and ignoring clients. In-service days that focus on both didactic presentation of communication strategies and role-playing–specific scenarios would be a first step to eliminating situations of enacted stigma in the workplace.

One way to increase visibility and heighten awareness about the impact of stigma is to encourage structured contact between healthcare professionals and affected individuals (Joachim & Acorn, 2000). This approach should be preceded by group work with a knowledgeable leader who can help identify and work through attitudes and reactions. For example, many nursing students do not like skilled nursing facilities (SNFs) because older adults are seen as unappealing. A gerontology nurse specialist spent time with such a group of students before they began working in the SNF. She showed slides of faces etched with character and told stories of interesting experiences these individuals had that helped the students see the elderly as human beings. A group discussion between the specialist and students confronted myths and stereotypical thinking regarding the stigma of aging. As a result, these students had a more positive experience at the SNF.

Knowledgeable preparation for contact with stigmatized individuals does not solve all problems; it is, however, one way to expose stigmatized reactions such as stereotyping, to examine them, and to provide information to caregivers. The group sessions described here may be appropriate for both nonprofessional and professional caregivers in the community or in agencies.

Implications for Community Education Programs

Educational programs that reduce the effects of stigma can be shared with the community at large. Many organizations, such as the American Cancer Society and the American Diabetes Association, provide speakers or literature for the community. Schools, scout troops, and church groups are ideal settings for sensitive introductions of individuals who have many positive values and characteristics but do not meet normal health expectations. For instance, individuals with HIV/AIDS have been the focus of group discussions in which children learn to see these people simply as other human beings. Educational programs, such as those that dispel the fears about mental illness, reduce the stigmatizing effects of that disease (Link et al., 1989).

Much of the stigma attached to chronic conditions still pervades society's attitudes and policies (Herek et al., 2003); yet, situations have changed. In the 1970s, an unprecedented and multilayered surge of activism grew among individuals with disabilities and their advocates and resulted in significant social and structural change. Individuals with disabilities began to speak out by publishing magazines, creating films, and organizing political action on both the local and national levels. Their actions greatly influenced a landmark change, namely, the Americans with Disabilities Act (ADA), which was signed into law in 1990. This legislation requires the government and the private sector to provide disabled individuals with opportunities for jobs and education, access to transportation, and access to public buildings.

The media can also be influenced to present a more positive portrayal of people with chronic conditions. Providers and others can write to television networks that show individuals with disabilities functioning well and commend them for these portrayals. Likewise, people can be encouraged to voice their displeasure and to point out inaccuracies surrounding chronic conditions. In late fall 2010, the National Alliance on Mental Illness called for individuals to write and email a major television network and a popular television show's producer over a disparaging, stereotypical portrayal of a historical figure's mental illness.

Mass media campaigns designed to increase awareness of certain conditions or risk factors for disease can backfire in terms of preventing or reducing stigma. Clients with lung cancer not only perceived stigma of cancer in general (such as fear of disclosure, financial impact, body image changes, and effects on family and social relationships), but also the stigma that is associated with smoking and the shame of a self-inflicted disease, regardless of whether they stopped smoking or had never smoked. They experienced fear related to death as depicted by the mass media, families and friends avoiding contact, and being looked upon as being "dirty" in relation to smoking (Chapple, Ziebland, & McPherson, 2004).

Another study identified methods of health communication that were designed to increase public awareness but actually had the opposite effect of increasing public stigma (Wang, 1998). The health communication approaches conveyed individuals with obvious disabling characteristics with the accompanying message, "Don't be like this." Awareness was heightened at the expense of furthering the stigma of the disabled individual. Healthcare professionals who volunteer to serve on executive boards of healthcare agencies or support agencies can offer guidance to those developing marketing campaigns, public service announcements, and community education materials.

Recent social changes have suggested that internalization of stigma based on prevailing social norms may be changing for some health problems. Rehabilitation programs for substance abuse are now commonly covered by health insurance, in part as a result of active consumer demand, evidencing a change of social attitude (Garfinkel & Dorian, 2000). The impact of stigmatizing conditions in women's health, such as abortion and breast cancer with mastectomy, has been reduced (Bennett, 1997). These changes are, perhaps, evidence that visibility and disclosure may have a positive impact on the process of negative stereotyping.

OUTCOMES

Determining client outcomes, like many of the psychosocial concepts associated with chronic illnesses, is difficult. Some clients may be stigmatized on a regular basis but have been able to overcome the personal feelings associated with it. Therefore, client outcomes of stigma might be the *lack* of other common psychosocial effects of chronic illness. For example:

- The client is *not* socially isolated, but is continuing his or her daily and normal activities without difficulty.

- The client's self-esteem remains high despite the chronic illness and accompanying physical symptoms.
- Healthy relationships continue with family, friends, and supportive others.
- The client is *not* depressed and interacts appropriately with others.

STUDY QUESTIONS

Compare and contrast the concepts of felt stigma and enacted stigma. Are these two concepts mutually exclusive?

How does the process of labeling by others influence the perception of felt stigma and the incidence of enacted stigma?

Advanced practice nurses can implement strategies to decrease the incidence of enacted stigma in society. What might the advanced practice nurse do in each of the following roles to decrease stigma: nurse administrator, nurse educator, clinician?

As a change agent in your practice setting, what strategies can you readily implement to increase awareness of stigma among administrators, healthcare professionals, and support staff?

What strategies can you readily implement to decrease the perceptions of stigma by your clients?

Discuss the similarities and differences among prejudice, stereotyping, and labeling. What is the relationship to stigma?

INTERNET RESOURCES

Resources

Mental Health Issues

Achieve Solutions website: https://www.achieve solutions.net/achievesolutions/en//Home .do?contentId=21466

U.S. Department of Health and Human Services, Substance Abuse and Mental Health Services Administration stigma homepage: http://www .whatadifference.samhsa.gov/

Stigma.org links to mental health websites: www .stigma.org

Active Minds: Changing the Conversation on Mental Health (working to reduce the stigma of mental illness on college campuses): www .activeminds.org

National Alliance on Mental Illness Stigma Busters (click on Fight Stigma to sign up for StigmaBusters alerts and to access resources): www.nami.org

HIV/AIDS Issues

HRSA Care Action—Providing HIV/AIDS Care in a Changing Environment: hab.hrsa.gov. Resources include a literature review on HIV and stigma, clinical guidelines.

HIV & AIDS: Stigma and Discrimination: http:// www.avert.org/hiv-aids-stigma.htm (Note: Avert.org is also available on Facebook.)

For a full suite of assignments and additional learning activities, use the access code located in the front of your book and visit this exclusive website: **http://go.jblearning.com/larsen**. If you do not have an access code, you can obtain one at the site.

REFERENCES

Abel, E. (2007). Women with HIV and stigma. *Family and Community Health, 30*(Suppl 1), 104–106.

American Psychiatric Association. (2010, May 3). Openness by friends, family, celebrities reduces stigma of mental Illness survey (press@psych.org Release No. 10-33). Retrieved January 14, 2011, from: https://www.achievesolutions.net/achievesolutions/en/tlc/Content.do?contentId=21466

Baker, G. A., Brooks, J., Buck, D., & Jacoby, A. (2000). The stigma of epilepsy: A European perspective. *Epilepsia, 41*(1), 98–104.

Balfe, M., Brugha, R., O'Connell, E., McGee, H., O'Donovan, D. & Vaughan, D. (2010). Where do young women in Ireland want Chlamydia screening services to be located? *Health and Place, 16*(1), 16–24.

Bauer, H., Rodriguez, M., Quiroga, S., & Flores-Ortiz, Y. (2000). Barriers to health care for abused Latina and Asian immigrant women. *Journal of Health Care for the Poor and Underserved, 11*(1), 33–44.

Bennett, T. (1997). Women's health in maternal and child health: Time for a new tradition? *Maternal and Child Health Journal, 1*(3), 253–265.

Brandon, D., Khoo, R., Maglajlie, R., & Abuel-Ealeh, M. (2000). European snapshot homeless survey: Result of questions asked of passers-by in 11 European cities. *International Journal of Nursing Practice, 6*(1), 39–45.

Brunstein Klomek, A., Sourander, A., & Gould, M. (2010). The association of suicide and bullying in childhood to young adulthood: A review of cross-sectional and longitudinal research findings. *Canadian Journal of Psychiatry, 55*(5), 282–288.

Butler, R. N. (1975). Psychiatry and the elderly: An overview. *American Journal of Psychiatry, 132,* 893–900.

Camp, D. L., Finlay, W. M. L., & Lyons, E. (2002). Is low self-esteem an inevitable consequence of stigma? An example from women with chronic mental health problems. *Social Science and Medicine, 55*(5), 823–834.

Chapple, A., Ziebland, S., & McPherson, A. (2004). Stigma, shame, and blame experienced by patients with lung cancer: Qualitative study. *British Medical Journal, 328*(7454), 1470.

Cinnirella, M., & Loewenthal, K. M. (1999). Religion and ethnic group influences on beliefs about mental illness: A qualitative interview study. *British Journal of Medical Psychology, 72*(4), 505–524.

Connor, K. O., Copeland, V. C., Grote, N. K., Koeske, G., Rosen, D., Reynolds, C. F., et al. (2010). Mental health treatment seeking among older adults with depression: The impact of stigma and race. *American Journal of Geriatric Psychiatry, 18*(6), 531–543.

Corrigan, P., & Penn, D. (1999). Lessons from social psychology on discrediting psychiatric stigma. *American Psychology, 54*(9), 765–776.

Crisp, A., Gelder, M., Rix, S., Meltzer, H., et al. (2000). Stigmatization of people with mental illness. *British Journal of Psychiatry, 177,* 4–7.

Davies, M. R. (2000). The stigma of anxiety disorders. *International Journal of Clinical Practice, 54*(1), 44–47.

de Souza, E. A., & Salgado, P. C. (2006). A psychosocial view of anxiety and depression in epilepsy. *Epilepsy and Behavior, 8*(1), 232–238.

Distabile, P., Dubler, N., Solomon, L., & Klein, R. (1999). Self-reported legal needs of women with or at risk for HIV infection. The HER Study Group. *Journal of Urban Health, 76*(4), 435–447.

Dudley, J. (1983). *Living with stigma: The plight of the people who we label mentally retarded.* Springfield, IL: Charles C. Thomas.

Erikson, E. (1968). *Identity: Youth in crisis.* New York: W. W. Norton.

Fife, B., & Wright, E. (2000). The dimensionality of stigma: A comparison of its impact on the self of persons with HIV/AIDS and cancer. *Journal of Health and Social Behavior, 41*(1), 50–67.

Franks, W., Henwood, K., & Bowden, G. (2007). Promoting maternal mental health: Women's strategies for presenting a positive identity and the implications for mental health promotion. *Journal of Public Mental Health, 6*(2), 40–51.

Garfinkel, P. E., & Dorian, B. J. (2000). Psychiatry in the new millennium. *Canadian Journal of Psychiatry, 45*(1), 40–47.

Gary, F. A. (2005). Stigma: Barrier to mental health care among ethnic minorities. *Issues in Mental Health Nursing, 26*(10), 979–999.

Gewirtz, A., & Gossart-Walker, S. (2000). Home-based treatment for children and families affected by HIV and AIDS. Dealing with stigma, secrecy, disclosure, and loss. *Child and Adolescent Psychiatry Clinics of North America, 9*(2), 313–330.

Glasman, L. R., Weinhardt, L. S., DiFranceisco, W., & Hackl, K. L. (2010). Intentions to seek and accept an

HIV test among men of Mexican descent in the midwestern USA. *AIDS Care, 22*(6), 718–728.

Goffman, E. (1963). *Stigma: Notes on management of spoiled identity.* Englewood Cliffs, NJ: Prentice-Hall.

Grytten, N., & Maseide, P. (2005). What is expressed is not always what is felt: Coping with stigma and the embodiment of perceived illegitimacy of multiple sclerosis. *Chronic Illness, 1*(3), 231–243.

Halevy, A. (2000). AIDS, surgery, and the Americans with Disabilities Act. *Archives of surgery, 135*(1), 51–54.

Heckman, T. G., Anderson, E. S., Sikkema, K. J., Kochman, A., et al. (2004). Emotional distress in nonmetropolitan persons living with HIV disease enrolled in a telephone-delivered, coping improvement group intervention. *Health Psychology, 23*(1), 94–100.

Healthcare.gov (2010). U.S. Department of Health & Human Services. Retrieved January 7, 2011, from: http://www.healthcare.gov/law/introduction/index.html

Heijnders, M., & Van Der Meij, S. (2006). The fight against stigma: An overview of stigma-reduction strategies and interventions. *Psychology, Health & Medicine, 11*(3), 353–363.

Herek, G. M., Capitanio, J. P., & Widaman, K. F. (2003). Stigma, social risk, and health policy: Public attitudes toward HIV surveillance policies and the social construct of illness. *Health Psychology, 22*(5), 533–540.

Hess, T. M., Hinson, J. T., & Hodges, E. A. (2009). Moderators of and mechanisms underlying stereotype threat effects on older adults' memory performance. *Experimental Aging Research, 35*(2), 153–177.

Heukelbach, J., & Feldmeier, H. (2006). Scabies. *The Lancet, 367*, 1767–1774.

Hinduja, S. & Patchin, J.W. (2010). Bullying, cyberbullying, and suicide. *Archives of Suicide Research, 14*(3), 206–221.

Hodgson, I. (2006). Empathy, inclusion and enclaves: The culture of care of people with HIV/AIDS and nursing implications. *Journal of Advanced Nursing, 55*(3), 283–290.

Hynd, H. M. (1958). *On shame and the search for identity* (3rd ed.). New York: Harcourt Brace Jovanovich.

Jacoby, A. (1994). Felt versus enacted stigma: A concept revisited. *Social Science and Medicine, 8*(2), 269–274.

Joachim, G., & Acorn, S. (2000). Stigma of visible and invisible chronic conditions. *Journal of Advanced Nursing, 32*(1), 243–248.

Jolley, D. J., & Benbow, S.M. (2000). Stigma and Alzheimer's disease: Causes, consequences, and a constructive approach. *International Journal of Clinical Practice, 54*(2), 117–119.

Katz, I. (1981). *Stigma: A social psychological analysis.* Hillsdale, NJ: Lawrence Erlbaum Associates.

Keltner, K., Schwecke, L., & Bostrom, C. (2003). *Psychiatric nursing* (4th ed.). St. Louis: Mosby.

King, M., Dinos, S., Shaw, J., Watson, R., Stevens, S., Passetti, F., et al (2007). The stigma scale: Development of a standardized measure of the stigma of mental illness. *British Journal of Psychiatry, 190*, 248–254.

Kurzban, R. & Leary, M. R. (2001). Evolutionary origins of stigmatization: The functions of social exclusion. *Psychological Bulletin, 127*(2), 187–208.

Ladieu-Leviton, G., Adler, D., & Dembo, T. (1977). Studies in adjustment to visible injuries: Social acceptance of the injured. In R. Marinelli & A. Dell Orto (Eds.), *The psychological and social impact of the physical disability.* New York: Springer.

Liggins, J., & Hatcher, S. (2005). Stigma toward the mentally ill in the general hospital: A qualitative study. *General Hospital Psychiatry, 27*(5), 359–364.

Link, B. G. (1987). Understanding labeling effects in the area of mental disorders: An assessment of the effects of expectations of rejection. *American Sociological Review, 52*(1), 96–112.

Link, B. G., Cullen, F. T., Struening, E., Shrout, P. E., et al. (1989). A modified labeling theory approach to mental disorders: An empirical assessment. *American Sociological Review, 54*(3), 400–423.

Link, B. G., Struening, E. L., Rahav, M., Phelan, J. C., et al. (1997). On stigma and its consequences: Evidence from a longitudinal study of men with dual diagnoses of mental illness and substance abuse. *Journal of Health and Social Behavior, 38*(2), 177–190.

Link, B. G., & Phelan, J. C. (2001). Conceptualizing stigma. *Annual Review of Sociology, 27*, 363–385.

Magin, P., Adams, J., Heading, G., Pond, D., & Smith, W. (2007). Psychological sequelae of acne vulgaris: Results of a qualitative study. *Australian Family Physician, 52*, 978–979.

Markowitz, F. E. (1998). The effects of stigma on the psychological well-being and life satisfaction of persons with mental illness. *Journal of Health and Social Behavior, 39*, 335–347.

Merriam Webster. (2011a). Dictionary: Stigma. Retrieved July 24, 2011, from: http://www.merriam-webster.com/dictionary/stigma

Merriam Webster. (2011b). Thesaurus: Stigma. Retrieved July 24, 2011, from: http://www.merriam-webster.com/thesaurus/stigma

Miller, N., Noble, E., Jones, D., & Burn, D. (2006). Hard to swallow: Dysphagia in Parkinson's disease. *Age and Ageing, 35*(6), 614–618.

Murray, J., Banerjee, S., Byng, R., Tylee, A., Bhugra, D., & Macdonald, A. (2006). Primary care professionals' perceptions of depression in older people: A qualitative study. *Social Science and Medicine, 63*(5), 1363–1373.

O'Sullivan, M. (2006). Making radio waves. *A Life in the Day, 10*(2), 6–8.

Rehm, R. S., & Franck, L. S. (2000). Long-term goals and normalization strategies of children and families affected by HIV/AIDS. *Advances in Nursing Science, 23*(1), 69–82.

Ritchie, D., Amos, A. & Martin, C. (2010). Original investigation: "But it just has that sort of feel about it, aleper"-Stigma, smoke-free legislation and public health. *Nicotine and Tobacco Research, 12*(6), 622–629.

Ritson, E.B. (1999). Alcohol, drugs, and stigma. *International Journal of Clinical Practice, 53*(7), 549–551.

Roberts, L. W., Warner, T. D., & Trumpower, D. (2000). Medical students' evolving perspectives on their personal health care: Clinical and educational implications of a longitudinal study. *Comprehensive Psychiatry, 41*(4), 303–314.

Rohleder, P. (2010). Rehabilitation in practice: "They don't know how to defend themselves:" Talk about disability and HIV risk in South Africa. *Disability and Rehabilitation, 32*(10), 855–863.

Rogge, M. M., Greenwald, M., & Golden, A. (2004). Obesity, stigma, and civilized oppression. *Advances in Nursing Science, 27*(4), 301–315.

Roskes, E., Feldman, R., Arrington, S., & Leisher, M. (1999). A model program for the treatment of mentally ill offenders in the community. *Community Mental Health Journal, 35*(5), 461–472.

Rossi, L. A., Vila Vda, S., Zago, M. M. & Ferreira, E. (2005). The stigma of burns perceptions of burned patients' relatives when facing discharge from hospital. *Burns, 31*(1), 37–44.

Salisbury, K. M. (2000). National and state policies influencing the care of children affected by AIDS. *Child and Adolescent Psychiatry Clinics of North America, 9*(2), 425–449.

Sandelowski, M., & Barroso, J. (2003). Motherhood in the context of maternal HIV infection. *Research in Nursing and Health, 26*, 470–482.

Scambler, G. (2004). Reframing stigma: Felt and enacted stigma and challenges to the sociology of chronic and disabling conditions. *Social Theory and Health, 2*, 29–46.

Schomerus, G., Lucht, M., Holzinger, A., Matschinger, H., Carta, M. G. & Angermeyer, M. C. (2010, December 18 epub). The stigma of alcohol dependence compared with other mental disorders: A review of population studies. *Alcohol Alcohol, 46*(2), 105–112.

Schreiber, R., Stern, P. N., & Wilson, C. (2000). Being strong: How black West-Indian Canadian women manage depression and its stigma. *Journal of Nursing Scholarship, 32*(1), 39–45.

Shontz, E. (1977). Physical disability and personality: Theory and recent research. In R. Marinelli & A. Dell Orto (Eds.), *The psychological and social impact of physical disability*. New York: Springer.

Simpson, G., Mohr, R., & Redman, A. (2000). Cultural variations in the understanding of traumatic brain injury and brain injury rehabilitation. *Brain Injury, 14*(2), 125–140.

Stephens, C. & Flick, U. (2010). Health and ageing–challenges for health psychology research. *Journal of Health Psychology, 15*(5), 643–648.

Stewart, M., Keel, P., & Schiavo, R. S. (2006). Stigmatization of anorexia nervosa. *International Journal of Eating Disorders, 39*(4), 320–325.

Van Brakel, W. H. (2006). Measuring health-related stigma: A literature review. *Psychology of Health and Medicine, 11*(3), 307–334.

Wallhagen, M. I. (2010). The stigma of hearing loss. *The Gerontologist, 50*(1), 66–75.

Wang, C. (1998). Portraying stigmatized conditions: Disabling images in public health. *Journal of Health Communication, 3*(2), 149–159.

Wang, J., Iannotti, R. J., Luk, J. W., & Nansel, T. R. (2010). Co-occurrence of victimization from five subtypes of bullying: physical, verbal, social exclusion, spreading rumors, and cyber. *Journal of Pediatric Psychology, 35*(10), 1103–1112.

Werner, P. (2006). Lay perceptions regarding the competence of persons with Alzheimer's disease. *International Journal of Geriatric Psychiatry, 21*, 674–680.

Weston, H. J. (2003). Public honor, private shame, and HIV: Issues affecting sexual health service delivery in London's South Asian communities. *Health and Place, 9*(2), 109–117.

CHAPTER 4

Adaptation

Pamala D. Larsen and Faye I. Hummel

INTRODUCTION

Persons with chronic illness chart a life course to successfully navigate the challenges that are inherent within themselves, their relationships, or the setting in which they find themselves. Throughout the course of their illness, individuals must rely on a healthcare system in which pharmaceuticals, machines, and a wide array of technology have become the hallmarks of quality health care. Although the disease focus may be appropriate intermittently during the trajectory of a chronic illness to meet the physical needs of the individual, this perspective does not meet the social, psychological, and emotional needs of clients with chronic conditions. In other words, the disease focus of the healthcare system does not and cannot manage the illness experience of the client and family.

Early work by Visotsky, Hamburg, Goss, and Lebovits in 1961 in studying clients with polio posed some initial questions regarding adaptation. They asked their clients how it was possible to deal with this stressor, polio, and what coping behavior(s) could predict a favorable outcome. Fifty years later, the same questions are being asked. Although we have made progress in understanding certain components of adaptation, many questions remain unanswered.

The lens for viewing chronic illness is determined by numerous variables within the person

as well as how the healthcare professional and the setting providing care view the chronic condition. The elderly woman with arthritis who has been socialized to the primacy of medicine in the healthcare arena may rely solely on her physician-prescribed pharmaceutical treatment of her joint pain and fatigue. On the other hand, a young man with Hepatitis C gathers information from a wide variety of sources regarding the treatment and management of his chronic condition and maintains control of his treatment plan. The adaptation mechanism of the elderly woman and the young man are very different as well. Each individual brings to the illness their own uniqueness—personality traits, past experiences, culture, values—to influence the adaptation process in his or her own way.

Defining Adaptation

The terms *adjustment* and *adaptation* are used interchangeably in the literature (Stanton & Revenson, 2007) and will be in this chapter as well. Sharpe and Curran (2006) define adjustment as a response to a change in the environment that allows an organism to become more suitably adapted to that change (p. 1154). Most definitions of adjustment or adaptation, however, elude to the lack of a psychological disorder being present. An early description of adjustment (and a continuing one) is the absence of a diagnosed psychological disorder, psychological symptoms, or negative mood (Stanton, Revenson, & Tennen, 2007). Even in Visotsky's study in 1961 with clients with polio, there was a movement to discount that definition. While the presence or absence of a psychological disorder may be a part of adjustment, it is only one indicator of it.

Adjustment to illness has been operationalized as good quality of life, well-being, vitality, positive affect, life satisfaction, and global self-esteem (Sharpe & Curran, 2006). Conversely, *adjustment disorder* is defined as the development of clinically significant emotional or behavioral symptoms in response to an identifiable stress or stressor (American Psychological Association, 2000).

There is little consistency in the literature in defining adaptation or adjustment. Each author/researcher defines adaptation or adjustment differently based on their own theoretical framework or outcome measurement. As one example, Kiebles, Doerfler, and Keefer (2010) in their study of adjustment to inflammatory bowel disease defined adjustment as a composite of perceived disability, psychological functioning, and disease-specific and health-related quality of life (p. 1).

This chapter provides an overview of adaptation in individuals with chronic illness. With entire books devoted to coping and adaptation, the depth of this chapter is limited. However, classic sources and models are included, along with interventions appropriate for individuals and families with chronic illness.

IMPACT

Conceptualization of Adjustment

Stanton and Revenson (2007) identified five attributes of adjustment: 1) chronic illness necessitates adjustment in multiple life domains; 2) there are positive and negative outcomes of adjustment; 3) adjustment is dynamic; 4) adjustment can be described only within the context of each unique individual; and 5) heterogeneity is the rule rather than the exception in adjustment. Each of these concepts are further described in the sections that follow.

Chronic Illness Necessitates Adjustment in Multiple Life Domains

We know from caring for clients that adjustment is more than just physical; it crosses interpersonal, cognitive, emotional, and behavioral domains. Adjustment is a holistic event in the client, with all domains being interrelated. Therefore, a change in one domain may affect adjustment in another domain (Stanton & Revenson, 2007; Stanton, Collins, & Sworowski, 2001; Stewart, Ross, & Hartley, 2004). Cognitive adaptation might involve personal self-evaluation or self-reflection. Adap-tation in the behavioral domain includes returning to work or resuming the role of the "breadwinner" of the family. Anxiety, in the emotional domain, may affect the ability to socialize in the interpersonal domain or influence blood pressure in the physical domain. Emotional adaptation could be the absence of depression, and interpersonal adaptation may be the willingness to be "social" again. Again, each domain may affect the other.

Adjustment Involves Both Positive and Negative Outcome Dimensions

Typically we think of outcomes of chronic illness as being negative, as evidenced by distress, psychological dysfunction, relationships in disarray, and so forth. As stated previously, one definition of positive adjustment is the absence of a psychological disorder. However, there may be a positive side of chronic illness as well.

It is not unusual to hear individuals with chronic illness say things like, "having this disease has been the best thing that ever happened to me—it made me wake up to see what was important." There may be positive aspects of chronic disease, but how clients come to view it in this way is not known. Folkman, Moskowitz, Ozer, and Park (1997), in their study of HIV-positive and HIV-caregiving partners of men with AIDS, found that although study participants reported high levels of depressive symptoms, they also demonstrated positive morale and positive states of mind when compared with general population norms.

One way to describe these paradoxical findings is a concept called *response shift*. Sprangers and Schwartz (2000) coined this phrase to describe a change in the meaning of one's self-evaluation of a target construct as a result of 1) change in an individual's internal standards of measurement, 2) change in the individual's values, or 3) reconceptualization of the target construct (p. 12).

Although anecdotally we consider negative outcomes of chronic illness more common, research demonstrates that positive adjustment may more accurately represent the adjustment experience of most individuals with chronic disease (Stanton & Revenson, 2007).

Adjustment Is a Dynamic Process

Adjustment to chronic illness is neither linear nor lockstep (Stanton & Revenson, 2007, p. 568). As exacerbations occur—as in rheumatoid arthritis or multiple sclerosis, the cancer recurs, or the physical limitations of heart failure increase, each change requires readjustment or readaptation. In addition, changes may not be limited to

changes in one's physical condition that affect adaptation, but changes in the rest of the individual's life. A spouse loses his/her job, a child is seriously injured, or a parent is no longer able to care for him- or herself are examples of factors that affect the adaptation of the client with chronic illness.

Adjustment Can Be Viewed Only from within the Context of the Individual

There is variability in adaptation, and that is to be expected. From the context of the individual, the physical symptoms, the functional changes, and the uncertainty may or may not be pertinent to the individual. Each stressor of the illness has a different relevance for each individual, and as a result will elicit a different reaction from each individual. The context of each individual is different, whether it be his or her age, gender, ethnicity, or socioeconomic status. The 35-year-old married woman with three grade-school-aged children with newly diagnosed breast cancer has a different context than the 80-year-old woman with the same diagnosis. Although that is an extreme example, the variation that exists among individuals cannot be underestimated.

Heterogeneity Is the Rule, Not the Exception

Anecdotally we know that if we put 20 women of the same age with the same stage of breast cancer and same prognosis in a room, each of those individuals will adapt to their chronic condition differently. Some will be considered by most as "well adjusted," whereas others might be considered maladjusted. The remaining individuals may fall somewhere in the middle. The person's individual determinants and uniqueness affect the ability of the individual to adapt to the illness. Although commonalities exist among individuals with chronic illness, there is significant variability as well.

Differences in individual adjustment abound in the literature. Helgeson, Snyder, and Seltman (2004) in a study of women with breast cancer from 4 to 55 months after diagnosis found that 43% of the sample evidenced high and stable psychological quality of life, 18% had a somewhat lower quality of life, 26% evidenced low psychological functioning, and 12% had an immediate and substantial decline in psychological function.

Dew and colleagues (2005) identified five groups of distinct distress profiles in heart transplantation patients over several years. Groups evidenced: 1) consistently low distress; 2) consistent, significant levels of distress; 3) high distress for the initial 3 months; 4) high distress at 3 years; and 5) fluctuating distress.

The Self in Chronic Illness

Chronic illness changes the body and forces identity changes (Brink, 2009). Before illness, most individuals take their health for granted. Any disruption of normality may cause a threat to the self (Charmaz, 1995). Bury (1982) conceptualizes this as a biographical disruption. The meaning of the illness and biographical disruption vary in significance for the individual and family. One's self-concept and self-confidence may change due to chronic illness. Morea, Friend, and Bennett (2008) refer to the illness self-concept (ISC). The ISC, according to the authors, is the integration of illness into the self and, in turn, it affects the adjustment to chronic illness.

Brink (2009), in her study with patients who were post-myocardial infarction, identified two different behaviors in her model: self-modifying and self-protecting behaviors. For example, self-protecting behaviors may block lifestyle changes (p. 132). Individuals with self-modifying behavior reoriented themselves to the situation and accepted the consequences of the illness. Identifying a client's behavior can better help the healthcare professional in planning appropriate interventions.

Models

As researchers, we have a broad goal to understand the process of adaptation, predict outcomes, and by having predictive ability be able to modify interventions to meet the needs of our clients. A model that is able to perform all those activities is preferable for practice; however, a perfect model does not exist at this time. What follows are sample models from the literature.

Biomedical Model

The medical model provides a framework for assumptions about the nature of health and illness. The client is a complex set of anatomic parts and interrelated systems. Anatomic, physiologic, and/or biochemical failures translate into etiologies of ill health, thus promoting a disease-oriented approach to care. This theoretical perspective of chronic illness is reflected in the language and actions of healthcare professionals who refer to "the diabetic in room 328," rather than to Mrs. Sanchez, who has diabetes.

Pathophysiology, pharmacotherapy, and technology are emphasized and become prominent in the diagnosis and intervention of all illness and disease, albeit acute or chronic. Antonovsky (1979) considered the medical model a dichotomous model. If pathology is present, then there is illness, and wellness or health is not possible. Explanatory assumptions and theories are used for determining the cause of symptoms, and uniformity of causality and treatment of disease is inferred.

The biomedical paradigm tends to medicalize all human conditions in which symptoms can be controlled and cured with biomedical strategies. This model reduces the individual to a disease and fails to recognize the human aspects and experiences of the individual who happens to have a chronic illness (Sakalys, 2000), and diminishes social and cultural explanation of disease (Mirowsky & Ross, 2002). Physical complaints and signs or symptoms of disease become the hallmarks of interaction and discourse within the healthcare arena.

The relationship between the healthcare professional and the client with chronic illness is one of objectivity, biological pathology, diagnosis, and signs and symptoms, all of which require medical interventions. Healthcare professionals tend to shield themselves from the human aspects of chronic illness, while their skill sets, techniques, and procedures become the focus of interaction with the client (Freeth, 2007). Power and expertise are held exclusively by the healthcare system, and the interactions between the healthcare professional and the client are directive and unbalanced. The individual with chronic illness becomes disempowered to engage in his/her own healthcare decisions and relies solely on the healthcare professional.

The biomedical model is insufficient in providing health care to individuals with chronic illness (Waisbond, 2007), as it fails to acknowledge the breadth and depth of the illness experience. This model does not acknowledge the person with the chronic condition, who holds knowledge and expertise about the factors that influence his/her physical symptoms of chronic disease, in other words, the expert patient. For example, at the end of the month, Mrs. Jones becomes anxious that she will not have enough money to purchase her prescriptions for her hypertension. Although she is able to financially manage, Mrs. Jones's stress and worry exacerbate her hypertension. Mrs. Jones does not inform her physician that the probable cause of her elevated blood pressure is related to her stress. The physician responds to Mrs. Jones's hypertension with a change of medication to manage her symptoms. The quantification of all signs and symptoms of disease fails to address the total illness experience of the individual. With increased attention to genetic research and gene technologies, the biomedical theories of disease continue to be reinforced, with less emphasis on the individual's social context and experiences (Dixon-Woods, 2001).

Despite the limitations of the biomedical model in adaptation, its usefulness is apparent during the acute phase of chronic illness. Although the focus of the biomedical model is limited to disease and organic dysfunction, this model is central for adaptation to chronic illness, particularly at the time of diagnosis when individuals and families are overwhelmed with a new diagnosis and sorting out the facts about the illness. In addition, during periods of illness exacerbations, the biomedical model helps explain signs and symptoms and may provide a source of retreat and relief, depending on the stage of the chronic illness. There are times when individuals and families need current information about the chronic illness, signs and symptoms, the anticipated trajectory of the illness course, the array of treatment modalities, and traditional as well as alternative strategies. The biomedical model is the foundation for evidence-based healthcare practice and provides the gold standard for treatment and intervention. As a consequence, this model provides measurable goals for treatment and client outcomes relative to morbidity and mortality.

Chronic Care Model

The goal of chronic illness care is to manage symptoms and minimize disability rather than cure disease. The Chronic Care Model in which client self-management is a key component (Bodenheimer, Lorig, Holman, & Grumback, 2002) was developed to address deficiencies in the medical model of healthcare systems in managing chronic conditions. The Chronic Care Model first appeared in the literature in 1998 (Wagner, 1998) and was later refined by Wagner and colleagues (Wagner et al., 2001). Subsequent research of interventions with chronic illness has resulted in best practices and a national program for improving chronic illness care (Robert Wood Johnson Foundation, 2006–2011). The Chronic Care Model is proactive and is focused on keeping the person with chronic illness as healthy as possible. Within this model, six major elements interact to produce high-quality care and evidence-based interventions for persons with chronic conditions in health systems at the community, organization, practice, and individual levels. The six elements are: 1) the healthcare system or healthcare organization; 2) clinical information systems; 3) decision support; 4) delivery system design; 5) self-management support; and 6) community, including organizations and resources for clients with chronic illness (Wagner et al., 2001).

As new treatment modalities for chronic illness become available, it is imperative for the healthcare provider to evaluate these interventions in relation to the elements of the Chronic Care Model. In doing so, the healthcare provider is able to assume a leadership role in improving the care and outcomes for persons with chronic conditions (Dancer & Courtney, 2010).

The Chronic Care Model has been used in caring for individuals with a variety of chronic conditions. Diabetes, in particular, has provided much research to support the model's effectiveness. Diabetes care modeled after the Chronic Care Model improved the overall quality of care and outcomes. This care included self-management support for persons with diabetes through goal-setting, follow up, referrals to community resources, and support for delivery system redesign (Siminerio, Piatt, & Zgibor, 2005).

Lazarus and Folkman Model

Although there are other stress and coping models, none are more well known than the one developed by Richard Lazarus and Susan Folkman (1984). Their model, a cognitive-phenomenological theory of stress, views adaptation to chronic illness through adapting to stressors. It is a transactional model of stress and coping, meaning that antecedent variables, such as personality traits, past experiences, and disease and treatment variables, act via mediating variables, such as coping strategies, to facilitate outcomes, and, in this case, adaptation. Stressors are mediated by primary appraisal, which is the individual's gauge of the significance and importance of the stressor. Primary appraisal is influenced by the background, experiences, culture, ethnicity, and personality of the individual, and is, therefore, characterized by stability across situations (Folkman, Lazarus, Gruen, & DeLongis, 1986).

The second step of the model is secondary appraisal of the situation. The individual asks the question, "What can I do about this situation?" and this leads to the coping strategies used to manage the stressor. Secondary appraisal is influenced by the physical and social environment and may be context specific (Stewart et al., 2004). To adapt involves applying the coping strategies that are most appropriate to the situation. Individuals use both problem-focused coping and emotion-focused coping. Originally it was presumed by Lazarus and Folkman that the goal for all individuals was to utilize problem-focused coping, and that emotion-focused coping yielded poor adaptation to the stressor, in this case the illness. However, work since 1986 has supported that there is a place for emotion-focused coping as well as problem-focused coping (Stewart et al., 2004).

Engel's Biopsychosocial Model

Clearly a model that could address both the biological and psychosocial aspects of chronic disease would be a preferred one for health care. Engel (1977) was perhaps one of the earliest authors of such a model. The main theme of the model is the influence of biological, psychological, and social influences on the disease process. Engel's model outlined three ways in which a psychosocial factor could influence a health outcome: direct, indirect, and moderating. A direct effect would be a belief or value of the client that would preclude him or her from a specific medical intervention. An indirect effect would be defined through a mediational process (Stewart et al., 2004). An example would be an individual's current symptoms, for instance nausea and vomiting, decreasing the client's motivation to participate in a prescribed exercise regimen, and thereby decreasing physical functioning. A moderating effect alters the causal relationship between a psychosocial factor and a health outcome.

Livneh and Antonak Model

Livneh and Antonak (1997), working from previous models, proposed that variables associated with chronic illness could be organized into four main categories: 1) disability-related (e.g., type of condition—terminal vs. nonterminal); 2) sociodemographic factors of the individual (e.g., gender, age, ethnicity); 3) individual differences or personality (e.g., coping strategies, locus of control, personal meaning of the condition); and 4) social and environmental factors (e.g., social support, stigma). The interactions of these classes of variables significantly affected adaptation.

Livneh and Antonak (1997) also saw the adaptation process as different from adaptation itself. They theorized that the process of adaptation was fluid and dynamic, whereas adaptation status was the end result or outcome of the process (Stewart et al., 2004).

Common Sense Model of Self-Regulation

The Common Sense Model of Self-Regulation (Leventhal, Leventhal, & Cameron, 2001) posits that the client's illness beliefs and representations of that illness influence adaptation to the illness and health outcomes. According to the model, patients develop cognitive and emotional representations of their condition to "make sense" or find meaning in the illness. Leventhal and colleagues (2001) identified five dimensions that represent a client's view of their illness: 1) identity of the illness—connecting the symptoms with the illness and having an understanding of the illness; 2) timeline—duration and progression of the illness; 3) causes—perceived reason for the illness; 4) consequences—what will be the physical, psychosocial, and economic impact of the illness; and 5) controllability—can this disease be controlled? Cured? After identification of these dimensions, Leventhal and colleagues believe that coping and appraisal follow. There is significant evidence that an adaptive perception of a curable/controllable illness is related to better health and functioning (Hagger & Orbell, 2003).

The Common Sense Model has been used extensively as a framework in research in chronic illness. Several examples follow:

- Relationship of illness representations and the end-stage appraisal of outcomes in clients with chronic cardiovascular disease (Karademas, Kynigopoulou, Aghathangelou, & Anestis, 2010)
- Prediction of self-care behaviors in patients with end-stage renal disease (O'Connor, Jardine, & Millar, 2008)
- Prediction of disability by illness beliefs in clients with rheumatoid arthritis (Graves, Scott, Lempp, & Weinman, 2009)
- Relationship of illness representations, coping, and psychological adjustment in clients with Parkinson's disease (Evans & Norman, 2009).
- Illness beliefs and adherence behaviors in African American clients with hypertension (Hekler et al., 2008)

Moos and Holahan Model

Stewart and colleagues (2004) suggest that an ideal model for adaptation should address four criteria: 1) the reciprocal influences of biological, psychological, social, and behavioral variables of the client and the disease process; 2) be sufficiently broad to apply to clients with a wide range of chronic illnesses and conditions; 3) be able to address the influences of culture, gender, ethnicity, and life stage of the client; and 4) be able to predict the level of client adaptation, which will then lead to appropriate interventions for the client.

Currently a search of the literature does not identify any "ideal" models that can meet the preceding criteria. Moos and Holahan (2007), however, have developed a simple model that provides a framework to view adaptation. Because of its ease of use and understanding, more detail is provided on this model.

Moos and Holahan's framework (**Figure 4-1**) is a way of conceptualizing coping and integrating it into a broader model.

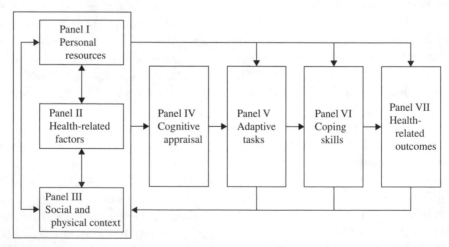

FIGURE 4-1   Conceptual Model of the Determinants of Health-Related Outcomes of Chronic Illness and Disability.
Source: Moos, R.H., & Holahan, C.J. (2007). Adaptive tasks and methods of coping with illness and disability. In E. Martz & H. Livneh (Eds.). *Coping with chronic illness and disability* (pp. 107–128). New York: Springer.

According to the model, there are five sets of factors that are associated with the selection of appropriate coping skills and the resulting health-related outcomes in this case, adaptation. The model includes three factors that influence cognitive appraisal: 1) personal resources (Panel I); 2) health-related factors (Panel II); and 3) the social and physical context (Panel III). Cognitive appraisal (Panel IV) then dictates what adaptive tasks (Panel V) need to be accomplished. Panels I through V mediate the choice of coping skills (Panel VI), leading to Panel VII, the outcome.

Personal Resources

This is a broad category that includes intellectual ability, ego and self-confidence, religion, and prior health-related and coping experiences. Demographic characteristics, such as age, gender, ethnicity, culture, and education are included in this category as well. Personal resources include personality—which may be viewed as either a risk factor or protective factor (Stanton et al., 2007)—locus of control, optimism, and autonomy. Individuals who have a more internal locus of control, higher self-confidence and self-efficacy, and a stronger sense of coherence are more likely to rely on problem solving than other aspects of approach coping (Moos & Holahan, 2007, p. 110).

Ethnic group membership is associated with many psychological processes such as identity, group pride, and discrimination (Stanton et al., 2007). Each ethnic group or culture may have different values and beliefs that affect illness perceptions that, in turn, may affect adaptation (see Chapter 13; Cohen & Welch, 2000). For some cultures, chronic disease and disability may produce stigma such that adaptation is not possible.

Zauszniewski, Chung, and Krafcik (2001) found greater resourcefulness in coping strategies among African American older adults with chronic illness than among white older adults. Degazon (1995), when exploring ethnic identification and coping strategies, found a significant relationship between the ethnic group with which the individual identified and the coping strategy used. Religion was key to coping with chronic illness for many African American older adults (Chin, Polonsky, Thomas, & Nerney, 2000). Loeb (2006) categorized coping strategies of African American older adults as: 1) dealing with it, 2) engaging in life, 3) exercising, 4) seeking information, 5) relying on God, 6) changing dietary patterns, 7) medicating, 8) self-monitoring, and 9) self-advocacy. These studies looked at coping specifically; however, the relationship of coping with adaptation is uncertain. In addition, it is clear that little is known about the implications of culture and ethnicity in disease-related adaptation (Stanton et al., 2007).

The uniqueness of each individual influences how the chronic condition is appraised, what coping strategies are used, and how and if adaptation can be achieved. For instance, pessimists report higher levels of hostility and depression on the day before coronary artery bypass graft surgery than do optimists (Maes, Leventhal, & deRidder, 1996). Clients who are optimists tend to cope in a more active, problem-oriented way, as opposed to pessimists who tend to use more avoidant or passive ways of coping. It is not clear how specifically these personality traits influence and affect coping. Carver, Scheier, and Weintraub (1989) have noted that the impact of personality characteristics on coping is modest, and that coping preferences exist independently of personality factors. Although coping preferences could be viewed as personality attributes, they may influence coping indirectly through their impact on appraisal (Maes et al., 1996).

Socioeconomic class affects health outcomes directly and through environmental mechanisms, including access to care and risky and protective health behaviors (Stanton et al., 2007). Although it can be conceptualized as a determinant of adaptation, the pattern is not unidirectional (p. 570). Chronic conditions often influence work patterns and work disability. Work-related disability and loss of a job can decrease an individual's socioeconomic status.

Health-Related Factors

These factors include the type of onset and progression of the chronic condition, the location of symptoms, the prognosis, and the type of disability. Disease- and treatment-related factors are often considered exogenous variables in adaptation (Stanton et al., 2001). A disease factor could be the stigma that the individual (and/or family) associates with the condition. Other disease factors could include a change in body image, declining mobility, extreme fatigue, and so forth. However, the existence and impact of disease factors may actually be influenced significantly by other determinants, such as ethnicity, socioeconomic status, and social support. Many studies do not reveal significant relationships of disease-related factors with adjustment (Stanton et al., 2001). The disease stage of a chronic condition is related inconsistently to adjustment (van't Spijker, Trijsburg, & Duivenvorrden, 1997).

The characteristics of the disease as well as the treatment characteristics contribute to the appraisal of the disease-related event. Surgery, monitoring of physical symptoms (e.g. blood glucose), diet, radiation, chemotherapy, and all of the side effects of treatment are important

components in how the client appraises the situation.

Social and Physical Context

This context includes the relationships between the individuals with the chronic disease, their family members, caregivers, and social network. A supportive social context can enhance self-efficacy, transforming appraisal of a health condition as a challenge rather than a threat, and enhance reliance on approach coping. When family members or friends do not convey interest, individuals with serious chronic conditions may avoid talking about their problem and be less likely to cope with the illness-related demands (Norton et al., 2005).

In general, social support is related to positive adaptation in several chronic diseases (Stanton et al., 2001). However, studies differ in how social support is conceptualized. Social support has been used as a coping strategy, a coping resource in the environment, and considered dependent on personality attributes and coping of the individual (Schreurs & deRidder, 1997). Interpersonal relationships can both aid and hinder adaptation to chronic illness. For women in particular, interpersonal relationships are vital components of their adjustment to major stressors (Revenson, 1994).

Cognitive Appraisal

Appraising the illness is the first step in deciding the adaptive tasks that need to be accomplished. This is also the step in the adaptation process where the illness is appraised as either a challenge or a threat. How the illness is appraised, whether it is controllable or threatening, determines appropriate adaptive tasks and subsequent coping strategies. Using Lazarus and Folkman's model, primary appraisal of the "threat" or "event" includes the appraisal of harm or loss that has already occurred, or threatened harm or loss (Folkman & Greer, 2000), and includes an evaluation of its personal significance (Walker, Jackson, & Littlejohn, 2004). Secondary appraisal occurs when one assesses the situation's controllability and compares to one's available coping resources.

The individual who appraises their diagnosis of colon cancer as a death sentence will make very different decisions regarding treatment than another individual who sees hope. With such different appraisals, coping and adjustment will be very different in these two individuals.

Adaptive Tasks

Moos and Holahan (2007) identified seven adaptive tasks. Three of the seven tasks are related to the health condition and its treatment, and the other four are more general and could apply to all life crises and transitions, not just chronic illness. The tasks include: 1) managing symptoms, 2) managing treatment, 3) forming relationships with healthcare providers, 4) managing emotions, 5) maintaining a positive self-image, 6) relating to family members and friends, and (7) preparing for an uncertain future (Moos & Holahan, 2007, p. 112–114).

CASE STUDY

It was 5 months after Dan was reunited with his wife and two daughters that he began to experience sleep disorders, night sweats, nightmares, and "flashbacks" of the horrors of war he had experienced while he was deployed to Iraq. There he had seen many of his buddies killed and injured. He, too, was injured by enemy fire but had healed and recovered. Dan found himself withdrawing from his family, and he no longer wanted to participate in his children's sporting events. He was experiencing conflict and difficulty at work. At a recent visit with his healthcare provider, Dan was diagnosed with post-traumatic stress disorder (PTSD). Dan was devastated. He believed he had left his fears and memories of violence in Iraq. Dan had assumed he would return to his previous happy life with his family. Doubts and questions about his future rushed over him. What would he and his family need to do to return to and maintain secure and safe relationships? Would he be able to return to work? Would he be able to enjoy his children's activities and events? Would his life ever return to "normal"? Where would all of this end?

Discussion Questions

1. What are Dan's personal resources, health-related factors, and social and physical factors that are contributing to his cognitive appraisal of the situation?
2. Compare and contrast the biomedical model and the Moos and Holahan model for adaptation for Dan and his chronic condition.
3. Discuss the role of the nurse for Dan and his family.

OVERVIEW OF COPING

Richard Lazarus's 1966 book, *Psychological Stress and Coping*, was an initial scholarly work that expanded how coping was conceptualized. Since that time, the coping literature has increased significantly, with researchers undertaking studies to understand why some individuals fare better than others when encountering stress in their lives (Folkman & Moskowitz, 2004). Coping is a process that unfolds in the context of a situation or condition that is appraised as personally significant, and as taxing or exceeding the individual's resources (Lazarus & Folkman, 1984). The coping process is initiated in response to the individual's appraisal that important goals have been harmed, lost, or threatened (Folkman & Moskowitz, 2004). What we have learned in the last 45 years is that coping is a complex, multidimensional process that is sensitive both to the environment and its demands and resources, and to personality traits that influence the appraisal of stress, in this case chronic illness, and the resources for coping (Folkman & Moskowitz, 2004). Coping is not a stand-alone concept or phenomenon, but embedded in a complex, dynamic process that involves the person, the environment, and the relationship between them.

Lazarus and Folkman (1984) described problem-focused and emotion-focused coping strategies. Problem-focused strategies alter person–environment relationships, and the purpose of emotion-focused strategies is to regulate internal states. Initially problem-focused strategies were seen as "better," or as able to influence health outcomes in a more positive manner. However, since Lazarus and Folkman posited their original work, that view has changed. Emotion-focused coping strategies may

specifically assist in developing and sustaining a sense of psychological well-being, despite unfavorable circumstances (Folkman & Greer, 2000).

Other theorists have used different terms to describe coping. In addition to problem-focused and emotion-focused coping, meaning-focused coping has been identified as a type of coping in which cognitive strategies are used to manage the meaning of the situation (Folkman & Moskowitz, 2004).

Shaw uses the terms *passive* coping, which includes avoidance, and *active* coping, which is nonavoidance coping (Shaw, 1999). This two-factor structure of coping is incorporated into the coping framework as an antecedent to the behavioral intention to cope as well as carry out the coping behavior. It is likely that individuals may have a number of coping responses at their disposal, although each individual may have their own preferred styles based on their personality attributes (Shaw, 1999).

An issue in studying coping is that the coping strategy needs to be evaluated in the specific context in which it is used (Folkman & Moskowitz, 2004). Coping strategies are not inherently good or bad, but instead their effectiveness depends on the context in which they are used. Evaluation of the effectiveness of coping requires first, selecting the appropriate outcomes, and second, paying attention to the fit between the coping and the situation (p. 754).

Adaptation/Adjustment

What do we know about adaptation? It is a complex construct (like coping), it is multidimensional, and it is holistic. However, it is rarely measured holistically in studies. Consensus does exist regarding the centrality of an individual's appraisal of their adjustment. It is the client's adjustment and perception, not the healthcare professional's (Stanton et al., 2001).

We also understand that emotionally supportive relationships set the stage for positive adjustment, whereas criticism, social constraints, and social isolation induce risk (Stanton et al., 2007). Active approach-oriented coping strategies manage disease-related challenges and may bolster adjustment, whereas concerted efforts to avoid disease-related thoughts and feelings are predictors of distress (p. 578). Two basic conclusions come from the descriptive research literature: most individuals appear to "adjust" well to chronic illness and there is considerable variability in adjustment both across studies and across individuals within single studies (Stanton et al., 2001).

In a review article on psychological adjustment to chronic disease, deRidder, Geenen, Kuijer, and van Middendorf (2008) identified five elements of successful adjustment: 1) successful performance of adaptive tasks; 2) absence of psychological disorders; 3) the presence of low negative affect and high positive affect; 4) adequate function status, for example, going to work; and 5) satisfaction and well-being in various life domains (p. 264). Some of these are easily "measured." For example, absence or presence of a psychological disorder could be ascertained with a degree of certainty. However, other conceptualizations cannot.

Maes and colleagues (1996) believe that definitions of adjustment are too simplistic, as many studies operationalize adjustment in terms of psychological outcomes and neglect the medical, cognitive, or social outcomes. Positive adjustment is not merely the absence of pathology. Typical indicators of adjustment in research are positive and negative effects and represent two very different dimensions. Therefore, using only lack of depressive symptoms to indicate adjustment will yield a partial picture of adjustment (Stanton et al., 2001). Maes and colleagues posit that although anxiety and depression are important markers of adjustment, assessment of everyday life behaviors and activities may be much more relevant (p. 243).

deRidder and colleagues' 2008 article appears to typify Maes and colleagues' concern. The primary emphasis is on psychological effects as noted by the title of the article, "Psychological Adjustment to Chronic Disease." Other factors in adaptation appear to be summarized in the subtitle "Satisfaction and Well-Being in Various Life Domains." The more appropriate term, from this author's point of view, is *psychosocial adaptation.* as it more clearly defines and describes the whole person than does *psychological adaptation*, which is too narrow.

One variable that was studied in the 1970s with Kobasa's work and into the late 1980s and early 1990s by Pollock, is the concept of hardiness. Brooks (2003) analyzed 125 articles published from 1966 to 2002 to determine the significance of hardiness in adaptation. This "personal resource," within Moos and Holahan's (2007) framework, demonstrated a significant relationship to psychological, psychosocial, and physiological adaptation. Higher levels of hardiness had positive outcomes in clients with chronic illness (Brooks, 2003, p. 11).

The current literature on hardiness is scarce; however, Brooks (2008) used a cross-sectional survey design involving 60 participants to look at the effect of health-related hardiness (HRH). Individuals who had higher HRH had better psychosocial adjustment to their illness. Additionally, individuals with higher HRH had a higher self-perception of their health status (Brooks, 2008, p. 112).

How coping is related specifically to adjustment has not been clearly described (Sharpe & Curran, 2006, p. 1154). Intellectually we believe that coping strategies do contribute to adaptation, and may be a mediator, but they probably interact with other factors in contributing to adaptation (Stanton & Revenson, 2007).

Berg and Upchurch (2007) have advanced a model that speaks to dyadic coping and adjustment. Their development–contextual model of couples coping with chronic illness views chronic illness as affecting the adjustment of both the client and the spouse such that coping strategies enacted by the patient are related to those enacted by the spouse and vice versa. In a sample of 190 couples with women having rheumatoid arthritis (RA), Sterba and colleagues (2008) demonstrated that couple congruence concerning women's personal control over RA and its cyclic nature predicted better psychological adjustment in women longitudinally (p. 221).

In the chronic pain literature acceptance is a more common concept than coping variables used to described how clients adapt to chronic pain. Acceptance includes responding to pain-related experiences without attempts at control or avoidance (Esteve, Ramirez-Maestre, & Lopez-Martinez, 2007).

Resilience

Resilience is linked to the constructs of coping and adaptation (Maluccio, 2002). While resilience captures a wide range of experiences, it is most notably understood as the ability to adapt in the face of adversity. Resilience helps people cope (Black & Ford-Giboe, 2004). Kralik, vanLoon, and Visentin (2006) utilized interactional processes inherent in participatory action research to explore the concept of resilience. In this collaborative inquiry, data were gathered through email discussion groups. Data analysis revealed resilience meant having a strong sense of self-worth, the ability to benefit from experiences, and the capacity to adapt. Resiliency is a process of reflection, learning, and action directed at overcoming adversity.

INTERVENTIONS

The literature provides an abundance of descriptive studies measuring coping and/or adaptation, but few interventional studies exist. It appears that we can measure coping or adaptation, but that we are unable to conceptualize those results into interventions or ways we can help clients better cope with or adapt to chronic illness.

Stanton and Revenson (2007) suggest that we improve the interpersonal context of our clients by teaching them to develop and maintain social ties, recognize and accept others' help and emotional encouragement, or change their appraisals of the support they are receiving. Psychosocial interventions are directed toward individual-level change and may include cognitive-behavioral, educational, and interpersonal support components. Support groups may provide emotional support as well as an educational focus. The education is expected to strengthen one's sense of control over the disease, reduce feelings of confusion, and enhance decision making (Stanton & Revenson, 2007, p. 221). The peer support provides emotional support and thus enhances self-esteem, minimizes aloneness, and may reinforce coping strategies.

An earlier study that is still referred to frequently in the literature is that of Folkman and colleagues' (1997) coping effectiveness training with HIV-positive men. This interventional study based on Lazarus and Folkman's (1984) stress and coping theory was effective in increasing the quality of life in these men. The training included: 1) appraisal training to disaggregate global stressors into specific coping tasks; 2) coping training to tailor application of strategies; and 3) social support training.

Nurses may be wise to capitalize on a client's religious beliefs and partner with clergy to effect adaptation (Loeb, 2006). Programs related to health education and screening, support groups, and physical activity that are based in a church may be helpful. Barg and Gullatte (2001) explain that church-based health programming can frame health information in a way that may better fit with a client's view of life, that is, their relationship with God.

From another perspective, Pakenham (2007) highlights the need for practitioners to facilitate clients' cognitive processing of the implications and meaning of their illness. A blend of cognitive-restructuring strategies, client-centered approaches, and existential approaches may be helpful to the client and family.

Cognitive-Behavioral Strategies

Cognitive-behavioral strategies can be used to teach coping skills to clients with chronic illness (Folkman & Moskowitz, 2004). Sharpe and Curran (2006) have also encouraged the use of cognitive-behavioral treatments (CBT), as the research literature is clear that CBT is effective in managing psychological distress associated with illness. Such programs include strategies with the aim of facilitating a realistic, but optimistic, attitude toward illness and/or facilitating more adaptive coping strategies. Programs typically include

education about the illness, goal setting and pacing, relaxation strategies and attention diversion skills, cognitive therapy, communication skills, and management of high-risk situations (such as exacerbations of the illness).

McAndrew and colleagues (2008) developed two interventions based on the Common Sense Model of Self-Regulation. The first intervention is a bottom-up concrete/behavioral approach that was used with clients with diabetes. The approach begins with a focus on behavior to create an overarching view of diabetes as a chronic condition that requires constant self-regulation. The second intervention is conceived as a top-down or abstract/cognitive strategy that provides clients who have asthma with a conceptual framework that focuses on asthma being present even when it is asymptomatic (p. 197). The authors suggest that clients may benefit from starting with one strategy or the other. However, it is expected that successful interventions will combine both approaches.

Emotional Intelligence

Emotional intelligence describes the ability to understand, perceive, use, and manage the emotions of self and others (McKenna, 2007). Emotional intelligence training includes six spheres of emotional competence: emotional openness/adaptation; the impact on and of others; self-esteem/identity; management of stress; communication skills/social functioning; and goal management and motivation. It is suggested that emotional self-management can affect the adjustment of individuals with chronic illness and this can be enabled by the use of emotional intelligence techniques by healthcare professionals (McKenna, 2007, p. 551).

Psychosocial Rehabilitation

Breast cancer survivors attended a 1-week psychosocial rehabilitation course consisting of moderate physical activity, lectures, group work, and addressing concerns about returning to work. The workshop was led by a multidisciplinary team. The researchers used the Common Sense Model of Self-Regulation as a framework for the study. Results demonstrated that illness perceptions of breast cancer survivors were not changed by a short psychosocial rehabilitation program (Jorgensen, Frederiksen, Boesen, Elsass, & Johansen, 2009).

Self-Management Programs

Based on the literature on chronic illness self-management, Swendeman, Ingram, and Rotheram-Borus (2009) identified three broad categories in chronic disease self-management. These categories included physical health, psychological functioning, and social relationships. Elements related to physical health were knowledge and behavior to maintain health status, whereas elements related to psychological functioning included self-efficacy and empowerment as well as emotional status and identity shifts. Social relationship elements related to collaborative partnerships with healthcare professionals and family members and social support. Self-management programs based on enhancing self-efficacy are highly successful in reducing symptoms and encouraging behavior change in many chronic illnesses (Newman, 2006). Self-efficacy could be considered a personal context variable and thus may be a determinant in the appraisal of the illness, the coping strategies used by the

individual, and the outcome (the physical, emotional, and social adaptation). Although self-efficacy is task- and situation-specific, programs that encourage that concept could influence adaptation.

Self-Help Groups

As common as self-help and self-support groups are for those with chronic illness, one would expect the research literature to be clear as to their value. Unfortunately, that is not the case. Anecdotal articles exist, but there are few research-based articles. In addition, research commonly looks at such support groups for a short period—6, 10, 12, and 15 weeks—whereas a chronic illness can be present for 30, 40, or 50 years. Therefore, the outcome that we might see in such studies is greatly diminished as the studies demonstrate outcomes at one point in time.

Dibb and Yardley (2006) investigated the role that social comparison might play in adaptation using a self-help group as the context. Social comparison proposes that individuals with similar problems compare each other's health status. Often this comparison occurs within self-help groups, which consist of individuals with similar circumstances. It has been suggested that downward comparison, where comparison is made with a person who is doing less well, will initiate positive affect as it increases self-esteem. Conversely, upward comparison with a person doing less well may result in hope (Dibb & Yardley, 2006, p. 1603). Results of the study with 301 clients with Ménière's disease demonstrated that positive social comparison was associated with better adjustment after controlling for other baseline variables, whereas negative social comparison was associated with worse adjustment over time.

Positive Life Skills

In a sample of 187 HIV-infected women, a positive life skills workshop was effective in increasing antiretroviral adherence, improving mental well-being, and reducing stress (Bova, Burwick, & Quinones, 2008). The workshop consisted of 10 weekly sessions with 6 to 15 women in each group. Workshop facilitators shared a vision of a safe, positive, and respectful environment for women to learn and experience. Part of the workshop involved reframing negative meanings.

SUMMARY

The literature on adjustment has been mostly spearheaded by the discipline of psychology. Thus the theme of that literature is psychological adaptation versus psychosocial adaptation. Unfortunately this narrow focus only addresses one component of adaptation. Psychosocial adaptation or adjustment better encompasses the totality of caring for the client and family. Examining the literature also demonstrates that there is a lack of studies that focus on clients from different ethnicities, cultures, and socioeconomic groups. Most studies have been done with white, middle class populations (deRidder et al., 2008). Thus the generalizability of these studies is limited. What is clear is that we have a long way to go in understanding, effecting, measuring, and influencing adaptation. With the increasing number of individuals with chronic disease, continuing research and study needs to be pursued in this area.

Evidence-Based Practice Box

Adaptation in chronic illness is a multidimensional construct. Adjustment to chronic illness requires attention to medical management of the disease as well as cognitive, emotional, behavioral, and psychological factors of daily life. Multiple sclerosis (MS) is a chronic illness noted for unpredictability of symptoms and progression of illness as well as variability in day-to-day symptoms. The chronic and uncertain nature of MS requires coping and adjustment not only for persons with MS but their families as well. Little research has been conducted to identify successful or unsuccessful adaptation to MS. Previous research has focused on the experience of caregivers rather than how couples work in concert to navigate alterations in their roles and responsibilities. Starks, Morris, Yorkston, Gray, & Johnson (2010) conducted a mixed methods study with couples in which one partner had MS. The purpose of the research was to identify strengths and adaptive coping behaviors as well as risk factors for relational stress. Data were collected through semi-structured interviews with eight couples to explore how these couples defined and identified their relationships, how they navigated role changes, and how they received external support. Data analysis was guided by a conceptual framework of family adaptation to chronic illness. Results included two patterns of

(continues)

adaptation to MS: "in sync" or "out of sync." Couples in sync were able to transition to managing MS as a chronic illness and continue to do things of importance to them, including work and leisure activities with family and friends. These couples were able to adjust their goals and expectations to the realities of their lives and maintain a collaborative problem-solving style. Couples out of sync had experienced loss of roles, identity, and self-worth as a result of the rapid progression of functional losses. Differences in personal styles in these couples shifted from being complementary to oppositional in the face of increased demands and struggles. This research identified mechanisms for adaptation that can assist healthcare professionals care for persons with MS and their families. This study provides a guide for healthcare professionals to assess the possible risk factors for relational strain in couples with MS and identify families who might benefit from referrals to family therapy or other relational support. Further, results from this research have applicability for persons with other chronic illnesses and their families and provide a resource for healthcare professionals for interventions to facilitate adaptation to chronic conditions.

Source: Starks, H., Morris, M. A., Yorkston, K. M., Gray, R. F., & Johnson, K. L. (2010). Being in- or out-of-sync: Couples' adaptation to change in multiple sclerosis. *Disability and Rehabilitation, 32*(3), 196–206.

STUDY QUESTIONS

Why is adaptation to chronic illness important to the client and family with chronic illness?

Describe how different personal resources could affect adaptation.

Compare and contrast the key concepts of the models discussed in this chapter. What are the overlaps in these models? What are the missing elements in these models that would facilitate adaptation?

Apply the adaptation framework of Moos and Holahan to one of your clients with chronic illness. What fits? What does not fit?

From your perspective, what is social support's relationship to adaptation? What is your experience with the role of social support in the adaptation of your clients?

Develop a generic teaching plan that addresses adaptation to chronic illness. What are key points that could then be individualized to clients?

For a full suite of assignments and additional learning activities, **WWW** use the access code located in the front of your book and visit this exclusive website: **http://go.jblearning.com/larsen**. If you do not have an access code, you can obtain one at the site.

REFERENCES

American Psychological Association. (2000). *Diagnostic and statistical manual IV (DSM-IV)*. New York: Author.

Antonovsky, A. (1979). *Health, stress, and coping*. San Francisco: Jossey-Bass.

Barg, F. K., & Gullatte, M. M. (2001). Cancer support groups: Meeting the needs of African Americans with cancer. *Seminars in Oncology Nursing, 17,* 171–178.

Berg, C. A., & Upchurch, R. (2007). A developmental-contextual model of couples coping with chronic illness across the adult life span [Electronic version]. *Psychological Bulletin, 133*(6), 920–954.

Black, C., & Ford-Giboe, M. (2004). Adolescent mothers: Resilience, family health work and health-promoting practices. *Journal of Advanced Nursing, 48*(4), 351–360.

Bodenheimer, T., Lorig, L., Holman, H., & Grumbach, K. (2002). Patient self-management of chronic disease in primary care. *Journal of the American Medical Association, 288*(19), 2469–2475.

Bova, C., Burwick, T. N., & Quinones, M. (2008). Improving women's adjustment to HIV infection: Results of the positive life skills workshop project [Electronic version]. *Journal of the Association of Nurses in AIDS Care, 19*(1), 58–65.

Brink, E. (2009). Adaptation positions and behavior among post-myocardial infarction patients. *Clinical Nursing Research, 18*(2), 119–135.

Brooks, M. (2003). Health-related hardiness and chronic illness: A synthesis of current research [Electronic version]. *Nursing Forum, 38*(3), 11–20.

Brooks, M. (2008). Health-related hardiness in individuals with chronic illnesses. *Clinical Nursing Research, 17*(2), 98–117.

Bury, M. (1982). Chronic ilness as biographical disruption. *Sociology of Health and Illness, 4,* 167–182.

Carver, C. S., Scheier, M. F., & Weintraub, J. K. (1989). Assessing coping strategies: A theoretically based approach. *Journal of Personality and Social Psychology, 56,* 267–283.

Charmaz, K. (1995). The body, identity, and self: Adapting to impairment. *Sociological Quarterly, 36,* 657–680.

Chin, M. H., Polansky, T. S., Thomas, V. D., & Nerney, M. P. (2000). Developing a conceptual framework for understanding illness and attitudes in older, urban African Americans with diabetes. *Diabetes Educator, 26,* 439–449.

Cohen, J. A., & Welch, L. M. (2000). Attitudes, beliefs, values and culture as mediators of stress. In V. Rice (Ed.), *Handbook of stress, coping and health: Implications for nursing research, theory and practice* (pp. 335–366). Thousand Oaks, CA: Sage.

Dancer, S., & Courtney, M. (2010). Improving diabetes patient outcomes: Framing research into the chronic

care model. *Journal of the American Academy of Nurse Practitioners, 22,* 580–585.

Degazon, C. E. (1995). Coping, diabetes, and the older African American. *Nursing Outlook, 43*(6), 254–259.

deRidder, D., Geenen, R., Kuijer, R., & van Middendorp, H. (2008). Psychological adjustment to chronic disease. *Lancet, 372,* 246–254.

Dew, M. A., Myaskovsky, L., Switzer, G. E., DiMartini, A. F., Schulberg, H. C. & Kormos, R. L. (2005). Profiles and predictors of the course of psychological distress across four years after heart transplantation [Electronic version]. *Psychological Medicine, 35,* 1215–1227.

Dibb, B., & Yardley, L. (2006). How does social comparison within a self-help group influence adjustment to chronic illness? A longitudinal study. *Social Science and Medicine, 63,* 1602–1613.

Dixon-Woods, A. (2001). Writing wrongs? An analysis of published discourses about the use of patient information leaflets. *Social Science & Medicine, 52,* 1432–1437.

Engel, G. L. (1977). Need for a new medical model. *Science, 196,* 129–136.

Esteve, R., Ramirez-Maestre, C., & Lopez-Martinez, A. E. (2007) Adjustment to chronic pain: The role of pain acceptance, coping strategies, and pain-related cognitions. *Annals of Behavioral Medicine, 33*(2), 179–188.

Evans, D., & Norman, P. (2009). Illness representations, coping and psychological adjustment to Parkinson's disease. *Psychology and Health, 24*(10), 1171–1196.

Folkman, S., & Greer, S. (2000). Promoting psychological well-being in the face of serious illness: When theory, research, and practice inform each other. *Psycho-Oncology, 9,* 11–19.

Folkman, S., & Moskowitz, J. T. (2004). Coping: Pitfalls and promise. *Annual Review of Psychology, 55,* 45–774.

Folkman. S., Lazarus, R. S., Gruen, R. J., & DeLongis, A. (1986). Appraisal, coping, health status, and psychological symptoms. *Journal of Personality and Social Psychology, 50*(3), 571–579.

Folkman, S., Moskowitz, J. T., Ozer, E. M., & Park, C. L. (1997). Positive meaningful events and coping in the context of HIV/AIDS. In B. H. Gottlieb (Ed.), *Coping with chronic stress* (pp. 293–314). New York: Plenum.

Freeth, R. (2007). Working within the medical model. *Healthcare Counseling & Psychotherapy Journal, 7*(4), 3–7.

Graves, H., Scott D. L., Lempp, H., & Weinman, J. (2009). Illness beliefs predict disability in rheumatoid arthritis. *Journal of Psychosomatic Research, 67,* 417–423.

Hagger, M. S., & Orbell, S. (2003). A meta-analytic review of the Common-Sense Model of illness representations. *Psychology and Health, 18*, 141–184.

Hekler, E., Lambert, J., Leventhal, E., Leventhal, H., Jahn, E., & Contrada, R. (2008). Commonsense illness beliefs, adherence behaviors and hypertension control among African Americans (2008). *Journal of Behavioral Medicine, 31*, 391–400.

Helgeson, V. S., Snyder, P., & Seltman, H. (2004). Psychological and physical adjustment to breast cancer over 4 years: Identifying distinct trajectories of change [Electronic version]. *Health Psychology, 23*, 3–15.

Jorgensen, I. L., Frederiksen, K., Boesen, E., Elsass, P., & Johansen, C. (2009). An exploratory study of associations between illness perceptions and adjustment and changes after psychosocial rehabilitation in survivors of breast cancer. *Acta Oncologica, 48*, 1119–1127.

Karademas, E. C., Kynigopoulou, E., Aghathangelou, E., & Anestis, D. (2010). The relation of illness representations to the 'end-stage' appraisal of outcomes through health status, and the moderating role of optimism. *Psychology and Health*, 1–17.

Kiebles, J. L., Doerfler, B., & Keefer, L. (2010). Preliminary evidence supporting a framework of psychological adjustment to inflammatory bowel disease. *Inflammatory Bowel Disease, 16*(10), 1685–1695.

Kobasa, S. C. (1979). Stressful life events, personality and health: An inquiry into hardiness. *Journal of Personal and Social Psychology, 37*(1), 1–11.

Kralik, D. vanLoon A., & Visentin, K. (2006). Resilience in the chronic illness experience. *Educational Action Research, 14*(2), 187–201.

Lazarus, R. S. (1966). *Psychological stress and the coping process*. New York: McGraw-Hill.

Lazarus, R. S., & Folkman, S. (1984). *Stress appraisal and coping*. New York: Springer.

Leventhal, H., Leventhal, E. A., & Cameron, L. (2001). Representations, procedures, and affect in illness self-regulation: A perceptual-cognitive model. In A. Baum, T. A., Revenson, & J. E. Singer. (Eds.), *Handbook of health psychology* (pp. 19–47). Mahwah, NJ: Lawrence Erlbaum Associates.

Livneh, H., & Antonak, R. F. (1997). *Psychosocial adaptation to chronic illness and disability*. Gaithersburg, MD: Aspen.

Loeb, S. (2006). African American older adults coping with chronic health conditions [Electronic version]. *Journal of Transcultural Nursing, 17*(2), 139–147.

Maes, S., Leventhal, H., & deRidder, D. (1996). Coping with chronic diseases. In M. Zeidner & N. S. Endler (Eds.), *Handbook of coping: Theory, research, applications* (pp. 221–251). New York: Wiley.

Maluccio, A. (2002). Resilience: A many-splendored construct? *American Journal of Orthopsychiatry, 72*(4), 596–599.

McAndrew, L. M., Musumeci-Szabo, T. J., Mora, P. A., Vileikyte, L., et al. (2008). Using the common sense model to design interventions for the prevention and management of chronic illness threats: From description to process. *British Journal of Health Psychology, 13*, 195–204.

McKenna, J. (2007). Emotional intelligence training in adjustment to physical disability and illness [Electronic version]. *International Journal of Therapy and Rehabilitation, 14*(12), 551–556.

Mirowsky, J., & Ross, C. (2002). Measurement for a human science [Electronic version]. *Journal of Health and Social Behavior, 43*, 152–170.

Moos, R. H., & Holahan, C. J. (2007). Adaptive tasks and methods of coping with illness and disability. In E. Martz & H. Livneh (Eds.), *Coping with chronic illness and disability* (pp. 107–128). New York: Springer.

Morea, J. M., Friend, R., & Bennett, R. M. (2008). Conceptualizing and measuring illness self-concept: A comparison with self-esteem and optimism in predicting fibromyalgia adjustment. *Research in Nursing and Health, 31*, 563–575.

Newman, A. (2006). Self-efficacy. In I. Lubkin & P. Larsen (Eds.). *Chronic illness: Impact and interventions* (6th ed., pp. 105–120). Sudbury, MA: Jones & Bartlett.

Norton, T. R., Manne, S. L., Rubin, S., Hernandez, E., et al. (2005). Ovarian cancer patients' psychological distress: The role of physical impairment, perceived unsupportive family and friend behavior, perceived control, and self-esteem [Electronic version]. *Health Psychology, 24*, 143–152.

O'Connor, S. M., Jardine, A. G., & Millar, K. (2008). The prediction of self-care behaviors in end-stage renal disease patients using Leventhal's Self-Regulatory Model. *Journal of Psychosomatic Research, 65*, 191–200.

Pakenham, K. I. (2007). Making sense of multiple sclerosis [Electronic version]. *Rehabilitation Psychology, 52*(4), 380–389.

Pollock, S. E. (1989). The hardiness characteristic: A motivating factor in adaptation. *Advances in Nursing Science, 11*(2), 53–62.

Revenson, T. (1994). Social support and marital coping with chronic illness. *Annals of Behavioral Medicine, 16*, 122–130.

Robert Wood Johnson Foundation (2006–2011). Improving chronic illness care. Retrieved September 15, 2011, from Robert Wood Johnson Foundation, http://www.improvingchroniccare.org

Sakalys, J. A. (2000). The political role of illness narratives. *Journal of Advanced Nursing, 31*(6), 1469–1475.

Schreurs, K. M. G., & deRidder, D. T. D. (1997). Integration of coping and social support perspectives: Implications for the study of adaptation to chronic diseases [Electronic version]. *Clinical Psychology Review, 17*, 89–112.

Sharpe, L., & Curran, L. (2006). Understanding the process of adjustment to illness [Electronic version]. *Social Science & Medicine, 62*, 1153–1166.

Shaw, C. (1999). A framework for the study of coping illness behavior and outcomes. *Journal of Advanced Nursing, 29*(5), 1246–1255.

Siminerio, L. M., Piatt, G., & Zgibor, J. D. (2005). Implementing the Chronic Care Model for improvements in diabetes care and education in a rural primary care practice. *Diabetes Educator, 31*(2), 225–234.

Sprangers, M. A. G., & Schwartz, C. E. (2000). Integrating response shift into health-related quality-of-life research: A theoretical model. In C.E. Schwartz & M. A. G. Sprangers (Eds.). *Adaptation to changing health: Response shift in quality-of-life research* (pp. 11–23). Washington, DC: American Psychological Association.

Stanton, A. L., Collins, C. A., & Sworowski, L. A. (2001). Adjustment to chronic illness: Theory and research. In A. Baum, T. A. Revenson, & J. E. Singer (Eds.). *Handbook of health psychology* (pp. 387–403). Mahwah, NJ: Lawrence Erlbaum.

Stanton, A. L., & Revenson, T. A. (2007). Adjustment to chronic disease: Progress and promise in research. In H. S. Friedman & R. C. Silver (Eds.), *Foundations of health psychology* (pp. 203–233). New York: Oxford.

Stanton, A. L., Revenson, T. A., & Tennen, H. (2007). Health psychology: Psychological adjustment to chronic disease [Electronic version]. *Annual Review of Psychology, 58*, 565–592.

Starks, H., Morris, M. A., Yorkston, K. M., Gray, R. F., & Johnson, K. L. (2010). Being in- or out-of-sync:

Couples' adaptation to change in multiple sclerosis. *Disability and Rehabilitation, 32*(3), 196–206.

Sterba, K. R., DeBellis, R. F., Lewis, M. A., DeVeillis, B. M., Jordan, J. M., & Baucom, D. H. (2008). Effects of couple illness perception congruence on psychological adjustment in women with rheumatoid arthritis. *Health Psychology* 27(2), 221–229.

Stewart, K. E., Ross, D., & Hartley, S. (2004). Patient adaptation to chronic illness. In T. J. Boll, J. M. Raczynski, & L. C. Leviton (Eds.), *Handbook of clinical health psychology, Vol. 2, Disorders of behavior and health* (pp. 405–421). Washington, DC: American Psychological Association.

Swendeman, D., Ingram, B. L., & Rotheram-Borus, M. J. (2009). Common elements in self-management of HIV and other chronic Illnesses: A integrative framework. *AIDS Care, 21*(10), 1321–1334.

van't Spijker, A., Trijsburg, R. W., & Duivenvorrden, H.J. (1997). Psychological sequelae of cancer diagnosis: A meta-analytical review of 58 studies after 1980 [Electronic version]. *Psychosomatic Medicine, 59*, 280–293.

Visotsky, H. M., Hamburg, D. A., Goss, M. E., & Lebovits, B. Z. (1961). Coping behavior under extreme stress: Observations of patients with severe poliomyelitis. *Archives of General Psychiatry, 5*, 27–52.

Wagner, E. H., (1998). Chronic disease management: What will it take to improve care for chronic illness? *Effective Clinical Practice, 1*, 2–4.

Wagner, E. H., Austin, B. T., Davis, C., Hindmarch, M., Schafer, J., & Bonomi, A., (2001). Improving chronic illness care: Translating evidence into action. *Health Affairs, 20*(6), 64–78.

Waisbond, S. (2007). Beyond the medical-informational model: Recasting the role of communication in tuberculosis control [Electronic version]. *Social Science & Medicine, 65*(10), 2130–2134.

Walker, J. G., Jackson, J. J., & Littlejohn, G. O. (2004). Models of adjustment to chronic illness: Using the example of rheumatoid arthritis [Electronic version]. *Clinical Psychology Review, 24*, 461–488.

Zauszniewski, J. A., Chung, C., & Krafcik, K. (2001). Social cognitive factors predicting the health of elders. *Western Journal of Nursing Research, 23*, 490–503.

CHAPTER 5

Social Isolation

Diana Luskin Biordi and Nicholas R. Nicholson

INTRODUCTION

Most of us actively seek human companionship or relationships. The lives of hermits or cloistered, solitary existences are extraordinary because they so vividly remind us that, usually, life is richer for the human contact we share. As valuable as life may be when we engage in a variety of relationships, time reserved for solitude is also necessary as we seek rest or contemplative opportunity in "our own space." The weaving together of individual possibilities for social engagement or solitude develops a certain uniqueness and texture in personal and community relationships. These distinctive personal configurations of engagement and disengagement have consequences for our work and social lives. It is critical, therefore, that healthcare professionals understand the value of social engagement and of solitude.

Isolation: A Working Definition

"Belonging" is a multidimensional social construct of relatedness to persons, places, or things, and is fundamental to personality and social well-being (Hill, 2006). If belonging is connectedness, then social isolation is the distancing of an individual, psychologically or physically, or both, from his or her network of desired or needed relationships with other persons. Therefore, social isolation is a loss of

place within one's group(s). The isolation may be voluntary or involuntary. In cognitively intact persons, social isolation can be identified as such by the isolate. While some may consider isolation as purely subjective, the various dimensions of isolation argue against this singular position, as will be seen in this chapter.

The literature portrays social isolation as typically accompanied by feelings related to loss or marginality. Apartness or aloneness, often described as solitude, may also be a part of the concept of social isolation, in that it is a distancing from one's network, but this state may be accompanied by more positive feelings and is often voluntarily initiated by the isolate. Some researchers debate whether apartness should be included in, or distinguished as a separate concept from, social isolation. As seen in the literature that follows, social isolation has several definitions and distinctions, dependent upon empirical research and the stance of the observer.

When Is Isolation a Problem?

Social isolation ranges from the voluntary isolate who seeks disengagement from social intercourse for a variety of reasons, to those whose isolation is involuntary or imposed by others. Privacy or being alone, if actively chosen, has the potential for enhancing the human psyche. On the other hand, involuntary social isolation occurs when an individual's demand for social contacts or communications exceeds the human or situational capability of others. Involuntary isolation is negatively viewed because the outcomes are the dissolution of social exchanges and the support they provide for the individual or their support system(s). Some persons, such as those with cognitive deficits, may not understand their involuntary isolation, but their parent, spouse, or significant other may indeed understand that involuntary social isolation can have a negative and profound impact on the caregiver and care recipient.

When social isolation is experienced negatively by an individual or his or her significant other, it becomes a problem that requires management. In fact, according to much of the literature, only physical functional disability ranks with social isolation in its impact on the client and the client's social support network (family, friends, fellow workers, and so forth). Therefore, social isolation is one of the two most important aspects of chronic illness to be managed in the plan of care.

Distinctions of Social Isolation

Social isolation is viewed from the perspective of the number, frequency, and quality of contacts; the longevity or durability of these contacts; and the negativism attributed to the isolation felt by the individual involved. Social isolation has been the subject of the humanities for hundreds of years. Who has not heard of John Donne's exclamation, "No man is an island," or, conversely, the philosophy of existentialism—that humans are ultimately alone? Yet the concept of social isolation has been systematically researched during only the last 50 years. Unlike some existentialists and social scientists, healthcare professionals, with their problem-oriented, clinical approach, tend to regard social isolation as negative rather than positive.

The Nature of Isolation

Isolation can occur at four layers of the social concept. The outermost social layer is community, where one feels integrated or isolated from the larger social structure. Next is the layer of organization (work, schools, churches), followed by a layer closer to the person, that is, confidantes (friends, family, significant others). Finally, the innermost layer is that of the person, who has the personality, the intellectual ability, or the senses with which to apprehend and interpret relationships (Lin, 1986).

In the healthcare literature, the primary focus is on the clinical dyad, so the examination of social isolation tends to be confined to the levels of confidante and person, and extended only to the organization and community for single clients, one at a time. For the healthcare professional, the most likely relationships are bound to expectations of individually centered reciprocity, mutuality, caring, and responsibility. On the other hand, health policy literature tends to focus on the reciprocity of community and organizations to populations of individuals, and so it deals with collective social isolation.

At the level of the clinical dyad, four patterns of social isolation or interaction have been identified; although these were originally formulated with older adults in mind, they can be analogized easily to younger persons by making them age-relative:

- Persons who have been integrated into social groups throughout their lifetime

- The "early isolate," who was isolated as an adult but is relatively active in old age
- The "recent isolate," who was active in early adulthood but is not in old age
- The "lifelong isolate," whose life is one of isolation

Feelings that Reflect Isolation

Social isolation can be characterized by feelings of boredom and marginality or exclusion (Weiss, 1973). Boredom occurs because of the lack of validation of one's work or daily routines; therefore, these tasks become only busy work. Marginality is the sense of being excluded from desired networks or groups. Other feelings ascribed to social isolation include loneliness, anger, despair, sadness, frustration, or, in some cases, relief.

Description and Characteristics of Social Isolation

The existence of social isolation increases our awareness of the need for humans to associate with each other in an authentic intimate relationship, whether characterized by caring or some other emotion, such as anger. When we speak of social isolation, we think first of the affected person; then we almost immediately consider that individual's relationships. This chapter will demonstrate that, as a process, social isolation may be a feature in a variety of illnesses and disabilities across the lifecycle.

As an ill person becomes more aware of the constricting social network and declining participation, he or she may feel sadness, anger, despair, or reduced self-esteem. These emotions factor into a changed social and personal identity, but are also separate issues for the person who is chronically ill. Moreover, depending on their own emotional and physical needs, friends and acquaintances may drop out of a person's social support system until only the most loyal remain (Tilden & Weinert, 1987). Families, however, are likely to remain in the social network. As the social network reaches its limitations, it may itself become needful of interventions, such as respite care for the parents of a child who is chronically ill or support groups for the siblings of children with cancer (Heiney et al., 1990).

Social Isolation versus Similar States of Human Apartness

Social isolation has been treated as a distinct phenomenon, or it has been combined or equated with other states relating to human apartness. The literature is replete with a variety of definitions of social isolation, many of which are interrelated, synonymous, or confused with other distinct but related phenomena.

Social Isolation and Alienation

Social isolation and alienation have been linked together or treated as synonymous in much of the healthcare literature, although these two concepts differ from one another. Alienation encompasses powerlessness, normlessness, isolation, self-estrangement, and meaninglessness (Seeman, 1959). Powerlessness refers to the belief held by an individual that one's own behaviors cannot elicit the results one desires or seeks. In normlessness, the individual has a strong belief that socially unapproved behaviors are necessary to achieve goals. Isolation means the inability to value highly held goals or beliefs that others usually value. Self-estrangement has come to mean the divorce of one's self from one's work or creative possibilities. Finally, meaninglessness is the sense that few significant predictions about the outcomes of behavior can be made. Thus, one can see that isolation is only one psychological state of alienation. However, authors frequently merge the finer points of one or more of the five dimensions of alienation and call the result isolation.

Social Isolation and Loneliness

Although social isolation is typically viewed today as a deprivation in social contacts, Peplau and Perlman (1986) suggest that it is loneliness, not social isolation, that occurs when an individual perceives her or his social relationships as not containing the desired quantity or quality of social contacts. In an even more subtle distinction, Hoeffer (1987) found that simply the perception of relative social isolation was more predictive of loneliness than actual isolation. Loneliness has been referred to as an alienation of the self and is sometimes seen as global, generalized, disagreeable, uncomfortable, and more terrible than anxiety (Austin, 1989). Loneliness differs from depression in that in loneliness, one attempts to integrate oneself into new relationships, whereas in depression, there is a surrendering of oneself to the distress (Weiss, 1973).

Nonetheless, loneliness does relate to social isolation. In fact, loneliness is the one concept most invoked when social isolation is considered (Dela Cruz, 1986; Hoeffer, 1987; Mullins & Dugan, 1990; Ryan & Patterson, 1987). However, to use social isolation and loneliness as interchangeable terms can be confusing. To maintain clarity, loneliness should be considered the subjective emotional state of the individual, whereas social isolation is the objective state of deprivation of social contact and content (Bennet, 1980). Therefore, loneliness refers to

the psychological state of the individual, whereas social isolation relates to the sociologic status. Although it is true that social isolation might lead to loneliness, loneliness is not, in itself, a necessary condition of social isolation. Both conditions can exist apart from each other.

Peplau and Perlman's (1986) view of loneliness is distinct from the current North American Nursing Diagnosis Association's (NANDA) nursing diagnosis of social isolation (Carpenito-Moyet, 2010). The NANDA diagnosis extends from the person to include the possibility that a group could also experience a "need or desire for increased involvement with others but is unable to make that contact" (p. 30). Attached to that must be feelings of rejection or aloneness, insecurity in social situations, a desire for more contact with people or lack of meaningful relationships. In the NANDA definition, the model combines psychological feelings with the sociologic state of isolation, and thus blurs the distinctions so carefully treated by others. As will be demonstrated in this chapter, social isolation becomes cause, process, or response, depending on analysis and circumstances. The complex sets of variables that figure into social isolation lend themselves to a variety of assessments, diagnoses, and interventions.

Social Isolation and Aloneness

Tightly linked with social isolation is the need for social support, which is the social context or environment that facilitates the survival of human beings (Lin, 1986) by offering social, emotional, and material support needed and received by an individual, especially one who is chronically ill. Although social support literature has focused on the instrumental and material benefits of support, recent literature on social isolation relates isolation more to the negative feeling state of aloneness. This feeling is associated with deficits in social support networks, diminished participation in these networks or in social relationships, or feelings of rejection or withdrawal.

Social Isolation as a Nursing Diagnosis

Social isolation is defined by NANDA (Carpenito-Moyet, 2010) as a state in which a client or group experiences or perceives a need or desire for increased involvement with others but is unable to make that contact. The NANDA definition has moved beyond the person to the possibility that a group experiences social isolation. Yet the defining characteristics are those of a *person's* subjective feelings of aloneness. In the current NANDA definition, only one of the major characteristics must be present for the diagnosis, and several minor characteristics are further described. Four major characteristics are noted: insecurity in social situations, a lack of meaningful relationships, expressed feelings of aloneness or rejection, and a desire for contact with more people. Of the 12 minor characteristics, most relate to uncommunicativeness, whether in affect or decision making, or expressions of withdrawals. These are mostly personal characteristics, and although some may be generalizable to a group, not all are.

In the NANDA description, social isolation is a *cause* or contributing factor to loneliness, but it is not a response of loneliness. Related to social isolation are several other factors, for example, diseases, social situations, or secondary sequelae to social factors or environments. The current nursing diagnosis of social isolation, combining as it does both psychological and sociologic states of isolation for both persons and groups, requires systematic empirical bases for refined distinctions of isolation. Nurses should continue to build on earlier studies (see Lien-Gieschen, [1993] for a validation study of major identifying characteristics of social isolation in the older adult) to empirically identify and distinguish the truly defining characteristics of social isolation. As it presently stands, the nursing diagnosis of social isolation is rather holistic and resonates strongly with earlier dimensions of the concepts of alienation and loneliness. Carpenito-Moyet (2010) suggests that nurses change diagnoses from social isolation to the diagnosis of loneliness or risk for loneliness, which is conceptually a clearer approach. However, the sociologic reality of social isolation remains, and can require intervention in its own right.

PROBLEMS AND ISSUES OF SOCIAL ISOLATION

Regardless of how social isolation occurs, the result is that basic needs for authentic intimacy remain unmet. Typically this is perceived as alienating or unpleasant, and the social isolation that occurs can lead to depression, loneliness, or other social and cognitive impairments that then exacerbate the isolation.

Several predisposing reasons for social isolation have been proposed: status-altering physical disabilities or illnesses; frailties associated with advanced age or developmental delays; personality or neurologic disorders; and environmental constraints, which often refer to physical surroundings but are also interpreted by some to include diminished personal or material resources (Tilden & Weinert, 1987).

The Isolation Process

A typical course of isolation that evolves as an illness or disability becomes more apparent in the change in social network relationships. Friends or families begin to withdraw from the isolated individual or the individual from them. This process may be slow or subtle, as with individuals with arthritis, or it may be rapid, as with the person with AIDS. Unfortunately, the process of isolation may not be based on accurate or rational information. For example, one woman with cancer reported that, at a party, she was served her drink in a plastic cup while everyone else had glasses (Spiegel, 1990).

Individuals with serious chronic illnesses come to perceive themselves as different from others and outside the mainstream of ordinary life (Williams & Bury, 1989). This perception of being different may be shared by others, who may then reject them, their disability, and their differentness. Part of this sense of being different can stem from the ongoing demands of the illness. For example, social relationships are interrupted because families and friends cannot adjust the erratic treatment to acceptable social activities. From such real events, or from social perceptions, social isolation can occur, either as a process or as an outcome.

Individuals with chronic illness often face their own mortality more explicitly than do others. For example, unmarried or younger clients with cancer express a loss of meaning in life, suggested to be due to cancer's threat to their lives as they grapple with the meaning of life; they may withdraw from their networks or the networks may withdraw from them (Noyes et al., 1990; Weisman & Worden, 1976–1977; Woods, Haberman, & Packard, 1993).

Even if death does not frighten those with chronic illness, it frequently frightens those in their social networks, which leads to guilt, and can lead to strained silences and withdrawal. In the case of individuals with cancer (Burnley, 1992; House, Landis, & Umberson, 1988; Reynolds & Kaplan, 1990) or heart disease (Kaplan et al., 1988; Orth-Gomer, Unden, & Edwards, 1988), social support is significant to their survival. For those who lack this social support, social isolation is not merely a metaphor for death but can hasten it.

Social Isolation and Stigma

Social isolation may occur as a result of stigma. Many persons will risk anonymity rather than expose themselves to a judgmental audience.

Because chronic illnesses can be stigmatizing, the concern about the possibility of revealing a discredited or discreditable self can slow or paralyze social interaction (see Chapter 3). In a study examining chronic sorrow in HIV-positive patients, stigma created social isolation. Women with children, particularly African American women, were more stigmatized and isolated than gay men because others perceived the women as associated with "dirty sex," contagion, and moral threat (Lichtenstein, Laska, & Clair, 2002). Therefore, social roles and the robustness of network support affect social isolation.

Individuals with chronic illness and their families grapple with how much information about the diagnosis they should share, with whom, and when (Gallo et al., 1991). If the illness is manageable or reasonably invisible, its presence may be hidden from all but a select few, often for years. Parents of children with chronic illnesses were reported to manage stressful encounters and uncertainty by disguising, withholding, or limiting information to others (Cohen, 1993), an action that may add to limiting their social network. Jessop and Stein

(1985) found that invisible illnesses of children with chronic illness led to greater difficulty in social interactions because of the uncertainty of ambiguity (disagreement about revealing or passing, or what courses of action to take). For example, parents of a child with cystic fibrosis may tell a teacher that the child is taking pills with meals because of a digestive disease (Cohen, 1993).

As siblings of children with cancer deal with the isolation of their brother or sister, they become vulnerable to being socially isolated themselves (Bendor, 1990). Social isolation not only burdens those with chronic illness, it also extends into family dynamics and requires the healthcare professional to consider how the family manages. Nurses must explicitly plan for the isolation in families with children who are chronically ill (Tamlyn & Arklie, 1986). Thus, with social isolation being a burden for the family, it requires the healthcare professional to consider how the family manages the illness and the isolation.

Where the stigmatized disability is quite obvious, as in the visibility of burn scars or the odor of colitis, the person who is chronically ill might venture only within small circles of understanding individuals (Gallo et al., 1991). Where employment is possible, it will often be work that does not require many social interactions, such as night work or jobs within protected environments (sheltered workshops, home offices). Regardless of what serves as reminders of the disability, the disability is incorporated into the isolate's sense of self; that is, it becomes part of his or her social and personal identity.

Social Isolation and Social Roles

Any weakening or diminishment of relationships or social roles might produce social isolation for individuals or their significant others. Clients who lose family, friends, and associated position and power are inclined to feelings of rejection, worthlessness, and loss of self-esteem (Ravish, 1985). These feelings become magnified by the client's culture if that culture values community (Litwin & Zoabi, 2003; Siplic & Kadis, 2002). An example of social isolation of both caregiver and care recipient occurred in a situation of a woman whose husband had Alzheimer's disease. The couple had been confined for more than 2 years in an apartment in a large city, from which her confused husband frequently wandered. Her comment, "I'm not like a wife and not like a single person either," reflected their dwindling social network and her loss of wifely privileges but not obligations. This ambiguity is common to many whose spouses are incapacitated. Moreover, after a spouse dies, the widow or widower often grieves as much for the loss of the role of a married person as for the loss of the spouse.

The loss of social roles can occur as a result of illness or disability, social changes throughout the lifespan (e.g., in school groups, with career moves, or in unaccepting communities), marital dissolution (through death or divorce), or secondary to ostracism incurred by membership in a "wrong" group. The loss of social roles and the resultant isolation of the individual have been useful analytic devices in the examination of issues of the aged, the widowed, the physically impaired, or in psychopathology.

The Older Adult and Social Isolation

Older age, with its many losses of physical and psychological health, social roles, mobility, economic status, and physical living arrangements, can contribute to decreasing social networks and increasing isolation (Creecy, Berg, & Wright, 1985; Howat, Iredell, Grenade,

Nedwetzky, & Collins, 2004; Ryan & Patterson, 1987; Trout, 1980; Victor et al., 2002). This will become even more of an issue as the number of older adults is expected to increase arithmetically and proportionately in the next 2 decades (Fowles & Greenberg, 2009). Older adults currently make up 12.9% of the overall U.S. population (Administration on Aging, 2010). The prevalence of social isolation in older adults has been approximated to be at 2–20% (Victor, Scambler, Bond, & Bowling, 2000) and even as high as 35% in assisted-living arrangements (Greaves & Farbus, 2006).

Social isolation has been linked with functional disability. One definition of functional disability is "the degree of difficulty or inability to independently perform basic activities of daily living (ADLs) or other tasks essential for independent living" (Mendes de Leon et al., 2001, p. S179). Social networks may influence the functional disability process by preventing decline or facilitating recovery (Mendes de Leon et al., 1999). Consequently, functional disability may impact social networks by preventing older adults from seeking engagement with other members. Network size and social interaction are significantly associated with functional disability risk (Mendes de Leon et al., 2001). Older adults who are more socially engaged report less functional disability (OR = 0.84, 95% CI 0.75–0.95) (Mendes de Leon, Glass, & Berkman, 2003), and those who are a strong part of a social network have been found to have reduced risk of functional disability (p < 0.01) (Mendes de Leon et al., 1999).

Social isolation has been shown to be a serious health risk for older adults (Findlay, 2003), with studies indicating a relationship between all-cause mortality (Ceria et al., 2001), coronary disease (Eng, Rimm, Fitzmaurice, & Kawachi, 2002), and cognitive impairments (Barnes, Mendes de Leon, Wilson, Bienias, & Evans, 2004; Holtzman et al., 2004; Zunzunegui, Alvarado, Del Ser, & Otero, 2003; Beland, Zunzunegui, Alvarado, Otero, & Del Ser, 2005). In a converse finding, older adults with extensive social networks were protected against dementia (Fratiglioni, Wang, Ericsson, Maytan, & Winblad, 2000; Fratiglioni, Paillard-Borg, & Winblad, 2004; Seidler, Bernhardt, Nienhaus, & Frolich, 2003; Wang, Karp, Winblad, & Fratiglioni, 2002). And, as described earlier, although low social engagement may not be a form of social isolation per se, it is a psychological isolator and thus a risk factor in social isolation (Howat et al., 2004). For example, depressive symptoms in older adults were shown to be decreased by social integration (Ramos & Wilmoth, 2003). Isolated older adults were shown to have increased risk for coronary heart disease (Brummett et al., 2001; Eng et al., 2002), and death related to congestive heart failure was predicted by social isolation (Murberg, 2004). Similarly, post-stroke outcomes, for example, additional strokes, myocardial infarction, or death, were predicted by pre-stroke isolation (Boden-Albala, Litwak, Elkind, Rundek, & Sacco, 2005). Isolated women before a diagnosis of breast cancer, when compared with socially integrated women, were found to have a 66% increase in all-cause mortality (Kroenke, Kubzansky, Schernhammer, Holmes, & Kawachi, 2006). Quality of life among breast cancer survivorship is impacted negatively by social isolation (Michael, Berkman, Colditz, Holmes, & Kawachi, 2002). Finally, and perhaps most relevant to health and cost outcomes, socially isolated older adults were found to be four to five times more likely to be re-hospitalized within a year from their previous hospitalization (Mistry et al., 2001).

The extent (from local to community and integrated to contained) and nature (positive or negative social relationships) of a social nework (Litwin, 1997; Wenger, Davies, Shahtahmasebi, & Scott, 1996) , affect health as well as social isolation (Seeman, 2000; Wenger, 1997). In fact, the quality of the social relationship may have more impact than the number of ties (Pinquart & Sorensen, 2001), which suggests that a few solid relationships may be more beneficial than many ties of poor quality.

CASE STUDY

Thomas is an 85-year-old man who has severe COPD, depression, and Type II diabetes. He currently smokes cigarettes and has smoked for the last 45 years. Thomas is a widower, but he has a live-in unmarried partner named Gretchen who has lived with him in their home for the past 8 years. Gretchen is very needy due to a recent Cerebral Vascular Accident (CVA), which left her with expressive aphasia and incontinence. Tom is a member of the local men's club and was in charge of fundraising until recently. He had to give up his position because he needed to be at home more to watch over Gretchen. When talking about his home situation, Thomas states, "I hate to give up all the time with my buddies. I've been a member for 50 years, but since she can't tell me she's wet, I have to check all the time. If I'm not at home, who's going to check?" Despite the fact that she is a lot of work physically and sometimes her inability to speak is discouraging, Thomas says he loves her company. He states that it is wonderful to have a constant companion even though direct conversations are extremely difficult, but you are unsure if this is really how he feels.

Prior to retirement, Thomas was a certified public accountant who worked for a local office. He enjoyed the interaction with his clients and was described as a very social person with numerous friends. He had made lots of new friends through his skills in bringing in high returns on taxes for his clients. In fact, the best man at his wedding, Frank, initially was his tax client. Frank had bought Thomas a steak dinner to thank him for saving him and his wife lots of money, after which, the two became best friends. The two men and their wives had shared many social occasions, but when Frank died years ago, Thomas became depressed and stopped wanting to go out socially. At that time, Thomas's wife of 50 years, Frances, had encouraged him to continue to go out and meet new people. He began to get out more and started to feel like his old self, when Frances died suddenly of a myocardial infarction. After her death Thomas refused to be social. He said, "What's the point of going out and meeting people, if they are just going to die on you? I'd rather stay in." He was also a man who had gone to church services every week and now doesn't go anymore; instead he watches the services on TV. Thomas says, "God knows I'm still dedicated, so I don't need to go out and chat about how great things are with a bunch of busybody church types—especially when things aren't that great at all." About a year after his wife Francis died, he met Gretchen in the supermarket, and they have been partners ever since—both are happy to stay in most of the time.

(continues)

CASE STUDY   (Continued)

Thomas was functioning at a moderate to high level, but recently had a fall secondary to shortness of breath related to emphysema and an acute syncopal episode. He was hospitalized for the shortness of breath, the mild abrasions from the fall, and to have a neurological work up. His respiratory status returned to baseline with the addition of a new inhaler, his neurological status checked out well and, thankfully, there were no broken bones. Because he is Gretchen's primary caretaker, her granddaughter flew in from out of town to take care of her until Thomas was released. He was released after 3 days in the hospital with an admission to the local visiting nurses' agency for an estimated time of 4 weeks of visits.

As you sit in the car, having completed your reading of Thomas' chart, you wonder how this man turned from a social accountant to someone who has been hospitalized for an injurious fall. Additionally, you wonder about how the many psychosocial factors play into his well-being and the well-being of Gretchen. Thomas has stopped seeing his friends, has stopped attending church, has had a decline in his overall health, has implied he doesn't really belong anywhere, and, aside from Gretchen, has a lack of fulfilling relationships—all leading to a possible diagnosis of social isolation. As you walk to the front door with your chart and admission paperwork, you see Thomas through the window silently crying by himself on the porch.

Discussion Questions

1. Given Thomas's history, identify the factors that put him most at risk for social isolation.
2. When considering nursing interventions for Thomas, what would be the number one health issue to address? In your opinion, is Thomas a social isolate? Why or why not?
3. Do you consider Gretchen, Thomas's live-in partner, a positive or negative influence on his life? Explain your answer.

Although much of the current research in social isolation with older adults has focused on community-dwelling adults, one growing segment of study is assisted-living arrangements, which is one of the fastest growing segments of senior housing (Hawes, Phillips, Rose, Holan, & Sherman, 2003). In assisted-living settings where there are many internal (to the setting) social networks, life satisfaction, quality of life, and perception of home were positively reported (Street, Burge, Quadagno, & Barrett, 2007). Assisted living has the potential to focus on health promotion and function maintenance, such as the identification of social isolation and appropriate interventions (Resnick, 2007).

Strictly speaking, social isolation is not confined to a place. The socially isolated are not necessarily homebound or place-bound, although that is typically the case. That being said, however, environments that are removed (such as rural locations) or those not conducive to safety (such as high-crime areas) can contribute to social isolation (Klinenberg, 2001). Social isolation as a function of location has been demonstrated, particularly for the older adult in urbanized settings, in a number of countries other than the United States (Klinenberg, 2001; Russell & Schofield, 1999). In these cases, elderly individuals cannot leave their homes because of lack of transportation or for fear of assault, so they increasingly isolate themselves from others. This situation is intensified by distrust, socioeconomic status, or locale, and it is worse if the older adult has a chronic illness compounding their constraints. Vehicular driving cessation may be an eventual reality as one ages. Limited or no driving confines activities outside the home (Marottoli et al., 2000) and thus limits interactions with others for the older adult.

One objective of planned senior housing is to provide individuals with a ready made social network within a community (Lawton, Kleban, & Carlson, 1973; Lawton, Greenbaum, & Liebowitz, 1980; Lawton, Moss, & Grimes, 1985), although this objective is not always met. The frail elderly are found to be less interactive with more mobile, healthier older adults, possibly because healthier older adults have few extra resources to expend on others who may have even fewer resources, or they may have better health and networks that are incongruent with, and less likely to cross, those of the frail elderly (Heumann, 1988).

Nursing home residents with chronic illness or sensory impairments tend to be more isolated than other elderly persons. In England, for instance, those in residential care who are ill or disabled are considered socially dead, impoverished by the inactive nature of institutionalization and unable to occupy any positive, valued role in the community (Watson, 1988). Stephens and Bernstein (1984) found that older, sicker residents were more socially isolated than

healthier residents. The investigators found that family and longer standing friendships served as better buffers to social isolation than did other residents. Impressionistically, however, the number of research citations about social isolation in England and Ireland, as well as in other European countries, seems to have increased since the 1980s and 1990s in contrast to the research in social isolation in the United States. More recent social isolation research in the United States focuses on policy that seems to incorporate the socially isolated individual into more viable social networks.

Social Isolation and Culture

As globalization and sensitivity to U.S. multiculturalism increases, with its concurrent absorption of multiethnic, multilingual, and multi-religious individuals into yet other cultures, there is an overlap into mainstream healthcare systems. This is especially true of cultural groups that have not assimilated into the dominant culture. Language differences and traditional living arrangements may impede social adaptation. In addition, many immigrants, especially those who are chronically ill, are less able to engage in support networks, given their long working hours, low-paying jobs, lack of health insurance, and changes in family lifestyles and living arrangements. Changes may occur over the second and third generations, but this is less true where the immigrants' home cultures are geographically close, such as Mexican Americans who live along the U.S.–Mexican border, or when reminders of traditions are more visible (Jones, Bond, & Cason, 1998).

An extensive literature review on health care and its relationship with culture demonstrated two overarching issues: 1) the definitions of culture are conceptually broad and/or indistinct, and 2) mainstream health care struggles to integrate these multicultural groups with varying degrees of success. When one speaks of "culture," many concepts are mixed, or even confused (Habayeb, 1995). The dominant white society in the United States and its healthcare system is secular, individualistic, technology- and science-oriented, and tends to be male dominated (Borman & Biordi, 1992; Smith, 1996). Other European-based cultures have similar situations. Social isolation must be viewed from the client's cultural definition of the number, frequency, and quality of contacts, the longevity or durability of these contacts, and the negativism attributed to the isolation felt by the individual involved.

Studies conducted since 1990 indicate how women, minority groups, the poor, and others have not received the same care as the dominant male Caucasian middle or upper classes (Fiscella et al., 2000). Fortunately, current cultural healthcare literature indicates a greater awareness of cultural groups and their values. One factor that may be influencing this change is that since 1990, other healthcare providers, including nurses, psychologists, case managers, and a variety of technical support personnel, have made significant advances in providing higher quality health care to formerly disenfranchised groups (Biordi, 2000).

Many ethnic and religious groups in the United States value community closeness, family kinship, geographic proximity, and social communication. They seek acknowledgment of their right to mainstream or alternative care (Cheng, 1997; Helton, 1995; Keller & Stevens, 1997; Kim, 1998; Kreps & Kreps, 1997). The task of attempting to deliver "tailored," culturally competent care to so many groups is overwhelming and lacks an integrating strategy that

appeals across all groups. One can now find a large number of articles targeting mainstream healthcare providers that provide hints, tips, or insights into cultural groups.

Social Components of Social Isolation

Mere numbers of people surrounding someone do not cure negative social isolation; an individual can be socially isolated even in a crowd if one's significant social network is lost. This situation is true for such groups as those living or working in sheltered-care workshops, residents in long-term care facilities, or people in prisons. What is critical to social isolation is that, because of situations imposed on them, individuals perceive themselves as disconnected from meaningful discourse with people important to them.

Associated with social isolation is reciprocity or mutuality, that is, the amount of give and take that can occur between isolated individuals and their social networks. Throughout the years, much evidence has accumulated to indicate that informal networks of social support offer significant emotional assistance, information, and material resources for a number of different populations. These support systems appear to foster good health, help maintain appropriate behaviors, and alleviate stress (Cobb, 1979; DiMatteo & Hays, 1981; Stephens & Bernstein, 1984).

Examining reciprocity in the relationships of social networks focuses not only on social roles and the content of the exchange, but also on the level of agreement between the isolated person and his or her "others" in the network (Goodman, 1984; Randers, Mattiasson, & Olson, 2003). The incongruence between respondents in a social network regarding their exchanges can help alert the healthcare professional to the level of emotional or material need or exhaustion that exists in either respondent. For example, the senior author observed, during a home visit by a nurse, that a homebound older woman complained that her children had done very little for her. However, it was discovered that the children visited every day, brought meals, shopped for their mother, and managed her financial affairs. In this case, the elderly mother felt isolated despite her children's visits and assistance.

Demographics and Social Isolation

Few studies focus directly on demographic variables and social isolation; typically, this topic is embedded in other research questions across a variety of illnesses. Nevertheless, when these disparate studies are taken together, the impact of demographics on social isolation in the individual with chronic illness is evident. Issues of gender, marital status, family position and context, and socioeconomic standing (such as education or employment) have been shown to affect social isolation.

Socioeconomic Factors

Changes in socioeconomic status, such as employment status, have been correlated with social isolation. The lack of employment of both caregiver and care recipient, cited in much of the caregiver literature, can have an adverse effect. A study of caregivers of frail elderly veterans noted that these caregivers are more at risk for physical, emotional, and financial strain than are other populations, because disabled elderly veterans receive fewer long-term care services than do other elderly populations (Dorfman, Homes, & Berlin, 1996).

Unemployment of the older adult is just one component of the maturational continuum; parents worry about the potential for employment and insurance for their children with chronic illnesses (Cohen, 1993; Wang & Barnard, 2004). Lower income status, especially when coupled with less education, negatively influences health status and is associated with both a limiting social network and greater loneliness, which, in turn, impacts health status and social isolation (Cox, Spiro, & Sullivan, 1988; Williams & Bury, 1989). For instance, almost half of the head-injured clients in one study could not work, which then affected their families' economic status and increased their social isolation (Kinsella, Ford, & Moran, 1989). Financial concerns were found to be a reason for older adults not to participate socially, thus leading to increased risk of social isolation. The study by Howat and colleagues (2004) used focus groups and interviews with adults aged 65 and older to help explain factors that contribute to social isolation, in addition to identifying barriers and facilitators to social participation.

In addition to problems of employment potential, there are economic and social concerns over the costs incurred by health care, employment discrimination, subsequent inability to secure insurance, and loss of potential friendship networks at work—all of which are factors in increasing social isolation or reducing social interactions. In fact, economics exaggerates the costs of chronic illness. People with disabilities suffer disproportionately in the labor market, which then affects their connections with family and community social networks (Christ, 1987). This is particularly evident in the examination of those with mental illness and their social isolation (Chinman, Weingarten, Stayner, & Davidson, 2001; Melle, Friis, Hauff, & Vaglum, 2000).

General Family Factors

As chronic illness persists, and tasks must be managed, relationships are drained, leaving individuals with chronic illness at high risk for social isolation (Berkman, 1983; Tilden & Weinert, 1987). When isolation does occur, it can be a long-term reality for the individual and family. However, if there is social support and involvement, people with chronic illnesses tend toward psychological well-being. Particularly important is the adequacy, more than the avaiability, of social relationships (Wright, 1995; Zimmer, 1995).

There is evidence that social isolation does not necessarily occur in every situation. In fact, the negative impact of social isolation on families with children who are chronically ill has been questioned. One study, which used a large community-based, random sample, found that families with children who are chronically ill did not experience a greater degree of social isolation than those with healthy children, nor did they function differently, except for modest increases in maternal dysfunction (Cadman et al., 1991). Cadman and his associates argue that prior studies were subject to biases because the families in those studies were in the clinic populations of the hospital or agency. By definition, such populations were receiving care for illnesses or responses to illnesses and hence were experiencing an unusual aggregate of problems, which is why they were at the clinic or hospital. Therefore, such families were not representative of families throughout the community.

In another study, classroom teachers evaluated children with cancer or sickle cell disease with a matched sample of controls. The authors found that the children who were chronically ill were remarkably resilient in the classroom setting, although those who survived their brain tumors and could attend regular classes were perceived as more sensitive and isolated (Noll et al., 1992). On the other hand, adolescents with chronic illnesses have been marginalized, which predisposes them to feelings of isolation and low self-worth (DiNapoli & Murphy, 2002).

Similarly, some studies of older adults found that isolation does not always occur with increasing age (Victor et al., 2002). Although childless older individuals tend to be more socially isolated than those with children, when adult children live nearby, older people frequently interact with at least one of them (Mullins & Dugan, 1990). Interestingly, older African American women, even if they lived alone, tended to have more visits from their children than did older African American men; the difference was not explained by needs, resources, or child/gender availability (Spitz & Miner, 1992). It is also interesting to note that older people tend to be less influenced by their children than by contacts with other relatives, friends, and associates (Berkman, 1983; Ryan & Patterson, 1987). One study found no relationship between the elders' emotional well-being and the frequency of interaction with their children (Lee & Ellithorpe, 1982).

Findings indicate that in every group from age 30 to older than 70 years of age, primarily those with the fewest social and community ties were nearly three times as likely to die as those with more ties (Berkman, 1983). In other words, maintaining social contacts enhanced longevity. These individuals tended to be widowers or widows and lacked membership in formal groups (Berkman, 1983), thereby limiting their social contacts. In another study, the older adults who lived in senior housing complexes showed little difference in friendship patterns and life satisfaction (Poulin, 1984). Both of these studies found that living alone, being single, or not having family does not necessarily imply social isolation. Rather, if older people have social networks, many developed throughout a lifetime, and if these networks remain available to them, they are provided with support when needed (Berkman, 1983).

Gender and Marital Status

Typically, women have more extensive and varied social networks than do men (Antonucci, 1985). However, if one spouse has a chronic illness, married couples spend more time together and less time with networks and activities outside the home (DesRosier, Catanzaro, & Piller, 1992; Foxall, Eckberg, & Griffith, 1986). Although gender differences in caregiving occur (Miller, 1990; Tilden & Weinert, 1987), women caregivers indicate greater isolation, increased loneliness, and decreased life satisfaction than do men. Yet both genders show psychological improvement if social contacts, by telephone or in person, increase (Foxall et al., 1986). After the death of a spouse, it has been suggested that men have higher psychological distress (Umberson, Wortman, & Kessler, 1992) and increased mortality rates (Stroebe & Stroebe, 1983) when compared to women.

Although women caregivers may have professional, community, and social networks to aid them in coping with their disabled spouses, over time, they reduce their links to these potential supports. Physical work, social costs and barriers, preparation time for care and outings, and other demands of caregiving become so extreme that women curtail access to and use of support networks external to home. As these caregivers narrow their use of social networks, they unwittingly isolate their spouse with chronic illness as well. Although women reported needing personal or psychological time alone for relief, the subject of their isolation, the person with chronic illness, also became their greatest confidante as the pair struggled in their joint isolation (DesRosier et al., 1992).

Illness Factors and Social Isolation

Chronic illness is multidimensional, and persons with chronic illness and their networks must assume a variety of tasks: managing treatment regimens, controlling symptoms, preventing and managing crises, reordering time, managing the illness trajectory, dealing with healthcare professionals, normalizing life, preserving a reasonable self-image, keeping emotional balance, managing social isolation, funding the costs of health care, and preparing for an uncertain future (Strauss et al., 1984) (see Chapter 2). As people with chronic illnesses struggle to understand their body failure and maintain personal and social identities, they may become fatigued, sicker, or lose hope more readily. Should this happen, they may more easily withdraw from their social networks. Individuals who have four or more chronic illnesses were shown to be at risk for social isolation (Havens & Hall, 2001).

It has been suggested that isolation not only influences the individual's social network (Newman et al., 1989), but also can lead to depression and even suicide (Lyons, 1982; Trout, 1980), particularly in the elderly (Frierson, 1991). Women whose illnesses required more physical demands on themselves and greater symptom management reported greater depression but no effect on their relationship with their partner. Women who had concerns about the meaning of their illness reported greater marital distress and lower satisfaction with their family network (Woods et al.,1993).

Persons with HIV or AIDS had psychological effects that depended not only on the diagnosis, but also on the age of the person. Older individuals showed significant differences in a number of variables, including social isolation (Catalan, 1998). In addition, HIV-negative men who cared for their partners or friends often lived in social isolation with their care recipients (Mallinson, 1999).

In the case of individuals with severe head injuries, it was not the chronic physical disability that disrupted family cohesion as much as the resulting social impairment (Kinsella et al., 1989). The greatest burden identified was social isolation brought on by the impaired self-control of the head-injured person and their inability to learn from social experience. However, the social isolation was particularly burdensome for the families, because the head injury reduced the client's capacity for recognition of and reflection on the deficiencies in social relationships and precluded formation of new close relationships. Consequently, although friendships and employment possibilities were reduced for the client, the real impact was felt by the constrained family (Kinsella et al., 1989).

Healthcare Perspectives

People with chronic illnesses struggle to understand their body failure and its effect on their activities and lives (Corbin & Strauss, 1987). In doing so, they also struggle to maintain their sense of personal and social identity, often in the face of altered self-image and enormous financial, psychological, and social obstacles. If individuals with chronic illness lose hope or become otherwise incapacitated, they may withdraw from their social networks, isolating themselves and others important to them.

Frequently, the daily management of illness means working with healthcare professionals who often do not recognize the inconspicuous but daily struggles of the person's realities of a "new" body, the issues of care, and the development of a new self-identity (Corbin & Strauss, 1987; Dropkin, 1989; Hopper, 1981).

With increased technology, the aging of the population, and changes in economics, chronic illness has begun to assume major proportions in the United States. Concomitantly, the literature contains more articles describing various chronic illnesses, the strategies used to manage them, and issues of social and psychological well-being, including social isolation. More recently, the literature has been extended to consider how chronic illnesses and related technologies are impacted by culture.

The impact of prevailing paradigms of care interventions held by various constituencies is evident. For example, most healthcare professionals still see clients only episodically, using the medical model of "cure" and remaining within the model of the dominant healthcare system. But, in the case of children with cancer, the child focuses on the meaning of his or her impairment (which varies by age); the parents focus first on the immediate concern with their child's longevity and cure, and later on the impairment and long-term effects; the healthcare professional focuses on client survival; the mental health professional focuses on identifying and minimizing impact, impairments, and social barriers; and the public (third-party payers, employers, schoolmates, partners) focuses on contributions and cost. All of these views center on the interaction and exchange, as well as the specific responsibilities and obligations, incurred by the various networks that touch them. Interactions are intensified by the potential withdrawal of any party from the network (Christ, 1987).

Given the variety of care-versus-cure paradigms, the real, daily micro-impositions of chronic illness on social identity and social networks are often lost. The compassion felt by many healthcare professionals is evident in the increasing number of articles available and the attempts to present evidence of the isolation felt by clients and their networks. Nevertheless, these articles may not be explicit; therefore, the proposed interventions for the isolate are unclear, irrelevant, or even discouraging. For example, when discussing facial disfigurement, one article noted that the healthcare professional expected evidence of the client's image integration as early as 1 week post-surgery (Dropkin, 1989). That same article suggested and reiterated that, although the surgery was necessary for removal of the cancer, the resulting defect was confined to a relatively small aspect of the anatomy and that the alteration in appearance or function did not change the person (Dropkin, 1989). The terminology and the interventions in this article focused on the acute postoperative period and did not take into account what disfigured clients were likely to feel later than 1 week post-surgery or that the word "defect" gives a strong clue to the understanding that the disfiguring surgery is obviously and emotionally charged toward the negative.

For a clearer view of the impact of such surgery as seen by the client, Gamba and colleagues (1992) asked postsurgical patients, grouped by the extent of their facial disfigurement, questions about their self-image, relationship with their partner and social network, and overall impact of the therapy. Those with extensive disfigurement reported that it was "like putting up with something undesirable" (p. 221), and many patients were unable to touch or look at themselves. Those with extensive disfigurement also reported more social isolation, poor self-image, and/or a worsened sexual relationship with their partner, even though they maintained satisfactory relationships with their children. In another study, reported in the Gamba article, half of the individuals who underwent hemi-mandibulectomy for head and neck cancers became social recluses, compared with 11% of patients who had laryngectomies. As can be seen, in more than one study, respondents attached a negative meaning to their disfiguring surgery and its results.

Such findings take into account the client's personal meaning of illness and treatment and their effects on social isolation, demonstrating that the isolating treatment or illness (e.g., disfigurement) often is not associated with objective disability. In fact, others have found that the degree of isolation is not directly proportional to the extent of disability (Creed, 1990; Maddox, 1985; Newman et al., 1989). It is important that healthcare professionals not ignore or discount the meaning of illness to the client, regardless of any professional opinion about objective disability or the desirability of treatment.

INTERVENTIONS: COUNTERACTING SOCIAL ISOLATION

In social isolation, the interventions of choice need to remain at the discretion of the client or caregiver. As can be seen from this chapter, writers focus largely on definitions and correlates of social isolation and relatively less on interventions. When interventions are reported, they often relate to the aggregate, such as the policy-related interventions of community housing. The results of many of these larger-scale interventions have been noted in this chapter. Other interventions are mentioned herein, although the list is not all inclusive.

Because the situation of each person with chronic illness is unique, interventions can be expected to vary (see Holley [2007] for examples). Nonetheless, certain useful techniques and strategies can be generalized (Dela Cruz, 1986). Basically, these strategies require that a balance of responsibilities be developed between the healthcare professional and the client, with the following aims:

- Increasing the moral autonomy or freedom of choice of the isolate
- Increasing social interaction at a level acceptable to the client
- Using repetitive and recognizable strategies that are validated with the client, which correlate to reducing particular isolating behaviors

The approach to interventions can also be matched, layer by layer, to the social layering model presented earlier in this chapter, that is, from community, to organization, to network, to person. Therefore, interventions might be cast as ranging from community-based empowerment (transportation-system improvements, for example), work-related enhancements (computer telecare), network and family support group enhancements (nursing), case management, neighborhood watches, or client–professional clinical treatments or care. Examples of these are discussed in this chapter.

Another point to remember is that evaluation is a key principle in any problem-solving system, such as the evaluation found in the nursing process. Throughout the assessment and intervention phases, the healthcare professional should explicitly consider how effective the intervention is or was. The effect of cultural and social differences should be taken into account. The willingness and flexibility to change an ineffective strategy is the mark of the competent professional.

Assessment of Social Isolation

When social isolation occurs, a systematic assessment can help determine proposed interventions, which the professional must validate with the client before taking action. Guiding people, rather than forcing them to go along with interventions, requires the healthcare professional to offer a rationale for the proposed interventions. One must ask if one is giving reasonable rationales, assurances, or support. At the same time, the professional should remember that some cultures value the authority and the expertise of other family members over that of the individual. Consequently, the healthcare professional may have to provide a rationale for suggested interventions to the ranking authority within the support group. Frequently, this is a male figure, often older, who is considered most deserving of any explanation. Other cultures may be matriarchal, so it would be a woman who is the ranking authority.

The key to assessing social isolation is to observe for three distinct features: 1) negativity, 2) involuntary or other imposed solitude, and 3) declining quality and numbers within the isolate's social networks. Social isolation must be distinguished from other conditions such as loneliness or depression, both of which are often accompanied by anxiety, desperation, self-pity, boredom, and signs of attempts to fill a void, such as overeating, substance abuse, excessive shopping, or kleptomania. In addition, loneliness is often associated with losses, whereas depression is frequently regarded as anger turned inward. Because social isolation, loneliness, and depression can all be destructive, the healthcare professional must be resourceful in assessing which issue predominates at any particular point in time.

Properly conducted, an assessment yields its own suggestions for responsive intervention. For instance, the assessment may indicate that the client is a lifelong isolate and that future isolation is a desired and comfortable lifestyle. In this case, the professional's best intervention is to remain available and observant but noninterfering.

If, on the other hand, the client has become isolated and wants or needs relief, then the intervention should be constructed along lines consistent with his or her current needs and history. In a study designed to be culturally sensitive, Norbeck, DeJoseph, and Smith (1996) applied a standardized intervention using designated individuals for person-to-person and telephone contacts for pregnant African American women who lacked social support networks. Their study showed significantly reduced low-birth-weight infants.

In another example, if the healthcare professional discovers that a support network is lax in calling or contacting a client, the provider can help the client and support network rebuild bridges to each other. Keep in mind that there are usually support groups to which those in a social network can be referred for aid. As an illustration, if the network is overwhelmed, information can be provided about respite programs. Interventions such as these will help members of the social network maintain energy levels necessary to help their chronically ill relative or friend.

Assessment typically involves the clinical dyad of caregiver and client. It is at this level that assessment is critical to the development of appropriate and effective interventions. Without an adequate and sensitive assessment, interventions are likely to be ineffective or incomplete.

Measurement of Social Isolation

The major issue in measuring social isolation is that the instrumentation does not fully capture the conceptual definition of social isolation. For example, social isolation, as described in this chapter, has no specific instrument of measurement. Some researchers have used instruments that define social isolation as an extreme lack of social networks or support, whereas others use a group of questions that purport to measure social isolation. The closely related concept of social networks has two frequently used research measures that may be useful when assessing social isolation. Because there is some conceptual overlap of both constructs, specifically the number of social contacts, measures used to assess social networks may serve as a useful initial assessment for social isolation.

A review of the literature found that the two most commonly used and reported research measures of social networks were the Lubben Social Network Scale (LSNS) (Lubben, 1988) and the Berkman-Syme Social Network Index (SNI) (Berkman & Syme, 1979). Both of these tools measure, essentially, the amount of contact one has with others.

The SNI was cited in 209 articles and the LSNS was cited in 38 articles found in MEDLINE, CINAHL, EMBASE, and PsycINFO. The SNI is a nontheoretical summed aggregation of several items that examined a range of social ties and networks and how they directly affected people. Both the relative importance and the number of social contacts are aggregated into four weighted sources. The Lubben Social Network Scale was developed to measure social networks among older adults (Lubben, 1988) and is based on the SNI and its original questionnaire. The LSNS has 10 equally weighted items, which place individuals into four quartiles with a cut-off score for social isolation. Reliability and validity have been examined (Lubben, 1988; Lubben & Gironda, 1996; Rubenstein, Josephson, & Robbins, 1994). The LSNS is typically administered prospectively during data collection, and is difficult to use in secondary data analysis, although this has been attempted (Lubben, Weiler, & Chi, 1989).

Given the state of the science, it is suggested that when measuring social isolation, the researcher choose from the SNI or LSNS dependent upon one's research purpose and question, and also use semi-structured interviews or questionnaires to confirm a diagnosis of social isolation. The SNI or LSNS score will give some indication as to whether the individual may be at risk for social isolation warranting further assessment through interview. Once social isolation is identified in an older adult, it is important to use evidence-based recommendations as interventions to decrease negative health-related consequences.

Management of Self: Identity Development

The need for an ongoing identity leads an individual to seek a level where he or she can overcome, avoid, or internalize stigma and, concomitantly, manage resulting social isolation. Social networks can be affected by stigma. Managing various concerns requires people who are chronically ill to develop a new sense of self consistent with their disabilities. This "new" life is intertwined with the lives of members of their social networks, which may now include both healthcare professionals and other persons with chronic illnesses. Lessons must be learned to deal with new body demands and associated behaviors. Consequently, the individual with chronic illness must redevelop an identity with norms different from previous ones.

The willingness to change to different and unknown norms is just a first step, one that often takes great courage and time. For instance, one study indicated that clients with pronounced physical, financial, and medical care problems following head and neck surgery exhibited prolonged social isolation 1 year post-surgery (Krouse, Krouse, & Fabian, 1989). Although no single study has indicated the time necessary for such identity transformations, anecdotal information suggests that it can last several years, and indeed, for some, it is a lifelong experience.

Identity Transformation

Clarifying how networks form and function is a significant contribution to the management of the struggles of the client who is chronically ill and isolated. The perceptive healthcare worker should know that much of the management done by the chronically ill and their networks is not seen or well understood by healthcare professionals today (Corbin & Strauss, 1987). However, we can use Charmaz's (1987) findings as guides for assessing the likely identity level of the individual as we try to understand potential withdrawal or actual isolation.

Charmaz (1987), using mostly middle-aged women, developed a framework of hierarchical identity transformations that is useful in diagnosing a chronically ill individual's proclivity to social networking and in discovering which social network might be most appropriate. This hierarchy of identity takes into account a reconstruction toward a desired future self, based on past and present selves, and reflects the individual's relative difficulty in achieving specific aspirations. Charmaz's analysis progresses toward a "salvaged self" that retains a past identity based on important values or attributes while still acknowledging dependency.

Initially, the individual takes on a supernormal identity, which assumes an ability to retain all previous success values, social acclamation, struggles, and competition. At this identity level, the individual who is chronically ill attempts to participate more intensely than those in a non-impaired world despite the limitations of illness. The next identity level that the person moves to is the restored self, with the expectation of eventually returning to the previous self, despite the chronic illness or its severity. Healthcare workers might identify this self with the psychological state of denial, but in terms of identity, the individual has simply assumed that there is no discontinuation with a former self. At the third level, the contingent personal identity, one defines oneself in terms of potential risk and failure, indicating the individual still has not come to terms with a future self but has begun to realize that the supernormal identity will no longer be viable. Finally, the level of the salvaged self is reached, whereby the individual attempts to define the self as worthwhile, despite recognizing that present circumstances invalidate any previous identity (Charmaz, 1987).

Not only does social isolation relate to stigma; it can develop as an individual loses hope of sustaining aspirations for a normal or supernormal self, which are now unrealistic. As persons with chronic illness act out regret, disappointment, and anger, their significant others and healthcare professionals may react in kind, perpetuating a downward spiral of loss,

anger, and subsequent greater social isolation. The idea of identity hierarchies thus alerts the caregiver to a process in which shifts in identity are expected.

The reactions, health advice, and the experiences of individuals with chronic illness must be taken into account in managing that particular identity, and also the various factors that help shape it. Both the social network and adapted norms now available play a role at each stage in identity transformation. At the supernormal identity level, individuals who are chronically ill were in only limited contact with healthcare professionals but presumably in greater contact with healthier individuals who acted as their referents; at the level of the salvaged self, a home health agency typically was used (Charmaz, 1987).

Integrating Culture into Health Care

Isolation, by its very definition, must include a cultural screening through which desired social contacts are defined. When one speaks of social isolation among unique ethnic groups, the number, type, and quality of contact must be sifted through a particularistic screen of that person's culture. Not only the clients', but also the provider's communication patterns, roles, relationships, and traditions are important elements to consider for both assessment and intervention (Barker, 1994; Cheng, 1997; Groce & Zola, 1993; Hill, 2006; Kim, 1998; Margolin, 2006; Treolar, 1999; Welch, 1998).

Some feel that matching culturally similar providers to clients would be a way to meet needs with effective interventions (Welch, 1998). However, healthcare educators and service providers recognize the issues of a smaller supply of providers and the greater numbers of clients in a struggling dominant healthcare system coping with multiculturalism. To meet supply and demand issues, as well as cultural needs, the idea of cultural competence is being promoted. Education about cultures is being advanced as the key to effective interventions that intersect the values of two disparate groups of individuals (Davidhizar, Bechtel, & Giger, 1998; Jones, Bond, & Cason, 1998; McNamara et al., 1997; Smith, 1996). Cultural education not only results in outcomes of culturally relevant compliance (Davidhizar et al., 1998) but also helps alleviate the isolation of individuals with chronic illness (Barker, 1994; Hildebrandt, 1997; Treolar, 1999).

For those who find that such culturally based education is unavailable, and assuming there are more groups and more traditions than can possibly be understood by a single healthcare provider, a fail-safe strategy remains. This approach requires the provider to approach each person, regardless of their cultural milieu, with respect and dignity, in an explicit good-faith effort to inquire, understand, and be responsive to the client's culture, needs, and person. The provider must set aside prejudices and stereotypes and instead use an authentic sensitive inquiry into the client's beliefs and well-being (Browne, 1997; Treolar, 1999).

By seeking to understand differences, one can find pleasure in the differences and move beyond them to enjoy the similarities of us all. This approach is undergirded by a culture of "caring," and moves toward a model of actively participating groups exchanging concerns of identity, egalitarianism, and needed care (Browne, 1997; Catlin, 1998; Keller & Stevens, 1997; Treolar, 1999). In so doing, social isolation can be managed within the context most

comfortable to the client, who is the raison d'être of the healthcare professional.

Respite

The need for respite has been cited as one of the greatest necessities for isolated older adults with illness and their caregivers, many of whom are themselves elderly (Miller, 1990; Subcommittee on Human Services, 1987). Its purpose is to relieve caregivers for a period of time so that they may engage in activities that help sustain them or their loved ones, the care recipients. Respite involves four elements: 1) purpose, 2) time, 3) activities, and 4) place. The time may be in short blocks or for a longer (but still relatively short-term) period, both of which temporarily relieve the caregiver of responsibility. Activities may be practical, such as grocery shopping; psychological, such as providing time for self-replenishment or recreation; or physical, such as providing time for rest or medical/nursing attention.

Respite may occur in the home or elsewhere, such as senior centers, daycare centers, or long-term care facilities. Senior centers usually accommodate persons who are more independent and flexible, often offering social gathering places and events, meals, and health assessment/exercise/maintenance activities. Daycare centers typically host individuals with more diminished functioning. Other places, such as long-term care facilities, manage clients with an even greater inability to function.

Finally, respite may be delivered by paid or unpaid persons who may be friends, professionals, family, employees, or neighbors. Although many care recipients welcome relief for their caregiver, some may fear abandonment. The family caregiver and professional must work together to assure the care recipient that he or she will not be abandoned (Biordi, 1993). Therefore, the professional has a great deal of latitude in using the four elements to devise interventions tailored to the flexible needs of an isolated caregiver and care recipient.

Support Groups and Other Mutual Aid

Support groups, or even peer counselors (Holley, 2007), have been identified for a wide variety of chronic illnesses and conditions, such as breast cancer (Reach to Recovery), bereavement (Widow to Widow), and alcoholism (Alcoholics Anonymous), or for other conditions such as multiple sclerosis (MS) or blindness. These groups or individuals assist those with chronic illness or disabilities to cope with their illness and the associated changes in identities and social roles of their chronic illness or disability. Such counseling can help enhance one's self-esteem, provide alternative meanings of the illness, suggest ways to cope, assist in specific interventions that have helped others, or offer services or care for either the isolate or caregiver (Holley, 2007). Almost every large city or county has lists of resources that can be accessed: health departments, social work centers, schools, and libraries. Even the telephone book's yellow pages can assist in finding support groups or other resources. The Internet is also a source of information about support groups and resource listings. Some resources list group entry requirements or qualifications. Because of their variety and number, support groups are not always available in every community, so healthcare professionals may find themselves in the position of developing a group. Therefore, as part of a community

assessment, the healthcare professional should not only note the groups currently available, but also identify someone who might be willing to develop a needed group. The healthcare professional also may have to help find a meeting place, refer clients to the group, assist clients in discussing barriers to their care, and, if necessary, develop structured activities (such as exercise regimens for arthritic individuals). In addition, the use of motivational devices, such as pictures, videos, audio recordings, reminiscence therapy, or games, may be helpful in developing discussion. Demonstrations of specific illness-related regimens, such as exercises, clothing aids, or body mechanics, are also useful to support groups.

Professionals should be alert to problems the isolate may have in integrating into groups, such as resistance to meeting new people, low self-esteem, apprehension over participation in new activities, or the problems of transportation, building access, and inconvenient meeting times (Matteson, McConnell, & Linton, 1997).

Social activity groups are one way of integrating isolated institutionalized individuals or of reversing hospital-induced confusion; such groups could be recreational therapy groups or those developed particularly to address a special interest (e.g., parents facing the imminent death of a child). Given the limited financial resources typical of most persons who are chronically ill, support groups that are not costly to the chronically ill or their families are more likely to be welcomed.

Spiritual Well-Being

For many, religious or spiritual beliefs offer an important social connection and give great meaning to life. Spiritual well-being typically affirms the unity of the person with his or her environment, often expressed in oneness with his or her god(s) (Matteson et al., 1997). Consequently, assuring isolates some means of connection to their religious support may help them find newer meaning in life or illness and provide them with other people with whom to share that meaning. The healthcare professional should assess the meaning of spirituality or religion to the individual, the kind of spiritual meeting place he or she finds most comforting, and the types of religious support available in the community. Religious groups range from formal gatherings to religiously aided social groups.

Frequently, the official gathering places of religious or spiritual groups, for example, churches, temples, or mosques, have outreach or social groups that will make visits, arrange for social outings, or develop pen pals or other means of human connectedness. The nurse or other healthcare professional may have to initiate contact with these groups to assist in developing the necessary outreach between them and the isolate.

Rebuilding Family Networks

Keeping, or rebuilding, family networks has much to offer. However, families that have disintegrated may have a history of fragile relationships. The healthcare professional must assess these networks carefully to develop truly effective interventions.

The professional must also take into account the client's type of isolation (lifelong versus recent) and the wishes of the isolate: With whom (if anyone) in the family does the isolate wish contact? How often? What members of the family exist, and which care about the isolate? What is their relationship to the isolate—parent, sibling, child, friend-as-family,

other relative? The professional can then make contact with the individuals indicated to be most accommodating to the isolate, explain the situation, make future plans to bring them and the isolate together, and afterward assess the outcome. However, it may not be possible to bring uninterested family members back into the isolate's social network.

For family members who are interested and willing, rebuilding networks means the professional must take into account the location or proximity of family members to the isolate. If they live near each other, and because a "space of one's own" is a critical human need, a balance of territorial and personal needs must be managed if the isolate is to be reintegrated. Should the isolate and family agree to live together, the family's physical environment will require assessment for safety, access, and territorial space. Not only are factors such as sleeping space and heat and ventilation important, but personal space and having one's own possessions are as important to the family members as they are to the ill person. Teaching the family and isolate how to respect each other's privacy (such as by getting permission to enter a room or look through personal belongings, speaking directly to one another, and so forth) is a way to help them bridge their differences.

Understanding Family Relationships

The nature of the relationship between family and isolate must be understood. The family's meanings and actions attached to love, power, and conflict, and observations of the frequency of controlling strategies by various individuals will inform the professional of potential interventions. For example, some clients who live alone were found to be more likely to be satisfied with support when they were feeling depressed, whereas clients living with others were more sat-isfied with supporters who cared about them (Foxall et al., 1994).

In some families, love is thought to indicate close togetherness, whereas, in other families, love is thought to provide members with inde-pendence. Love and power can be developed and thought of either as a pyramidal (top-down) set of relationships or as an egalitarian circle. Conflict may be a means of connection or of distancing and can be expressed by shouting and insults or by quiet assertion.

Community Resources to Keep Families Together

Using community resources, such as support groups, is a way to help keep a family together. Families draw on each other's experiences as models for coping. For example, families in which there is a child with cancer find ways to help their child cope with the isolation induced by chemotherapy. When necessary, the health-care professional may wish to refer the isolate and family to psychiatric or specialty nurses, counselors, psychiatrists, or social workers to help them overcome their disintegration. Successful implementation of the wide range of family-related interventions requires sensitive perceptions of the needs not only of the isolate, but also of the various family members with whom that individual must interact.

Two interesting community resources that could help alert families to potential problem situations for isolates are the post office and newspaper delivery services. If these delivery persons observe a build-up of uncollected mail or newspapers, they can call or check the house to see if there is an older adult isolate in distress. Families who are concerned about their isolated family member can provide their post office,

regular mail carrier, or news delivery service with information about the isolate that can be used in the event of a problem. Nurses and social workers can also contact mail and news services or help families make these contacts. This intervention can be expanded to include any regular visitor, such as a rental manager, janitor, or neighbor, who might be willing to check on the welfare of the isolate.

In some communities, employees at banks and stores also react to older individuals who may be isolated. Should there be unusual finan-cial activities or changes in shopping patterns, the individual can be contacted to make sure that everything is satisfactory. Although, in some communities, mail and newspaper services and banks and stores are not involved with people in their areas, these resources are valuable and should be expanded throughout the country.

Communication Technologies

Telephone

The telephone is a method used to counteract the effects of place-boundedness. Although, findings of its effectiveness are equivocal (Kivett, 1979; Praderas & MacDonald, 1986), the telephone is considered almost a necessity in reducing the isolation of a place-bound indi-vidual. In literature other than that of the socially isolated, nurses using telephone contact reduced health problems and costs of readmis-sion for patients (Norbeck et al., 1996).

Computers

For many persons, including homebound older adults or people with disabilities, computers have helped offset social isolation and loneliness through features such as access to the Internet, which allows the person to reach family and friends or to find new friends, activities, and other common interests. Computers can also be used to provide fun activities, such as games. In the United States, computers are more widely available than elsewhere, and more so among those within higher socioeconomic status and the more highly educated. Increasingly, online groups offer support, such as that described for breast cancer patients (Hoybye, Johansen, & Tjornhoj-Thomsen, 2005).

Evidence-Based Practice Box

Methodologically rigorous, evidence-based practice research about social isolation is difficult to find. One such study, however, was undertaken by Fyrand and colleagues. This study examines the effect of a social network intervention on 264 women participants with rheumatoid arthritis (RA). Participants were randomized into three groups, that is, one intervention and two control groups. These were labeled as the Intervention Group, the Attention Control Group, and the No-Treatment Control Group.

The *research questions* guiding this study were: "To what extent, if any, will network intervention influence (1) the total size of the patients' social network, (2) the amount of the patients' daily emotional support, and (3) the patients' social functioning" (Fyrand, 2003, p. 72). The *intervention* in this study consisted of two separate but related sessions: 1) a Preparatory Assessment session and 2) the Network Meeting. If the participants

were randomized into the attention control group, they were given the opportunity to attend a single 2-hour meeting in which they were presented information about RA from a panel of experts who also responded to their questions about RA. The third control group had no intervention or meeting.

Three *findings* indicated that 1) the intervention group experienced a statistically significant increase in their social network size; 2) at time 2 in the study, emotional social support was higher for the intervention group; and (3) less social dysfunction occurred in the intervention group.

The *intervention* basically assessed a patient participant's social network and then helped the patient and the social network to assist the patient in socially functional problem solving about the illness. Through the meeting process in the intervention group, a change in attitude was observed when the patient developed an increased awareness of the need for social network members. In addition, the network members often would share problems about their own lives, which normalized any feelings of stigma experienced by the patient. The authors call this a "response shift," where both parties change their self-evaluation and make a concerted effort to support each other (p. 83).

During the preparatory assessment session, three important areas were covered: 1) information about the research project, 2) the relationship between health and social networks, and 3) how the patient experienced chronic illness. During this 2-hour preparatory assessment, the researchers mapped the participant's present social network. The social network map helped the participants to obtain a deeper analysis of the makeup of their social networks, and allowed the researcher and participant to make decisions about which member of the network should be invited to the network meeting (the second element of this intervention). In this initial preparatory session, participant patients also discussed, in depth, how their chronic disease (RA) impacted their lives. As feelings were explored, researchers took great care to ensure that the participants had adequate time and attention regarding these important topics.

The network meeting consisted of network members, typically the friends and family who were listed in the preparatory assessment, getting together to problem solve. An average of seven network members, in addition to a network research therapist, attended for an average of 2 hours. The research network therapist acted as a leader and catalyst of the group, mobilizing the participant and the group of network members to dialogue about the participant patient's problem-solving process. The group leader opened the meeting with the expectations of the meeting and a presentation of the topics that were deemed important, as derived from the preparatory meeting. The general goal for the group was to

share how they viewed the participant's life with RA and to describe their hopes and expectations of the meetings. The goal for the participant was to elicit free discussion of those topics that were of highest importance. A consensus was formed within the group about how to best solve the problems raised, with the further intention to develop trust and involvement between members of the network. In addition to the participant learning how to best present problems to social network members, the aim of the network meeting was to help the participant and members change dysfunctional network behaviors. The researchers suggested that by clustering the network members and the participant together in a single room the network and participant would better sense their collective power and the participant could re-bond with any hitherto damaged social network relationships.

This article lays out a sensible intervention that targets social network members. Through a pair of relatively short meetings, the researchers created an exportable, effective intervention that reduced social isolation and rehabilitated, to some extent, dysfunctional social networks. Furthermore, not only is this intervention brief, but it also does not require technology that requires extra training. It does require that the network therapist be a professional, such as a nurse, social worker, or psychologist, who is skilled in group therapy and mapping social networks. Therefore, this cost-effective intervention can be easily conducted in a variety of settings with a variety of patients who have social networks willing to meet together for a minimum of only 4 hours.

Source: Fyrand, L. (2003). The effect of social network intervention for women with rheumatoid arthritis. *Family Process, 42*(1), p. 71.

Advances in computer technology have created special attachments, such as cameras, breath tubes, or special keyboards and font sizes, which customize computers to the needs of the isolated or disabled, including those with visual impairment (Imel, 1999; Salem, 1998). In parts of the United States, outreach efforts are increasing, as projects aim to reduce the social isolation of the homebound by providing computers and Internet access to caregivers and care receivers. The use of information and other communication technologies has been helpful in alleviating barriers to the return to work for those with spinal cord injuries and the resulting disabilities (Bricout, 2004). Telecommuting enables home-based work, and has proven effective for those with mobility or transportation limitations, or those whose illnesses or disabilities necessitate rest periods incompatible with typical work environments. Computers have also been used to relieve isolation or loneliness, and assist in the management of chronic illness and support groups located in rural environments (Clark, 2002; Hill & Weinert, 2004; Johnson & Ashton, 2003; Weinert, Cudney, & Winters, 2005).

Whether connecting via the Internet, using word processing, corresponding via email, taking classes, or joining social networking sites,

computers also allow isolates to actively fill many hours of otherwise empty time, bringing a measure of relief to tedium while expanding their intellectual and social lives. The caveat, of course, is that the use of the computer, and especially the Internet, could itself be an isolating factor for many individuals. This creates a danger of virtual reality overrunning actual reality, in which case, isolates compound their isolation. That having been said, however, the computer offers many more advantages than disadvantages in the possibilities for overcoming some elements of isolation.

Touch

In cultures where touch is important, families and professionals must learn the use and comfort of touch. American studies indicate that the elderly are the least likely group to be touched, and yet they find touch very comforting. Pets may be useful alternatives to human touch and human interaction; pet therapy is increasingly used as an intervention in families, communities, and group settings such as nursing homes (Banks, 1998; Collins, Fitzgerald, Sachs-Ericsson, Scherer, Cooper, & Boninger, 2006). Feeling loved and having it demonstrated through touch can do much to reduce isolation and its often concomitant lowered self-esteem. Because some individuals find touch uncomfortable, professionals must assess (by simply asking or observing flinching, grimacing, or resignation) the family's or isolate's responsiveness to touch.

Behavior Modification

Behavior modification is a technique that is best used by skilled professionals. It involves the systematic analysis of responses and their antecedent cues and consequences; the use of cognitive therapy to change awareness, perceptions, and behaviors; and the specification of realistic, measurable goals or actual behaviors. In addition, reward structures and understanding support persons are necessary in the definition of the problem and its solution. Consistency is needed to develop stable patterns of responses. The timeframe of such modification can vary with the problem.

Behavior modification is particularly useful for addressing specific problems, for example, the isolate who is fearful of going outside the house. It is also an important intervention when the environment can be held stable, such as in an institutional setting. Matteson and colleagues (1997) note that where groups are small or the motivation intense, successful behavioral interventions have been instituted for the socially isolated in institutions as well as in the home.

OUTCOMES _____

Ideally, the reduction of social isolation and the maintenance of the integrity of the person who is chronically ill and his or her caregiver(s) are preferred outcomes of interventions. However, so many factors can affect social isolation, its assessment, and intervention that it is difficult to draw simple linear relationships between structure, process, and outcomes. As shown throughout this chapter, a professional must be sensitive to, and prioritize, interventions within the cultural milieu in which the client and support network reside.

Handling the emotionally charged issues surrounding every social isolate requires that professionals recognize in their clients, as well as in themselves, those values that most drive their relationships, and build solutions that best deliver culturally and personally competent care toward a better life for their clients.

STUDY QUESTIONS   **WWW**

Is loneliness the same thing as social isolation? Why or why not?

How might the distance that a manually powered or an electrically powered wheelchair can go relate to social isolation?

List six characteristics that identify a client who may be at risk for social isolation. What criteria did you use to develop these characteristics?

Suppose another healthcare professional said about a very new client, "Oh, we must make certain that Mrs. Jones has company. She's a widow, you know." With regard to social isolation, what arguments could you make, pro or con, about this statement?

Develop at least five questions you could use to assess and validate social isolation in a client. Consider how you might approach identity levels, actual isolation, network assessment, and feelings of the isolate. Add other priorities as you wish, but offer rationales for each of them.

Name three community resources you could use to reduce the social isolation of clients.

What two principles should guide a healthcare professional when developing any intervention with an isolated client? Why are these important?

(continues)

Study Questions (Cont.)   WWW

Suppose a client said to you, "I have had arthritis in my fingers and hands for a long time now. I simply can't do what I used to do. I now have new handles for my kitchen cabinets because the knobs hurt my hands, and new clothes especially made for people like me who can't work buttons. My daughter was shopping and she saw them and told me about them. Now I feel better when I get together with them to see my grandchildren." At what stage of identity might you expect this client to be? Why? Is this person an isolate? Explain your answer.

A gay teenager is your client. He has recently "come out" and is now depressed because his schoolmates shun him, his parents are going through a grief reaction to his announcement, and he has few other friends who share his interests or sexual orientation. Is he at risk for social isolation? Loneliness? How would you assess his social network? What interventions, if any, would you recommend? Explain your answers.

For a full suite of assignments and additional learning activities,   WWW
use the access code located in the front of your book and visit this exclusive website: **http://go.jblearning.com/larsen**. If you do not have an access code, you can obtain one at the site.

REFERENCES

Administration on Aging (2010). A profile of older Americans: 2010. Retrieved September 13, 2011 from http://www.aoa.gov/AoARoot/Aging_Statistics/Profile/2010/2.aspx

Antonucci, T. (1985). Social support: Theoretical advances, recent findings, and pressing issues. In I. G. Sarason & B. R. Sarason (Eds.), *Social support: Theory, research, and application*. Boston: Martinus Nyhoff.

Austin, D. (1989). Becoming immune to loneliness: Helping the elderly fill a void. *Journal of Gerontological Nursing, 15*(9), 25–28.

Banks, M. R. (1998). *The effects of animal-assisted therapy on loneliness in an elderly population in long-term care facilities*. Louisiana State University Health Sciences Center School of Nursing.

Barker, J. C. (1994). Recognizing cultural differences: Health care providers and elderly patients. *Gerontology & Geriatric Education, 15*(1), 9–21.

Barnes, L. L., Mendes de Leon, C. F., Wilson, R. S., Bienias, J. L., & Evans, D. A. (2004). Social resources and cognitive decline in a population of older African Americans and whites. *Neurology, 63*(12), 2322–2326.

Beland, F., Zunzunegui, M. V., Alvarado, B., Otero, A., & Del Ser, T. (2005). Trajectories of cognitive decline and social relations. *The Journals of Gerontology. Series B, Psychological Sciences and Social Sciences, 60*(6), P320–P330.

Bendor, S. (1990). Anxiety and isolation in siblings of pediatric cancer patients: The need for prevention. *Social Work in Health Care, 14*(3), 17–35.

Bennet, R. (1980). *Aging, isolation, and resocialization*. New York: VanNostrand Reinhold.

Berkman, L. (1983). The assessment of social networks and social support in the elderly. *Journal of the American Geriatrics Society, 31*(12), 743–749.

Berkman, L. F., & Syme, S. L. (1979). Social networks, host resistance, and mortality: A nine-year follow-up study of Alameda County residents. *American Journal of Epidemiology, 109*(2), 186–204.

Biordi, D. (1993). [In-home care and respite care as self-care] Unpublished data.

Biordi, D. (2000). Research agenda: Emerging issues in the management of health and illness. *Seminars for Nurse Managers, 8*, 205–211.

Boden-Albala, B., Litwak, E., Elkind, M.S., Rundek, T., & Sacco, R.L. (2005). Social isolation and outcomes post stroke. *Neurology, 64*(11), 1888–1892.

Borman, J., & Biordi, D. (1992). Female nurse executives: Finally, at an advantage. *Journal of Nursing Administration, 22*(9), 37–41.

Bricout, J. C. (2004). Using telework to enhance return to work outcomes for individuals with spinal cord injuries. *Neurorehabilitation, 19*(2), 147–159.

Browne, A. J. (1997). The concept analysis of respect applying the hybrid model in cross-cultural settings. *Western Journal of Nursing Research, 19*(6), 762–780.

Brummett, B. H., Barefoot, J. C., Siegler, I. C., Clapp-Channing, N. E., Lytle, B. L., Bosworth, H. B., et al. (2001). Characteristics of socially isolated patients with coronary artery disease who are at elevated risk for mortality. *Psychosomatic Medicine, 63*(2), 267–272.

Burnley, I. H. (1992). Mortality from selected cancers in NSW and Sydney, Australia. *Social Science and Medicine, 35*(2), 195–208.

Cadman, D., Rosenbaum, P., Boyle, M., & Offord, D. (1991). Children with chronic illness: Family and parent demographic characteristics and psychosocial adjustment. *Pediatrics, 87*(6), 884–889.

Carpenito-Moyet, L. J. (2010). *Nursing diagnosis* (13th ed.). Philadelphia: Wolters Kluwer/Lippincott Williams & Wilkins.

Catalan, J. (1998). Mental health problems in older adults with HIV referred to a psychological-medicine unit. *AIDS Care: Psychological and Socio-medical Aspects of AIDS/HIV, 10*(2), 105–112.

Catlin, A. J. (1998). Editor's choice. When cultures clash, comments on a brilliant new book. *The spirit catches you and you fall down.* New York: Farrar, Straus, and Giroux.

Ceria, C. D., Masaki, K. H., Rodriguez, B. L., Chen, R., Yano, K., & Curb, J. D. (2001). The relationship of psychosocial factors to total mortality among older Japanese-American men: The Honolulu heart program. *Journal of the American Geriatrics Society, 49*(6), 725–731.

Charmaz, K. (1987). Struggling for a self: Identity levels of the chronically ill. In J. Roth & P. Conrad (Eds.), *Research in the sociology of health care.* Greenwich, CT: JAI Press.

Cheng, B. K. (1997). Cultural clash between providers of majority culture and patients of Chinese culture. *Journal of Long Term Home Health Care, 16*(2), 39–43.

Chinman, M. J., Weingarten, R., Stayner, D., & Davidson, L. (2001). Chronicity reconsidered: Improving person-environment fit through a consumer-run service. *Community Mental Health Journal, 37*(3), 215–229.

Christ, G. (1987). Social consequences of the cancer experience. *The American Journal of Pediatric Hematology/Oncology, 9*(1), 84–88.

Clark, D. J. (2002). Older adults living through and with their computers. *Computers, Informatics, Nursing, 20*(3), 117–124.

Cobb, S. (1979). Social support and health through the life course. In M. W. Riley (Ed.), *Aging from birth to death.* Boulder, CO: Westview Press.

Cohen, M. (1993). The unknown and the unknowable – Managing sustained uncertainty. *Western Journal of Nursing Research, 15*(1), 77–96.

Collins, D., Fitzgerald, S., Sachs-Ericsson, N., Scherer, M., Cooper, R., & Boninger, M. (2006). Psychosocial well-being and community participation of service dog partners. *Disability and Rehabilitation, 1*(1), 41–48.

Corbin, J., & Strauss, A. (1987). Accompaniments of chronic illness: Changes in body, self, biography, and biographical time. In J. Roth & P. Conrad (Eds.), *Research in the sociology of health care.* Greenwich, CT: JAI Press.

Cox, C., Spiro, M., & Sullivan, J. (1988). Social risk factors: Impact on elders' perceived health status. *Journal of Community Health Nursing, 5*(1), 59–73.

Creecy, R., Berg, W., & Wright, L. (1985). Loneliness among the elderly: A causal approach. *Journal of Gerontology, 40*(4), 487–493.

Creed, F. (1990). Psychological disorders in rheumatoid arthritis: A growing consensus? *Annual Rheumatic Disorders, 49*, 808–812.

Davidhizar, R., Bechtel, G. L., & Giger, J. N. (1998). Model helps CMs deliver multicultural care: Addressing cultural issues boosts compliance. *Case Management Advisor, 9*(6), 97–100.

Dela Cruz, L. (1986). On loneliness and the elderly. *Journal of Gerontological Nursing, 12*(11), 22–27.

DesRosier, M., Catanzaro, M., & Piller, J. (1992). Living with chronic illness: Social support and the well spouse perspective. *Rehabilitation Nursing, 17*(2), 87–91.

DiMatteo, M. R., & Hays, R. (1981). Social support and serious illness. In B. H. Gottlieb (Ed.), *Social networks and social support.* Beverly Hills, CA: Sage.

DiNapoli, P., & Murphy, D. (2002). The marginalization of chronically ill adolescents. *The Nursing Clinics of North America, 37*(3), 565–572.

Dorfman, L., Homes, C., & Berlin, K. (1996). Wife caregivers of frail elderly veterans: Correlates of caregiver satisfaction and caregiver strain. *Family Relations, 45*, 46–55.

Dropkin, M. (1989). Coping with disfigurement and dysfunction. *Seminars in Oncology Nursing, 5*(3), 213–219.

Eng, P. M., Rimm, E. B., Fitzmaurice, G., & Kawachi, I. (2002). Social ties and change in social ties in relation to subsequent total and cause-specific mortality and coronary heart disease incidence in men. *American Journal of Epidemiology, 155*(8), 700–709.

Findlay, R. (2003). Interventions to reduce social isolation amongst older people: Where is the evidence? *Aging & Society, 23*, 647–658.

Fiscella, K., Franks, M., Gold, M., & Clancy, D. (2000). Social support, disability, and depression: A longitudinal study of rheumatoid arthritis. *Journal of the American Medical Association*, 283, 2579–2584.

Fowles, D., & Greenberg, S. (2009). *A profile of older Americans: 2009*. Retrieved September 15, 2011, from www.aoa.gov/aoaroot/aging_statistics/profile/2009/18.aspx

Foxall, M., Barron, C., Dollen, K., Shull, K., et al. (1994). Low vision elders: Living arrangements, loneliness, and social support. *Journal of Gerontological Nursing, 20*, 6–14.

Foxall, M., Eckberg, J., & Griffith, N. (1986). Spousal adjustment to chronic illness. *Rehabilitation Nursing, 11*, 13–16.

Fratiglioni, L., Paillard-Borg, S., & Winblad, B. (2004). An active and socially integrated lifestyle in late life might protect against dementia. *Lancet Neurolology, 3*(6), 343–353.

Fratiglioni, L., Wang, H. X., Ericsson, K., Maytan, M., & Winblad, B. (2000). Influence of social network on occurrence of dementia: A community-based longitudinal study. *Lancet, 355*(9212), 1315–1319.

Frierson, R. L. (1991). Suicide attempts by the old and the very old. *Archives of Internal Medicine, 151*(1), 141–144.

Fyrand, L. (2003). The effect of social network intervention for women with rheumatoid arthritis. *Family Process, 42*(1), 71.

Gallo, A. M., Breitmayer, B. J., Knafl, K. A., & Zoeller, L. H. (1991). Stigma in childhood chronic illness: A well sibling perspective. *Pediatric Nursing, 17*(1), 21–25.

Gamba, A., Romano, M., Grosso, I., Tamburini, M., Cantu, G., Molinari, R., et al. (1992). Psychosocial adjustment of patients surgically treated for head and neck cancer. *Head and Neck, 14*(3), 218–223.

Goodman, C. (1984). Natural helping among older adults. *The Gerontologist, 24*(2), 138–143.

Greaves, C. J., & Farbus, L. (2006). Effects of creative and social activity on the health and well-being of socially isolated older people: Outcomes from a multi-method observational study. *Journal of the Royal Society of Health, 126*(3), 134–142.

Groce, N. E., & Zola, I. (1993). Multiculturalism, chronic illness, and disability. *Pediatrics, 91*(5), 32–39.

Habayeb, G. L. (1995). Cultural diversity: A nursing concept not yet reliably defined. *Nursing Outlook, 43*(5), 224–227.

Havens, B., & Hall, M. (2001). Social isolation, loneliness, and the health of older adults in Manitoba, Canada. *Indian Journal of Gerontology, 1*(15), 126–144.

Hawes, C., Phillips, C. D., Rose, M., Holan, S., & Sherman, M. (2003). A national survey of assisted living facilities. *The Gerontologist, 43*(6), 875–882.

Heiney, S., Goon-Johnson, K., Ettinger, R., & Ettinger, S. (1990). The effects of group therapy on siblings of pediatric oncology patients. *Journal of Pediatric Oncology Nursing, 7*(3), 95–100.

Helton, L. R. (1995). Intervention with Appalachians: Strategies for a culturally specific practice. *Journal of Cultural Diversity, 2*(1), 20–26.

Heumann, L. (1988). Assisting the frail elderly living in subsidized housing for the independent elderly: A profile of the management and its support priorities. *The Gerontologist, 28*, 625–631.

Hildebrandt, E. (1997). Have I angered my ancestors? Influences of culture on health care with elderly black South Africans as an example. *Journal of Multicultural Nursing and Health, 3*(1), 40–49.

Hill, D. L. (2006). Sense of belonging as connectedness, American Indian worldview and mental health. *Archives of Psychiatric Nursing, 20*(5), 210–216.

Hill, W. G., & Weinert, C. (2004). An evaluation of an online intervention to provide social support and health education. *Computers, Informatics, Nursing, 22*(5), 282–288.

Hoeffer, B. (1987). A causal model of loneliness among older single women. *Archives of Psychiatric Nursing, 1*(5), 366–373.

Holley, U. A. (2007). Social isolation: A practical guide for nurses assisting clients with chronic illness. *Rehabilitation Nursing, 32*(2), 51–56.

Holtzman, R. E., Rebok, G. W., Saczynski, J. S., Kouzis, A. C., Wilcox Doyle, K., & Eaton, W. W. (2004). Social network characteristics and cognition in middle-aged and older adults. *The Journals of Gerontology, Series B, Psychological Sciences and Social Sciences, 59*(6), P278–P284.

Hopper, S. (1981). Diabetes as a stigmatized condition: The case of low income clinic patients in the United States. *Social Science and Medicine, 15*, 11–19.

House, J., Landis, K., & Umberson, D. (1988). Social relationships and health. *Science, 241*, 540–544.

Howat, P., Iredell, H., Grenade, L., Nedwetzky, A., & Collins, J. (2004). Reducing social isolation amongst older people implications for health professionals. *Geriaction, 22*(1), 13–20.

Hoybye, M. T., Johansen, C., & Tjomboj-Thomsen, T. (2005). Online interaction: Effects of storytelling in an internet breast cancer support group. *Psychooncology, 14*(3), 211–220.

Imel, S. (1999) *Seniors in cyberspace. Trends and issues alerts*. Washington, DC: Office of Educational Research and Improvement (ED). EDD00036.

Jessop, D., & Stein, R. (1985). Uncertainty and its relation to the psychological and social correlates of chronic illness in children. *Social Science and Medicine, 20*(10), 993–999.

Johnson, D., & Ashton, C. (2003). Effects of computer-mediated communication on social support and loneliness for isolated persons with disabilities. *American Journal of Recreational Therapy, 2*(3), 23–32.

Jones, M. D., Bond, M. L., & Cason, C. L. (1998). Where does culture fit in outcomes management? *Journal of Nursing Care Quality, 13*(1), 41–51.

Kaplan, G., Salonen, J., Cohen, R., Brand, R., et al. (1988). Social connections and mortality from all causes and from cardiovascular disease: Prospective evidence from Eastern Finland. *American Journal of Epidemiology, 128*(2), 370–380.

Keller, C. S., & Stevens, K. R. (1997). Cultural considerations in promoting wellness. *Journal of Cardiovascular Nursing, 11*(3), 15–25.

Kim, L. S. (1998). Long term care for the Korean American elderly: An exploration for a better way of services. *Journal of Long Term Home Health Care, 16*(2), 35–38.

Kinsella, G., Ford, B., & Moran, C. (1989). Survival of social relationships following head injury. *International Disability Studies, 11*(1), 9–14.

Kivett, V. (1979). Discriminators of loneliness among the rural elderly: Implications for interventions. *The Gerontologist, 19*(1), 108–115.

Klinenberg, E. (2001). Dying alone: The social production of urban isolation. *Ethnography, 2*(4), 501–531.

Kreps, G., & Kreps, M. (1997). Amishing "medical care." *Journal of Multicultural Nursing & Health, 3*(2), 44–47.

Kroenke, C. H., Kubzansky, L. D., Schernhammer, E. S., Holmes, M. D., & Kawachi, I. (2006). Social networks, social support, and survival after breast cancer diagnosis. *Journal of Clinical Oncology, 24*(7), 1105–1111.

Krouse, J., Krouse, H., & Fabian, R. (1989). Adaptation to surgery for head and neck cancer. *Laryngoscope, 99*, 789–794.

Lawton, M., Greenbaum, M., & Liebowitz, B. (1980). The lifespan of housing environments for the aging. *The Gerontologist, 20*, 56–64.

Lawton, M., Kleban, M., & Carlson, D. (1973). The inner-city resident: To move or not to move. *The Gerontologist, 13*, 443–448.

Lawton, M., Moss, M., & Grimes, M. (1985). The changing service need of older tenants in planned housing. *The Gerontologist, 25*, 258–264.

Lee, G. R., & Ellithorpe, E. (1982). Intergenerational exchange and subjective well-being among the elderly. *Journal of Marriage and the Family, 44*, 217–224.

Lichtenstein, B., Laska, M. K., & Clair, J. M. (2002). Chronic sorrow in the HIV-positive patient: Issues of race, gender, and social support. *AIDS Patient Care and STDs, 16*(1), 27–38.

Lien-Gieschen, T. (1993). Validation of social isolation related to maturational age: Elderly. *Nursing Diagnosis, 4*(1), 37–43.

Lin, N. (1986). Conceptualizing social support. In N. Lin, A. Dean, & W. Ensel (Eds.), *Social support, life events, and depression*. New York: Academic Press.

Litwin, H. (1997). Support network type and health service utilization. *Research on Aging, 19*(3), 274–299.

Litwin, H., & Zoabi, S. (2003). Modernization and elder abuse in an Arab-Israeli context. *Research on Aging, 25*(3), 224–246.

Lubben, J. (1988). Assessing social networks among elderly populations. *Family Community Health, 11*(3), 42–52.

Lubben, J., & Gironda, M. (1996). Assessing social support networks among older people in the United States. In H. Litwin (Ed.), *The social networks of older people: A cross-national analysis* (pp. 144). Westport, CT: Praeger.

Lubben, J., Weiler, P., & Chi, I. (1989). Gender and ethnic differences in the health practices of the elderly poor. *Journal of Clinical Epidemiology, 42*(8), 725–733.

Lyons, M. J. (1982). Psychological concomitants of the environment influencing suicidal behavior in middle and later life. *Dissertation Abstracts International, 43*, 1620B.

Maddox, G. L. (1985). Intervention strategies to enhance well-being in later life: The status and prospect of guided change. *Health Services Research, 19*, 1007–1032.

Mallinson, R. K. (1999). The lived experiences of AIDS-related multiple losses by HIV-negative gay men. *Journal of the Association of Nurses in AIDS Care, 10*(5), 22–31.

Margolin, S. (2006). African American youths with internalizing difficulties: Relation to social support and activity involvement. *Children and Schools, 28*(3), 135–144.

Marottoli, R. A., deLeon, C. F. M., Glass, T. A., Williams, C. S., Cooney, L. M., & Berkman, L. F. (2000). Consequences of driving cessation: Decreased out-of-home activity levels. *Journal of Gerontology Series B: Psychological Sciences and Social Sciences, 55*(6), S334–S340.

Matteson, M. A., McConnell, E. S., & Linton, A. (1997). *Gerontological nursing: Concepts and practice* (2nd ed.). Philadelphia: Saunders.

McNamara, B., Martin, K., Waddel, C., & Yuen, K. (1997). Palliative care in a multicultural society: Perceptions of health care professionals. *Palliative Medicine, 11*(5), 359–367.

Melle, I., Friis, S., Hauff, E., & Vaglum, P. (2000). Social functioning of patients with schizophrenia in high income welfare societies. *Psychiatric Services, 51*(2), 223–228.

Mendes de Leon, C. F., Glass, T. A., & Berkman, L. F. (2003). Social engagement and disability in a community population of older adults: The New Haven EPESE. *American Journal of Epidemiology, 157*(7), 633–642.

Mendes de Leon, C. F., Glass, T. A., Beckett, L. A., Seeman, T. E., Evans, D. A., & Berkman, L. F. (1999). Social networks and disability transitions across eight intervals of yearly data in the new haven EPESE. *The Journals of Gerontology. Series B, Psychological Sciences and Social Sciences, 54*(3), S162–S172.

Mendes de Leon, C. F., Gold, D., Glass, T., Kaplan, L., & George, L. (2001). Disability as a function of social networks and support in elderly African Americans and whites: The Duke EPESE 1986–1992. *The Journals of Gerontology. Series B, Psychological Sciences and Social Sciences, 56B*(3), S179–S190.

Michael, Y. L., Berkman, L. F., Colditz, G. A., Holmes, M. D., & Kawachi, I. (2002). Social networks and health-related quality of life in breast cancer survivors: A prospective study. *Journal of Psychosomatic Research, 52*(5), 285–293.

Miller, B. (1990). Gender differences in spouse caregiver strain: Socialization and role explanations. *Journal of Marriage and the Family, 52*, 311–322.

Mistry, R., Rosansky, J., McGuire, J., McDermott, C., Jarvik, L., & UPBEAT Collaborative Group. (2001). Social isolation predicts rehospitalization in a group of older American veterans enrolled in the UPBEAT program. *International Journal of Geriatric Psychiatry, 16*(10), 950–959.

Mullins, L., & Dugan, E. (1990). The influence of depression, and family and friendship relations, on residents' loneliness in congregate housing. *The Gerontologist, 30*(3), 377–384.

Murberg, T. A. (2004). Long-term effect of social relationships on mortality in patients with congestive heart failure. *International Journal of Psychiatry in Medicine, 34*(3), 207–217.

Newman, S. P., Fitzpatrick, R., Lamb, R., & Shipley, M. (1989). The origins of depressed mood in rheumatoid arthritis. *The Journal of Rheumatology, 16*(6), 740–744.

Noll, R., Ris, M. D., Davies, W. H., Burkowski, W., et al. (1992). Social interactions between children with cancer or sickle cell disease and their peers: Teacher ratings. *Developmental and Behavioral Pediatrics, 13*(3), 187–193.

Norbeck, J., DeJoseph, J., & Smith, R. (1996). A randomized trial of an empirically derived social support intervention to prevent low birthweight among African-American women. *Social Science and Medicine, 43*, 947–954.

Noyes, R., Kathol, R., Debelius-Enemark, P., Williams, J., et al. (1990). Distress associated with cancer as measured by the illness distress scale. *Psychosomatics, 31*(3), 321–330.

Orth-Gomer, K., Unden, A., & Edwards, M. (1988). Social isolation and mortality in ischemic heart disease: A 10-year follow-up study of 150 middle aged men. *Acta Med Scan, 224* (3), 205–215.

Peplau, L. A., & Perlman, D. (Eds.). (1986). *Loneliness: A sourcebook of current theory, research, and therapy.* New York: John Wiley & Sons.

Pinquart, M., & Sorensen, J. (2001). Influences on loneliness in older adults: A meta-analysis. *Basic and Applied Social Psychology, 23*(4), 245–266.

Poulin, J. (1984). Age segregation and the interpersonal involvement and morale of the aged. *The Gerontologist, 24*(3), 266–269.

Praderas, K., & MacDonald, M. (1986). Telephone conversational skills training with socially isolated, impaired nursing home residents. *Journal of Applied Behavior Analysis, 19*(4), 337–348.

Ramos, M., & Wilmoth, J. (2003). Social relationships and depressive symptoms among older adults in southern Brazil. *Journal of Gerontology, Series B, Psychological Sciences and Social Sciences, 58*(4), S253–S261.

Randers, I., Mattiasson A., & Olson T. H. (2003). The "social self": The 11th category of integrity—implications for enhancing geriatric nursing care. *Journal of Applied Gerontology, 22*(2), 289–309.

Ravish, T. (1985). Prevent isolation before it starts. *Journal of Gerontological Nursing, 11*(10), 10–13.

Resnick, B. (2007). Assisted living: The perfect place for nursing. *Geriatric Nursing, 28*(1), 7–8.

Reynolds, P., & Kaplan, G. (1990). Social connections and risk for cancer: Prospective evidence from the Alameda County study. *Behavioral Medicine, 16*(3), 101–110.

Rubenstein, L. Z., Josephson, K. R., & Robbins, A. S. (1994). Falls in the nursing home. *Annals of Internal Medicine, 121*(6), 442–451.

Russell, C., & Schofield, T. (1999). Social isolation in old age: A qualitative exploration of service providers' perceptions. *Ageing and Society, 19*(1), 69–91.

Ryan, M., & Patterson, J. (1987). Loneliness in the elderly. *Journal of Gerontological Nursing, 13*(5), 6–12.

Salem, P. (1998). Paradoxical impacts of electronic communication technologies. Paper presented at the International Communication Association/National Communication Association Conference, Rome, Italy, July 15–17, 1998.

Seeman, M. (1959). On the meaning of alienation. *American Sociological Review, 24*, 783–791.

Seeman, T. E. (2000). Health promoting effects of friends and family on health outcomes in older adults. *American Journal of Health Promotion, 14*(6), 362–370.

Seidler, A., Bernhardt, T., Nienhaus, A., & Frolich, L. (2003). Association between the psychosocial network and dementia—A case-control study. *Journal of Psychiatric Research, 37*(2), 89–98.

Siplic F., & Kadis, D. (2002). The psychosocial aspect of aging. *Socialno Delo, 41*(5), 295–300.

Smith, J. W. (1996). Cultural and spiritual issues in palliative care. *Journal of Cancer Care, 5*(4), 173–178.

Spiegel, D. (1990). Facilitating emotional coping during treatment. *Cancer, 66*, 1422–1426.

Spitz, G., & Miner, S. (1992). Gender differences in adult child contact among Black elderly parents. *The Gerontologist, 43*, 213–218.

Stephens, M., & Bernstein, M. (1984). Social support and well-being among residents of planned housing. *The Gerontologist, 24*, 144–148.

Strauss, A., Corbin, J., Fagerhaugh, S., Glaser, B., et al. (1984). *Chronic illness and the quality of life* (2nd ed.). St. Louis: Mosby.

Street, D., Burge, S., Quadagno, J., & Barrett, A. (2007). The salience of social relationships for resident well-being in assisted living. *The Journals of Gerontology, Series B, Psychological Sciences and Social Sciences, 62*(2), S129–S134.

Stroebe, M., & Stroebe, W. (1983). Who suffers more? Sex differences in health risks of the widowed. *Psychological Bulletin, 93*(2), 279.

Subcommittee on Human Services of the Select Committee on Aging: U.S. House of Representatives (1987). Exploding the myths: Caregiving in America (Committee Print No. 99-611). Washington, DC: US Government Printing Office.

Umberson, D., Wortman, C., & Kessler, R. (1992). Widowhood and depression: Explaining long-term gender differences in vulnerability. *Journal of Health and Social Behavior, 33*(1), 10.

Tamlyn, D., & Arklie, M. (1986). A theoretical framework for standard care plans: A nursing approach for
working with chronically ill children and their families. *Issues in Comprehensive Pediatric Nursing,
9*, 39–45.

Tilden, V., & Weinert, C. (1987). Social support and the
chronically ill individual. *Nursing Clinics of North
America, 22*(3), 613–620.

Treolar, L. L. (1999). People with disabilities—the same,
but different: Implications for health care practice.
Journal of Transcultural Nursing, 10(4), 358–364.

Trout, D. (1980). The role of social isolation in suicide.
Suicide and Life Threatening Behavior, 10, 10–22.

Victor, C. R., Scambler, S., Bond, J. & Bowling, A.
(2000). Being alone in later life: Loneliness, isolation, and living alone in later life. *Reviews in Clinical
Gerontology, 10*, 407–417.

Victor, C., Scambler, S. J., Shah, S., Cook D. G., Harris, T.,
Rink, E., et al. (2002). Has loneliness amongst older
people increased? An investigation into variations
among cohorts. *Ageing and Society, 22*(5), 585–597.

Wang, K. W., & Barnard, A. (2004). Technology-
dependent children and their families: A review.
Journal of Advanced Nursing, 45(1), 34–46.

Wang, H. X., Karp, A., Winblad, B., & Fratiglioni, L.
(2002). Late-life engagement in social and leisure
activities is associated with a decreased risk of dementia: A longitudinal study from the Kungsholmen
Project. *American Journal of Epidemiology, 155*(12),
1081–1087.

Watson, E. (1988). Dead to the world. *Nursing Times,
84*(21), 52–54.

Weinert, C., Cudney, S., & Winters, C. (2005). Social
support in cyberspace: The next generation.
Computers, Informatics, Nursing, 23(1), 7–15.

Weisman, A. D., & Worden, J. W. (1976–1977). The existential plight in cancer: Significance of the first 100
days. *International Journal of Psychiatry in
Medicine, 7*, 1–15.

Weiss, R. S. (1973). *Loneliness: The experience of emotional and social isolation.* Cambridge, MA:
Massachusetts Institute of Technology Press.

Welch, C. M. (1998). The adult health and development
program: Bridging the racial gap. *International
Electronic Journal of Health Education, 1*(3), 178–181.

Wenger, G. C. (1997). Social networks and the prediction
of elderly people at risk. *Aging and Mental Health,
1*(4), 311.

Wenger, G. C., Davies, R., Shahtahmasebi, S., & Scott,
A. (1996). Social isolation and loneliness in old age:
Review and model refinement. *Aging & Society, 16*,
333–358.

Williams, S., & Bury, M. (1989). Impairment, disability,
and handicap in chronic respiratory illness. *Social
Science and Medicine, 29*(5), 609–616.

Woods, N., Haberman, M., & Packard, N. (1993).
Demands of illness and individual, dyadic, and fam-
ily adaptation in chronic illness. *Western Journal of
Nursing Research, 15*(1), 10–30.

Wright, L. (1995). Human development in the context
of aging and chronic illness: The role of attachment
in Alzheimer's disease and stroke. *International
Journal of Aging and Human Development, 44*,
133–150.

Zimmer, M. (1995). Activity participation and well being
among older people with arthritis. *The Gerontologist,
351*, 463–471.

Zunzunegui, M. V., Alvarado, B. E., Del Ser, T., &
Otero, A. (2003). Social networks, social integration, and social engagement determine cognitive
decline in community-dwelling Spanish older
adults. *The Journals of Gerontology, Series B,
Psychological Sciences and Social Sciences, 58*(2),
S93–S100.

CHAPTER 6

Body Image

Diana Luskin Biordi and Patricia McCann Galon

INTRODUCTION

Of all the prisms through which culture can be viewed, body image is one of the most prevalent and profound. From the abstract concepts of beauty, sexuality, and community to the tangibles of health, mobility, and communication, the ideal of the perfect body prevails. Against that culturally normed model of the perfect body, one forms an image of one's own body that is reflective of the culture and social interactions. The perfect body changes from culture to culture and across time. Models of ancient Greeks, for example, show muscular young men and women with broad shoulders, small waists, and narrow pelvises, whereas today's prevalent American model is waif-like thinness with body tone for women and defined muscularity for men. When and how an individual differs from the cultural norm requires social and emotional management to explain. Therefore, individuals use a frame of reference for their own bodies, which is shaped by the prevailing body norm of the culture, and perhaps, by subcultures within the larger culture. If one's body image differs from the body norm, social and physical rationalizations come into play. Insofar as those rationalizations themselves are exaggerated from yet other norms, healthcare interventions may be required.

One's mental image of one's physical self is one's body image. Individual body images may change over time, depending on life tasks such as learning one's gender role, performing a job or sport, creating a family, body or brain chemistry and structure, or aging. In chronic illness, body image is both a modifier of, and is modified by, the illness. Chronic illness, in its capacity to change the body, typically necessitates revisitations to one's body image. These revisitations are modified by the psychology of the individual and his or her perceptions of an ideal. That is, the individual will have to decide, consciously or unconsciously, whether to persevere in meeting an ideal body image (the culturally defined perfect body), reformulate or readjust the ideal to conform to his or her own attributes, or reject the ideal.

Significant research in body image has occurred only recently, despite being a common subject in the literature since the late 1800s. In fact, since 2004, an entire journal has been devoted to *Body Image* (published by Elsevier). In nursing, there appears to be a large gap between an initial spate of studies in the 1970s to those of the 1990s, with a substantial increase in research since 2000. Most of the literature examining body image is found in practice disciplines such as nursing, medicine (e.g., neurology), bioengineering, psychology, and vocational counseling. This literature focuses on neurologic and psychological studies of person and gender, health studies on chronic illness (particularly, cancer), and most recently bariatric studies on obesity. In addition, some body image studies focus on plastic surgery or reconstruction, which are increasingly used by a number of persons for cosmetic reasons and/or as interventions for illness, accidents, obesity, or for other treatments (Frederick, Lever, & Peplau, 2007). The current emphasis on youth and beauty in American culture and the anti-obesity objectives of the nation (through the campaigns of First Lady Michelle Obama; see also *Healthy People 2020*) are expected to spur more research on body image.

Definitions of Body Image

Body image is defined and referred to in two ways. The most prevalent definition of body image is the psychological view, in which body image is the mental image of one's physical self, including attitudes and perceptions of one's physical appearance, state of health, skills, and sexuality. Another term with the same definition is *body schema*.

Body image is how one perceives one's own body, including its attractiveness, and how that body image influences interactions and others' reactions. Therefore, body image is not only the way people perceive themselves but, equally important, the way they think others see them. Consequently, body image is a major delimiter of social interactions, and as such has a profound effect on physical health, social interaction, psychological development, and interpersonal relationships. Moreover, because body image is conceptual, even if it is expressed inferentially, as in anorexia nervosa, most of the literature describes body image from information taken from cognitively intact, communicative human beings. Issues of profoundly retarded individuals and their body images, for example, are more likely examined from the perspective of others as they regard the person's body and whether it deviates from norms, as well as the reactions of others to the person.

The second way in which body image is used is more neurologic and technical. In this definition, body image has been shown to relate to the association of brain areas, particularly the *motor cortex*, with portions of the body, such as the limbs or lips. Particular parts of the brain are also associated with the sense of the body in space and that the self is localized, or embodied, within body borders (Blanke, 2007). Embodiment is important to the models of the self or self-consciousness, and also, more tangibly, of body parts properly belonging to one's person. Abnormalities in embodiment can lead to such distress as "amputation desire" or "amputation envy," in which persons are profoundly frustrated by their sense that one of their body parts (limbs) does not "belong" to them, and actively seek its removal to satisfy their sense of body/embodiment (Mueller, 2007–2008). Voluntary movement of body limbs, or sensations, often of pain, have been shown to be linked to limbs, teeth, or breasts, when certain brain areas or neurons are invoked. Thus, body image is defined and discussed in the theory, empiricism, and language of brain, neuropathology, neurology, anatomy, and/or physiology (Lewis, 1983; Mueller, 2007–2008; Ramachandran, 2004; Ramachandran & Rogers-Ramachandran, 2007).

It is interesting that the symptoms of the psychiatric diagnosis, body dysmorphic disorder (BDD), also are characterized as both psychological and neuropathological. Persons with BDD, a chronic disorder, suffer distress and functional impairment due to a preoccupation with even a slight defect in their appearance. The preoccupation can progress to a delusional state. BDD is a fairly common disorder with an estimated prevalence of about 0.7–1.7 % of the population, but it often goes unrecognized. Persons with BDD often seek plastic surgery or dermatologic treatment for this "abnormality" but are never satisfied with the results and thus may seek repeated procedures (Feusner, Yaryura-Tobias, & Saxena, 2008). In addition they believe they are mocked by others for their defect and see themselves as generally less healthy and capable than the rest of the population (Didie, Kuniega-Pietrzak, & Phillips, 2010).

One can develop BDD in response to brain trauma or disease in the central nervous system, especially in the temporal lobe area. About 8% of persons with BDD can identify relatives with obsessive compulsive disorder or BDD, indicating inheritability. Phillips and Hollander (2008) suggest that persons with BDD have fundamental differences in visual processing with a focus on the specific rather than on an overall picture, both in consideration of the self and their environment. It is also speculated based on neuropsychological evaluation that emotional arousal may contribute to the attentional bias (concentration on defect) and social anxiety associated with the disorder.

Body image is referred to in two other ways in the literature. First, body image is conceptualized as a *final product* or end state—a state of being, such as, "Charles's body image is that of a muscular young man." Second, body image can be portrayed as a *process*—a continuous examination by the self or others, whereby one's body is defined and redefined. In both of these conceptualizations, there are a number of factors that influence body image. Furthermore, the attitudes and perceptions about one's body guide evaluation and investment in body image, which affect physical and psychosocial functioning. Attitudes about body image are related to one's self-esteem, interpersonal functioning, eating and exercise patterns, self-care activities, and sexual behaviors (Cash & Fleming, 2002; Peelen & Downing, 2007).

In summary, body image is theorized as conceptual and neurologic, with each concept feeding into the other. Body image is one's perception of one's body and its interactions with others. It includes a sense of ownership and boundaries of one's body, the image of which is constructed psychologically and through the neurologic system of the brain—through proprioception (the sense of the body in space), vision, and the vestibular system. Body image can be thought of as both a process and an end product, and one's body image affects physical and psychosocial functioning.

Historical Foundations of Body Image

Although body image has been discussed in the literature since the 1880s, it was not until Schilder presented his work in 1935 that a new understanding of this concept arose. In *The Image and Appearance of the Human Body*, Schilder (1950) explored the dimensions of body image: "The image of the human body means the picture of our own body which we form in our mind, that is to say the way in which the body appears to ourselves" (p. 11). He believed that the perception of one's body is based on a three-dimensional image that comprises physiologic, psychological, and social experiences.

Schilder's work affected subsequent researchers, even into the 21st century. Critiquing Schilder's broad and complex theory, Cash and Pruzinsky (1990) claim that Schilder's chief contribution was not just the idea of body image, but the idea that body image has "central pertinence not only for the pathologic but also everyday events of life" (p. 9). Later, Cash and Pruzinsky (2002) assert that Schilder "single handedly moved the study of body image beyond the exclusive domain of neuropathology" (p. 4).

Most current discussions now frame body image as having a perceptual component, a psychological component, and a social component (Cash & Fleming, 2002; Thompson & Gardner, 2002; Thompson & Van Den Berg, 2002). For example, with regard to eating and weight disorders, the perceptual component is the accuracy of the person's body size estimation, the psychological component is the person's attitudes or feelings toward their own body, and the social component might be the cultural context in which body image is assessed.

Like others, Thompson and Gardner (2002), and Cash and Fleming (2002) argue that body image is not a simple perceptual phenomenon, but is highly influenced by cognitive, affective, attitudinal, and other variables. Thompson has been attributed as the impetus in the 1990s to a more clinically and physiologically based concept of body image, particularly in examining eating disorders (Cash & Pruzinsky, 2002). Building on his work, research later focused on cultural overlays, including feminist critiques of the 1990s, and later, the effects of family or ethnicity on

body image. More recent work in the 2000s is refocusing on the physiologic basis of body image, while attending to more evidence-based interventions on body image and its effects (Cash & Pruzinsky, 2004).

Currently, major empirical analyses of body image focus on neurology, particularly those studies involving the brain and associated visual, vestibular, vascular, and proprioceptor stimuli. Impactful studies by Ramachandran and Rogers-Ramachandran (2007) indicate that body image can be shaped and changed by the brain. Using vision and proprioceptor cues, they were able to map where in the brain (somatosensory, motor, and parietal cortices) cues were received to fashion a virtual sense of body that did not correspond to actuality. The idea that body image can be so profoundly shaped by the brain has important implications for theory and for treatment. In a related set of studies, Ramachandran (2004) indicates that when motor signals are sent to muscles, duplicate signals are sent to the brain's parietal lobes, giving a sense of real limbs when there are actually amputations, leading to the phenomenon of phantom limb syndrome. Therefore, as is known in the field of prosthetics, amputees who are unable to incorporate a change in body image that genuinely indicates a lost limb were shown to be unable to use prosthetics effectively.

Of particular importance to healthcare professionals in chronic illness is the empirically derived idea that the perceptual elements of body image are complex. Fisher (1986) found that people not only compartmentalized their body image, but also differed in how they did so. Some localized their body image, whereas others had a more global view of their body. For instance, people with serious body defects might approach their bodies as separate regions, specifically isolating the defective region so that it will not influence their overall evaluation of self. Fisher believed that this ability suggests "important defensive and maturational significance in how differentiated one's approach to one's body is" (p. 635). He also argued that the rubric of body image itself is vague, representing a number of dimensions of the same and different constructs. New neurologic data (Ramachandran [2004]; Ramachandran and Rogers-Ramachandran [2007]) indicate that certain brain regions governing specific body parts play a role in whether body images can be sustained or demarcated as separate. For example, clients with left-sided hemiplegia caused by a stroke often experience a dissociation from their paralyzed limbs.

Factors in the Definition of Body Image

Definitions of body image, although varied, share similarities. Common to many of the definitions is the belief that body image develops in response to multiple sensory inputs (visual, tactile, proprioceptive, and kinesthetic). Therefore, although physicality is included in one's body image, body image is subjective and dynamic because it is influenced by multiple factors (Cash, 2002; Pruzinsky, 2004). Body image is brought into the immediate focus of the individual by pain, physical or psychological illness, age, or weight (Krueger, 2002). Kinesthetic perceptions of function, sensation, and mobility are also part of our image. For example, children without sensation of body parts (e.g., spina bifida) often do not include in their art those body parts where they lack sensation.

Body image also includes feelings and thoughts. How one thinks and feels about one's body will influence social relationships and other psychological characteristics. Furthermore, how people feel and think about their bodies influences the way they perceive the world (Cash & Fleming, 2002).

Nezlek (1999) found three factors were included in the definition of body image. These included body attractiveness, social attractiveness (how attractive people believed others found them to be), and general attractiveness. For both men and women, self-perceptions of body attractiveness and social attractiveness were positively related to intimacy. Because body attractiveness is an important function of body image, this concept frequently is confused with body image itself; however, body image encompasses more than attractiveness.

Many definitions of body image today involve the notions of the real and the ideal. Theorists would argue that the ideal image of one's self and the real image must be compatible, or dissonance results. A discrepancy between the real and the ideal body image may lead to conflicts that adversely affect personality, interactions, and health. For example, "normative discontent" refers to the pervasive negative feelings women and girls experience when they negatively distort their appearance, experience body image dissatisfaction, or overevaluate appearance in defining a sense of self (Striegel-Moore & Franko, 2002).

For the healthcare professional, definitions of body image indicate the complexity of the concept, but more importantly, emphasize how significantly the client's cultural, social, historical, and biological factors affect body image. Perhaps even more important to healthcare professionals and their professionally derived norms is that body image and the factors affecting it are not merely cosmetic. A client's perceptions and attitudes about his or her body can affect health, social adjustment, interpersonal relationships, and general well-being. These perceptions are profoundly affected by chronic illness, as shown in this text.

Perhaps because body image is so vital to issues of ordinary health as well as chronic illness, it has come to be associated with, or even confused with, several other terms. The terms *body image*, *self-concept*, and *self-esteem* are frequently used interchangeably. Body image is not the same as body attractiveness but is related to both attractiveness and to self-esteem. Body image is a mental image of one's physical self, moderated by one's psychology and the social environment, and as is being discovered, by certain physiologic parameters of the brain. Body image, thus, is an integral component of self-concept. Self-concept is the total perception an individual holds of self—who one believes one is, how one believes one looks, and how one feels about one's self (Mock, 1993). Research extends self-concept to include not only ongoing perceptions of one's self, but also the idea that self-concept so mediates and regulates behavior that it is one of the most significant regulators of behavior (Markus & Wurf, 1987). Self-concept also is used to describe roles in which one casts the self, which can further stretch, and perhaps muddy, the concept. Finally, self-esteem is related to "the evaluative component of an individual's self-concept" (Corwyn, 2000, p. 357).

Factors Influencing Adjustment to Body Image

Meaning and Significance

As critical as each influence may be to the individual's adaptation, it is most important that the meaning of the event to the individual be understood. Knowing that clients may compartmentalize both the meaning and the body's parts, the healthcare professional must recognize and accept how each client assesses the changes occurring in his or her body, their importance, and the way that the client chooses to incorporate (or not) changes into their body image. Thus, treatment of chronic illness and by association body image, functionality, or appearance cannot be far removed from the meaning attributed to such by the client or significant other.

In most cultures, body parts carry emotional attribution quite aside from functionality or appearance. The hands, for instance, are critical portrayals of the meanings and metaphysics of religions, whether shown invitingly open, in clasped position, or thumbs and forefingers together. Similarly, the mind is associated with the brain and all the significance attached to it in a knowledge society, whereas the heart is universally seen as the font of emotions. The heart is, to many, the symbol of love, courage, and life, and the seat of joy, hate, and sorrow. Indeed, in some cultures, the heart is seen as the location of the soul. Consider the emotional significance, then, that damage to the heart would engender in the body image of the affected client. Most nurses have been taught about clients who, after sustaining a myocardial infarction, are so anxious that they become a "cardiac cripple," owing to their fear of death from exercise or normal activity. Clearly, the self-image of such clients has sustained a serious insult. Dementia creates issues of self-image not only for the person undergoing the change, but also for significant others in the interactions and subsequent reappraisals. How many times have nurses heard families say that they "no longer know their loved one" as the disease progresses?

To counter the insult to body image and functionality, and knowing likely prognoses, the healthcare professional must reassure the client and family about their perceptions of body image and help them reconcile to the present and future realities of the situation. That is, the healthcare professional should make efforts to reconcile the ideal body image of the client with the current attributes of the person and encourage the client to move toward a more realistic body image, while recognizing that, for the client, losing their desired body image can create a grieving process that must also be managed.

Body image and the insults to functionality from chronic illness cannot be isolated from the meaning and significance the client gives to them. Furthermore, the meaning and significance to family members or significant others can also play an important role in the client's response. These are crucial factors to consider in offering and performing effective and sensitive care. Of all the aspects of body image in chronic illness, the appreciation and understanding of the meaning and significance to the client are areas to which nursing can most contribute. The client's meaning and significance of the change in body image must not be overlooked or down played. Nursing's empathic and holistic approach can be of great value in this arena of health care.

The cause of the person's chronic illness and associated insult to one's body image can be an important coping factor. If the change was caused by an accident, healthcare mismanagement, or personal negligence, the person may harbor unresolved anger, blame, and shame. The person may also be guarded about sharing and discussing such matters, which confounds recovery and makes it more difficult. On the other hand, if the cause was recommended or was a life-saving intervention, the person perceives the body image insult as an unavoidable consequence and a relatively small price to pay (Rybarczyk & Behel, 2002).

Another important factor the nurse must not forget is the "fifth vital sign," or pain. If pain is associated with the cause of the body image change, the meaning and significance of the altered body image can be negatively influenced. Pain may also nourish a persisting and even worsening negative body image and impair recovery in functionality (Rybarczyk & Behel, 2002). Hence, it is essential to assess the person for pain and discomfort, and to treat accordingly.

Influence of Time

The length of time during which body changes occur may influence one's body image and subsequent psychological adjustment (White, 2002). Changes in body image may occur slowly, over a lifetime, or quickly, within hours or days. Although some might argue that more time gives individuals greater opportunity to reformulate a body image, the fact remains that some individuals will never adapt their body image to the ideal they hold or their current attributes. A person with type 2 diabetes may have a slow progression of changes and ample time for denial and grief resolution, whereas trauma and sudden illness, such as head trauma, stroke, or certain surgeries, may lead to abrupt changes in the body and in body image. Individuals who experience sudden traumatic illnesses have no warning, and thus little opportunity to adjust to the changes (Bello & McIntire, 1995). A classic example is the lag between limb amputations and phantom pain, where clients are confused about whether they still have the appendage. To adjust to rapid change, the client must grieve the loss as well as physically adjust to the changes.

The client who cannot cope with the dysfunction is at high risk for infection, noncompliance with therapeutic care, depression, social isolation, and obsession with or denial of the changes in body image (Dropkin, 1989).

The permanence of the change in appearance also affects adjustment to changes in body image. A person may better cope with changes in appearance that are temporary (i.e., temporary ileostomy) more so than those that are permanent (i.e., limb amputation). However, adjusting to body image changes depends partly on the meaning the individual ascribes to the changes and, in some cases, the length of time during which the change occurs (White, 2002).

Social Influences

Each sociocultural group establishes its own norms governing the acceptable, especially in terms of physical appearance and personality attributes (Jackson, 2002). Societies can hold a persistent, pervasive view with standards that dictate ideal physical appearance and role performance. These standards, although some with caveats, serve all members of that social group, including those who have chronic illness and those who do not.

Groups target their social influence and affect the self-images of individuals. Family relationships are often important to the person with a chronic illness and can impact their initial perception of their own body image when they become chronically ill. Negative family reactions about appearance, behavior, performance, and body image have been linked with recurrent poor body image consequences (Byely, Archibald, Graber, & Brooks-Gunn, 1999; Kearney-Cooke, 2002). Peers are also important mediating groups, particularly for those who are uncertain how to structure their lifestyles (e.g., adolescents). On one hand, peers can help shape conformance to a model. An example is the currently popular view of the muscle-bound, minimal-body-fat male model that is popular among young people (Olivardia, Pope, & Hudson, 2000). On the other hand, peer groups can call into question the appropriateness of such modeling for their own age group (e.g., older adults' perception of the aforementioned male model).

Persons with disfigurements are often, with little choice in the matter, forced to deal with their body image and the prevailing societal view. Depending on the visibility of the disfigurement and the coping of the disfigured person, sanctions such as staring, whispering, or shunning can negatively affect body image and personal value (Pruzinsky, 2002; Rumsey, 2002).

Untoward issues of body image often begin early in life. There is evidence now that in the United States and Britain, both girls and boys as young as 6 years old are overly conscious of their body weight and would begin dieting in an attempt to meet social norms of idealized thin and handsome young men and women. These young children, especially girls, are reported to be influenced by parental models and fashion magazines toward a desired thinness (Fornari & Dancyge, 2006; McCabe, Ricciardelli, & Lina, 2005; Lowes & Tiggemann, 2003). The body image issues that begin in early years often persist throughout adolescence and into adulthood (Striegel-Moore & Franko, 2002).

The effect of society and environment on body image is reciprocal. Societal reactions can affect body image, but the individual is not entirely passive and so can react in opposition to such standards. Nevertheless, societal influences weigh heavily on behavior and body image, frequently leading to stereotypical assignments that affect individual body image adjustments. For example, persons with craniofacial disfigurement, or those who are chronically obese, have been subjected to societal reactions and expectations of ideal beauty throughout their lives. Over the years, having been constantly compared with the "ideal" beautiful or thin person, the individual with chronic illness has had to manage their own responses as well as those of others in the obvious discrepancy between an ideal body and their own real bodies.

Cultural Influences

Many aspects of culture affect body image. A cultural map has been suggested by Helman (1995) in which the members of a particular cultural or social group share a view of the body. This cultural map tells individuals how their body is structured and how it functions, includes ideal body definitions, and identifies "private" and "public" body parts as well as differentiating between a "healthy" and an "unhealthy" body (Helman, 1995).

The perceptions of health and illness and their effects on body image vary from culture to culture. In Altabe's (1998) study on ideal physical traits and body image, ethnic groups were similar in their identification of ideal body traits but different in assigning values to the body traits (e.g., valuing skin color or breast size). Findings indicated that African Americans had the most positive self-view and body image, whereas Asian Americans placed the least importance on physical appearance. Some non-Caucasians had a more positive body image than did Caucasians.

African Americans view health as a feeling of well-being, the ability to fulfill role expectations, and experiencing an environment free of pain and excessive stress. In the United States,

the Latino cultural perception of health is being and looking clean, feeling happy, getting adequate rest, and being able to function in expected roles. An imbalance in the emotional, physical, and social arenas may produce illness. Hispanic individuals often do not seek health care until they are very sick, and those with chronic illness may view themselves as victims of malevolent forces, attributed to God or punishment. Native Americans view health as a balancing of mind, body, spirit, and nature. The practice of medicine is viewed as cooperative and offers choice and individual involvement in the pursuit of health.

Southeast Asian cultural health beliefs focus on the concept of yin and yang (balance) and maintaining this balance to achieve wellness. Additionally, obesity was once viewed as a sign of contentment and socioeconomic status in this culture. South Asians are particularly prone to subsequent cardiac and diabetic conditions because of lack of exercise, cultural emphases on high caloric foods, and religious and genetic influences (Pella, Thomas, Tomlinson, & Singh, 2003).

Influence of Healthcare Team Members

The care given to persons with a chronic disease or disability has a direct influence on their ability to adapt to societal pressures. Members of the healthcare team, although subject to the norms of the larger society, also have perceptions of illness and certain disabilities shaped by such professional norms as objectivity, compassion, and moral judgment. When caring for an individual with chronic illness, reactions from the healthcare team are important in the clients' adjustment and acceptance of body image.

Healthcare team members must understand that they are often the first person to see the changes engendered by the chronic illness or treatment. Their reactions often set the stage for body image expectations of their clients. Seeing their caregiver's reactions may reinforce body images for clients that continue for a long period of time, whether those images are positive or negative. Healthcare team members, therefore, must learn to manage their demeanor, voice, tone, and body reactions, avoiding any obvious rejections or trivialization of clients with chronic illness. One of the goals of the healthcare team should be to assist clients in having and/or maintaining a positive image and acceptance of self. For example, the client who has recently undergone breast reconstructive surgery following a mastectomy may have problematic body image issues. The support and guidance by healthcare team members in helping the client with information about surgery, pain relief, self-care, positive reinforcement, family relationships, and emotional support are important to building a positive body image (Van Deusen, 1993). Assessing concerns related to appearance and allowing clients to express fears, beliefs, thoughts, and life experiences also contribute to adjustment to body image changes (White, 2002).

Age

Erik Erikson's classic developmental theory is useful in examining phases of psychosocial development, particularly as this theory examines various stages throughout the lifespan that encourage or inhibit body image and personal feelings of value (Erikson, 1963). In younger age groups, conflicts about industry versus inferiority are changed into feelings of worth and competence (Cash & Pruzinsky, 1990). If there were negative effects during early developmental stages, altered or poor body image may result.

It is thought that younger children may be able to adapt more easily to changing body images because they have not fully come to recognize or appreciate their body image, unlike an adolescent or adult. Because their bodies are constantly changing, and because they are attending to their peers, adolescents can have an especially difficult time adapting to body image changes brought on by chronic illness. Patients with juvenile diabetes or adolescents with visible physical disfigurements, such as skin or neurologic diseases, frequently act out their frustrations via risky behaviors, depression, or withdrawal.

In a qualitative study of young males (18–25 years of age) and body image, Bottamini and Ste-Marie (2006) found that males are often reluctant to acknowledge their investment in body image as they believe it is seen as a more appropriate preoccupation of women. Nevertheless, these young men see attractiveness and the resultant positive body image they project as important in the work world because they believe an employer would associate a good physique with the ability to persevere. The authors hypothesize that body image awareness in men has increased with the decline of males as breadwinners due to women's expanding roles and earning capacity. Muscularity is not typically attained by women (at least to the same degree), so muscularity is seen as a last bastion of male prowess.

Body image in an adult has likely been well established and serves as an identity base. Adaptation to changes in body image can be more difficult to accept in older age groups because illness challenges their fundamental identity. Older adults' acceptance of body image changes tends to be related more to the ability to be useful in society, loss of independence and health status, and, possibly, attractiveness to others (Krauss-Whitbourne & Skultety, 2002).

Older adults may still feel young at heart, but as their bodies age, they are subject to changes in skin, hair, posture, strength, or speed of action, which are compounded by various chronic illnesses such as cardiac, respiratory, orthopedic, visual, or hearing problems. They may feel young, but their outer appearances demonstrate their age and associated conditions in a culture that values the young. The elderly often want to maintain an accepted social body image, so it is important to consider these issues when possible body image disturbances arise.

Gender

The gender of a person may influence his or her response to a change in body image. Although both genders are subject to norms of beauty, women and girls are reported to be more affected by breaches of the norms of beauty than boys and men are (Emslie, Hunt, & McIntyre, 2001). Women with burns, for example, generally have a more negative body image than do men with burns, although the effect of burns on body image depends on the locus of the burn and the percentage of body surface involved (Orr, Reznikoff, & Smith, 1989; Thombs et al., 2008). It is important to note, however, that females tend to have negative body image perceptions more often than males across age and cultures; therefore, women may experience more disturbances in body images than males when faced with a chronic illness (Striegel-Moore & Franko, 2002).

Typically, the male gender is associated with a "masculine, strong" appearance, and the female gender is associated with a "feminine, softer" appearance. Role behaviors are less strictly segregated now than in the 1950s, 1960s, and 1970s, yet, many older clients were socialized to gender roles during those years and have strong expectations of clear role behaviors. Men were expected to be strong, active, rational, and silent, whereas women were expected to be indirect, passive, capable, and emotional. These views have an impact on their self-image and the differences engendered by chronic illness. Older men with chronic illness or widowers who need assistance in learning to cook, or women learning to be more assertive even as their bodies are less conducive to these activities, often must change their body image. Often they do so gracefully, as we hear in the admonition, "Growing old is not for sissies." However, it behooves healthcare professionals—many of whom were not born in the times generating the social norms governing the body images of the older adults—to learn about the histories of those individuals whose chronic illnesses they treat. By doing so, the healthcare professional can become more empathetic and understand the possible contributions to the body images of their clients. This is particularly important, for example, for older women with diabetes who feel the need to be good cooks to accommodate their self-image as competent women, but whose diets must now be strictly managed. Another example is men with hypertension taking medication that limits libido or sexual performance.

Prior Experience and Coping Mechanisms

Body image is thought to be individually developed through each person's concept of his or her "ideal" perception and based on his or her previous experiences within society as well (Cash & Pruzinsky, 2002). Because past experiences, positive or negative, can substantially affect present circumstances, understanding how a client is likely to perceive an event, and cope with it, is one of the more important assessments performed by the healthcare professional. This awareness is particularly beneficial to the individual who has not had much exposure to the healthcare system and may require advocacy by the healthcare professional.

Coping mechanisms already developed by the individual through support from family, the healthcare team, or the client's social group are helpful in promoting adaptation to changes in body image during chronic illness. Understanding the individual's perception of body image before and during a diagnosis of chronic illness can be helpful to the healthcare professional in easing the client's adjustment to body image changes. Knowing that body image is an inferential diagnosis is helpful for the healthcare professional to discern whether clients are persevering, reformulating, or rejecting their body image.

The anxiety associated with the diagnosis of a chronic illness influences a person's coping style. Such crises can present the opportunity for personal growth or for overwhelming loss. Often, in the initial phase of chronic illness, clients will display an over-reliance on their typical coping mechanisms, even if those methods are not particularly effective in the current circumstances. At the same time, early in the trajectory of chronic illness, the person's ability to develop alternative coping mechanisms may be compromised. Identifying previously functional defenses as well as new, potentially helpful coping styles can be the first step taken by the healthcare professional in the outgoing assessment and management of body image alterations in persons with chronic illness.

ASSESSMENT OF BODY IMAGE

Evidenced-based practice guidelines are not yet available for the assessment or treatment of impaired body image. Yet, there are many assessment techniques from which the sensitive

or skilled healthcare professional may derive interventions. Practice in psychological assessment is useful. The focus in this section, therefore, is on assessment.

Assessing the behaviors of individuals who have experienced an alteration in function or change leading to a disruption in body image is vital in planning appropriate interventions. This assessment leads to a determination of perceptions and meanings associated with the change that is unique to the client, and allows recognition of barriers to health. Such an assessment requires the observation and interviewing of the client to determine the nature and meaning of the threat. Only after such an assessment and validation of its correctness may the healthcare professional provide interventions.

A key to a successful assessment is a therapeutic relationship with the client. Trust, sensitivity to the client's thoughts and feelings, and provision of accurate and realistic support all help to build and strengthen the therapeutic relationship between the client and provider (Hayslip, Cooper, Dougherty, & Cook, 1997).

A complete assessment of a client's experience and meaning of change is facilitated by asking questions related to the client's perception of the experience, knowledge of the illness and its effects, and others' perceptions of the client's illness. Accounting for these factors in the assessment process creates a client-centered knowledge base for choosing appropriate interventions. In addition, assessing the client's psychosocial history and support systems allows the provider to elicit greater support for the client in areas already known to the client.

Assessing a client's unique influencing factors is essential in planning interventions. Knowing how much value is placed on the appearance or functioning of the body helps the healthcare professional to determine the impact of the image disruption. Assessing self-esteem and the client's perceived attitudes of others is also important in discovering the meaning and impact of the disruption to the client. Ascertaining the phase of recovery of the client is essential, and is particularly important in planning specific client-centered interventions. Knowing when to implement educational, supportive, or rehabilitative interventions makes these interventions most useful.

Questions that might help the healthcare professional assess whether a client has a poor body image, particularly because of illness or injury, might focus on hiding or denial. Denial of one's self, self-effacement, or denial of the injury's severity is one hint of a poor self-image. A more typical indication of poor self-image or self-esteem is hiding, physically or mentally, from others. Actions such as avoiding others, avoiding close contact (such as undressing in front of others or sexual intimacy), avoiding displays of the injury or scars, or feelings of shame or embarrassment when discussing the injury or illness, are important clues to self-image.

CASE STUDY

Mary Ellen is a 36-year-old, single mother of two children, a girl age 8 years and a boy age 10. Mary Ellen is 5 feet 6 inches and weighs 302 pounds (BMI 48.7, which is considered very obese). Her mother and two sisters are also obese. Mary Ellen was never thin in childhood or adolescence and was occasionally teased at school, but more serious problems did not occur until adulthood. After her pregnancies and a painful divorce she has progressively gained weight. She has tried numerous diets with limited success, subsequently regaining even more weight. She is becoming increasingly unhappy for a number of reasons which include her daughter's burgeoning weight, her inability to keep up with her son's involvement in sports (climbing into the stands at games, long walks to the baseball field from parking), and hints that her son is ashamed of her appearance. She believes her obesity has also influenced her work life. She is an accountant with a public accounting firm, and she is no longer assigned the better projects that lead to promotion because those choice assignments involve going to client offices. On her last assignment she had difficulty fitting into the chairs at the client's site and was certain there was snickering by both the client and her coworker. Realizing these stresses trigger binge eating and additional guilt, Mary Ellen feels increasingly unable to manage her life. She has reluctantly decided to seek medical attention to learn about bariatric surgery. She dreads seeing a healthcare practitioner; in the past she has felt rejected by providers because of her lack of success in managing her weight.

Discussion Questions

1. In assisting patients like Mary Ellen, nurses must examine their own attitudes about obesity. Do you consider it a chronic disease, an unhealthy lifestyle choice, a sign of weakness or overindulgence, or a food addiction? Do you consider obesity with a "live and let live" attitude or some other conceptualization/belief about the condition? How do your views influence your approach and recommendations to Mary Ellen?

(continues)

CASE STUDY   (Continued)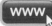

2. Do you think you are obliged to tell Mary Ellen your views as you counsel her, because
   they inform your recommendations? That is, Mary Ellen may want to "consider the
   source" and actively choose to accept in whole or in part what you suggest. What are your
   obligations as a healthcare professional involved in Mary Ellen's care?
3. The stigmatization of obesity is often considered "the last acceptable prejudice." Because
   obese persons in our society are socialized the same as the rest of society, how might that
   influence body image for persons with obesity?
4. What are Mary Ellen's strengths? What opportunities do you see to assist her to improve
   her body image and perceptions of self-efficacy?

In some instances, it may be necessary to use a standardized assessment tool to measure body disturbances and number and types of support systems. Many tools are available for this use (Cash & Pruzinsky, 2002). Tools about body disturbances generally have questions on general appearance, body competence, others' reaction to appearance, value of appearance, and so forth. These tools have incorporated related concepts to body image, such as self-esteem and self-concept, and are able to measure affective, cognitive, and behavioral components of body image (Thompson & Van Den Berg, 2002).

Incorporating families into assessment is encouraged. This can be done by interviewing, observing, and taking note of both verbal and nonverbal interactions within the family system (Wright & Leahey, 2000). Assessing family meanings of the chronic illness, perceived losses, and stresses placed on the family because of the illness are important in planning interventions.

BODY IMAGE ISSUES IMPORTANT TO CHRONIC ILLNESS

Chronic illness has many challenges, one of which includes the adaptation to changes in body image. The process of adaptation depends on many factors, but primary among those are the external changes to the person, functional limitations, the changes' significance and importance to the person, the time over which the change (and losses) have occurred, social influences, and the impact of culture.

External Changes

Important external factors that influence body image are the visibility and functional significance of the body part involved, the importance of physical appearance to the individual, and the rate at which the change occurred (Rybarczyk & Behel, 2002). For example, epilepsy is a chronic disease that illustrates all of these factors. Epileptic seizures, such as tonic–clonic seizures, can affect the entire body; the seizures are easily observed and happen suddenly. Epilepsy may also prevent the client from maintaining a job, driving a car, or engaging in sports or popular activities such as swimming. Typically epilepsy's onset is acute. The person does not have time to prepare for accepting this chronic disease. A seizure occurs and the person's life is changed from that moment forward. This can make it more challenging to accept and live "normally" with the image of "being an epileptic," and potentially having a very visible, sudden, and dysfunctional (possibly dangerous) experience. The severity of insult to appearance and functional significance, and the degree of importance to the person, must be considered on an individual basis. For example, some persons may find epilepsy a minor nuisance while others might find mild psoriasis traumatizing, because the latter is more visible. It is essential to assess the meaning and significance of the change to the person.

Another common example is the obese client. Obesity is now listed as one of the leading health indicators that is problematic in the United States (*Healthy People 2020*), and because of its close ties to body image, it deserves increased consideration in this discussion. Obesity is typically a nonacute, slowly progressing condition, which has come to be viewed as a major risk factor in several chronic illnesses, such as diabetes, heart disease, and osteoarthritis. Obesity is also considered déclassé in Western culture, often viewed as an indicator of overindulgence and sloth, and frequently associated with lower classes. Although the obesity risk has been challenged (Campos, 2005; Flegal, Graubard, Williamson, & Gail, 2007), most healthcare professionals still believe obesity must be medically managed. Today there are public health campaigns to reduce obesity, beginning in childhood. Obese persons are reacting to the medicalization and stigmatization of obesity: Since 1969 an organization called the National Association to Advance Fat Acceptance (NAAFA) has existed to argue for the dignity, equality, and civil rights of obese persons (see www.naafa.org). The organization, however, both explicitly and implicitly acknowledges that a person's body image can be negatively and

powerfully influenced by obesity and others' reactions to it.

The stigmatization of obesity is considerable in the United States and throughout the world, despite its seemingly relentless increase in prevalence (Centers for Disease Control and Prevention, 2008a; World Health Organization, 2011). There is evidence that weight is perhaps the most important factor in evaluating female attractiveness (Swami & Tovee, 2005; Tovee, Rhinehart, Emery, & Cornelissen, 1998). Fairburn & Brownell (2002) posit that the anti-obesity sentiment originates in the Euro-American ideal of individualism in which the bad situations in which people find themselves are the result of their own doing. There is a widespread myth that obesity is the result of personal failings and a lack of self-discipline, although scientific evidence suggests that body weight is determined by a complex interaction of biological and environmental factors that are at best only partially controlled by the individual. There is also evidence that the greater the degree of deviation from the socially perceived ideal body weight the greater the degree of stigmatization, suggesting that the more obese a person becomes the more they are stigmatized (Swami et al., 2008).

Mental illnesses can also influence body image, and yet, many healthcare professionals overlook this aspect of chronic mental illness. For instance, a person with schizophrenia may have a negatively altered body image as part of the disturbed thinking caused by the illness and/or from the perceived change the illness has on the behavior and presentation of the person. Furthermore, the medication used to treat schizophrenia can affect body image because of its neurological side effects (movement disorders), weight gain, and sexual dysfunction.

Therefore, ignoring the potential side effects in treating individuals with mental illness is likely to affect not only medication compliance but also physical self-image.

External changes and their rapidity of change are important in assessing body image. Healthcare professionals should not assume, but verify with the client, what the current body image is, and what it means to the client. Each person is unique, and, therefore, each experience with chronic illness and its impact on body image is unique.

Appearance

The physical appearance of a disease is frequently a change for which clients are unprepared. Given the possibility of perseverance, reformulation, or rejection of changes, further studies are needed of the ways in which body image and its accompanying variables affect acceptance by others. Empirical evidence and anecdotal data exist to guide us in considering suitable interventions. For example, when appearance also draws attention to a disease's underlying cause, clients and their significant others are often ostracized, particularly when the disease is one that carries a stigma (see Chapter 3). Many clients with AIDS develop Kaposi's sarcoma (KS), a common and sometimes disfiguring tumor related to HIV. Because the skin is a common site for KS, the characteristic purple hue of KS is easily visible, and is considered by many patients as a "public signature" of HIV (deMoore, Hennessey, Kunz, Ferrando, & Rabkin, 2000). In more severe cases of illness, in which the body is catastrophically debilitated, as in amyotrophic lateral sclerosis (ALS), Helman (1995) notes that the entire body image may accommodate the body as separated from the sense of self—that is, "It is my body that is diseased, but not me."

Visibility and Invisibility

Chronic illness and its treatment provide visible, outward changes in appearance and invisible, internal changes. Both types of change can significantly affect individuals' perceptions of themselves. In an adult, it is suggested that the more visible or extensive the body alteration, the more likely it is to be perceived as a threat to one's body image. Loss of hair, scarring, edema, amputations, and disfigurement are common examples in the body image literature. In reading the life accounts of severely disfigured persons, many choose to work at unusual times (nights) and in jobs in which they have little contact with others (see Chapter 5). In a meta-analysis of 12 articles that met their inclusion criteria, Bessel and Moss (2007) reported that truly efficacious interventions are lacking for adults with visible differences in appearance. In a related study, Thompson and Kent (2001) reported that persons with disfigurements shape their self-image by interactions with others in social contexts, and that interventions are available. Like Bessel and Moss, they note that reports and interventions were not methodologically rigorous or informed by theory.

In another study of patients with severe burns and their adjustment to disfigurement, Thombs and colleagues (2008) found that over time, women, more than men, suffered dissatisfaction with body image, particularly with larger burns, and that their dissatisfaction interfered with psychological functioning over time. The findings of these studies argue a need for more research of a longitudinal and qualitative nature, toward a better understanding of the processes and outcomes of visible differences and their impact on body image.

The matter of body image and incorporation of changes seems to be more ambiguous in children. Children are strongly subject to the norms imposed by their peers, with their self-image being readily influenced. A visible change or disfigurement in a child could ostracize the child from his or her peer group. Of particular strength and importance to children, especially for those with "stigmatized" body images, are the family members or healthcare professionals who can support the child's acceptance of the body image changes. Puberty is one time of life in normal development in which personal identity and body image are strongly affected. It is during this time then that parents and adults who work with children should support healthy body images and intervene when a child begins to develop poor body images (see, for example, Fornari & Dancyge, 2006). The diagnosis of a chronic illness, with or without visible body changes, can profoundly affect the adolescent at this vulnerable time in his or her life.

When a change is not markedly visible, as when an ostomy is created, or its treatment (e.g., colostomy appliances) is introduced, persons with chronic illness must take previously "invisible" body parts and make them "visible" (Helman, 1995). This dynamic is further compounded when the new intervention is preferentially hidden from others. Such procedures and the management of visible and hidden change likely lead to dramatic changes in an individual's lifestyle and self-image. For example, clients with a stoma must periodically empty the appliance bag, learn to change it, irrigate the stoma when needed, cope with social matters such as dressing to fit the appliance, and manage social etiquette with problems of leaking, odors, and the noises resulting from involuntary discharge into the appliance. The person dealing with such challenges may keep this hidden, and limit social functioning to avoid possible embarrassment (Kirkpatrick, 1986). Since the late 1980s, in a movement begun by former First Lady Betty Ford when she announced her decision to manage alcoholism and breast cancer, many are now openly announcing illnesses and treatments that were previously hidden. Nonetheless, the visibility or invisibility of an illness, injury, or treatment regimen must be managed, and in that management exists the potential to enhance or diminish body images held by the individual.

Functional Limitations

Functionality is something that is conceptualized as "external," in that functionality is usually a visible part of enactment of one's role—though some functions, such sexual function, are carried out privately. Function is the ability of a body part to conduct its usual purpose. The ability to function in a meaningful way is essential to a sense of well-being; consequently, any limitation of functional ability may alter one's concept of body image. Most clients and their significant others are not prepared for the appearance and functional limitations associated with chronic illness.

The function of a body part and its importance and visibility are critical to one's body image. The leg, because of its functional importance in mobility and a person's life, is more likely to be a more important part of body image than, say, a toe (Brown, 1977). Loss of a toe, for example, is likely to be viewed as less problematic than loss of a leg, because much function can be retained by compensatory body parts and also because a toe is less visible. Therefore, one might expect different accommodations in body image to such amputations, even as it is recognized that perception of loss and its impact vary from person to person and culture to culture.

The roles of worker, gendered persona, and sexual being are three important facets of body image. Chronic illness or treatment can threaten the client's ability to perform each of these roles. Furthermore, the stage of one's life can make a major difference in the perception of the strength of the threat or its incorporation into one's body image. A teenager, perhaps, is likely to regard work or sexual function and their concomitant body image differently than would a seasoned elder who has had different experiences and usually, changed body appearance and function.

Loss of sexual function for most persons, particularly those who are sexually active, is often perceived as a profound loss. Women with breast removal from cancer, or men and women with genital cancers, frequently avoid sexual situations after treatments (Golden & Golden, 1986). The male client may feel especially vulnerable if he thinks sexuality or provider role is compromised by chronic illness. Testicular cancer is the most common cancer in young men ages 18 to 35 and typically results in the removal of the diseased testicle. Older men with prostate cancer may require the removal of both testicles, with a resultant loss of libido and virility and compromised perception of "manhood." Although implants can be used, the perception of functional loss can strongly persist. The nurse can be, and may often be, the main source of professional support and education, and thus assists clients with the sensitive issues involved with body image.

INTERVENTIONS

Interventions, particularly those of assessment, have been described throughout this chapter. Interventions are used to help clients manage their own reactions and the reactions of others to changes in body structure, function, or appearance as the result of chronic illness.

These changes are frequently interpreted as setting one apart and as different from one's peers (see Chapter 3), leading to self-doubt, inhibited participation in social activities, and a disruption of perceptions of self. Finding appropriate interventions for clients experiencing an altered body image can aid the client in healing and adapting to changes in body image (Norris, Connell, & Spelic, 1998).

Adapting to changes in body image resulting from chronic illness is a dynamic process. On a daily basis, clients are faced with thoughts and reminders of their illness and changes to their bodies. During periods of exacerbation, remission, and rehabilitation, clients are grieving the loss of their former selves, living with the uncertainty of their chronic illness, and learning to create new images of self (Cohen, Kahn, & Steeves, 1998). Knowing that the process is continually changing, with steps forward and backward, helps the nurse to support clients as they adapt to changes in body image.

Interventions are chosen after careful assessment of the client. As mentioned previously, a therapeutic relationship with the client is an essential beginning to the process. Before successful intervention can occur, the following must be addressed: acknowledgment of barriers to communication, feelings about the illness, changes the illness caused, and personal biases on the part of the healthcare professional. Accurate knowledge about the disease process and the client's response are also necessary if the healthcare professional is to assist the client. In addition, the healthcare professional must be able to recognize that body image changes will require a supportive, accepting, and consistent relationship that can withstand setbacks and emotional tension. It is important to be aware of the client's attitude and participation in the recovery process. This may involve professional rehabilitation, including physical and occupational therapy, or it may involve informal self- or family-directed interventions. The healthcare professional who is knowledgeable about evidence-based practice, guidelines, and treatment regimens can be influential in acknowledging subtle progress that the client may or may not be aware of and supporting the benefit of rehabilitation as part of the overall recovery process. Through evidence-based practice, the knowledgeable healthcare professional can provide not only quality care in the chronic illness, but also begin helping the client toward forming a more balanced and realistic body image.

Communication

Providing opportunities for clients to express feelings and thoughts about the changes they are experiencing can be beneficial to both clients and healthcare professionals. It allows clients to speak and be heard, and also allows careful assessment of the clients' thoughts and feelings. Assumptions should not be made about the meaning of experiences relating to changes in body image (Cohen, Kahn, & Steeves, 1998). In addition, ensuring client comfort in expressing both positive and negative feelings and emotions helps strengthen the therapeutic relationship and facilitate the journey to wholeness. Allowing family members to express their thoughts, feelings, and concerns is also beneficial and should be incorporated into the recovery process.

Talk therapy, either individual or group, can be of much benefit in the recovery process. Cognitive-behavioral therapy has a proven record—that is, it is evidence-based practice—in helping clients change their dysfunctional thinking and related behaviors associated with chronic illness and negative body image (Peterson et al., 2004; Rumsey & Harcourt, 2004; Rybarczyk & Behel, 2002; Veale, 2004).

There is some evidence that healthcare professionals who have had similar life experiences may be perceived as more credible sources of information and inspiration to clients experiencing difficulty coping with illnesses. In the substance abuse treatment system, providers often are in recovery themselves. In a qualitative study of self-perceptions of obesity, Thomas, Mosely, Stallings, Nichols-English, and Wagner (2008) found that obese women overwhelmingly preferred to work with healthcare professionals who had experienced weight problems themselves over those who were thin and had not had the personal experience of being overweight. The degree of self-disclosure by healthcare professionals is a matter governed by boundary considerations and personal choice; however, some degree of self-disclosure to those suffering from body image difficulties may enhance communication.

Self-Help Groups

Self-help groups for clients experiencing body image changes may help to buffer the stressors created by the changes. Providing clients with opportunities to share experiences with others in similar situations can be therapeutic for some individuals. Self-help or support groups offer important emotional, social, and spiritual fellowship, as well as education about the focus of the support group. Before encouraging support groups as an intervention, it is important to assess the willingness of individuals to participate in a group setting. Support groups that are most helpful are those where the members are encouraged, but not forced, to share information, and where the leader can lead the discussions to bring out salient points intelligently, empathetically, and fairly. Groups should be avoided that are unstable, promote products or purchases, or that charge inordinate fees. Groups that encourage gripe sessions, allow individuals to dominate a discussion, or that demand cult-like allegiances or sharing of information clients don't wish to share should also be avoided (Centers for Disease Control and Prevention, 2008b). Some individuals are not comfortable in a group setting, especially when they are dealing with a body image disruption. For those who find it helpful, the benefits are many. Seeing others on the road to recovery, helping those who are struggling, developing friendships, or finding where they themselves are in the journey can help with the healing process (Corey & Corey, 1997). Furthermore, these groups provide an opportunity for clients to begin socializing with others in a safe and nonthreatening environment.

Evidence-Based Practice Box

Many women in all age groups harbor negative body images, especially related to weight and the self-perception of physical attractiveness (Frederick, Peplau, & Lever, 2006). Women suffer low self-esteem and even depression as a result of a negative body image. Arbour and Ginis (2008) recognized that exercise can positively influence body image and that walking was one of the most acceptable physical activities for adult women across the lifespan. Because of the multiple demands of family and home to women, they are particularly attracted to "lifestyle activity" as an exercise regimen. Lifestyle activities are those that can be incorporated into everyday life with minimal

disruption. Arbour and Ginis (2008) conducted a randomized clinical trial to examine whether walking as a lifestyle activity, measured in the number of steps recorded on a pedometer during an 11-week period, would mediate change in the body image of previously sedentary women.

The women who participated and completed the assigned activities of the study were largely white and middle aged. In the control group (n = 25) the women simply self-monitored steps daily using a pedometer, while the experimental group (n = 17) monitored their steps but also developed an action plan. Defined as self-regulatory strategies that entail formation of strong mental associations between a situational cue and a specific behavioral response, action plans assist motivated individuals to generate specific regimens to move good intentions into actual behavior (Gollwitzer, 1999).

Using the Adult Body Satisfaction Questionnaire (ABSQ), Arbour and Ginis measured two subscales of the ABSQ that represented two aspects of body image that they speculated could be influenced by exercise. These included satisfaction with physical functioning and satisfaction with physical appearance. Measurements were done during the first and the 11th week of the intervention. The ABSQ is considered a reliable instrument to measure body image with an alpha of 0.85 in this study. Steps were measured using a standard pedometer.

Post-testing verified that the intervention (action planning) predicted the mediator (the number of steps), which in turn was associated with higher scores on the satisfaction with physical functioning subscale of the ABSQ. Analysis indicated that 41% of the effect of the intervention on the satisfaction with physical functioning was mediated by the number of steps taken. However, results did not support a similar relationship among the variables related to satisfaction with physical appearance.

The authors note the benefits of this relatively simple yet effective activity-enhancing intervention. Thus exercise not only positively influences physical health in women but may support aspects of a more positive body image.

Sources: Arbour, K., & Ginis K. (2008). Improving body image one step at a time: Greater pedometer step counts produce greater body image improvements. *Body Image, 5,* 331–336.

Frederick, D., Peplau, L.,& Lever, J. (2006). The swimsuit issue: Correlates of body image in a sample of 52,677 heterosexual adults. *Body Image, 4,* 413–419.

Gollwitzer, P. (1999). Implementation Intentions: Strong effects of simple plans. *American Psychologist, 54,* 493–503.

Spiegel and colleagues' (2008) research indicate that breast cancer patients who participated in a support group lived, on average, 18 months longer than those who did not belong to a support group. Subsequent research could not duplicate those findings, but women who have joined support groups have shown other benefits, primarily experiencing less depression, distress, anxiety, and pain, and importantly, obtaining information about their disease and its treatment.

In another survey of 367 women with advanced breast cancer, almost as many clients got their information from the Internet (39%) as from their doctors (42%) (Y-ME National Breast Cancer Organization, 2007). These data indicate that healthcare professionals must find more meaningful ways to convey needed information to this group of patients. Because of the findings on support groups and because of the needs of clients with breast cancer, support groups have found a place in therapeutic regimens. Almost all oncology centers can direct patients to such groups, as patients increasingly find them a useful adjunct and information site as they manage work, family, sexuality, and uncertain cancer prognoses.

Nurses and other healthcare professionals can locate a variety of support groups, or even begin one themselves as a therapeutic intervention. The Internet is an excellent tool for locating support groups and the resources needed to begin or maintain support groups; there are also many Web-based support groups. One site alone included almost 500 different support groups listed alphabetically, all relating to various illnesses or states of life (e.g., divorce, parenting). Nurses, by virtue of their place in the healthcare delivery system, are poised to address both physical and psychosocial needs of patients, and are able to deliver information in helpful ways: Support groups are one intervention that nurses can develop to help patients meet their needs for information and emotional support.

Education and Anticipatory Guidance

This intervention is effective only when the client has indicated a readiness to learn. Knowledge of disease processes, information about symptoms, and methods of treatment are important educational topics for the client. In providing education, it is important to consider the preferred learning style (e.g., visual, auditory, and/or practice) of the client (Cohen, Kahn, & Steeves, 1998). The benefits of client education and anticipatory guidance should be stressed to stimulate and support the client's readiness to learn (see Chapter 15).

Self-Care

Encouraging clients to participate in the activities of daily living that are meaningful to them helps restore feelings of normalcy. Whether engaging in personal grooming activities, such as applying cosmetics, jewelry, or hair accessories, caring for one's self can be an effective intervention. Self-care will help the client incorporate the change in body image into the normal functioning of daily living. This intervention may also help the client become less sensitive to physical appearances and learn to manage everyday activities (Norris, Connell, & Spelic, 1998). Regular exercise can be helpful to improve body image as well as support physical health and function (Wetterhahn, Hanson, & Levy, 2002; see Chapter 14).

Prostheses

The oldest prosthesis known of is a large wooden toe that was found attached by leather thongs to the foot of an ancient Egyptian female mummy. This well carved prosthesis, unhidden by a sandal, aided the woman in walking and maintaining balance ("A Ticklish Matter," 2007). Prostheses vary in sophistication and availability. Most healthcare professionals are familiar with prosthetic eyes, hearing aids, various

"limbs" (e.g., hand, foot, leg, arm), or breast, penile, or testicular implants. In amputations, the age of the client presents unusual concerns. The prosthetic hand, foot, or knee of a child, for example, may require, for the child's adequate social development, that the prosthetic stand up to repeated use in play—for example, in swimming, it must withstand the effects of water, sand, chlorine, and/or salt. Adults may wish to maintain a physically normal appearance and avoid the functional "hook" hand prosthesis. In older adults whose gait problems may be exacerbated by joint problems, the "fit" of a prosthesis, as in a hip replacement, is a special concern. The rehabilitation required after hip replacement is particularly necessary, and its success has much to do with subsequent body image improvement related to increased mobility.

Spinal cord injury has sparked research that focuses on current knowledge of spinal cord treatment, electrical stimulation, mechanisms of secondary damage, and possibilities for regeneration of nerves. Bioengineering, electric-powered prostheses, invasive and noninvasive sensors to control prostheses, and use of brain waves or pupillary contraction to power computers for communication are currently being used or being tested. Their success is a huge event for the affected person, and this specialized area of knowledge typically requires focus and specialization by healthcare professionals.

The use of prostheses and the unique technologies to power these prostheses will continue to expand in the future. It is important to understand that the field of prosthetics requires knowledge about the illness as well as the care with which clients implement and maintain their prosthetics and the impact of prosthetics on body image.

OUTCOMES

Body image, the physical aspect of self-concept, is closely linked with the concept of self-esteem in the Nursing Outcomes Classification (NOC) (Moorhead, Johnson, Maas, & Swanson, 2008). Disturbances of self-concept along with personal identity disturbance, chronic low self-esteem, and situational low self-esteem are considered part of what Carpenito-Moyet (2008) globally calls disturbed self-concept. Alterations in self-concept can occur because of an immediate problem, such as sudden disfiguration from surgery or burns, or can be related to long-term changes resulting from disease processes, therapies, dietary and medication management, or from lifestyle changes or an uncertain future.

Defining characteristics of alterations in self-concept can be multiple: denial, withdrawal of the individual, refusal to be part of the care required, refusal to look at the body part involved or let immediate family look at it, refusal to discuss rehabilitation efforts, signs and symptoms of grieving, self-destructive behavior such as alcohol or drug abuse, and hostility toward healthy individuals. One's sense of femininity or masculinity may also be threatened, which can lead to difficulty in sexual functioning, and, combined, these changes can lead to social anxiety, self-consciousness, and depression (Carpenito-Moyet, 2008; White, 2002).

The NOC diagnosis of Disturbed Body Image includes an assessment of the patients' sense of congruence between body reality, body ideal, and body presentation; their description of the affected body part; their willingness to touch the affected body part; their satisfaction with body appearance or body function; and their willingness to use strategies to adjust to their new status and changes in bodily appearance or function. These adjustments would occur with bodily changes that were the result of injury, surgery, or life trajectories (e.g. adolescence, aging) (Moorhead et al., 2008). The ultimate therapeutic goal for patients is successful adaptation to their own body appearance and function, and we would argue that the definition of success should be defined by the patients themselves and supported by the healthcare professional.

STUDY QUESTIONS   WWW

What are the general themes of body image discourse? How did this chapter help you in furthering the discussion or in understanding everyday concerns about body image?

What elements would you include in an educational intervention for a patient group with body image issues? Justify your choices.

Name three concepts related to body image and explain their relationship.

Describe how you would assess a client with a changed body image.

Discuss how age, gender, and culture can affect body image.

How often in your own friendships do issues of body image come up in conversation?

INTERNET RESOURCES

Albert Einstein Sociedade Beneficente Israelita Brasileira Mental Help page (in Portugese): www.mentalhelp.com

American Heart Association on Obesity: http://www.heart.org/HEARTORG/GettingHealthy/WeightManagement/Obesity/Obesity-Information_UCM_307908_Article.jsp

Daily Strength Support Group Resource: www.dailystrength.com

Kids Health: http://kidshealth.org/parent/general/body/overweight_obesity.html

U.S. Department of Health and Human Services Women's Health: http://womenshealth.gov/

Weight-control Information Network: www.win.niddk.nih.gov/publications/health_risks.htm

For a full suite of assignments and additional learning activities, **WWW** use the access code located in the front of your book and visit this exclusive website: **http://go.jblearning.com/larsen**. If you do not have an access code, you can obtain one at the site.

REFERENCES

A ticklish matter: Photograph and caption. (2007, July 28). *Pittsburgh Post-Gazette*.

Altabe, M. (1998). Ethnicity and body image: Quantitative and qualitative analysis. *International Journal of Eating Disorders, 23*, 153–159.

Arbour, K., & Ginis K. (2008). Improving body image one step at a time: Greater pedometer step counts produce greater body image improvements. *Body Image, 5,* 331–336.

Bello, L., & McIntire, S. (1995). Body image disturbance in young adults with cancer. *Cancer Nursing, 18*(2), 138–143.

Bessell, A., & Moss, T. P. (2007). Evaluating the effectiveness of psychosocial interventions for individuals with visible differences: A systematic review of the empirical literature. *Body Image, 4*(3), 227–238.

Blanke, O. (2007). I and me: Self-portraiture in brain damage. *Frontiers of Neurology and Neuroscience, 22,* 14–29.

Bottamini, G & Ste-Marie, D. (2006). Male voices on body image. *International Journal of Men's Health. 5*(2), 109–132.

Brown, M. S. (1977). The nursing process and distortions or changes in body image. In F. L. Bower (Ed.), *Distortions in body image in illness and disability* (pp. 1–19). New York: Wiley.

Byely, L., Archibald, A., Graber, J., & Brooks-Gunn, J. (1999). A prospective study of familial and social influences on girls' body image and dieting. *International Journal of Eating Disorders, 28*, 155–164.

Campos, P. (2005). *The diet myth: Why America's obsession with weight is hazardous to your health.* New York: Gotham.

Carpenito-Moyet, L. (2008). *Handbook of nursing diagnosis* (12th ed.). Philadelphia: Lippincott, Williams & Wilkins.

Cash, T. F. (2002). Cognitive behavioral perspectives on body image. In T. Cash & T. Pruzinsky (Eds.), *Body image: A handbook of theory, research, and clinical progress* (pp. 38–46). New York: Guilford Press.

Cash, T. F., & Fleming, E. C. (2002). The impact of body image experiences: Development of the body image quality of life inventory. *International Journal of Eating Disorders, 31*, 455–460.

Cash, T. F., & Pruzinsky, T. (1990). *Body images: Development, deviance, and change.* New York: Guilford Press.

Cash, T. F., & Pruzinsky, T. (2002). Understanding body image: Historical and contemporary perspectives. In T. Cash & T. Pruzinsky (Eds.), *Body image: A handbook of theory, research, and clinical progress* (pp. 30–37). New York: Guilford Press.

Cash, T., & Pruzinsky, T. (2004). *Body image: A handbook of theory, research, and clinical practice.* New York: Guilford Press.

Centers for Disease Control and Prevention. (2008a). Prevalence of overweight, obese, and extreme obesity among adults: United States trends 1976–1980 through 2005–2006. Retrieved August 2, 2011, from: http://www.cdc.gov/nchs/data/hestat/overweight/overweight_adult.pdf

Centers for Disease Control and Prevention. (2008b). Chronic fatigue syndrome: Support groups. Retrieved August 2, 2011, from: http://www.cdc.gov/cfs/general/treatment/options.html

Cohen, M. Z., Kahn, D. L., & Steeves, R. H. (1998). Beyond body image: The experience of breast cancer. *Oncology Nursing Forum, 25*(5), 835–841.

Corey, M., & Corey, G. (1997). *Groups: Process and practice* (5th ed.). Boston: Brooks/Cole.

Corwyn, R. F. (2000). The factor structure of global self-esteem among adolescents and adults. *Journal of Research and Personality, 34,* 357–379.

deMoore, G. M., Hennessey, P., Kunz, N. M., Ferrando, S.J., & Rabkin, J. G. (2000). Kaposi's sarcoma: The scarlet letter of AIDS. The psychological effects of a skin disease. *Psychosomatics, 41*(4), 360–363.

Didie. E., Kuniega-Pietrzak, T., & Phillips, K. (2010). Body image in patients with body dysmorphic disorder: Evaluations of and investment in appearance, health, illness, and fitness. *Body Image, 7,* 66–69.

Dropkin, M. J. (1989). Coping with disfigurement and dysfunction after head and neck cancer surgery: A conceptual framework. *Seminars in Oncology Nursing, 5*(3), 213–219.

Emslie, C., Hunt, K., & Macintyre, S. (2001). Perceptions of body image among working men and women. *Epidemiology and Community Health, 55,* 406–407.

Erikson, E. (1963). *Childhood and society* (2nd ed.). New York: Norton.

Fairburn, C., & Brownell K. (2002). *Eating disorders and obesity: A comprehensive handbook.* (2nd ed.). New York: Guilford Press.

Feusner, J., Yaryura-Tobias, J. & Saxena, S. (2008). The pathophysiology of body dysmorphic disorder. *Body Image, 5,* 3–12.

Fisher, S. (1986). *Development and structure of the body image* (Vol. 2). Hillsdale, NJ: Lawrence Erlbaum Associates.

Flegal, K. M., Graubard, B. I., Williamson, D. F., & Gail, M. H. (2007). Cause-specific excess deaths associated with underweight, overweight, and obesity. *Journal of the American Medical Association, 298*(17), 2028–2037.

Fornari, V., & Dancyge, I. F. (2006). Physical and cognitive changes associated with puberty. In T. Jaffa & B. McDermott (Eds.), *Eating Disorders in Children and Adolescents*, (pp. 57–69). Cambridge: Cambridge University Press.

Frederick, D. A, Lever, J., & Peplau, L. A. (2007). Interest in cosmetic surgery and body image: Views of men and women across the lifespan. *Plastic & Reconstructive Surgery, 120*(5), 1407–1415.

Frederick, D., Peplau, L., & Lever, J. (2006). The swimsuit issue: Correlates of body image in a sample of 52,677 heterosexual adults. *Body Image, 4,* 413–419.

Golden, J. S., & Golden, M. (1986). Cancer and sex. In J. M. Vaeth (Ed.), *Body image, self-esteem, and sexuality in cancer patients* (2nd ed., pp. 68–76). Basel, Switzerland : Karger.

Gollwitzer, P. (1999). Implementation Intentions: Strong effects of simple plans. *American Psychologist, 54,* 493–503.

Hayslip, B., Cooper, C. C., Dougherty, L. M., & Cook, D. D. (1997). Body image in adulthood: A projective approach. *Journal of Personality Assessment, 68*(3), 628–649.

Healthy People 2020. (2011).Topics and objectives: Nutrition and weight status. Retrieved August 2, 2011, from: http://www.healthypeople.gov/2020

Helman, C. G. (1995). The body image in health and disease: Exploring patients' maps of body and self. *Patient Education and Counseling, 26,* 169–175.

Jackson, L. A. (2002). Physical attractiveness: A sociocultural perspective. In T. Cash & T. Pruzinsky (Eds.), *Body image: A handbook of theory, research, and clinical progress* (pp. 13–21). New York: Guilford Press.

Kearney-Cooke, A. (2002). Familial influences on body image development. In T. Cash & T. Pruzinsky (Eds.), *Body image: A handbook of theory, research, and clinical progress* (pp. 99–107). New York: Guilford Press.

Kirkpatrick, J. R. (1986). The stoma patient and his return to society. In J. M. Vaeth (Ed.), *Body image, self-esteem, and sexuality in cancer patients* (2nd ed., pp. 24–27). Basel, Switzerland: Karger.

Krauss-Whitbourne, S., & Skultety, K. (2002). Body image development: Adulthood and aging. In T. Cash & T. Pruzinsky (Eds.), *Body image: A handbook of theory, research, and clinical progress* (pp. 83–90). New York: Guilford Press.

Krueger, D. W. (2002). Psychodynamic perspectives on body image. In T. Cash & T. Pruzinsky (Eds.), *Body image: A handbook of theory, research, and clinical progress* (pp. 30–37). New York: Guilford Press.

Lewis, J. (1983). *Something hidden: A biography of Wilder Penfield.* Halifax, Nova Scotia: Goodread Biographies.

Lowes, J., & Tiggemann, M. (2003). Body dissatisfaction, dieting awareness, and the impact of parental influence in young children. *British Journal of Health Psychology, 8,* 135.

Markus, H., & Wurf, E. (1987). The dynamic self-concept: A social psychological perspective. *Annual Review of Psychology, 38,* 299–337.

McCabe, M., & Ricciardelli, P., & Lina A. (2005). A prospective study of pressures from parents, peers, and the media on extreme weight change behaviours among adolescent boys and girls. *Behaviour Research and Therapy, 43,* 653–668.

Mock, V. (1993). Body image in women treated for breast cancer. *Nursing Research, 42*(3), 153–157.

Moorhead, S., Johnson, M., Maas, M. & Swanson, E., (Eds.), (2008). *Nursing outcomes classification (NOC)* (4th ed.). St. Louis: C.V. Mosby Co.

Mueller, S. (2007–2008). Amputee envy. *Scientific American Mind, 18*(6), 60–65.

National Association to Advance Fat Acceptance (NAAFA). (2011). Homepage. Retrieved August 2, 2011, from: http://www.naafaonline.com/dev2/

Nezlek, J. B. (1999). Body image and day-to-day social interaction. *Journal of Personality, 67*(5), 793–817.

Norris, J., Connell, M. K., & Spelic, S. S. (1998). A grounded theory of reimaging. *Advances in Nursing Science, 20*(3), 1–12.

Olivardia, R., Pope, H. J., & Hudson, J. I. (2000). Muscle dysmorphia in male weightlifters: A case control study. *American Journal of Psychiatry, 157,* 1291–1296.

Orr, D. A., Reznikoff, M., & Smith, G. M. (1989). Body image, self-esteem, and depression in burn-injured adolescents and young adults. *Journal of Burn Care and Rehabilitation, 10*(5), 454–461.

Peelen, M., & Downing, P. E. (2007). The neural basis of visual body perception. *Nature Reviews Neuroscience, 8*(8), 636–648.

Pella, D., Thomas, N., Tomlinson, B., & Singh, R.(2003). Prevention of coronary artery disease: The South Asian paradox. *The Lancet, 361*(9351), 79.

Peterson, C. B, Wimmer, S., Ackard, D. M., Crosby, R., Cavanagh, L. C., Engbloom, S., et al. (2004). Changes in body image during cognitive–behavioral treatment in women with bulimia nervosa. *Body Image, 1*(2), 139–153.

Phillips, K.,. & Hollander, E. (2008). Treating body dysmorphic disorder with medication: Evidence, misperceptions, medication, and a suggested approach. *Body Image, 5, 3–12.*

Pruzinsky, T. (2002). Body image adaptation to reconstructive surgery for acquired disfigurement. In T. Cash & T. Pruzinsky (Eds.), *Body image: A handbook of theory, research, and clinical progress* (pp. 440–449). New York: Guilford Press.

Pruzinsky, T. (2004). Enhancing quality of life in medical populations: A vision for body image assessment and rehabilitation as standards of care. *Body Image, 1,* 71–81.

Ramachandran, V. S. (2004). *A brief tour of human consciousness.* New York: Pearson Education.

Ramachandran, V. S., & Rogers-Ramachandran, D. (2007). It's all done with mirrors. *Scientific American Mind, 18*(4), 16–18.

Rumsey, N. (2002). Body image and congenital conditions with visible differences. In T. Cash & T. Pruzinsky (Eds.), *Body image: A handbook of theory, research, and clinical progress* (pp. 226–233). New York: Guilford Press.

Rumsey, N., & Harcourt, D. (2004). Body image and disfigurement: Issues and interventions. *Body Image, 1,* 83–97.

Rybarczyk, B., & Behel, J. (2002). Rehabilitation medicine and body image. In T. Cash & T. Pruzinsky (Eds.), *Body image: A handbook of theory, research, and clinical progress* (pp. 387–394). New York: Guilford Press.

Schilder, P. (1950). *The image and appearance of the human body.* New York: International Universities Press.

Spiegel D., Butler L. D., Giese-Davis J., Koopman C., Miller E., Dimiceli S., et al. (2008). Reply to effects of supportive-expressive group therapy on survival of patients with metastatic breast cancer: A randomized prospective trial. *Cancer, 112*(2), 444.

Striegel-Moore, R., & Franko, D. (2002). Body image issues among girls and women. In T. Cash & T. Pruzinsky (Eds.), *Body image: A handbook of theory, research, and clinical progress* (pp. 183–191). New York: Guilford Press.

Swami, V., Furnham, A., Amin, R., Chaudri, J., Jundi, S., Miller, R., et al. (2008). Lonelier, lazier, and teased:

The stigmatizing effect of body size. *The Journal of Social Psychology, 148*(5), 577–593.

Swami, V., & Tovee, M. (2005). Female physical attractiveness in Britain and Malaysia: A cross cultural study. *Body Image, 2*, 115–128.

Thomas, A., Mosely, G., Stallings, R., Nichols-English, G., & Wagner, P. (2008). Perceptions of obesity. Black and white differences. *Journal of Cultural Diversity, 15*(4), 174–180.

Thombs, B. D., Notes, L. D., Lawrence, J. W., Magyar-Russell, G., Bresnick, M. G., Faurerbach, J. A., et al. (2008). From survival to socialization: A longitudinal study of body image in survivors of severe burn injury. *Journal of Psychosomatic Research, 64*(2), 205–212.

Thompson, J., & Gardner, R. (2002). Measuring perceptual body image in adolescents and adults. In T. Cash & T. Pruzinsky (Eds.), *Body image: A handbook of theory, research, and clinical progress* (pp. 142–154). New York: Guilford Press.

Thompson, A., & Kent, G. (2001). Adjusting to disfigurement: Process involved in dealing with being visibly different. *Clinical Psychology Review, 21*(5), 663–682.

Thompson, J., & Van Den Berg, P. (2002). Measuring body image attitudes among adolescents and adults. In T. Cash & T. Pruzinsky (Eds.), *Body image: A handbook of theory, research, and clinical progress* (pp. 155–162). New York: Guilford Press.

Tovee, M., Reinhardt, S., Emery, J., & Cornelissen, P. (1998). Optimum body mass index and maximum sexual attractiveness. *Lancet, 352*, 548.

Van Deusen, J. (1993). *Body image and perceptual dysfunction in adults*. Philadelphia: W. B. Saunders.

Veale, D. (2004). Advances in cognitive behavioural model of body dysmorphic disorder. *Body Image, 1*(1), 113–125.

Wetterhahn, K., Hanson, C., & Levy, C. (2002). Effect of participation in physical activity on body image of amputees. *American Journal of Physical Medicine and Rehabilitation, 81*(3), 194–201.

White, C. A. (2002). Body image issues in oncology. In T. Cash & T. Pruzinsky (Eds.), *Body image: A handbook of theory, research, and clinical progress* (pp. 379–386). New York: Guilford Press.

World Health Organization. (2011). Obesity and overweight: Fact sheet N311. Retrieved August 2, 2011, from: http://www.who.int/mediacentre/factsheets/fs311/en/index.html

Wright, L., & Leahey, M. (2000). *Nurses and families: A guide to family assessment and intervention* (3rd ed.). Philadelphia: F.A. Davis.

Y-ME National Breast Cancer Organization. (2007). Survey underscores importance of emotional, educational needs among women with advanced breast cancer. *Science Daily*. Retrieved August 2, 2011, from: http://www.sciencedaily.com/releases/2007/12/071216104300.htm

CHAPTER 7

Uncertainty

The words of the radiologist, "it's breast cancer," rang through my head over and over again as I sat in silence, alone, trying to make sense of this dreadful news. I couldn't believe my body had forsaken me. I felt betrayed. Why me? Would I survive? Could this be true? What if . . . ? Uncertainty built inside me, like a violent thunderstorm on a hot summer day. Uncertainty drenched me to my very core. That dark cloud of uncertainty follows me, even on the sunniest of days.

—Rita, 59-year-old female with breast cancer

Faye I. Hummel

INTRODUCTION

Uncertainty in chronic illness is pervasive. Chronic illness is marked by unpredictable changes in physical, cognitive, social, and lifestyle functions. Chronic illness restricts the terrain of the sufferer to local and familiar territory where one is least likely to be exposed to the gaze and questions of others (Goffman, 1963). With chronic illness, the timing, duration, and severity of symptoms are erratic. Misgivings about what one may be able to achieve in the present or in the future persist. Doubt about the success of treatment to slow disease progression and modify the disease course erodes self-confidence and generates stress and anxiety.

Chronic illness brings a prolonged state of impending adversity. The legend of Damocles' sword illuminates the insidious nature of uncertainty and chronic illness. In this tale, Damocles spoke of his sovereign's wealth and happiness, and as a result, Dionysius invited him to a great banquet at which Damocles was seated beneath a sharp sword suspended by a single hair (Encyclopedia Britannica, 2011). Damocles' sword symbolizes the precarious nature of everyday life for persons with chronic illness. On any given day, an individual with chronic illness may need to forego cherished or longed for activities, experience loss of freedom due to limitations and special needs, or be unable to purchase prescribed treatments and pharmaceuticals. Everyday life changes dramatically and is filled with unknowns. Uncertainty in chronic illness has been described as a cognitive stressor marked by a loss of control and a perception of doubt. Uncertainty impedes coping and adjustment to chronic illness, increases psychological and emotional distress, and diminishes quality of life.

The Nature of Uncertainty

Uncertainty arises when "details of situations are ambiguous, complex, unpredictable, or probabilistic; when information is unavailable or inconsistent; and when people feel insecure in their own state of knowledge or the state of knowledge in general" (Brashers, 2001, p. 478). Uncertainty is derived from one's self-perception of cognition. Thus, a person who believes him/herself to be uncertain is uncertain. Further, uncertainty may be experienced in relation to probability of an event. When the likelihood of an event is 0% or 100%, uncertainty is lowest. If there are multiple alternatives with equal probability, then uncertainty is highest (Brashers, 2001). Attributes of probability, perception, and temporality are present in every situation of uncertainty (McCormick, 2002).

Uncertainty is a hallmark of acute and chronic illness. Uncertainty is experienced by those with chronic illness who may fear rejection and social isolation; some may be concerned with diagnosis and treatment, while others may worry about recurrence of their illness even with improved physical health. An understanding of the nature of uncertainty enhances one's ability to describe and explain influences on behavior and develop interventions to improve people's lives (Brashers, 2001).

Uncertainty in Chronic Illness Is Certain

The dynamic nature of chronic illness makes uncertainty a part of life (Mishel, 1999). In acute illness, individuals act to decrease uncertainty, whereas individuals with chronic conditions seek to manage uncertainty. Even though uncertainty is experienced in the present, uncertainty is based on past experiences and assumptions for the future (Penrod, 2001). Embedded within the illness experience are ambiguity, inconsistency, vagueness, unpredictability, unfamiliarity, and the unknown, all creating uncertainty (Mishel, 1984). Persons with chronic illness experience situations and symptoms for which they have no experience or knowledge, thus triggering uncertainty. Uncertainty is a psychological state in which individuals initially perceive it and respond relative to how they believe it will impact them. As such, uncertainty is a neutral experience, neither good nor bad (Brashers, 2001; Mishel, 1988). The assessment of uncertainty as beneficial or harmful determines one's affective response to uncertainty (Mishel, 1988).

Uncertainty is the inability of an individual to understand the meaning of illness-related events such as disease process or treatment (Mishel, 1988) and one's perception of ambiguity, complexity, inconsistency, and unpredictability associated with illness and illness-related events (Mishel, 1984, 1990). Vague prognosis, lack of illness-related information, and unpredictability of symptoms and complications lead to uncertainty (Mishel, 1984, 1988).

When certainty exists, the future is taken for granted. When uncertainty exists, the future becomes the focus, with attempts to capture a clear vision of what was never clear to begin with (McCormick, 2002). Persons with chronic conditions do not know how their chronic illness will impact the future. They may feel good one day and incapacitated the next. They receive inconsistent information from healthcare providers and information sources about disease management and necessary lifestyle changes. Uncertainty clouds one's ability to determine if aches and pains are associated with the disease process or are benign.

Building on Mishel's (1981, 1988, 1990) theoretical work on uncertainty in acute and chronic illnesses, scholars have identified similar experiences of uncertainty in many chronic illnesses. Uncertainty is a universal phenomenon among chronic illnesses including cancer (Clayton, Mishel, & Belyea, 2006; Sammarco & Konecny, 2010); peritoneal dialysis (Madarv & Bar-Tal, 2009); Parkinson's disease (Sanders-Dewey, Mullins, & Chaney, 2001); multiple sclerosis (McNulty, Livneh, & Wilson, 2004); chronic pain (Johnson, Zautra, & Davis, 2006); organ transplantation (Lasker, Sogolow, Olenik, Sass, &Weinrieb, 2010; Martin, Stone, Scott, & Brashers, 2010); and HIV/AIDS (Brashers et al., 2003). Uncertainty influences the way in which individuals respond to a diagnosis, deal with illness symptoms, manage treatment regimens, and maintain social relationships.

Illness uncertainty influences coping with and adapting to fibromyalgia. Johnson and colleagues (2006) examined the role of uncertainty in coping with pain in 51 women with fibromyalgia. They found women who were experiencing greater pain levels and high illness uncertainty had more difficulty coping with their disease. Women with endometriosis reported uncertainty and emotional distress as a result of the complexity and impact of endometriosis on their lives (Lemaire, 2004). In persons undergoing home peritoneal dialysis, uncertainty was positively associated with self-rated illness severity (Madar & Bar-Tal, 2009).

Uncertainty is present across the illness trajectory, during events of diagnosis, treatment, and prognosis (Mishel, 1981, 1984, 1988). A longitudinal study examined uncertainty and anxiety in 127 women with suspected breast cancer during the diagnostic period. Results demonstrated that uncertainty and anxiety were significantly higher before the diagnosis than after the diagnosis. Uncertainty and anxiety were significantly lower for women diagnosed with benign disease than for those women with malignant diagnosis (Liao, Chen, Chen, & Chen, 2008).

Uncertainty was measured in three groups of adolescents and young adults with cancer at specific times in their cancer experience: newly diagnosed, diagnosed 1 to 4 years, and diagnosed 5 or more years. Overall level of uncertainty remained unchanged among the three groups, although differences did exist in the specific concerns related to uncertainty (Decker, Haase, & Bell, 2007). Women who had undergone surgery for ovarian malignancies reported that anxiety and depression played an important role in uncertainty throughout their illness (Schulman-Green, Ercolano, Dowd, Schwartz, & McCorkle, 2008).

Martin and colleagues (2010) identified sources of uncertainty across the transplantation trajectory. Thirty-eight participants who were waiting for or who had received an organ transplant were interviewed. During all phases of the transplant experience, participants reported medical, personal, and social forms of uncertainty. Denny (2009), in a qualitative study of 31 women with endometriosis, found uncertainty exists around diagnosis, disease course, and the future. In a longitudinal, descriptive study of persons with an implantable cardioverter defibrillator, twenty-one male participants—who were educated, married, and white—demonstrated that uncertainty did not change significantly over time (Mauro, 2010).

Uncertainty is pervasive and can persist for long periods of time even after life-saving procedures and treatments are complete (Martin et al., 2010; Mauro, 2010). Persson and Hellstrom (2002) reported uncertainty as a theme that emerged from interviews with nine patients after ostomy surgery. Similarly, uncertainty of cancer recurrence was highlighted by persons with colorectal cancer (Simpson & Whyte, 2006). For breast cancer survivors, survivor uncertainty persists long after treatment completion due to fear of recurrence (Dirksen & Erickson, 2002) and erodes quality of life (Sammarco & Konecny, 2008). Gil and colleagues (2004) examined the sources of uncertainty in 244 older African American and Caucasian long-term breast cancer survivors. They found the most important triggers for uncertainty were hearing about someone else's cancer and their own new aches and pains. Among breast cancer patients, uncertainty affects the illness experience, adaptation, quality of life, and sense of hope (Sammarco, 2001).

From the moment of my diagnosis of breast cancer to this very day two years later, uncertainty has been constant and consistent. First it was doubt about surgery and treatment. Were my healthcare providers competent? Did I have enough information to make the right decisions? Would I be able to handle all that was ahead of me? Even during the first year of being "cancer free," I always felt as though the other shoe was going to drop. And sure enough, results from a follow-up mammogram fueled my cancer fears. The biopsy showed no further breast

cancer, I was relieved but . . . I simply can't subdue the nagging doubt and fear that cancer will return at any time. Uncertainty, a constant reminder there simply is no guarantee with cancer.

—*Rita*

Older adults report less intolerance of uncertainty compared to their younger counterparts (Basevitz, Pushkar, Chaikelson, Conway, & Dalton, 2008). Uncertainty appears to decrease with age. Older people in Taiwan report less illness uncertainty than when they were younger (Lien, Lin, Kuo, & Chen, 2009). Younger Taiwanese women with breast cancer reported higher uncertainty due to concerns with changes in their physical condition, careers, and family roles (Liao et al., 2008).

Other uncertainty differences were noted in the literature. Sammarco and Konecny (2010) reported higher levels of uncertainty in Latina breast cancer survivors compared to Caucasian breast cancer survivors. Level of education affects uncertainty and stress; for example in one study (Madar & Bar-Tal, 2009), educated patients were better able to manage levels/feelings of uncertainty. The ability of patients to process information influences uncertainty.

Current research supports a positive association between symptom severity and uncertainty in chronic illness. Mullins and colleagues (2001) found a relationship between illness intrusiveness and uncertainty among persons with multiple sclerosis. Kang (2006) reported similar findings with adults diagnosed with atrial fibrillation. Those with greater symptom severity perceived more uncertainty. Wolfe-Christensen, Isenberg, Mullins, Carpentier, and Almstrom (2008) found a similar relationship among college students with asthma. Mullins, Chaney, Balderson, and Hommel (2000) found with increased illness severity, uncertainty had a significant effect on depression in young adults with long-standing asthma.

Uncertainty and Social Networks

Illness uncertainty affects the individual with chronic illness as well as those within his/her social network, including caregivers, family members, and friends. Members of a social network of someone with a chronic illness face their own feelings and fears of uncertainty and unpredictability (Mitchell, Courtney, & Coyer, 2003; Northouse et al., 2002; Donovan-Kicken & Bute, 2008) and may experience discomfort and anxiety about how to act and what to say to the person with chronic illness. Adults with a parent with probable Alzheimer's disease reported uncertainty about the medical aspects of Alzheimer's disease, including etiology, symptoms, treatment, and prognosis. They reported uncertainty about their own predisposition for Alzheimer's disease as well as conflicting caregiver roles and their financial responsibilities. Social sources of uncertainty experienced by these families included unpredictability of social reactions and social interactions, including family dynamics (Stone & Jones, 2009).

In a qualitative study investigating the experiences of informal caregivers, including spouses and adult children of stroke survivors, Greenwood, Mackenzie, Wilson, and Cloud (2009) reported uncertainty as a central theme. Reich, Olmsted, and van Puymbroeck (2006) reported uncertainty significantly impacted the partner relationships of patients with fibromyalgia.

Uncertainty among family and friends of someone with a chronic illness is managed by seeking information from a variety of sources including the Internet, professional and mainstream publications, healthcare providers, support groups, and other members in their social network (Donovan-Kicken & Bute, 2008).

Sources of Uncertainty

Uncertainty permeates all aspects of one's life including diagnosis, treatment, and prognosis. Medical uncertainty has been associated with insufficient information about diagnosis, ambiguous symptoms and disease trajectory, and complex treatments and interventions (Mishel, 1988, 1990). In research conducted with persons with HIV disease, Brashers and colleagues (2003) extended Mishel's (1990) model of uncertainty in illness to include not only medical uncertainty but also personal and social sources of uncertainty. Sources of medical uncertainty identified by persons with HIV disease were ambiguity with their HIV diagnosis and associated diagnostic tests as well as unpredictability and multiplicity of opportunistic infections. Personal sources of uncertainty were related to the invisibility of their chronic illness, social roles, and precarious financial situations due to the expense of necessary medications (Brashers et al., 2003). Families coping with Alzheimer's disease reported similar sources of uncertainty. Interviews with participants in Sammarco and Konecny's (2010) examination of the experiences of adult children of a parent with Alzheimer's disease revealed medical, personal, and social sources of uncertainty.

CASE STUDY

Jim, age 70, lives with his wife, Nancy, age 68. Both Jim and Nancy are retired. They have been married for 25 years and have no children. Both are in excellent physical health. They have many friends and have been active in social and community organizations and events. They enjoy sports and travel frequently. Two years ago, with little notice, Jim began having difficulty remembering minor things, such as where he put his keys, or what he had for breakfast. He thought these changes were probably just a sign of "old age." But with time, Jim experienced even more difficulty with his memory and after a number of tests and physician visits, he was diagnosed with Alzheimer's disease. This devastating news was confusing and overwhelming. Jim and Nancy were consumed with questions, and worries and stress. Jim began pharmacological treatment for his Alzheimer's disease. When one drug failed to slow his symptoms, he tried another. As Jim's cognitive abilities continued to slowly erode, he experienced more frustration, anxiety, and depression with associated fatigue and loss of appetite. Nancy has been very attentive to Jim's needs and provides psychological and behavioral support. She has cut back on her social activities to minimize the time Jim is home alone. They now see their friends less frequently and often decline invitations for social gatherings. Nancy and Jim are reluctant to travel despite a long planned trip to Mexico.

Discussion Questions

1. Discuss how uncertainty is manifested in Alzheimer's disease for Jim. Discuss for Nancy.
2. Explore the issue of uncertainty for a chronic illness using the four constructs of uncertainty (ambiguity, complexity, inconsistency, and unpredictability).
3. How is uncertainty different and similar for the person with chronic illness compared to the caregiver? Compared to others in the social network?
4. Design an action plan to assist persons with chronic illnesses and their families to manage uncertainty and promote quality of life.

THEORETICAL UNDERPINNINGS OF UNCERTAINTY _____

Early work on uncertainty distinguished clinical from functional uncertainty (Davis, 1960). McIntosh (1974, 1976) examined uncertainty in persons with cancer and other chronic conditions. Mishel (1981) posited uncertainty as one's inability to form a cognitive schema, which is created when stimuli are recognized and classified, a process that gives meaning to an event. Based on Lazarus and Folkman's (1984) stress and coping framework, Mishel (1988) developed a middle range theory of uncertainty to explain how people with illness cognitively process illness-related stimuli to construct meaning for illness events. This theory purports that uncertainty occurs when there is difficulty constructing a cognitive schema—a person's subjective interpretation—of illness events. Mishel subsequently extended her theory to uncertainty in chronic illness. Mishel (1990) recognized those with acute illness experienced time-limited uncertainty whereas those with chronic conditions experienced uncertainty throughout their lives. Mishel's theory progressed from predicting, controlling, and eliminating uncertainty to include managing and accepting uncertainty as a way of life in chronic illness.

Mishel (1988) identified the primary antecedent of uncertainty as stimuli frame. Stimuli frame has three components: symptom pattern, event familiarity, and event congruence. Symptom pattern is the consistency of symptoms to form a pattern. Event familiarity is the degree to which a situation is habitual, repetitive, or contains recognizable cues and is determined by time and experience in a healthcare environment (Mishel, 1988, p. 225). Event congruence is the consistency between the expected and actual experience with an illness-related event. Events are reliable and stable, subsequently facilitating interpretation and understanding. These three components of the stimuli frame reduce uncertainty (Mishel, 1988).

The stimuli frame is influenced by two variables: cognitive capacity and structure providers. Cognitive capacity is the ability of the person to process information. Limited cognitive capacity due to information overload, ability of a person to process information, and the physiologic factors that may impair cognitive ability diminish the ability to recognize the symptom pattern, event familiarity, and event congruence. The second variable, structural providers, are the resources used to interpret the stimuli frame. Structure providers reduce uncertainty by assisting in the interpretation of an illness event or by helping identify symptom patterns, event familiarity, and event congruence. Structure providers include credible authority, social support, and education (Mishel, 1988). Credible authority is the degree to which a person has trust and confidence in his/her healthcare provider. Social support is the ability of the person to express his/her thoughts and feelings with those (e.g., family, social network) who are also experiencing the disease. Together these variables support development of a cognitive schema for interpretation of illness events, and thus reduce uncertainty (Mishel, 1988).

Persons with chronic illness cannot assign a definite value to objects or events or predict outcomes with accuracy (Bailey et al., 2009). If one does not have sufficient cues to structure or categorize an illness event, uncertainty arises. Inconsistent symptom patterns, lack of familiarity with healthcare providers and procedures, and unanticipated illness experiences contribute to one's uncertainty. Further, one's stimulus frame is influenced by his or her cognitive capacity and structure providers such as education, social support, and credible authority which assist the individual in interpreting the stimulus frame. One's cognitive capacity may be impaired by illness-related factors such as pain or medication, creating difficulty in constructing meaning from the stimuli cues. On the other hand, receiving assurance from a trusted and competent healthcare provider about some aspect of his or her chronic condition can diminish uncertainty.

Illness uncertainty has four forms: 1) ambiguity about the illness; 2) complexity of the treatment and healthcare system; 3) inadequate information about the disease and its seriousness; and 4) unpredictability about the disease and its trajectory (Mishel, 1988). Uncertainty may lead to psychological distress if coping responses are insufficient to resolve or manage uncertainty.

Uncertainty is neutral until it is assessed to be a danger or an opportunity. Illness events perceived as a danger imply harm. Uncertainty is perceived as a threat to well-being based on previous personal experiences. With perceived harm, coping strategies are implemented to reduce uncertainty. Uncertain events evaluated as opportunity imply a positive outcome. Appraisal of uncertainty as an opportunity is explained as construction of a positive meaning for an event based on one's personal beliefs or purposeful misrepresentation (Mishel, 1990). In the case of uncertainty as an opportunity, strategies to maintain uncertainty are initiated. If coping strategies are effective, adaptation will occur (Mishel, 1988).

Mishel and Braden (1988) tested the theoretical variables of uncertainty with 61 women with gynecological cancer. Their research found that these women had low levels of uncertainty. Further, they found significant relationships between uncertainty and theory variables, symptom patterns, event familiarity, credible authority, social support, and education. Mast (1998) explored the antecedents of uncertainty in research with 109 survivors of breast cancer. As a result, antecedent variables proposed by Mishel (1988) were modified to include symptom distress, concurrent illness, and fear of recurrence. Wallace (2005) conducted research to examine the antecedents associated with uncertainty in 19 men with prostate cancer who were undergoing watchful-waiting management. Study results revealed significant relationships between level of education, length of illness, and uncertainty, lending support to Mishel's (1988) Uncertainty in Illness Model and enhancing understanding of factors that influence uncertainty.

Ambiguity and subsequent uncertainty can generate stress and inhibit effective coping (Lazarus & Folkman, 1984). Uncertainty is one of the greatest challenges in successfully adapting to chronic illness. Individuals with a variety of chronic illnesses experiencing increased levels of uncertainty experience diminished levels of adjustment (McNulty et al., 2004). In a sample of 50 individuals with multiple sclerosis (MS), researchers examined the contributions of illness uncertainty and spiritual well-being to psychosocial adaptation. Spiritual well-being influenced adaptation to MS and mitigated the impact of uncertainty on adaptation (McNulty et al., 2004).

Bailey and colleagues (2009) examined the constructs of ambiguity, complexity, inconsistency, and unpredictability in 126 persons undergoing a watchful-waiting protocol for individuals with chronic hepatitis C. Ambiguity was identified as a primary construct of illness uncertainty having the strongest relationships with depressive symptoms, quality of life, and fatigue. Persons with chronic hepatitis C responded to ambiguity by limiting their investment of energy in future activities, acting on information they perceived important, and favoring nonthreatening explanations of symptoms. These results give healthcare providers parameters for assisting persons with chronic illness self-management interventions.

Uncertainty as Opportunity

Mishel (1988) proposed reconceptualization of uncertainty from a deficit to a source of personal growth. Uncertainty outcomes are not always negative. Uncertainty can be a useful coping mechanism for persons with chronic illness. Sometimes not knowing is better than knowing (Greenwood et al., 2009).

> March was our "ignorance is bliss" month. Radiation and chemotherapy were over in February, and although the effects of the treatment had been brutal, we felt that better days surely were coming. R's next PET scan wasn't scheduled until mid-April, giving us 6 weeks of respite from treatment, albeit uncertainty as well as respite. However, it served as a healing time for us mentally. The future might be bright or bleak, as we were uncertain what the PET scan would show, but somehow, not knowing was OK. We were able to move cancer to the side for awhile.
>
> —*Jenny, wife of a 63-year-old man with*
> *Stage III esophageal cancer*

Uncertainty can provide the opportunity for persons with chronic illness to reevaluate their lives and establish priorities. The literature reflects evidence of positive reappraisal including increased tolerance and appreciation for others, greater self-acceptance, increased optimism and joy in life (McCormick, 2002), getting a second chance in life, and enjoying the simple pleasures and small things in life. In the case of a potentially negative outcome, uncertainty can be more desirable than certainty. Maintaining a level of uncertainty can help an individual with a chronic illness to preserve hope (Brashers, Goldsmith, & Hsieh, 2002; Mishel, 1988).

Uncertainty as Harm

The chronic illness experience can trigger perceptions of harm that increase illness uncertainty. Factors that promote uncertainty are discussed in this section.

Stress and Uncertainty

Uncertainty is a significant psychological stressor, particularly in a cultural context that values predictability and control (Mishel, 1990). It is also associated with decreased quality of life (Mishel, 1983, 1999) and diminished coping with illness symptoms (Johnson et al., 2006). Other psychological dimensions of chronic illness are fear and anxiety, coping, and worry. Chronic psychological stress of living with a chronic illness is associated with anticipation of an unwanted decline. The inability to make a prediction about one's disease course is stressful. For example, uncertainty is significantly associated with decreased perceived control and increased psychological distress in adolescents with type 1 diabetes (Hoff, Mullins, Chaney, Hartman, & Domek, 2002). This can result in psychological distress if coping responses are not sufficient to resolve the uncertainty.

A high degree of uncertainty is related to increased emotional distress, anxiety, and depression (McCormick, 2002). Persons with MS who reported greater uncertainty about their chronic illness were less hopeful and had more negative moods (Wineman, Schwetz, Zeller, & Cyphert, 2003). In 44 dyads composed of individuals with Parkinson's disease and their caregivers, uncertainty in illness did not predict distress for persons with the disease; however, uncertainty emerged as a significant predictor of distress for their caregivers. Caregivers reported stress as they faced an uncertain future regarding their caregiver responsibilities and tasks (Sanders-Dewey et al., 2001). Addressing psychological issues in chronic illness is vital to diminishing uncertainty and increasing quality of life (Lasker et al., 2010).

Anxiety

Increased illness uncertainty was associated with greater anxiety in a sample of 56 older adolescents with childhood-onset asthma (Hommel et al., 2003). Fifty research studies were examined to synthesize the state of the science on uncertainty in relation to women undergoing diagnostic evaluation for suspected breast cancer. All studies reported anxiety persisting throughout the diagnostic period until the final diagnosis (Montgomery, 2010).

Loss of Control

One's perception of self-control impacts illness uncertainty (Mishel, 1997). A decline in self-efficacy and sense of mastery may contribute to a lack of confidence in making decisions about treatment and daily activities. Because of uncertainty, persons with chronic conditions frequently put their lives on hold. Loss of control is a component of uncertainty. Mishel (1988) hypothesized that persons with high internal locus of control would be more likely to perceive uncertainty as an opportunity, but people with an external locus of control would appraise uncertainty as a threat or danger. If the person's external locus of control is related to a strong belief in a higher power, then uncertainty may not necessarily be viewed as a threat or danger by the individual (McCormick, 2002).

Waiting

Waiting is a hallmark of the healthcare system. Waiting creates a loss of control for those who must wait for treatment decisions, test results, appointments, and so forth. Waiting produces anxiety, depression, panic, and uncertainty (Bailey, Wallace, & Mishel, 2007; Mishel, 1999; Wallace, 2003). Waiting is "a grueling experience of unsure stillness" (Bournes & Mitchell, 2002, p. 62). For women suspected of having breast cancer, waiting is limbo (Montgomery, 2010). In a qualitative research study with 21 women and 5 men who had been affected by cancer, waiting emerged as a theme. Waiting was described by many of the informants "as the worst part of the cancer experience: waiting for diagnosis, waiting for treatment, waiting for remission, and waiting for relapse" (Mulcahy, Parry, & Glover, 2010, p. 1065–1066). Waiting became a feature of the cancer experience, exacerbating the constant uncertainty at each stage of the cancer journey.

McCormick, McClement, and Naimark (2005) explored the experience of waiting for coronary artery bypass surgery. Telephone interviews were conducted with 25 participants. The study authors concluded that lengthy waits resulted in significant psychological disturbance, including anxiety and uncertainty about the future.

Watchful waiting is a protocol often used in chronic conditions. Watchful waiting is observation, expectant management, active monitoring, or deferred treatment (Wallace, Bailey, O'Rourke, & Galbraith, 2004). Watchful waiting provokes uncertainty. Without active treatment, many persons with chronic conditions are left worrying about how their illness will unfold in the future; for example, the person may wonder: "Is the cancer growing while we wait?" As such, these persons must not only manage their lives with a chronic illness but deal with uncertainty about disease progression (Bailey et al., 2009).

Lack of Information

Information may increase or decrease uncertainty. Information about a particular chronic illness may or may not be readily available to clients and their social network. Information from various sources may lack consistency and may be contradictory. Additionally, individuals who seek information may not have the cognitive abilities to comprehend, integrate, and apply the information. Health information can be challenging and difficult to understand. Frequently, health information contains medical jargon that is not easily understood. Healthcare providers may provide unsolicited and unwanted advice to individuals in an attempt to manage the uncertainty.

Compounding these issues with the availability of information, outcomes in chronic illness are difficult to predict. There aren't clear milestones in the chronic illness trajectory due to individual differences and responses to the illness and treatment. Due to this unpredictability, it is challenging for the healthcare provider to provide an accurate progression of disease or timeline, thus adding to uncertainty.

In a correlational study with 71 patients undergoing peritoneal dialysis, Madar and Bar-Tal (2009) examined factors of severity and duration of disease, credible authority of healthcare providers, social support and education, and levels of uncertainty and stress. Patients' self-rated health, level of education, and their perception of their doctors as credible authorities contributed significantly to explaining patients' uncertainty. Uncertainty and stress were influenced by the patient's level of education. Factors associated with a patient's ability to process information most influenced their uncertainty.

Patients need healthcare providers to deliver the desired level and amount of information to the patient as well as assess the psychological and physical qualities that potentially contribute to uncertainty. The level of education of the person with chronic illness affects the time needed for that individual to construct meaning and context for the events in chronic illness. Persons with more education, more social support, and more trust in healthcare providers experience less uncertainty (Mishel, 1988).

Evidence-Based Practice Box

Illness uncertainty continues long after cancer diagnosis and treatment. Older women who have survived breast cancer experience ongoing illness uncertainty, fears about cancer recurrence, and symptoms from treatment side effects. Vicarious experiences such as hearing about cancer in a friend, having unfamiliar aches and pains, and media coverage about cancer can trigger feelings of uncertainty. Based on the theory of uncertainty in illness (Mishel, 1988, 1997), an uncertainty management intervention for older long-term breast cancer survivors was developed. The intervention consisted of cognitive-behavioral messages delivered by audiotapes and a self-help manual. Four hundred eighty-three recurrence-free women (342 white and 141 African American women) were randomly assigned to either the intervention or usual care (control) group. Nurses guided women through the intervention during four weekly telephone sessions and

(continues)

focused on one of four skills: relaxation, pleasant imagery, calming self-talk, and distraction. The nurses guided the women through the self-help manual that contained educational material and resources. Results indicated that the intervention in uncertainty management resulted in improvements in cognitive reframing (viewing their situation in a more positive light), cancer knowledge, and a variety of coping skills. At 20 months post-intervention, women continued to demonstrate benefits from the intervention in terms of decline in illness uncertainty and improved personal growth. Cognitive-behavioral interventions are beneficial to women with chronic illness. These interventions improve knowledge and behavioral skills and help foster a more positive appraisal of illness. This research supports the importance of nurses to assist persons with chronic illness in identifying appropriate sources of information and in developing behavioral skills.

Sources: Gil, K. M., Mishel, M. H., Belyea, M., Germino, B., Porter, L. S., & Clayton, M. (2006). Benefits of the uncertainty management intervention for African American and white older breast cancer survivors: 20-month outcomes. *International Journal of Behavioral Medicine, 13*(4), 286–294.

Gil, K. M., Mishel, M. H., Germino, B., Porter, L. S., Carlton-LaNey, I., & Belyea, M. (2005). Uncertainty management intervention for older African American and Caucasian long-term breast cancer survivors. *Journal of Psychosocial Oncology*, 23, 3–21.

INTERVENTIONS

Certainty and predictability of outcomes are valued in Western society. When persons face chronic conditions with uncertain outcomes, they search for a cure (Mishel, 1990). The goal of nursing interventions is to reduce uncertainty in persons with chronic illness and promote self-confidence in their abilities, thus increasing certainty in their daily lives. There are a number of factors that have been demonstrated to enhance self-confidence and promote certainty. Social support that enables the person with a chronic illness to rely on others including family members, friends, or healthcare professionals enhances self-confidence and certainty. Education and information given at the right time, at the right place, and at the right educational level are essential to enhancing certainty. Trust and confidence in one's healthcare provider are essential in managing chronic illness.

Chronic illness is complex and often poorly understood as there are no cures, and treatment effectiveness varies. Predicting outcomes is difficult and increases uncertainty. Despite extensive research and practice knowledge about the trajectory of chronic illness, individual characteristics and diversity of symptom experiences produce unpredictability. Uncertainty looms large with limited information about the course of the disease and treatment options. Negative effects of uncertainty can be ameliorated by anticipating and understanding patients' individual needs along their illness trajectory.

Managing uncertainty is complex and dynamic and requires thoughtful and vigilant assessment by the healthcare provider. For some, lack of information may stimulate uncertainty. Others may embrace uncertainty and not desire more information, because more information might bring bad news. Some may embrace a watch-and-wait perspective rather than seek information about the future. Negative effects of uncertainty can be ameliorated by anticipating and understanding a patient's needs along their illness trajectory.

Strategies to maximize perceptions of confidence and control are essential to the management of uncertainty. Cognitive, emotive, and behavioral strategies act in concert to alter a patient's perception of uncertainty. First, however, an assessment of the psychological and physical factors that potentially contribute to uncertainty is essential. Persons experiencing chronic illness need healthcare professionals to provide the desired level and amount of information to them and their social network. Interventions to manage uncertainty across the chronic illness trajectory include strategies to 1) control emotion, 2) restructure life to incorporate the unpredictability of symptoms and promote normalization of life, and 3) understand the illness to better formulate an illness schema (Mishel, 1999). The strategies for management of illness uncertainty discussed in this section are based on Mishel's (1988) Uncertainty Theory. See **Figure 7-1**.

Cognitive Strategies

Uncertainty can be reduced by cognitive strategies that provide and process facts, assist with problem solving, and address knowledge deficits. Uncertainty can be diminished by providing clients and families with information and skills needed to alter their perception of stress. Meaning can be enhanced through personalized plans of care and appropriate educational interventions. Nurses can reduce uncertainty with "structural resources" that include education, social support, and care from healthcare providers who are credible sources of confidence and authority (Donovan-Kicken & Bute, 2008; Mishel, 1988, 1999).

Education

Increased availability of education that adds to patient and family knowledge reduces uncertainty (Clayton et al., 2006; Donovan-Kicken & Bute, 2008). Information reduces uncertainty and facilitates understanding of the chronic disease (Mishel, 1988). However, it is important to note individual differences. For some persons with chronic illness, their uncertainty can be reduced by seeking out information and taking action based on that

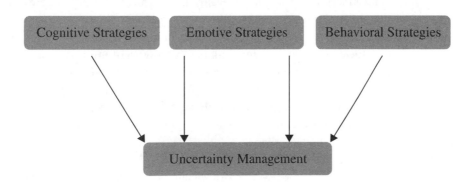

FIGURE 7-1 Adaptation to Uncertainty.

information. Others use avoidance to protect themselves from undesirable information.

Education for clients and their social support network has long been the hallmark of quality health care. Regardless of the inevitability of disease progression and physical deterioration intrinsic to chronic illness, education is an effective tool to promote a sense of control and manage uncertainty. Unfortunately, it is often difficult to ascertain the amount of information that individuals want or can process. As healthcare providers, we often provide more information, particularly in the beginning of a disease process, than the person with chronic illness and family can absorb. More is not always better. A thorough assessment of the needs of the individual and family, taking into account their educational background, past life experiences and cultural beliefs, form the basis for educational interventions.

The healthcare provider should be aware that for some patients, health information does not decrease uncertainty. Not knowing may be less threatening and less stressful than potentially bad news (Brashers et al., 2002; Brashers, Neidig, & Goldsmith, 2004). For other persons, having adequate information enables them to cope, participate in healthcare decisions, and deal with illness uncertainty. The premise that individuals with chronic illness and their families desire information and options for their treatment and care is a valued feature of Western healthcare practice. However, for many in diverse social groups, healthcare decisions are within the purview of others, whether they are family members or healthcare providers. Healthcare providers must assess when informational support is appropriate. The role of education in reducing uncertainty is complex (Clayton et al. 2006).

The literature on treatment decision making suggests those who resist assuming this active role may be overwhelmed, misinformed as to the treatment options, and, in general, lack the capacity to participate. In a qualitative study with five women diagnosed with breast cancer, in-depth interviews revealed patients' ambivalence in making treatment decisions were efforts to recast identities and positions of patients and physicians in the cancer care organization. Patients seek not only information but interpretation of information by their oncologists (Sinding et al., 2010).

Cultural values and beliefs must be considered in education. Persons from family-centered cultures may be reluctant to assume responsibility for seeking information about their chronic disease and treatment and rely on family members to take charge. In family-centered cultures, families interact with healthcare providers to seek information and may handle information in such a manner as to shield the person with the chronic illness from negative information that may result in the loss of hope (Brashers et al., 2002).

Nurses play a pivotal role by providing the right education in the right manner and at the appropriate point in the illness trajectory. Nurses may assist individuals in identifying credible sources of information that match the cognitive processing ability of the client. Healthcare providers need to be aware of local and national sources of information and support related to chronic conditions. Many chronic conditions have voluntary agencies with resources that provide information and other social support. Professional organizations are excellent resources for persons with a chronic condition and also for healthcare providers.

Know Thy Illness

Knowledge of self-management programs that incorporate information about the chronic disease is essential for the individual and family.

Identification of triggers that exacerbate illness symptoms and the activities that help modify and manage those symptoms are also important aspects of self-management.

Persons with chronic illness experience uncertainty when making decisions regarding treatment options and subsequent interventions. Nurses need to be aware of this uncertainty and provide support and information to help make informed decisions (Guadalupe, 2010).

Symptom Management

Individuals often have difficulty managing chronic illness symptoms (O'Neill & Morrow, 2001). Nursing assessment and intervention must include attention to symptom management. Individuals may need assistance in setting priorities for activities of daily living, strategies to diminish illness symptoms such as fatigue or pain, and fostering a plan of care that engenders confidence and normalcy to the highest degree possible. Interventions need to focus on physiological and emotional response to illness.

Designing and Adapting Routines

Individuals with chronic illness are unable to make predictions about the impact of illness on their lives. To help facilitate predictability, healthcare providers can assist the client and family to focus on planning for the short term and for events with immediate consequences. Individuals can make decisions and make plans despite uncertainty. People can cushion the effects of uncertainty by developing a structure or routine that encourages familiar and recognizable patterns of behavior.

Social Support

Social support plays an important role in uncertainty and adaptation. Social support can provide stable relationships where people can openly express emotions and feelings and find reassurance of their humanness and worthiness. Supportive others assist those with chronic conditions to reappraise uncertainty as opportunity or inconsequential and to incorporate uncertainty as a normal part of life. Social support directly and indirectly reduces uncertainty (Mishel, 1988; Lien et al., 2009) and promotes coping with chronic illness. Social support facilitates information seeking and avoidance and encourages reappraisal of uncertainty (Brashers et al., 2004). When persons with chronic illness have the opportunity to discuss and reflect on their illness, they gain insight and clarity about their situation and achieve more certainty (Bar-Tel, Barnoy, & Zisser, 2005). Active and reflective listening by nurses are key strategies to promote opportunity for persons with chronic illness to reflect and gain understanding of their illness experience.

Healthcare providers must be aware of the importance of social support in not only reducing uncertainty but enhancing quality of life. In Latina breast cancer survivors, perceived social support and uncertainty played a pivotal role in managing and maintaining quality of life. Perceived social support promoted quality of life while uncertainty diminished quality of life (Sammarco & Konecny, 2008). Sammarco and Konecny (2010) examined the differences between Latina and Caucasian breast cancer survivors and their perceived social support, uncertainty, and quality of life. Caucasians reported significantly higher levels of perceived social support and quality of life than their Latina counterparts. Healthcare providers must be aware of these differences and integrate cultural values and demographic differences into their plans of care in addressing quality of life.

Advice giving is a form of social support that may or may not be helpful. Advice giving is an effective support intervention when the advice is appropriate, relevant, and presented in a positive manner. However, when giving advice to persons with chronic illness, healthcare providers need to assess whether the individual wants their advice. If the individual is not receptive to advice, then other forms of support such as active listening or emotional support may be more appropriate (Thompson & O'Hair, 2008).

The nurse may need to assist the client in establishing a helpful social network. In addition to family members and friends, nurses and other healthcare providers are an important source of social support. Brashers and colleagues (2004) examined the effect of social support on management of uncertainty in persons living with HIV or AIDS. They found social support helps people with HIV and AIDS through information gathering and avoiding; providing instrumental support, skill development, acceptance, and validation; allowing venting; and encouraging shifts in perspective.

Emotive Strategies

Emotive intervention strategies alter feelings of uncertainty. Management programs that enhance coping and improve overall well-being are effective in persons with chronic illness (Gil et al., 2006).

Normalization

An emotive method to manage uncertainty in chronic illness is to restructure life to incorporate the unpredictability of chronic illness symptom onset, severity, and duration. Living in the present, one day at a time, reduces uncertainty. Activities of daily living are designed to incorporate realistic expectations and include a contingency plan.

Control Emotion

Strategies to control emotion are used by persons with chronic illnesses to control uncertainty. Healthcare professionals must assist clients and their families with viewing uncertainty as an opportunity. Uncertainty can be used to move from a perspective of limited choice to that of multiple opportunities (Mishel, 1990).

Formulate Cognitive Schema

Mishel (1999) suggested forming illness schema as a management method for uncertainty. Nurses can work with clients with chronic illness to construct personal scenarios of their illness that include the beginning of the illness, the progression of the illness, and how recovery will occur. This provides clients with an opportunity to integrate incongruent events into an individualized illness framework that provides meaning and understanding. Promoting self-care behaviors facilitates redefining an uncertain situation into one that is manageable.

Trust and Confidence in Healthcare Providers

Chronic illness requires attention to issues of life and death and wellness and illness, as well as daily management of symptoms and treatment. Trust and confidence in healthcare providers plays a significant role in reducing uncertainty in persons with chronic illness (Madar & Bar-Tal, 2009).

Becoming Engaged

Becoming engaged in support groups and other support resources allows persons with chronic illness to have a sense of control over their illness. When people are engaged in the decisions regarding the management of their condition and are more informed about their options, they have a greater sense of control. However, patients may experience obstacles in becoming engaged in support services and groups because of fatigue, illness, or lack of confidence and resources. Nurses need to assess the client for the capability and desire to become engaged. Available and appropriate resources need to be identified and referred to the client and family.

Mindfulness

Mindfulness is an attribute of consciousness associated with psychological well-being. Brown and Ryan (2003) report a relationship between mindfulness and positive emotional states. Mindfulness-based stress reduction employs techniques that help individuals cope with clinical and nonclinical problems (Grossman, Niemann, Schmidt, & Walach, 2004) and mitigate the negative effects of illness uncertainty. An intervention study of persons with cancer demonstrated that increased mindfulness over time resulted in decreases in mood disturbances and stress (Brown & Ryan, 2003). Mindfulness techniques are accessible to everyone and do not require financial resources or special equipment. Nurses can assist their clients with chronic illness to identify appropriate and acceptable mindfulness strategies to incorporate in their activities of daily living. These activities focus on outcomes such as acceptance and living in the present, and recognition and acknowledgment of negative thoughts, feelings, or coping difficulties. Mindfulness exercises to reduce the negative effects of uncertainty include meditation, deep breathing exercises, and listening to music.

Cognitive Reframing

Cognitive reframing techniques are powerful tools that assist clients with chronic illness to deal with and manage symptoms, reduce uncertainty, and find meaning in life as it changes. Cognitive reframing seeks to alter one's cognitive schema and identify other ways of interpreting present and future situations and circumstances. Cognitive reframing in essence puts a new perspective on a situation while acknowledging the reality of the situation.

Bailey and colleagues (2004) evaluated the effectiveness of an intervention to help men cognitively reframe and manage the uncertainty of watchful waiting. Those in the intervention group received weekly calls from a nurse and those in the control group received usual care. Intervention participants reported greater improvement in the quality of their life and their future quality of life compared to the control group, thus documenting the effectiveness of cognitive reframing in reducing uncertainty.

Nurses can teach clients reframing strategies by helping them examine their expectations and exploring ways to set realistic expectations for themselves. Nurses can assist clients with acknowledging their changing needs and making modifications, substitutions, and adaptations when necessary and appropriate to accommodate their changing needs. Cognitive reframing requires ongoing attention and repetition, thus nurses must provide ongoing encouragement and support for clients to use this technique successfully. Cognitive reframing techniques help persons with chronic illness rethink their perceptions of uncertainty and can impact mood and hopefulness.

Behavioral Strategies

Healthcare providers must be alert to expressions of uncertainty. These expressions can be ascertained in language and in behavior such as withdrawing from self-care activities or social interaction.

Activities of Daily Living

A focus on daily routines and expectations reduces uncertainty and diminishes anxiety. Living in the present with a "today focus" rather than a "tomorrow focus" helps reduce uncertainty. (Greenwood et al., 2009).

Managing Unpredictability: Anticipatory Guidance

In anticipation of progressive disability, nurses may refer persons to rehabilitative therapies for interventions designed to enhance and prolong independence in their daily activities, occupation, and relationships. Members of the interdisciplinary team should be used to help the client and family deal with financial or vocational issues that may contribute to uncertainty. Individuals may seek out advice from others who had the same condition to assist them in anticipating an effective way to engage in health promotion and maintenance activities.

OUTCOMES

Uncertainty is chronic and persists over the trajectory of disease. Accepting uncertainty is an adaptive mechanism (Mishel, 1990). Negative effects of uncertainty can be ameliorated by anticipating and understanding individual needs across the disease course. Nurses and other healthcare professionals can work with persons with chronic illness to modify negative outcomes of the illness experience and promote positive perceptions of uncertainty.

Nurses are valuable partners of persons with chronic conditions and their families in assisting them to cope with uncertain experiences by providing positive communication and support. Nursing assessments and interventions directed toward reducing uncertainty can improve quality of life and adaptation to living with chronic conditions (Elphee, 2008). Assessment of uncertainty needs to be included as an element of all nursing assessments of persons with chronic illness. Theory-based nursing interventions designed to educate and support persons with chronic illness to integrate and manage uncertainty across their disease trajectory are essential. Unacknowledged and unaddressed uncertainty can erode quality of life for those with chronic conditions and for those in their social network.

STUDY QUESTIONS   WWW

Describe the social and cultural factors related to uncertainty in chronic illness.

Apply Mishel's Theory of Uncertainty to one of your clients with a chronic condition.

How does cognitive reframing assist a client with uncertainty?

Describe how one would assess a patient and family for their educational/informational needs.

The primary antecedent of Mishel's theory is the stimuli frame. Describe its components and how they influence uncertainty.

Seeing uncertainty as "harm" is understandable, but how can uncertainty be seen as an opportunity?

For a full suite of assignments and additional learning activities, use the access code located in the front of your book and visit this exclusive website: **http://go.jblearning.com/larsen**. If you do not have an access code, you can obtain one at the site.

REFERENCES

Bailey, D. E., Landerman, L., Barroso, J., Bixby, P., Mishel, M. H., Muir, A. J., et al. (2009). Uncertainty, symptoms, and quality of life in persons with chronic hepatitis C. *Psychosomatics, 50*(2), 138–146.

Bailey, D. E., Mishel, M. H., Belyea, M., Stewart, J. L., & Mohler, J. (2004).Uncertainty intervention for watchful waiting in prostate cancer. *Cancer Nursing, 27*(5), 339–346.

Bailey, D. E., Wallace, M., & Mishel, M. H. (2007). Watching, waiting and uncertainty in prostate cancer. *Journal of Clinical Nursing, 16,* 734–741.

Bar-Tel, Y., Barnoy, S., & Zisser, B. (2005). Whose informational needs are considered? A comparison between cancer patients and their spouses' perceptions of their own and their partners' knowledge and informational needs. *Social Science & Medicine, 60*(7), 1459–1465.

Basevitz, P., Pushkar, D., Chaikelson, J., Conway, M., & Dalton, C. (2008). Age-related differences in worry and related processes. *International Journal of Aging and Human Development, 66*(4), 283–305.

Bournes, D. A., & Mitchell, G. J. (2002). Waiting: The experience of persons in a critical care waiting room. *Research in Nursing & Health, 25,* 58–67.

Brashers, D. E. (2001). Communication and uncertainty management. *Journal of Communication, 51,* 477–497.

Brashers, D. E., Goldsmith, D. J., & Hsieh, E. (2002). Information seeking and avoiding in health contexts. *Human Communication Research, 28,* 258–271.

Brashers, D. E., Neidig, J. L., & Goldsmith, D. J. (2004). Social support and the management of uncertainty for people living with HIV or AIDS. *Health Communication, 16,* 305–331.

Brashers, D. E., Neidig, J. L., Russell, J. A., Cardillo, L. W., Haas, S. M., Dobbs, L. K., et al. (2003). The medical, personal, and social causes of uncertainty in HIV illness. *Issues in Mental Health Nursing, 24,* 497–522.

Brown, K. W., & Ryan, R., M. (2003). The benefits of being present: Mindfulness and its role in psychological well-being. *Journal of Personality and Social Psychology, 84*(4), 822–848.

Clayton, M. F., Mishel, M. H., & Belyea, M. (2006). Testing a model of symptoms, communication, uncertainty and well-being in older breast cancer survivors. *Research in Nursing and Health, 29,* 18–39.

Davis, F. (1960). Uncertainty in medical prognosis clinical and functional. *American Journal of Sociology, 66,* 41–47.

Decker, C. L., Haase, J. E., & Bell, C. J. (2007). Uncertainty in adolescents and young adults with cancer. *Oncology Nursing Forum, 34*(3), 681–688.

Denny, E. (2009). "I never know from one day to another how I will feel": Pain and uncertainty in women with endometriosis. *Qualitative Health Research, 19*(7), 985–995.

Dirksen, S., & Erickson, J. (2002).Well-being in Hispanic and non-Hispanic Caucasian survivors of breast cancer. *Oncology Nursing Forum, 29,* 820–826.

Donovan-Kicken, E., & Bute, J. J. (2008). Uncertainty of social network members in the case of communication-debilitating illness or injury. *Qualitative Health Research, 18*(1), 5–18.

Elphee, E. E. (2008). Understanding the concept of uncertainty in patients with indolent lymphoma. *Oncology Nursing Forum, 35*(3), 449–454.

Encyclopedia Britannica. (2011). Damocles. Retrieved March 1, 2011, from: http://www.britannica.com/EBchecked/topic/150566/Damocles

Gil, K., Mishel, M. Belyea, M., Germino, B., Porter, L., & Clayton, M. (2006). Benefits of the uncertainty management intervention for African American and Caucasian older breast cancer survivors: 20-month outcomes. *International Journal of Behavioral Medicine, 13,* 286–294.

Gil, K. M., Mishel, M. H., Belyea, M., Germino, B., Porter, LaNey, I. C., & Stewart, J. (2004). Triggers of uncertainty about recurrence and long-term treatment side effects in older African American and Caucasian breast cancer survivors. *Oncology Nursing Forum, 31*(3), 633–639.

Gil, K. M., Mishel, M. H., Germino, B., Porter, L. S., Carlton-LaNey, I., & Belyea, M. (2005). Uncertainty management intervention for older African American and Caucasian long-term breast cancer survivors. *Journal of Psychosocial Oncology, 23,* 3–21.

Goffman, E. (1963). Stigma: *Notes on the management of spoiled identity.* New York: Simon and Schuster.

Greenwood, N., Mackenzie, A., Wilson, N., & Cloud, G. (2009). Managing uncertainty in life after stroke: A qualitative study of the experiences of established and new informal carers in the first 3 months after discharge. *International Journal of Nursing Studies, 46,* 1122–1133.

Grossman, P., Niemann, L., Schmidt, S., & Walach, H. (2004). Mindfulness-based stress reduction and health benefits: A meta-analysis. *Journal of Psychosomatic Research, 57*(1), 35–43.

Guadalupe, K. (2010). Understanding a meningioma diagnosis using Mishel's theory of uncertainty in illness. *British Journal of Neuroscience Nursing, 6*(2), 77–82.

Hoff, A. L., Mullins, L. L., Chaney, M. J., Hartman, V. L., Domek, D. (2002). Illness uncertainty, perceived control, and psychological distress among adolescents with type 1 diabetes. *Research and Theory for Nursing Practice, 16*(4), 223–236.

Hommel, K. A., Chaney, J. M., Wagner, J. L., White, M. M., Hoff, A. L., & Mullins, L. L. (2003). Anxiety and depression in older adolescents with long-standing asthma: The role of illness uncertainty. *Children's Health Care, 32*(1), 51–63.

Johnson, L. M., Zautra, A. J., & Davis, M. C. (2006). The role of illness uncertainty on coping with fibromyalgia symptoms. *Health Psychology, 25*(6), 696–703.

Kang, Y. (2006). Effect of uncertainty on depression in patients with newly diagnosed atrial fibrillation. *Progress in Cardiovascular Nursing, 21*(2), 83–88.

Lasker, J. N., Sogolow, E. D., Olenik, J. M., Sass, D. A., & Weinrieb, R. M. (2010). Uncertainty and liver transplantation: Women with primary biliary cirrhosis before and after transplant. *Women & Health, 50,* 359–375.

Lazarus, R. S., & Folkman, S. (1984). *Stress, appraisal, and coping.* New York: Springer.

Lemaire, G. S. (2004). More than just menstrual cramps: Symptoms and uncertainty among women with endometriosis. *Journal of Obstetric, Gynecologic, and Neonatal Nursing, 33,* 71–79.

Liao, M. N., Chen, M. F., Chen, S. C., Chen, P. L. (2008). Uncertainty and anxiety during the diagnostic period for women with suspected breast cancer. *Cancer Nursing, 31*(4), 274–283.

Lien, C. Y., Lin, H. R., Kuo, I. T., & Chen, M. L. (2009). Perceived uncertainty, social support and psychological adjustment in older patients with cancer being treated with surgery. *Journal of Clinical Nursing, 18,* 2311–2319.

Madar, H., & Bar-Tal, Y. (2009). The experience of uncertainty among patients having peritoneal dialysis. *Journal of Advanced Nursing, 65*(8), 1664–1669.

Martin, S. C., Stone, A. M., Scott, A. M., & Brashers, D. E. (2010). Medical, personal, and social forms of uncertainty across the transplantation trajectory. *Qualitative Health Research, 20,* 182–196.

Mast, M. E. (1998). Survivors of breast cancer: Illness uncertainty, positive reappraisal and emotional distress. *Oncology Nursing Forum, 25,* 555–562.

Mauro, A. M. (2010). Long-term follow-up study of uncertainty and psychosocial adjustment among implantable cardioverter defibrillator recipients. *International Journal of Nursing Studies, 47*(9), 1080–1088.

McCormick, K. M. (2002). A concept analysis of uncertainty in illness. *Journal of Nursing Scholarship, 34*(2), 127–131.

McCormick, K. M., McClement, S., & Naimark, B. J. (2005). A qualitative analysis of the experience of uncertainty while awaiting coronary artery bypass surgery. *Canadian Journal of Cardiovascular Nursing, 15*(1), 10–22.

McIntosh, J. (1974). Processes of communication, Information seeking and control associated with cancer: A selective review of the literature. *Social Science & Medicine, 8,* 167–187.

McIntosh, J. (1976). Patients' awareness and desire for information about diagnosed but undisclosed malignant disease. *Lancet, 2,* 300–303.

McNulty, K., Livneh, H., & Wilson, L. M. (2004). Perceived uncertainty, spiritual well-being, and psychosocial adaptation in individuals with multiple sclerosis. *Rehabilitation Psychology, 49*(2), 91–99.

Mishel, M. H. (1981). The measurement of uncertainty in illness. *Nursing Research, 30*(5), 258–263.

Mishel, M. H. (1984). Perceived uncertainty and stress in illness. *Research in Nursing and Health, 7*(3), 163–171.

Mishel, M. H. (1988). Uncertainty in illness. *Image: Journal of Nursing Scholarship, 20*, 225–232.

Mishel, M. H. (1990). Reconceptualization of the uncertainty in illness theory. *Image: Journal of Nursing Scholarship, 22*, 256–262.

Mishel, M. H. (1997). Uncertainty in acute illness. *Annual Review of Nursing Research, 15*, 57–80.

Mishel, M. H. (1999). Uncertainty in chronic illness. *Annual Review of Nursing Research, 17*, 269–294.

Mishel, M. H., & Braden, C. J. (1988). Finding meaning: Antecedents of uncertainty. *Nursing Research, 37*, 98–103.

Mitchell, M. L., Courtney, M., & Coyer, F. (2003). Understanding uncertainty and minimizing families' anxiety at the time of transfer from intensive care. *Nursing and Health Sciences, 5*, 207–217.

Montgomery, M. (2010). Uncertainty during breast diagnostic evaluation: State of the science. *Oncology Nursing Forum, 37*(1), 77–83.

Mulcahy, C. M., Parry, D. C., & Glover, T. D. (2010). The "patient patient": The trauma of waiting and the power of resistance for people living with cancer. *Qualitative Health Research, 20*(8), 1062–1075.

Mullins, L. L., Chaney, J. M., Balderson, B., & Hommel, K. A. (2000). The relationship of illness uncertainty, illness intrusiveness, and asthma severity to depression in young adults with long-standing asthma. *International Journal of Rehabilitation and Health, 5*(3), 177–185.

Mullins, L. L., Cote, M. P., Fuemmeler, B. F., Jean, V. M., Beatty, W. W., & Paul, R. H. (2001). Illness intrusiveness, uncertainty, and distress in individuals with multiple sclerosis. *Rehabilitation Psychology, 46*(2), 139–153.

Northouse, L. L., Mood, D., Kershaw, T., Schafenacker, A., Mellon, S., Walker, J., et al. (2002). Quality of life of women with recurrent breast cancer and their family members. *Journal of Clinical Oncology, 20*, 4050–4064.

O'Neill, E. W., & Morrow, L. L. (2001). The symptom experience of women with chronic Illness. *Journal of Advanced Nursing, 33*, 257–268.

Penrod. J. (2001). Refinement of the concept of uncertainty. *Journal of Advanced Nursing, 34*, 238–245.

Persson. E., & Hellstrom, A. (2002). Experiences of Swedish men and women 6 to 12 weeks after ostomy surgery. *Journal of Wound, Ostomy and Continence Nursing, 29*(2), 103–108.

Reich, J. W., Olmsted, M. E., & van Puymbroeck, C. M. (2006). Illness uncertainty, partner caregiver burden and support, and relationship satisfaction in fibromyalgia and osteoarthritis patients. *Arthritis & Rheumatism, 55*(1), 86–93.

Sammarco, A. (2001). Perceived social support, uncertainty, and quality of life of younger breast cancer survivors. *Cancer Nursing, 24*(3), 212–219.

Sammarco, A., & Konecny, L. (2008). Quality of life, social support and uncertainty among Latina breast cancer survivors. *Oncology Nursing Forum, 35*, 844–849.

Sammarco, A., & Konecny, L. M. (2010). Quality of life, social support, and uncertainty among Latina and Caucasian breast cancer survivors: A comparative study. *Oncology Nursing Forum, 37*(1), 93–99.

Sanders-Dewey, J. E. J., Mullins, L. L., & Chaney, J. M. (2001). Coping style, perceived uncertainty in illness, and distress in individuals with Parkinson's disease and their caregivers. *Rehabilitation Psychology, 46*, 363–381.

Schulman-Green, D., Ercolano, E., Dowd, M., Schwartz, P., & McCorkle, R. (2008). Quality of life among women after surgery for ovarian cancer. *Palliative Support Care, 6*(3), 239–247.

Simpson, M. F., & Whyte, F. (2006). Patients' experiences of completing treatment for colorectal cancer in a Scottish district general hospital. *European Journal of Cancer Care, 15*(2), 172–182.

Sinding, C., Hudak, P., Wiernikowski, J., Aronson, J., Miller, P., Gould, J., et al. (2010). "I like to be an informed person but…" negotiating responsibility for treatment decisions in cancer care. *Social Science & Medicine, 71*, 1094-1101.

Stone, A. M., & Jones, C. L. (2009). Sources of uncertainty: Experiences of Alzheimer's disease. *Issues in Mental Health Nursing, 30*, 677–686.

Thompson, S., & O'Hair, H. D. (2008). Advice-giving and the management of uncertainty for cancer survivors. *Health Communication, 23,* 340–348.

Wallace, M. (2003). Uncertainty and quality of life of oler men who undergo watchful waiting for prostate cancer. *Oncology Nursing Forum, 30,* 303–309.

Wallace, M. (2005). Finding more meaning: The antecedents of uncertainty revisited. *Journal of Clinical Nursing, 14,* 863–868.

Wallace, M., Bailey, D., O'Rourke, M., & Galbraith, M. (2004). The watchful waiting management option for older men with prostate cancer: State of the science. *Oncology Nursing Forum, 31*(6), 1057–1064.

Wineman, N. M., Schwetz, K. M., Zeller, R., & Cyphert, J. (2003). Longitudinal analysis of illness uncertainty, coping, hopefulness, and mood during participation in a clinical drug trail. *Journal of Neuroscience Nursing, 35*(2), 100–107.

Wolfe-Christensen, C., Isenberg, J. C., Mullins, L. L., Carpentier, M. Y., & Almstrom, C. (2008). Objective versus subjective ratings of asthma severity: Differential predictors of illness uncertainty and psychological distress in college students with asthma. *Children's Health Care, 37,* 183–195.

CHAPTER 8

Quality of Life

Victoria Schirm

INTRODUCTION

This chapter focuses on quality of life for the more than 133 million Americans who live with chronic illness and their families. Emphasis is on nursing practice issues related to the leading causes of death in the United States (Centers for Disease Control and Prevention [CDC], 2010a). This approach aligns with the focus of the National Institute of Nursing Research (NINR) 2006–2010 strategic plan (NINR, 2006). NINR is leading the way in promoting research in the development of nursing interventions for clients and families, focusing particularly on health promotion, quality of life, and end-of-life care. This chapter includes theoretical conceptualizations and clinical research findings that demonstrate the unique contribution of nursing in assessment, intervention, and outcomes evaluation of quality of life in chronic illness.

Nursing practice and nursing research are well positioned to meet the challenge of identifying, testing, and applying interventions that promote quality of life for survivors of acute illness who are now disabled or otherwise living with a chronic condition. Application of research findings to an individual's quality of life enables nurses in clinical practice to plan and deliver evidence-based care.

Nursing interventions guided by the best available evidence can then be individualized to the values and preferences of the client, thereby ensuring better adherence to a plan that must be a lifelong commitment. Client participation in clinical decision making about the effect that treatments may have on quality of life can be used to monitor therapy over the long term.

Quality of life evaluations can also be used to scrutinize the appropriateness of treatments and show progress toward attainment of treatment goals and responses to therapy. Objective knowledge about desired treatment outcomes for chronic illness that incorporate quality of life domains (improved health and function, pain and symptom control, or prolonged life) can be considered against expected, negative treatment effects such as financial burdens, anxiety, and disrupted lives.

Quality of life assessments provide a way to evaluate the impact of chronic illness on clients and their families. The complex interrelationships of the associated burdens of chronic illness are appreciated more fully when the client's overall quality of life is known. In chronic illness research, quality of life is studied to identify and evaluate specific problems and needs of clients with illness or disability. In the larger arena of the healthcare system, quality of life evaluations are used to monitor the extent to which delivered services address client needs. Outcomes that promote quality of life are valued, particularly when positive results are achieved with efficiency and cost savings. This chapter demonstrates that managing the effects of chronic illness and enhancing quality of life is a multifaceted, complex endeavor.

Defining Quality of Life

Defining quality of life has never been easy. Each individual's unique circumstances and experiences shape quality of life, and this subjective component is an important defining element in quality of life. At the same time, objective indicators of what constitutes quality of life are needed to assess outcomes. The general or global meaning of quality of life and an overall sense of well-being may be anchored to an individual's social and economic conditions, living arrangements, and community environment as well as culture, personal values, happiness, life satisfaction, and spiritual well-being.

The more specific health-related quality of life generally refers to perceived physical and mental health over time. Healthcare providers typically use quality of life measures to learn about an individual's illness and its effect on daily life. In the public health arena, quality of life is evaluated to identify and track different population groups. This information can aid in supporting policies as well as in the development of interventions that enhance quality of life (CDC, 2010b).

Regardless of whether one is referring to global quality of life or health-related quality of life, the subjective or individual perspective is important to the definition. Rene Dubos's (1959) definition addresses the subjective nature and the multidimensionality of quality of life:

Men naturally desire health and happiness . . . The kind of health that men desire most is not necessarily a state in which they experience physical vigor and a sense of well-being, not even one giving them a long life. It is, instead, the condition best suited to reach goals that each individual formulates for himself. (p. 228)

The World Health Organization (WHO, 1948) definition of health as "a state of complete physical, mental, and social well-being and not merely the absence of disease or infirmity" recognizes the multidimensionality of health that is inclusive of a personal evaluation of one's circumstances. Nurses involved in chronic illness care have a stake in understanding distinctions and overlaps in quality of life, health-related quality of life, and self-perceived health.

CONCEPTUALIZING AND MEASURING QUALITY OF LIFE

Key to understanding quality of life are the theoretical frameworks or models that influence the patient and family's illness trajectory. Additionally, if increased or "better" quality of life is a patient outcome, the need to quantitatively measure quality of life is necessary.

Theoretical Frameworks

Theories, frameworks, or models in chronic illness explain the complex interrelationships among factors that influence the illness trajectory on quality of life. Such conceptualizations are important not only to generate new evidence for best nursing practice, but also to test and evaluate existing interventions that may affect quality of life in chronic illness. This section presents the literature on quality of life as a theoretical framework or conceptualization, and quality of life as an outcome influenced by various factors depicted in an explanatory model. Examples from the nursing literature are given that use quality of life as a specific outcome of nursing interventions for persons with chronic illness.

Plummer and Molzahn (2009) conducted a critical appraisal of nursing theories to examine quality of life as embedded within the theorists' original frameworks. They evaluated four attributes of quality of life as depicted by nurse theorists (Imogene King, Madeleine Leininger, Rosemarie Parse, Hildegard Peplau, and Martha Rogers): contextual, subjective, intangible, and health related. Plummer and Molzahn concluded there is merit in considering quality of life as more useful to nursing than the term *health*. In relation to nursing practice, they proposed that quality of life is valuable because it considers connections between the intangible and subjective aspects of the client's environment. They recommended that further research be done to develop a better understanding of quality of life for differing client populations.

Naef and Bournes (2009) reviewed quality of life in a similar fashion, comparing and contrasting it to the lived experience of waiting. Their purpose was to derive knowledge for nursing practice and research. Although Naef and Bournes limited their study to clients awaiting lung transplantation, they concluded that the concept of waiting has commonalities with quality of life outcomes for other clients. To this end, they noted that the framework offers guidance to nursing practice as well as nursing research in that living in the context of waiting influences quality of life.

Understanding the theoretical underpinnings of quality of life in the context of chronic illness informs nursing research and nursing practice.

For example, Weinert, Cudney, and Spring (2008) describe their conceptual model of adaptation in chronic illness. Their evolving Women to Women Conceptual Model for Adaptation to Chronic Illness consists of three constructs: environmental stimuli, psychosocial response, and illness management. Quality of life is a component of the model, defined and measured according to the WHO definition of physical health, psychological well-being, social relationships, and environment. The purpose of the model is to provide a conceptualization that increases understanding of adaptation to chronic illness and gives direction to development of appropriate nursing interventions. Weinert and colleagues note that adaptation to chronic illness is related to psychosocial responses, self-management skills, and enhanced quality of life.

Some quality of life theoretical frameworks have been posited from an ethical perspective. Allmark (2005) suggests that ethical theories are relevant to answering moral questions, especially regarding issues of quality of life versus quantity of life. An ethical framework is useful in clinical nursing practice because it gives guidance to ways that individuals' voices can be discerned; enhances development of decision making in routine clinical practice; and considers the client's beliefs, values, and preferences in the context of complex questions (Allmark, 2005).

Hirskyj (2007) considers ethical ramifications of resource allocations associated with the quality-adjusted life years (QALY) concept. QALY is an outcome measure that can be used to determine the efficacy of nursing care as measured by not only the quantity of life (length of life) but also the quality of life. The QALY framework provides a means to estimate and reveal client's values, beliefs, and preferences in relation to care outcomes. Although nurses may be hesitant to use formulas in providing holistic care, especially in the context of resource allocation, the QALY concept is supported by evidence that suggests better clinical outcomes are achieved with cost-effective care. QALY offers a systematic, evidence-based model to practice nursing care and meet the individual needs of clients (Hirskyj, 2007). These frameworks provide a context in which to consider the ethical issues that surround quality of life outcomes in chronic illness.

Other researchers have expanded the knowledge base and theory development in understanding quality of life in chronic illness by investigating clients' priorities and perceptions. Carter, MacLeod, Brander, and McPherson (2004) found that clients' perspectives with regard to quality of life in terminal illness are important components. A framework that considers quality of life outcomes from clients' perspectives, as opposed to models developed by experts emphasizing a good death, can lead to interventions that are more client centered. For example, knowing that "being in charge" is more important to a dying person's quality of life than "having a good death" can support development of appropriate interventions that facilitate client control within the context of the illness.

Theoretical models have also been constructed to elicit variables that can significantly influence and predict quality of life for the many older adults who live with chronic illness (Low & Molzahn, 2007). Such models are helpful in understanding the complex interrelationships among physical functioning, perceived health, and emotional and mental well-being to quality of life as an outcome of nursing care. Low and Molzahn found that good health, financial stability, and meaning and purpose in life have substantial positive effects on the quality of life of older adults. This model provides conceptual links among several variables—financial resources, health, physical function, meaning and purpose in life, emotional support, and environment—to quality of life. The underpinnings of this model provide direction for improving the quality of life of older adults through development of nursing interventions that promote activities of daily living, provide emotional support, or enhance the environment.

The structure, process, and outcome framework originally developed by Donabedian (1988) to assess quality of healthcare delivery guided a randomized clinical trial of a discharge intervention for hospitalized older adults with hip fractures (Huang & Liang, 2005). A structured discharge plan that was systematically implemented by an advanced practice nurse was used to evaluate several outcomes, including quality of life, after hospital discharge of elders who had sustained a hip fracture as a result of a fall.

In another study (Suhonen, Välimäki, Katajisto, & Leino-Kilpi, 2005), a model of individualized nursing care was used to evaluate outcomes of satisfaction, autonomy, and health-related quality of life in hospitalized clients. This model testing demonstrated a positive association between clients' perceptions of care given by nurses and their ratings of satisfaction with care, ability to make decisions about care, and health-related quality of life. This affirmation of individualized nursing care as explicated in the model provides supporting data for evidence-based nursing practice.

Saunders and Cookman (2005) explored the theoretical underpinnings of depression related to hepatitis C virus infection to gain a better understanding of quality of life in this client population where the illness is often chronic. The symptom experience, stigma associated with the illness, and uncertain illness trajectory were described as multidimensional components of hepatitis C–related depression. Saunders and Cookman proposed that the conceptualization provides a model for developing nursing interventions that are likely to be effective for maximizing quality of life outcomes in this special population.

Theoretical frameworks also have been advanced to explain the changing dimensions of cancer care. Once viewed as an acute, life-limiting illness, cancer in most instances is now managed as a chronic illness. Cancer nursing with children is one area where the science of nursing is embedded within the art of nursing practice (Cantrell, 2007). This conceptualization views quality of life as foundational to the experiences of children and adolescents with cancer. For good quality of life to be an outcome, the values, beliefs, and wishes of children and their families as well as the values and expertise of the oncology nurse must be acknowledged and applied with the best available scientific evidence. One without the other is not sufficient to produce health-related quality of life in pediatric oncology.

Clark (2004) used quality of life as the conceptual basis to determine how psychiatric nurses assess and provide care to clients with serious mental illness residing in community settings. Three themes emerged as ways in which quality of life influenced psychiatric nursing practice. One was that quality of life defined the goal of care in that it permeated everything nurses did. The second was that the nurse's

concern for quality of life focused interventions on the person and away from the mental illness. The third theme was that quality of life formed the foundation of the nurse–client relationship, where the focus is the individual client's perspective as opposed to management of a disease or symptoms.

Measuring Quality of Life

As described in the previous section, theoretical frameworks provide a systematic approach to studying quality of life. Regardless of whether quality of life is conceptualized as a complex set of relationships that influence the chronic illness trajectory, or viewed as an outcome of the illness itself, an appropriate measure of quality of life is crucial. Valid and reliable measures are needed to capture accurately the elements or concepts that characterize quality of life. Quality of life has a subjective component as defined by the individual's unique situation that reflects happiness and life satisfaction (CDC, 2010c). This general quality of life includes health as well as culture, values, beliefs, and environment. The more specific health-related quality of life is usually defined in relationship to health and physical function, and emotional and mental well-being. Elements that contribute to the more general or global quality of life may not be considered in assessments about health-related quality of life. At the same time, reference to health-related quality of life may suggest illness or disease.

Nurses, in particular, have a stake in understanding the distinctions and the overlaps in the quality of life dimensions. When used as a framework, the dimensions of quality of life provide a context for assessing nursing's contribution to improved care outcomes for clients with chronic illness. In clinical practice, nurses can use standardized quality of life assessments to plan, implement, and evaluate evidence-based care for clients with chronic illnesses. Measurement is a first step in the process because accurate and appropriate assessment of symptom status has the potential for better care management and evaluation of nursing intervention effectiveness. To this end, Sousa, Ryu, Kwok, Cook, and West (2007) created a model and validated a measure to assess the impact of rheumatoid arthritis on quality of life. They found two factors, arthritic pain and general symptoms, to be confirmatory and predictive of quality of life evaluations. They surmised that nursing interventions aimed at assessing pain and managing overall symptoms have the most potential to enhance quality of life and function for individuals with rheumatoid arthritis.

The CDC (2010c) is concerned with quality of life as a health outcome. Traditional illness outcome measures of morbidity and mortality are limiting, in that they do not consider risks, burdens, resource needs, or declines associated with illness, particularly as they relate to chronic conditions. To this end, the CDC created the "Healthy Days" measure that evaluates one's perception of well-being via four items: self-rated health, number of days of illness or injury, number of days of emotional distress, and days unable to do self-care or work. The four-item measure was expanded to include 10 additional questions eliciting responses on individuals' days of activity limitations, pain, depression, anxiety, sleeplessness, and feeling energized.

The WHO (2004) has also developed a standardized tool to measure quality of life and health from the individual's perspective. In contrast to the CDC measure, the WHO quality of life measure has 26 items that assess an individual's feelings of satisfaction and enjoyment with life, limitations due to pain, capacity for work, ability to perform activities of daily living and to get around, access to health care, and satisfaction with relationships. Both the CDC and the WHO tools have the common objective to quantify and standardize measurement of quality of life. These tools are intended to measure health and well-being in healthy populations as well as to detect illness conditions that could benefit from early intervention and treatment.

Increasingly, nursing as a discipline has recognized that it too needs to focus on measurable outcomes related to interventions. The measurement of quality of life, including health-related quality of life, has become one such standardized assessment as an indicator for outcomes of nursing care. Quality of life determinations that use consistent measures provide an objective assessment of clients' care needs. Measures that include appropriate determinants that contribute to or influence quality of life can be used by nurses to give care based on the best available evidence.

Context of Quality of Life in Chronic Illness

Quality of life in chronic illness can be viewed within the context of health and functioning, psychological and spiritual well-being, societal roles, and economic status. These multiple dimensions provide a practical way to discuss the background that contributes to quality of life for individuals living with chronic illness.

Considerable overlap exists among these components. For example, health and function is multifaceted and may include perceived health, energy level, pain experiences, stress levels, independence, capacity to meet responsibilities, access to and use of health care, and usefulness to others. This view of health and function together as a quality of life component shows that reliance on any one clinical parameter may not capture the client's overall picture of health and well-being. People with chronic illness may report a good perceived quality of life, but clinically they have objective symptoms. Thus knowledge of how symptoms affect clients' health and function can lead to a better understanding of their quality of life in chronic illness. Typically, the presence of symptoms prompts an individual to seek health care—for example, weakness and poor coordination in the individual with multiple sclerosis. In addition, people with chronic illness are subjected to symptoms from the iatrogenic effects of their treatments. Regardless of the origin, physically distressing symptoms affect health and function and, ultimately, one's quality of life. Moreover, symptoms and the distress they cause result in varying reports about health and function as perceived by clients. Healthcare professionals and family members sometimes report conflicting views about a person's health and function, thereby producing quality of life ratings that may differ. Treatment decisions may be impacted by such ratings, demonstrating the importance of using quality of life assessments that consider clients' perspectives of their health and function.

The complexity of health and function in chronic illness suggests that neither good health nor optimal function is a necessary or sufficient condition for quality of life. Psychological and spiritual components are part of quality of life, and include intangibles such as happiness, peace of mind, and a belief system. Considerable overlap exists between psychological and spiritual well-being. Psychological well-being may be thought of as an essential component of quality of life that influences overall adjustment to chronic illness. More directly, spirituality has been advanced as an important element in quality of life measurement across different cultures (Moreira-Almeida & Koenig, 2006). At the same time, caution is urged—spirituality is different from religiosity as well as different from meaning in life, hope, and peace. Most definitions take into consideration that spirituality affects all aspects of a person's well-being. Persons living with a chronic illness sometimes must make significant life changes in order to maintain quality of life. For many individuals with chronic illness, there may be an increased reliance on psychological and spiritual resources and on the social and emotional support offered by friends and confidantes. Spirituality that included components of life satisfaction, less stress, and meaning in life was the basis for a study of women with cancer (López, McCaffrey, Quinn Griffin, & Fitzpatrick 2009). For these women, family activities, listening to music, and helping others were the most frequently used spiritual practices. López and colleagues concluded that it is beneficial to support women in their ongoing spiritual practices as they deal with a chronic illness.

Supportive care or the lack of it influences how individuals manage and cope with stress. Indeed, most people know the positive effect of having "moral support" and companionship at times of difficulty. Family health and relationships are a large part of this aspect of quality of life. Any illness affecting a family member inevitably affects other family members, resulting in a changed quality of life for them as well. For example, when family members become primary caregivers of a member with chronic illness, there are role changes, additional responsibilities, and increased stressors that have varying effects on quality of life. Without a doubt, the overwhelming nature of chronic illness affects the quality of life not only for the client, but also for family members. Therefore, nursing interventions to promote quality of life in chronic illness are frequently aimed at caregivers. It is reasonable to expect that when caregivers are helped to manage their stress and anxiety, both the caregiver and the client realize better quality of life.

The social and cultural context of quality of life are far reaching components, as is evidenced by the manner in which organizations such as the WHO and the CDC define and measure quality of life. Unique cultural interpretations can influence perceived quality of life. Social conditions, expectations of individual behaviors, and cultural regulations affect and contribute to quality of life. Social support and cultural influences are intertwined frequently with economic aspects. Chronic illness affects the financial resources of individuals and their families. The negative impact causes psychological and emotional burdens, and drains financial assets. The reasons for financial strain and its effects vary. Frequently, a chronic illness requires individuals to decrease, suspend, or end their work, leading to a reduction or loss of income. Furthermore, if the care recipient requires much assistance or supervision, the primary family caregiver may also have to terminate employment. Therefore, a family with a member with chronic illness faces an increased financial burden resulting from the unemployment of two members. These situations contribute to an adverse quality of life through decreased workforce participation, and ultimately cause lost productivity, which further increases the overall cost of chronic illness.

Individuals with chronic illness also suffer financially because of the additional expenses incurred with medical insurance rates or out-of-pocket expenses for items not covered by insurance. Transportation to medical or treatment appointments, for example, or the extra cost of special dietary foods or supplements can add up quickly. The desperately ill person who has found little benefit from traditional therapies may spend large amounts of money on alternative forms of treatment to improve their health. The combined effect on quality of life associated with decreased income and increased expenses may not always be obvious. Therefore, nurses must be aware of how this financial burden may contribute to decreased quality of life. For example, clients may take fewer medications because they cannot afford to take the prescribed amount, or the family caregiver may be overtaxed by the caregiving burden because the family cannot afford assistance.

The following case study illustrates many aspects of quality of life in living with a chronic illness, including health and function, psychosocial elements, socioeconomic components, and the meaning of support from family and friends. The story narrative transitions across the many trajectories of living with a chronic illness.

CASE STUDY

Quality of Life in Multiple Phases of Chronic Illness

Terry, a 53-year-old wife and mother of two, who received a diagnosis of breast cancer, was already facing the challenges of living with multiple sclerosis (MS). She had made numerous adjustments in her life because of MS. She was aware of the progressive decline that accompanies her type of MS, and had given up any notion of working outside the home when she received the MS diagnosis initially. She felt overwhelmed at the prospect of coping with the burden of another life-altering illness. This dual diagnosis truly required individualized treatment not only because of the symptom variability of MS, but also because unexpected relapses may occur with the added stress of surgery, chemotherapy, and radiation for her breast cancer. Terry worked diligently to surround herself with support. Most of the time she was her best advocate for keeping all care providers informed of her situation. In a sense she was striving for health care that was person-centered, coordinated, comprehensive, and compassionate. This was no easy task in a healthcare delivery system dominated by a focus on acute, episodic, and fragmented care. MS has forced Terry to face undesirable challenges in her life, and she felt she was making great strides in living with it. She is concerned that her cancer diagnosis will now superimpose added stress on her and her families' ability to maintain quality of life.

Discussion Questions

1. What barriers do you see that may be factors in maintaining quality of life for Terry?
2. What nursing interventions could be used to promote self-care and provide educational resources to Terry?
3. Discuss the issues that Terry and her family face in dealing with the complexity of her situation.
4. Describe the process to promote collaboration among healthcare providers that could enhance quality of life for Terry.
5. What potential quality of life issues are likely to arise and what assessments and interventions would be appropriate?

Although chronic illness usually involves great financial costs, caution is warranted in assuming that a positive relationship exists between a good quality of life and an adequate income. The high degree of subjectivity in quality of life and the existence of many interrelated components suggest that other aspects may influence one's quality of life. The interrelatedness of these various quality of life aspects is evident in the literature that reports results of interventions in chronic illness conditions (Jonas-Simpson, Mitchell, Fisher, Jones, & Linscott, 2006; Baird & Sands, 2006; Crone, 2007).

EVIDENCE-BASED INTERVENTIONS TO PROMOTE QUALITY OF LIFE ___

Evidence-based nursing practice has the most potential to enhance quality of life in chronic illness. The best available research evidence combined with nursing expertise and consideration of individual values and preferences enables effectiveness and efficiency in nursing care. Nurses cannot afford to base practice solely on tradition or experience, or even on knowledge of experts or highly rated textbooks. Increasingly, nursing interventions are seen as having a direct impact on patient outcomes. In chronic illness care, this pivotal nursing role raises the bar to practice nursing that is systematic, produces outcomes that contribute to cost effectiveness, and enhances quality care. As a result of the efforts of nurse researchers and the NINR initiatives, interventions with known efficacy are being implemented to promote quality of life in chronic illness.

This section reviews nursing interventions in chronic illness that promote and evaluate quality of life as an outcome. Overall, a reasonable outcome of any nursing intervention is improved quality of life for clients. In chronic illness, this goal is even more salient. Nurses as essential healthcare professionals to clients with chronic illness can be instrumental in planning, carrying out, and evaluating care that promotes quality of life. For clients, enhancing their quality of life amid the debilitating effects of a long-term illness becomes an especially relevant outcome. Moreover, quality of life from the client's context is a reasonable outcome measure of the effectiveness of clinical interventions. The review includes nursing and related investigations on quality of life outcomes for clients and families who have conditions that are the leading causes of death, such as heart disease

and cancer. Also included are studies that address quality of life as an outcome in chronic conditions such as arthritis, mental illness, and functional decline associated with aging. A review of the quality of life research for those at end of life is presented as well. These investigations provide examples of ways that nurses can intervene effectively to promote quality of life for clients and their families living with a chronic illness, disability, or other condition.

Evidence-Based Guidelines

Clinical practice guidelines provide easily accessed and current, evidence-based information about recommendations, strategies, or information for care and decision making in specific clinical conditions (Coopey, Nix, & Clancy, 2006). Guidelines about interventions specific to promoting quality of life are embedded in some guidelines, and many guidelines include nurses as the intended users. Four guidelines are presented in **Table 8-1**: 1) self-management in chronic care, 2) advance care planning with cancer patients, 3) clinical practice for quality palliative care, and 4) family preparedness and end-of-life support for nursing home residents. These and other evidence-based guidelines are readily available at the National Guideline Clearinghouse (Agency for Healthcare Research and Quality, 2011). Guidelines can be used by nurses to evaluate quality of life as it is influenced by clinical decision making and intervening in chronic illness situations. For example, the evidence-based guideline for chronic care self-management was developed for counseling, evaluation, and management of families who have children with chronic illnesses. This guideline, created by an expert panel at a major children's hospital, specifically targets families of children with chronic illness. Intended users include advanced practice nurses, among others.

Table 8-1   Comparison of Guidelines That Measure Quality of Life Outcomes

	Evidence-based care guideline for chronic care: self-management (2007)	Advance care planning with cancer patients (2008)	Clinical practice guidelines for quality palliative care (2004; revised 2009)	Family preparedness and end-of-life support before the death of a nursing home resident (2002; revised 2009)
Guideline Title				
Guideline Developer(s)	Cincinnati Children's Hospital Medical Center	Program in evidence-based Care	National Consensus Project	University of Iowa College of Nursing, John A. Hartford Foundation Center of Geriatric Nursing Excellence
Disease/ Condition(s)	Chronic illness/ condition	Cancer	Chronic, debilitating, and life-threatening illnesses	Bereavement
Clinical Specialty	Family practice, internal medicine, nursing, nutrition, pediatrics, physical medicine, rehabilitation, psychology	Oncology	Family Practice, Geriatrics, Internal Medicine, Nursing, Nutrition, Pediatrics, Psychiatry, Psychology,	Family Practice, Geriatrics, Psychology
Intended Users	Advanced practice nurses, allied health personnel, dietitians, healthcare providers, nurses, patients, pharmacists, physicians, psychologists/non-physician behavioral health clinicians, social workers	Advanced practice nurses, nurses, physician assistants, physicians	Advanced practice nurses, allied health personnel, dietitians, healthcare providers, health plans, hospitals, managed care organizations, nurses, pharmacists, physician assistants, physicians, psychologists/ non-physician behavioral health clinicians, social workers, speech-language pathologists, utilization management	Advanced practice nurses, nurses, social workers

(Continues)

Table 8-1   Comparison of Guidelines That Measure Quality of Life Outcomes (continued)

Guideline Title	Evidence-based care guideline for chronic care: self-management (2007)	Advance care planning with cancer patients (2008)	Clinical practice guidelines for quality palliative care (2004; revised 2009)	Family preparedness and end-of-life support before the death of a nursing home resident (2002; revised 2009)
Guideline Objective(s)	To provide evidence-based recommendations for self-management by families of children with chronic conditions in order to improve health outcomes and quality of life	To evaluate advance care planning (ACP) impact on cancer patient outcomes; key elements of ACP for cancer patients; and barriers to engaging in and following through on ACP with cancer patients	To serve as a comprehensive description of what constitutes comprehensive, high-quality palliative care services, as well as a resource for practitioners addressing the palliative care needs of patients and families in primary treatment settings	To provide guidelines for end-of-life support of family members before the death of a nursing home resident
Client Population	Children with chronic conditions and their families	Cancer patients are the relevant population; non-cancer patients with chronic or life-threatening illnesses	Patients of all ages, who are living with a persistent or recurring condition adversely affecting daily functioning Family members or other individuals who provide support	All family members and significant others with an attachment to a nursing home resident nearing end of life
Major Outcomes Considered	Self-efficacy; health-related quality of life; healthcare utilization; parent/patient satisfaction; missed days from usual activities; cost specific disease measures	Meeting patient or substitute preferences; healthcare resource use	Patient and caregiver quality of life; incidence of ethical or legal problems arising from end-of-life care Rate of use of end-of-life support programs	Preparedness for death of a loved one

Table 8-1   Comparison of Guidelines That Measure Quality of Life Outcomes (continued)

Guideline Title	Evidence-based care guideline for chronic care: self-management (2007)	Advance care planning with cancer patients (2008)	Clinical practice guidelines for quality palliative care (2004; revised 2009	Family preparedness and end-of-life support before the death of a nursing home resident (2002; revised 2009)
Methods Used to Access the Quality and Strength of the Evidence	Not stated	Expert consensus	Not stated	Weighting according to a rating scheme
Methods Used to Formulate the Recommendations	Expert consensus (Delphi Expert consensus and nominal group techniques)	Available evidence from published literature, environmental scan, and expert opinion to reach consensus	Consensus process involving: American Academy of Hospice and Palliative Medicine; Center to Advance Palliative Care; Hospice and Palliative Nurses Association; National Hospice and Palliative Care Organization	Not applicable

Source: Agency for Healthcare Research and Quality. (2010). National Guidelines Clearinghouse. Retrieved January 25, 2011, from: www.guidelines.gov

Clinical areas where children with chronic illness and their families are cared for are the practice areas in which these guidelines are most likely to be used. As an outcome, health-related quality of life is one measure that healthcare professionals can use to evaluate the effects of their interventions on client outcomes.

The accessibility and ease of use related to evidence-based guidelines provide an efficient and effective manner for nurses to intervene and evaluate quality of life for clients and their families with chronic illness. At the same time, it is important that the user evaluate the relevance, currency, and validity of guidelines for measurement of intended

outcomes. Consequently, along with guideline use, nurses must be aware of the recent quality of life research and measurement to apply the best available evidence at the client-care level. Therefore, it is important to consider specific practice characteristics that may influence guideline effectiveness and the time and effort that might be required to implement recommendations (Coopey et al., 2006). The guideline should reflect the nurses' clinical knowledge and experience as well as the clients' values and preferences (Clark, Donovan, & Schoettker, 2006).

Using guidelines from the National Guideline Clearinghouse offers assurances that the recommendations, strategies, and information are based on systematic literature reviews and scientific evidence. Guidelines offer recommendations for practice that are based on a specified level of evidence. For example, the table comparing evidence-based guidelines shows that expert consensus was the primary means to formulate the recommendations put forth in the guideline for advance care planning with cancer patients. A consensus process involving well recognized palliative care organizations was used to evaluate the quality of the recommendations in application of these guidelines to palliative care, with quality of life for client and family, incidence of ethical/legal issues, and use of end-of-life support programs as outcomes. For application in clinical practice, nurses could review the guidelines and assess the methods and rating scheme that were used in development. A determination can be made that if a recommendation is strong, the intervention is always indicated and acceptable, and, therefore, likely to positively influence quality of life for clients. On the other hand, nurses would need to use additional information in their decision-making process if the recommendation has a lower rating, such as "useful," "should be considered," or "not useful."

Interventions from the Research Literature to Promote Quality of Life

A review of nursing and health-related literature that report the effects of various interventions on quality of life as one outcome in chronic illness conditions is presented in this section. Much of the research is descriptive in nature; therefore, cause-and-effect relationships between nursing interventions and quality of life as an outcome are not well established. It is also difficult to collect data on outcomes that are sensitive and unique to nursing care interventions. Individuals with chronic illness are seen by a variety of healthcare professionals who may potentially affect their quality of life. Nevertheless, findings from many of the studies suggest that quality of life has usefulness as a nurse-sensitive quality indicator and as a measure of intervention effectiveness in chronic conditions. Doran and colleagues (2006) noted that linking outcomes to nursing interventions is necessary to determine and identify specific nursing interventions that improve health outcomes and provide the evidence base to improve nursing care in chronic illness.

Most of the reports view the quality of life of a client as an important outcome measure across several domains, and specific interventions have focused on outcomes such as stage of the disease, disability, and mortality rates. The view of outcomes in terms of morbidity and death discounts other aspects of health and function in chronic illness, such as the client's perceived health, pain experiences, stress levels, independence, capacity to meet responsibilities, access to and use of health care, and usefulness to others. These outcomes are important to clients who want to know how interventions are going to influence health and function. Clients also want guidance in choosing options that will produce the best outcomes. In addition, regulatory bodies and manufacturers of pharmaceuticals and technologic devices want guidance about product effectiveness on client outcomes, and in particular how an individual's quality of life is affected. The results of the research and of the other literature reviewed here show the many facets of client quality of life outcomes in chronic illness care.

Overview of Nursing Interventions

Nursing interventions can empower clients to practice healthy behaviors and enable them to be self-directed in their care and thereby contribute appreciably to quality of life. Feldman,

Murtaugh, Pezzin, McDonald, and Peng (2005) found that use of an email reminder improved self-care management and health-related quality of life for clients with heart failure. The email reminders provided evidence-based, condition-specific information to nurses as they cared for heart failure clients. These reminders were integrated into the assessment and routine teaching interventions that nurses carried out for clients. When compared with routine care, the basic email reminder to nurses that they should teach to the specific areas of medication knowledge, diet, and weight monitoring produced positive results in clients' quality of life. Moreover, Feldman and colleagues found that this basic teaching for heart failure generated results similar to that of a more intensive intervention that included more reminders and additional nursing time. The study is limited in so far as the sample was from one urban homecare agency. However, the results are useful in linking a nursing practice intervention to clients' quality of life, and thereby add to a better understanding of nursing interventions that are appropriate as well as cost effective.

Nursing-led management and intervention in chronic disease care has been investigated and evaluated in relation to client quality of life outcomes. These investigations are hampered frequently by an inability to produce conclusive results regarding nursing impact on quality of life. Results of one study provide evidence that nurse-mediated interventions have the potential to yield positive quality of life outcomes for clients with implantable cardioverter-defibrillators (Dickerson, Wu, & Kennedy, 2006). However, establishing a link via statistically significant results is more complicated. This situation frequently occurs as the result of multiple factors that affect quality of life, inability to isolate a single nursing intervention, or failure in the adequacy of the measurement (Dickerson et al., 2006). At the same time, the imperative to promote quality of life in chronic illness care requires continued nursing research. Taylor and colleagues (2005) acknowledged the urgency of the need for ongoing research in their systematic review of evidence effectiveness related to nursing's role in chronic obstructive pulmonary disease (COPD). As a chronic illness, COPD is a prime example of an escalating public health burden in terms of number of persons affected and the resources used. Nurses have been recognized as playing a critical role in chronic illness care of COPD. Taylor and colleagues called for reprioritization of nurse-led models of chronic illness care. The equivocal results of this study and many others investigating quality of life as an end result suggest the need for more carefully designed nursing interventions as well as measurement of additional outcomes.

Health and Function

Health and function as determinants of quality of life are used frequently with traditional clinical and disease indicators to evaluate outcomes for older adults with chronic illness. In clinical practice, these quality of life assessments can enhance understanding about treatment preferences and future care needs. For example, health-related quality of life was used as a predictor of potential need for future hospital care for older adults in a large primary care practice (Dorr et al., 2006). Dorr and colleagues found that consideration of quality of life may improve decision making about treatment preferences and intensity for care. Knowledge of an older person's capacity for self-care and functional abilities can maximize appropriate resources and need for care when critical situations arise. Many times the needed information about quality of life addressing psychosocial aspects of chronic illness is missing from assessments. The assessment data can be used to plan, carry out, and evaluate treatments. In situations in which treatments are known to cause extreme debility, changes should be considered for older clients based on quality of life outcomes.

Nursing care for elderly cancer survivors is one area where information about potential effects on quality of life can be used in clinical practice. Quality of life and related symptoms in elderly women with breast cancer are entangled frequently with other chronic health conditions or are attributed to aging. Heidrich, Egan, Hengudomsub, and Randolph (2006) found that poor social situations, a pessimistic outlook on life, and not knowing the reason for many distressing symptoms further contribute to decreased quality of life. In these situations, effective interventions may include helping older women better understand why they are experiencing symptoms and that depression, anxiety, or lack of energy may be caused by cancer and are not part of normal aging.

Clients need information about the reason for symptoms and to know that some symptoms are intertwined with chronic illness and compounded by the aging process. This knowledge can help older adults develop more effective coping strategies. Targeting intervention strategies also can be done more appropriately when quality of life outcomes are better identified. Awareness that women report worse quality of life compared to men because women tend to have a higher prevalence of chronic illness and related functional declines can lead to more proactive early detection and health promotion interventions (Orfila et al., 2006).

Frequently, lack of awareness about available help and treatments is an obstacle to better quality of life. In a study of bowel function and associated fecal incontinence among those older than 75 years of age, researchers found that decreased quality of life was influenced by the amount of dependence that symptoms caused (Stenzelius, Westergren, & Hallberg, 2007).

Appropriate assessment of bowel symptoms and the extent of dependency along with nurses' encouragement of clients to seek appropriate care are straightforward interventions that can have a positive impact on quality of life for older adults with bowel dysfunction.

Cancer Care

Nursing research related to care of clients with cancer and their families provides an excellent illustration of the complexity of measuring, intervening, and evaluating quality of life in chronic illness. Cancer is increasingly recognized as a chronic illness because of better survival rates that have resulted from effective treatments. With the increased survival following a diagnosis of cancer, quality of life emerges as a predominant issue. Identification, prevention, and management of the long-term effects of cancer and related treatments have received attention by nurse researchers. Bender, Ergÿn, Rosenzweig, Cohen, and Sereika (2005) identified the prevalence of symptoms experienced by women across three phases of breast cancer treatment. They assessed global quality of life, and evaluated how vasomotor, physical, psychosocial, and sexual components were experienced by women in the various phases of breast cancer care and treatment. Fatigue, cognitive impairments, and mood disturbances emerged as common symptoms experienced by the women, regardless of the phase of illness or treatment. Fatigue associated with cancer and related treatments was an especially bothersome symptom, suggesting that nursing interventions focused on alleviating and managing fatigue may promote better quality of life for women with breast cancer.

The positive effect on quality of life produced by interventions that prevent or lessen fatigue associated with cancer has been given attention in the nursing literature. Cancer-related fatigue is frequently measured as a quality of life component, and various interventions have been proposed to reduce fatigue. Mitchell, Beck, Hood, Moore, and Tanner (2007) conducted a systematic review of the literature and used a rating scheme to support the efficacy of different interventions to reduce fatigue associated with cancer care and treatment. For many interventions, effectiveness was not well established, owing to insufficient or poor quality data. These interventions included alternative therapies such as yoga, acupuncture, and nutritional supplements; drugs that may help alleviate fatigue; and psychotherapy. Strategies that teach clients to manage and balance activity, rest, and sleep were rated as likely to be effective, because the evidence is based on small, descriptive studies or expert consensus. Exercise was the one intervention that was recommended for practice because of the strength of the evidence and because the benefits outweighed the harm.

Other studies have also shown that exercise is a safe and effective intervention for reducing fatigue and promoting quality of life in cancer patients. Exercise combined with structured group sessions was effective, owing in part to the group cohesion and atmosphere, and the direct effects that exercise has on reducing fatigue (Losito, Murphy, & Thomas, 2006). This understanding and awareness of the evidence supporting nursing interventions for cancer care promotes best practices interventions for clients and their families. In particular, the growing body of evidence that cancer clients reap many benefits from exercise provides substantial rationale for nurses to promote and use physical activity as a means of improving health and quality of life for many clients with cancer (Hacker, 2009).

Quality of Life in Terminal Illness

Nurses' involvement as researchers and clinicians in end-of-life care has created heightened interest in measuring, promoting, and maintaining quality

of life as a nursing care outcome for clients at the end of life. Indeed, the primary objective of palliative and hospice care is to optimize quality of life for individuals and their families. In their review of the literature, Jocham, Dassen, Widdershoven, and Halfens (2006) found that research on nursing interventions in quality of life in palliative cancer care creates special challenges. A primary challenge is the methodological issues related to measurement of quality of life. Most often the aim of end-stage treatment is to control physical symptoms and promote psychological, social, and spiritual comfort. Hence, an individual's quality of life becomes anchored in other aspects of life, and traditional measures may not be accurate or appropriate. Despite the presence of a terminal illness, clients may continue to give rather favorable ratings to their situation, suggesting that other values, goals, and preferences are important to quality of life.

In older adults, measuring quality of life at end of life, likewise, is beset by methodological issues as it is difficult to quantify the experiences of clients and families. Gourdji, McVey, and Purden (2009) conducted a qualitative study on the meaning of quality of life in 10 individuals receiving palliative care. Responses of these individuals showed a strong desire to overcome the negative aspects of their situation, and find ways to fully engage in life. Based on the findings, Gourdji and colleagues recommended interventions that enable patients with terminal illness to continue doing the things they want to do, being helpful to others, and sharing a caring environment The aging process alters responses to illness, and disease and symptoms may not manifest in ways that nurses are familiar with in younger adults. Evidence-based activities that promote and maintain quality of life for terminally ill older adults include attention to age-related changes and the impact on sensory function and physiologic responses. Particular consideration should be given to pain assessment, medication management, and assessments of depression and cognitive status (Amella, 2003). Others have shown that by asking seriously ill clients what they view as quality of life is instructive in helping decide on treatment plans, making advance directives, or prioritizing activities (Vig & Pearlman, 2003).

Psychosocial and Other Supportive Interventions

Nursing studies have focused on interventions to promote quality of life when technology and other well established treatments fail or when these tools and machinery are insufficient to maintain health and function. Facing suffering on a daily basis and the need to find meaning and purpose in living with a chronic disability challenges healthcare professionals to address a client's needs in other than physical ways. Psychosocial well-being, including health and functionality, contributes immensely to one's quality of life in chronic illness. This type of well-being can be characterized as the capacity to view oneself in a positive manner as well as see the world as meaningful, manageable, and logical. The capacity to view self in a positive manner, despite serious physical symptoms that accompany chronic illness, has been shown to be moderated by a strong sense of coherence (Delgado, 2007). In some situations, the simple act of listening to a client's burdens and feelings promotes quality of life. This response comes about through the contentment, respect, and nurturance that are shown by the nurse who listens without judgment (Jonas-Simpson et al., 2006). Interventions that enable better understanding and use of coping skills can be supportive of quality of life for clients and families experiencing chronic illness. Clients who were

post-myocardial infarction and who reported quality of life improvements used optimistic, self-reliant, and confrontational coping strategies most frequently over a 1-year period (Kristofferzon, Löfmark, & Carlsson, 2005).

In addition to psychosocial-related activities that augment chronic illness care, evidence-based alternative interventions can likewise be part of the client's care routine. Interventions such as guided imagery and relaxation therapy have the potential to supplement traditional medical and health care that chronically ill clients need. The combination of guided imagery and relaxation techniques improved health-related quality of life for women with osteoarthritis by alleviating pain intensity and increasing mobility. Moreover, this intervention is easily taught and readily available to clients (Baird & Sands, 2006).

Clients with chronic mental illness are another group that can benefit from interventions that augment prescribed medication and counseling therapies. Crone (2007) reported that physical activity programs enabled mentally ill individuals to have positive emotional experiences, increased social interaction, and enhanced well-being. Nurses can be instrumental in facilitating development and referral to programs that help increase physical activity for clients with mental illnesses, and thereby promote quality of life. Individuals with other chronic conditions also have benefited from exercise programs. Knowing the stage of a client's readiness to engage in exercise is an additional factor that can give nurses information to tailor education more specifically (Lee, Chang, Liou, & Chang, 2006).

Interventions for Family Quality of Life

Nursing interventions to promote quality of life are, likewise, important to family members and others who are caregivers to clients living with a chronic illness. Consequently, it is important to know how caregivers experience quality of life. In general, chronic illness affects quality of life for the entire family. Therefore, family assessment and intervention is necessary. The level of the nurse's involvement with the family will determine the extent of the interventions. Most nurses can meet the basic need that families of clients with chronic illness have for factual information. This information may include education about the disease, treatments, and prognosis. Being available to answer questions and to give practical advice is important. Intervening at this fundamental level establishes trust with families that helps foster continued support. Nurses can invite family members to participate in care activities as appropriate. Families with complex problems may need referral to a specialist. Appropriate use of support groups can create an added network for clients and relieve some of the family burden that may be present (Sutton & Erlen, 2006). The nurse is often in a position to evaluate how such supportive interventions may affect quality of life. A safe and supportive environment can facilitate family sharing of feelings about the illness. Support groups can be suggested that would be appropriate for clients and their family caregivers. The nurse is one of the members of a collaborative healthcare team that is needed to maintain and promote optimum quality of life for clients with chronic illness and their families.

The complex trajectory of chronic illness poses difficulties in making a strict separation of interventions for quality of life for both clients and family members. It is reasonable, therefore, to expect that nursing interventions with families can be as helpful as interventions that directly promote health and function in the individual with chronic illness. Moreover, inclusion of the family may strengthen the adjustments that

clients with chronic illness must make during the course of illness. As family members increasingly are relied on to provide time-consuming health care, their health and well-being directly affect care outcomes for the chronically ill member. As a result, defining and assessing quality of life is not limited to the client, but should include specific measures that enable nurses to assess and meet the needs of family caregivers (Kitrungrote & Cohen, 2006).

A study of the effects of mental illness on families offers insights into strategies that nurses can use to promote quality of life for the caregivers (Walton-Moss, Gerson, & Rose, 2005). An important finding of the research is that nurses need to recognize the variability among families in how they respond to mental illness. All family members, regardless of where the relative with mental illness is within the illness trajectory, need to be listened to as they tell their stories and want help to communicate with their loved one. This nursing care is supportive of a family's quality of life when members are coping reasonably well or when they are overwhelmed by numerous challenges. Ultimately, the social and emotional support and financial resources of families impact quality of life. Knowledge about resources, services, and organizations for chronic illness conditions can help in making appropriate and timely referrals that will better maintain quality of life and well-being of clients and families.

Individuals and families shift perspectives on their quality of life as they progress through the illness trajectory. At various points, the illness may be primary; at other times, wellness may predominate. When illness is at the center, a situation that occurs most often with a new diagnosis, the focus is on suffering, loss, and burden. Families may become overwhelmed. When the focus is on wellness, this may provide an opportunity to refocus on aspects that engage the family and client to promote quality of life. The nurse who is aware of these shifts in chronic illness behavior is better equipped to support clients through appropriate interventions.

Quality of Life and Technologic Interventions

Nurses are becoming increasingly involved either directly as researchers or indirectly as research coordinators in clinical trials that evaluate quality of life as one outcome for clients receiving new products, devices, and drugs. Attention to and awareness of the effects that technologic advances have on clients' quality of life, therefore, becomes important in nursing care.

Measurement of client-related outcomes is a particularly important evaluation component in clinical trials, with quality of life being one such aspect. This approach provides insight regarding treatment effectiveness that can be determined only by clients. An individual's perspective about a drug or treatment effect provides corroboration with observable clinical data. This confirmation is important, because enhanced clinical outcomes such as better glucose control or decreased blood pressure may not necessarily correspond to improvements in function or well-being if the individual is experiencing side effects of the new treatment or drug. In addition, many clinical trials are investigating therapies that are expensive and carry with them uncertain outcomes with regard to quality of life (Grusenmeyer & Wong, 2007). In these instances it is important for clinicians to understand that extraordinary economic costs may be at issue with minimal impact on an individual's quality of life. Clients with life-threatening chronic illnesses also are confronted with choosing life-extending treatments at the expense of quality of life, as these treatments may cause debilitating

side effects. Periodic quality of life assessments throughout the course of treatment may offer a better discrimination between improvements versus deterioration in quality of life, and allow client preferences to be included in the decision to continue or forego the specific treatment (Bozcuk et al., 2006).

Another issue with technologic interventions that extend life is deciding when to forego continued treatment. For example, implantable cardioverter-defibrillators have become a well accepted, evidence-based practice for high-risk, life-threatening arrhythmias. Individuals with these devices are not only experiencing a better quality of life but also living longer. These issues bring to the forefront nurses' role in assessing and managing physical and psychological responses to the devices, and what to do when an individual needs end-of-life care. Care of clients and families in these situations requires nursing knowledge about the efficacy and cost effectiveness of interventions to promote quality of life (Dunbar, 2005).

Similar issues confront those receiving hemodialysis for end-stage renal disease. Hemodialysis frequently impacts quality of life throughout the course of the disease, such that physical and mental well-being are negatively affected. The concern at hand becomes identification of indicators that offer realistic appraisals of outcomes associated with the quality as well as the quantity of life (Cleary & Drennan, 2005).

OUTCOMES

Quality of life as an outcome of care is being increasingly addressed by all healthcare entities, including providers, payers, and consumers. In addition, the increased attention globally to chronic illness care makes it imperative that nurses address quality of life as a nurse-sensitive quality indicator.

Clearly as an outcome of nursing care, quality of life can be influenced by appropriately designed care interventions. Nurses are in a position, through research and clinical application of interventions, to make a difference in the lives of clients and families. They can apply evidence-based practices that relieve symptoms and provide comfort; these are actions that promote quality of life. Decision making to initiate, continue, modify, or withdraw treatments can be made by evaluating quality of life as an outcome. The efficacy of clinical nursing interventions and practice behaviors, likewise, can be evaluated based on their contribution to clients' quality of life. By evaluating the extent to which nursing interventions improve quality of life for clients and families, nurses are in a position to show the efficacy of what they do. That nurses can carry out interventions to promote quality of life becomes meaningful to cost-effective care as well.

Throughout this discussion, repeated emphasis has been given to interrelatedness and overlap of interventions that promote and maintain quality of life in a variety of chronic illness conditions. Physical, functional, and psychosocial components are related, especially in the context of chronic illness. As such they are significant determinants of one's quality of life. In many instances, these characteristics and the social and environmental context of the individual can influence quality of life negatively or positively, depending on the particular set of circumstances. The presence of resources, family support, and access to social and health services can have a powerful and affirming influence on quality of life, despite serious chronic illness disability.

Assessing outcomes of nursing interventions using quality of life as a measure contributes to a fuller description of the accountability nurses have in promoting quality care and outcomes. Knowledge of the individual circumstances that influence quality of life in chronic illness enables

better care planning. This targeting of interventions to the specific quality of life for individuals can lead to successful preventive and therapeutic approaches in caring for people with chronic illness. With an ever present awareness of the many components that influence quality of life in chronic illness, nurses can intervene more effectively.

STUDY QUESTIONS

What elements are a part of quality of life evaluations in chronic illness? Discuss how the perceptions of individual clients and healthcare professionals contribute to quality of life evaluations.

Identify a theoretical or conceptual framework that addresses quality of life as an outcome for clients and families with a chronic illness. Describe an intervention using that framework that demonstrates how nursing can make a difference in quality of life.

Describe the importance of quality of life as a nurse-sensitive quality indicator.

As an outcome of care, how is quality of life viewed by healthcare providers, consumers, agencies, and third-party payers?

Describe how nurses can use guidelines to promote evidence-based quality of life care to clients and families with chronic illness.

What interventions can nurses use to promote client and family quality of life at end of life?

Describe outcomes that indicate a good quality of life. How might quality of life outcomes change over time?

What potential ethical dilemmas arise when evaluating quality of life in chronic illness?

For a full suite of assignments and additional learning activities, **WWW** use the access code located in the front of your book and visit this exclusive website: **http://go.jblearning.com/larsen**. If you do not have an access code, you can obtain one at the site.

REFERENCES

Agency for Healthcare Research and Quality. (2011). National Guideline Clearinghouse. Retrieved January 25, 2011, from: www.guidelines.gov

Allmark, P. (2005). Can the study of ethics enhance nursing practice? *Journal of Advanced Nursing, 51*(6), 618–624.

Amella, E. J. (2003). Geriatrics and palliative care: Collaboration for quality of life until death. *Journal of Hospice and Palliative Nursing, 5*(1), 40–48.

Baird, C. L., & Sands, L. P. (2006). Effect of guided imagery with relaxation on health-related quality of life in older women with osteoarthritis. *Research in Nursing & Health, 29*, 442–451.

Bender, C. M., Ergÿn, F. S., Rosenzweig, M. Q., Cohen, S. M., & Sereika, S. M. (2005). Symptom clusters in breast cancer across 3 phases of the disease. *Cancer Nursing, 28*(3), 219–225.

Bozcuk, H., Dalmis, B., Samur, M., Ozdogan, M., Artac, M., & Savas, B. (2006). Quality of life in patients with advanced non-small cell lung cancer. *Cancer Nursing, 29*(2), 104–110.

Cantrell, M. A. (2007). The art of pediatric oncology nursing practice. *Journal of Pediatric Oncology Nursing, 24*(3), 132–138.

Carter, H., Macleod, R., Brander, P., & McPherson, K. (2004). Living with a terminal illness: Patients' priorities. *Journal of Advanced Nursing, 45*(6), 611–620.

Centers for Disease Control and Prevention. (2010a). Chronic diseases and health promotion. Retrieved August 6, 2011, from: http://www.cdc.gov/chronic-disease/overview/index.htm

Centers for Disease Control and Prevention. (2010b). Health-related quality of life. Retrieved August 6, 2011, from: http://www.cdc.gov/hrqol/

Centers for Disease Control and Prevention. (2010c). Health-related quality of life: Methods and measures. Retrieved August 6, 2011, from: http://www.cdc.gov/hrqol/methods.htm

Clark, E. H. (2004). Quality of life: A basis for clinical decision-making in community psychiatric care. *Journal of Psychiatric and Mental Health Nursing, 11*, 725–730.

Clark, E., Donovan, E. F., & Schoettker, P. (2006). From outdated to updated, keeping clinical guidelines valid. *International Journal for Quality in Health Care, 18*(3), 165–166.

Cleary, J., & Drennan, J. (2005). Quality of life of patients on haemodialysis for end-stage renal disease. *Journal of Advanced Nursing, 51*(6), 577–586.

Coopey, M., Nix, M. P., & Clancy, C. M. (2006). Translating research into evidence-based nursing practice and evaluating effectiveness. *Journal of Nursing Care Quality, 21*(3), 195–202.

Crone, D. (2007). Walking back to health: A qualitative investigation into service users' experiences of a walking project. *Issues in Mental Health Nursing, 28*, 167–183.

Delgado, C. (2007). Sense of coherence, spirituality, stress and quality of life in chronic illness. *Journal of Nursing Scholarship, 39*(3), 229–234.

Dickerson, S. S., Wu, Y. B., & Kennedy, M. C. (2006). A CNS-facilitated ICD support group: A clinical project evaluation. *Clinical Nurse Specialist 20*(3), 146–153.

Donabedian, A. (1988). Quality assessment and assurance: Unity of purpose diversity and means. *Inquiry, 25*, 173–192.

Doran, D. M., Harrison, M. B., Laschinger, H. S., Hirdes, J. P., Rukholm, E., Sidani, S., et al. (2006). Nursing-sensitive outcomes data collection in acute care and long-term-care settings. *Nursing Research, 55*(2S), S75–S81.

Dorr, D. A., Jones, S. S., Burns, L., Donnelly, S. M., Brunker, C. P., Wilcox, A., et al. (2006). Use of health-related, quality-of-life metrics to predict mortality and hospitalizations in community-dwelling seniors. *Journal of the American Geriatrics Society, 54*(4), 667–673.

Dubos, R. (1959). *Mirage of health: Utopias, progress, and biological change.* Garden City, NY: Doubleday.

Dunbar, S. B. (2005). Psychosocial issues of patients with implantable cardioverter defibrillators. *American Journal of Critical Care, 14*(4), 294–303.

Feldman, P. H., Murtaugh, C. M., Pezzin, L. E., McDonald, M. V., & Peng, T. R. (2005, June). Just-in-time evidence-based e-mail "reminders" in home health care: Impact on patient outcomes. *HSR: Health Services Research, 40*(3), 865–885.

Gourdji, I., McVey, L., & Purden, M. (2009). A quality end of life from a palliative care patient's perspective. *Journal of Palliative Care, 25*(1), 40–50.

Grusenmeyer, P. A., & Wong, Y. (2007). Interpreting the economic literature in oncology. *Journal of Clinical Oncology, 25*(2), 196–202.

Hacker, E. (2009). Exercise and quality of life: Strengthening the connections. *Clinical Journal of Oncology Nursing, 13*(1), 31–39.

Heidrich, S. M., Egan, J. J., Hengudomsub, P., & Randolph, S. M. (2006). Symptoms, symptom beliefs, and quality of life of older breast cancer survivors: A comparative study. *Oncology Nursing Forum, 33*(2), 315–322.

Hirskyj, P. (2007). QALY: An ethical issue that dare not speak its name. *Nursing Ethics, 14*(1), 72–82.

Huang, T., & Liang, S. (2005). Care of older people: A randomized clinical trial of the effectiveness of a discharge planning intervention in hospitalized elders with hip fracture due to falling. *Journal of Clinical Nursing, 14*, 1193–1201.

Jocham, H. R., Dassen, T., Widdershoven, G., & Halfens, R. (2006). Quality of life in palliative care cancer patients: A literature review. *Journal of Clinical Nursing, 15*, 1188–1195.

Jonas-Simpson, C. M., Mitchell, G. J., Fisher, A., Jones, G., & Linscott, J. (2006). The experience of being listened to: A qualitative study of older adults in long-term care settings. *Journal of Gerontological Nursing, 32*(1), 46–53.

Kitrungrote, L., & Cohen, M. Z. (2006). Quality of life of family caregivers of patients with cancer: A literature review. *Oncology Nursing Forum, 33*(3), 625–632.

Kristofferzon, M., Löfmark, R., & Carlsson, M. (2005). Issues and innovations in nursing practice: Coping, social support, and quality of life over time after myocardial infarction. *Journal of Advanced Nursing, 52*(2), 113–124.

Lee, P., Chang, W., Liou, T., & Chang, P. (2006). Issues and innovations in nursing practice: Stage of exercise and health-related quality of life among overweight and obese adults. *Journal of Advanced Nursing, 53*(3), 295–303.

López, A., McCaffrey, R., Griffin, M., & Fitzpatrick, J. (2009). Spiritual well-being and practices among women with gynecologic cancer. *Oncology Nursing Forum, 36*(3), 300–305.

Losito, J. M., Murphy, S. O., & Thomas, M. L. (2006). The effects of group exercise on fatigue and quality of life during cancer treatment. *Oncology Nursing Forum, 33*(4), 821–825.

Low, G., & Molzahn, A. E. (2007). Predictors of quality of life in old age: A cross-validation study. *Research in Nursing & Health, 30*, 141–150.

Mitchell, S. A., Beck, S. L., Hood, L. E., Moore, K., & Tanner, E. R. (2007). Putting evidence into practice: Evidence-based interventions for fatigue during and following cancer and its treatment. *Clinical Journal of Oncology Nursing, 11*(1), 99–113.

Moreira-Almeida, A., & Koenig, H.G. (2006). Retaining the meaning of the words religiousness and spirituality: A commentary on the WHOQOL-SRPB group's "A cross-cultural study of spirituality, religion, and personal beliefs as components of quality of life." *Social Science & Medicine, 63*, 843–845.

Naef, R., & Bournes, D. (2009). The lived experience of waiting: A Parse method study. *Nursing Science Quarterly, 22*(2), 141–153.

National Institute of Nursing Research. (2006). Changing practice, changing lives: NINR strategic plan (2006–2010). Retrieved August 6, 2011, from http://www.ninr.nih.gov/NR/rdonlyres/9021E5EB-B2BA-47EA-B5DB-1E4DB11B1289/4894/NINR_StrategicPlanWebsite.pdf

Orfila, F., Ferrer, M., Lamarca, R., Tebe, C., Domingo-Salvany, A., & Alonso, J. (2006). Gender differences in health-related quality of life among the elderly: The role of objective functional capacity and chronic conditions. *Social Science & Medicine, 63*, 2367–2380.

Plummer, M., & Molzahn, A. (2009). Quality of life in contemporary nursing theory: A concept analysis. *Nursing Science Quarterly, 22*(2), 134–140.

Saunders, J. C., & Cookman, C. A. (2005). A clarified conceptual meaning of hepatitis C-related depression. *Gastroenterology Nursing, 16*(46), 123–130.

Sousa, K. H., Ryu, E., Kwok, O., Cook, S. W., & West, S. G. (2007). Development of a model to measure symptom status in persons living with rheumatoid arthritis. *Nursing Research, 56*(6), 434–440.

Stenzelius, K., Westergren, A., & Hallberg, I. R. (2007). Bowel function among people over 75 years reporting faecal incontinence in relation to help seeking, dependency and quality of life. *Journal of Clinical Nursing, 16*, 458–468.

Suhonen, R., Välimäki, M., Katajisto, J., & Leino-Kilpi, H. (2005). Provision of individualized care improves hospital patient outcomes: An explanatory model using LISREL. *International Journal of Nursing Studies, 44*, 197–207.

Sutton, L. B., & Erlen, J. A. (2006). Effects of mutual dyad support on quality of life in women with breast cancer. *Cancer Nursing, 29*(6), 488–498.

Taylor, S. J. C., Candy, B., Bryar, R. M., Ramsay, J., Vrijhoef, H. J. M., Esmond, G., et al. (2005). Effectiveness of innovations in nurse led chronic disease management for patients with chronic obstructive pulmonary disease: Systematic review of evidence. *British Medical Journal, 331*(7515), 485.

Vig, E.K., & Pearlman, R.A. (2003). Quality of life while dying: A qualitative study of terminally ill older men. *Journal of the American Geriatrics Society, 51*(11), 1595–1601.

Walton-Moss, B., Gerson, L., & Rose, L. (2005). Effects of mental illness on family quality of life. *Issues in Mental Health Nursing, 26*, 627–642.

Weinert, C., Cudney, S., & Spring, A. (2008). Evolution of a conceptual model for adaptation to chronic illness. *Journal of Nursing Scholarship, 40*(4), 364–372.

World Health Organization. (1948). WHO definition of health. Retrieved August 6, 2011, from:https://apps.who.int/aboutwho/en/definition.html.

World Health Organization. (2004). The World Health Organization quality of life (WHOQOL)–BREF. Retrieved August 6, 2011, from: http://www.who.int/substance_abuse/research_tools/en/english_whoqol.pdf

CHAPTER 9

Adherence

Jill Berg, Lorraine S. Evangelista, Donna Carruthers, and Jacqueline M. Dunbar-Jacob

INTRODUCTION

Adherence of patients to prescribed treatment by their healthcare professionals has been discussed in the medical literature since the 1950s (Greene, 2004). The lack of agreement between healthcare recommendations and patient behavior has been defined as an issue of adherence or nonadherence (Haynes, 1979; Rand, 1993; World Health Organization [WHO], 2003). Early research identified this problem of discrepancy between an ordered treatment and the actual implementation of the treatment by the patient as a factor that affected patient outcomes (Sackett & Snow, 1979). In fact, a 1998 *New York Times* article proclaimed poor adherence in medicine as the world's "other drug problem" (cited in Lehane & McCarthy, 2009).

In 2001, the World Health Organization (WHO) convened a meeting on treatment adherence. Poor adherence to treatment of chronic diseases was identified to be 50% in developed countries, with lower rates of adherence in developing countries (WHO, 2003). Although preventable diseases are estimated to consume 70% of all medical care spending in the United States (Curry & Fitzgibbon, 2009), adherence to medical recommendations is poor across all chronic disease regimens, which further increases healthcare expenditures and prevents patients from achieving the full benefit of any intervention. In addition, most chronic disorders are treated with a plan of care that cncompasses a variety of components that may include medication, diet, and exercise. Therefore, patients are often asked to manage a complex treatment regimen.

Goals for *Healthy People 2020*

Overall goals for *Healthy People* (U.S. Department of Health and Human Services, 2010; the *Healthy People* goals were defined every decade from 2000 to 2010 to 2020; see www.healthypeople.gov) are to help Americans lead healthy and long lives and to reduce health disparities. There are nearly 600 objectives within 39 topic areas to be met by 2020, and many of the objectives in this document relate to behavior-change strategies. For example, for diabetes, many of the goals in *Healthy People 2020* refer to lifestyle changes and education to better manage the disease and avoid complications such as cardiovascular disease and death. Goals for *Healthy People 2020* include health behavior change such as adherence to chronic illness regimens and preventive behaviors such as screenings to detect risk factors for disease.

Adherence and Chronic Illness

The predominant pattern of illness has changed from acute to chronic as science and technology have advanced. With that technology, treatment regimens have become more complex. However, because of changes in managed health care, these complex regimens are implemented with limited or no supervision as the patient and/or family caregivers carry out these prescribed regimens at home. Therefore, practitioners must be concerned with the extent to which patients can implement the treatment plans they design, as well as the evaluation of the patient's responses.

Patient responsibility for managing chronic conditions has increased, but there is concern about adherence as it relates to medical outcomes and economic costs. For example, an individual who has insulin-dependent diabetes mellitus (IDDM) may have a computerized insulin pump and a blood-testing device. This individual may, at some point, be a candidate for hemodialysis or renal transplantation because of complications. All of these treatment modalities require adherence behaviors to ensure maximal benefit and minimal harm to the patient. According to DiMatteo (2004), the average rate of nonadherence to treatment across all diseases is 24.8%. If this rate was extrapolated to physician visits by individuals with diabetes, as many as 7.6 million visits would result in nonadherence.

The managed care environment has also had an impact on patient burden in chronic illness. Managed care's influence on health care has been demonstrated by earlier hospital discharges, shortened office visits, and decreasing home health referrals. In addition, recent literature indicates that as many as 46% of healthcare professionals do not prescribe adequate therapy for their patients (Rhiner & von Gunten, 2010; McGlynn et al., 2003). Therefore, patients and family members have had to shoulder more of the responsibility for the treatment regimen, often in isolation. Although disease management programs have been developed by health maintenance organizations (HMOs), few programs have been implemented and critically evaluated to date. Healthcare professionals working within a managed care system often have little time to address the management of chronic illness and adherence to the recommended regimen (McWlliam, 2009; Golin, Smith, & Reif, 2004; Miller, Hill, Kottke, & Ockene, 1997). Other findings suggest that healthcare professionals and agencies can make a difference in medical outcomes by means of integrating multidisciplinary interventions specifically aimed at assisting patients with managing their chronic disease through education, self-management instruction, prevention, and outreach strategies (Barnestine-Fonseca et al., 2011; McWilliam, 2009; Feachem, Sekhri, & White, 2002).

Literally hundreds of studies have examined adherence behavior, but unfortunately that research has not effected significant changes in behavior (Dunbar-Jacob & Schlenk, 2001; McDonald, Garg, & Haynes, 2002). Even in the 1980s, health behavior researchers such as Conrad (1985) asserted that it was reasonable to assume that a patient with chronic illness attempts to self-regulate in order to gain some control over something that is not always controllable. Rosenstock (1988) also noted that healthcare professionals should "encourage people to make informed decisions, but decisions of their own choice" (p. 72). He added that healthcare professionals are not always right, and there is always the potential for untoward side effects from ordered treatment. These assertions have not changed over the years, and, in fact, we have made little progress even in our understanding of adherence behavior. Furthermore, we have not successfully implemented interventions to ensure continuing adherence with chronic regimens.

Chronic illness regimens can be exceedingly complex, and resources to assist individuals with chronic illness are often limited. Therefore, it is important that the healthcare professional understands the variables that affect the ability of the person to adhere to a regimen. To facilitate understanding, this chapter addresses factors that have an impact on adherence behavior. A discussion of the theories and a description of techniques are also presented to provide a context for the behavioral changes that are required in treatment regimens. We will also present information on goals related to *Healthy People 2020*, as well as evidence-based guidelines and their relationship to adherence behaviors. Finally, interventions to improve adherence are presented, along with case studies to illustrate key strategies.

CASE STUDY

Mrs. W is a 74-year-old woman with a history of ischemic heart disease, hypertension, and hyperlipidemia. She comes in to the clinic for a routine physical exam. She presents with complaints of shortness of breath on exertion that has been progressively getting worse over the last few months. During the physical exam you notice a weight gain of 15 pounds since her last annual physical exam and some swelling in her ankles. She informs you that her daughter who used to cook her meals moved out of state 3 months ago and she has had to eat out more often or eat frozen or canned meals that she buys at the grocery store. She also tells you that she and her daughter used to walk regularly every afternoon, but since her daughter left, she has not had the energy or motivation to go on her afternoon walks or to go out shopping. She also tells you she has not been sleeping well and finds herself crying uncontrollably and attributes this to her missing her daughter so much.

After 3 months, Mrs. W returns for a follow-up visit. She seems to be happier and tells you that she is going out with a retired businessman who has helped her cope with her daughter leaving. She tells you she has stopped taking her antidepressants and the other pills that the doctor prescribed the last time she was at the clinic because she feels better and doesn't think she needs them anymore. You also notice that she has not lost any weight and admits that she has not been exercising as much as she should.

Discussion Questions

1. Would you, the healthcare provider, label Mrs. W as nonadherent? Why or why not?
2. Suggest several lifestyle modifications that may benefit Mrs. W.
3. How might Mrs. W's perspective of her illness differ from the perspective of her provider?
4. How can you, a healthcare provider, help Mrs. W to develop a course of action to which she is likely to adhere?
5. How would you suggest that Mrs. W's boyfriend help with her recent health problems and new treatment regimens?
6. Suggest possible measures of adherence behaviors that you might use to assess Mrs. W's adherence.

Definition of Terms and Historical Perspectives

Greene (2004) addresses the first use of terms related to patients following recommended treatment regimens. He credits medical sociology and further describes the evolution of terms as well as the development of a discipline concerned with health behavior. There were a variety of labels associated with these behaviors, and patients were labeled as "uncooperative, noncompliant, poorly controlled, resistant, devious, incorrigible, irresponsible, and careless" (Greene, 2004, p. 330). Early descriptions of patients having difficulty following treatment regimens reflected societal attitudes related to tuberculosis in patients who were poor and foreign born. Eventually, the terms used to describe behavior included compliance, adherence, and concordance.

In 1974 a group of scientists gathered in Canada to discuss compliance with therapeutic regimens (Greene, 2004). The term *compliance* was chosen after some careful debate (well described in the Greene essay). Compliance was used as an umbrella term for all behavior related to healthcare recommendations, particularly in light of the shift from acute to chronic disease seen in the last half of the 20th century.

Adherence and nonadherence are generally used as synonyms for the original terms *compliance* and *noncompliance*. The term *adherence* has eventually been adopted instead of the term compliance on the global stage of healthcare delivery. An example of an interesting classic presentation in the meaning and use of these words was presented by Barofsky (1978), who proposed a continuum of self-care with three levels of patient response to healthcare

recommendations: compliance, adherence, and therapeutic alliance. In his model, compliance is linked with coercion; adherence, to conformity; and a therapeutic alliance with provider–patient interactions to self-care. Misselbrook (1998) used the term *concordance* to indicate the partnership between practitioner and patient in achieving health outcomes. Medication adherence has been divided into two main concepts: adherence and persistence. Adherence refers to the intensity of drug use during the duration of therapy, while persistence refers to overall duration (Bosworth, 2010).The literature reveals different schools of thought related to adherence. One school supports the notion that it is impossible to ever have patients completely adhere to medical regimens. A contradictory school of thought suggests that it is possible, through education or other means, to have patients adhere to their regimen requirements. These contrary schools of thought may be dependent on how a health plan was formulated (Dunbar, 1980). If a plan is formulated by a partnership between the patient and the healthcare professional, the possibility of the patient "adhering" to the plan increases. Adherence also implies a biopsychosocial approach as it focuses on actual medication-taking behavior and its measurement, stresses the importance of the relationship between the patient and provider, and addresses the patient's motivation, health beliefs, and habits (Lehane & McCarthy, 2009). Should the patient be expected to follow a plan created exclusively by the healthcare professional, without input by the patient, then the patient may or may not "comply." The WHO has adopted adherence as the term of choice and suggests that it is necessary to incorporate the agreement of the patient with the prescribed treatment plan (McWilliam, 2009; WHO, 2003).

Creer and Levstek (1996) as well as Dunbar-Jacob (1993) questioned the extent to which we "blame the patient" for their adherence behavior. Part of the responsibility, they assert, belongs to healthcare professionals, and there are instances when nonadherence is wise, given the regimen. Trostle (1997) argued that there is too much emphasis placed on the authority physicians have in recommending healthcare regimens. He further asserted that nonadherence is viewed as "nonconformity with medical advice" (p. 116) and suggested that we look broadly at the behaviors that are being engaged in by patients within the context of their illness. He also cautioned that attempts to motivate patients to comply could be considered coercive and manipulative. In any event, healthcare professionals often make decisions about the effectiveness of treatments without knowing whether the patient is actually following the treatment or in agreement with their healthcare professional (McWilliam, 2009; Rand, 2004).

In order to provide efficacious treatment of chronic disease, healthcare professionals face two challenges. First, we must ascertain whether patients are following the regimen, and secondly we must find effective ways of helping patients to overcome barriers in carrying out complex regimens.

Components of Adherence

The relevance of adherence to the total wellness–illness continuum was first described by Marston, a nurse, in 1970. Marston considered adherence to be self-care behaviors that individuals undertake to promote health, to prevent illness, or to follow recommendations for treatment and rehabilitation in diagnosed illnesses. She is notable in the history of treatment adherence as the first reviewer of literature in the field (Greene, 2004).

It may be helpful, however, to consider adherence as more than self-care behaviors; rather, it is behavior that is often shared, because patients cannot always implement their medical regimens without the participation of others, even though the delineation of responsibilities is not always clear. Sackett and Haynes (1976) outlined three necessary ingredients before labeling a patient as noncompliant: 1) a correct diagnosis must be made, 2) the recommended treatment must be determined to be efficacious, and 3) the patient must be informed and willing. For example, Greenley, Josie, and Drotar (2006) note that there are misunderstandings about the responsibility for asthma treatment regimens in inner-city children, and that this misunderstanding often leads to nonadherence. This is especially true when there is a change in the dependence/independence status of the patient, as with the teenager who assumes greater responsibility for management of his or her healthcare regimen or the older adult who now requires more supervision and assistance by family members.

In the classic book *Chronic Illness and the Quality of Life*, Strauss and colleagues (1984) noted that family members often take on assisting or controlling roles in influencing patients to adhere to medical regimens. Stephens, Rook, Frank, Khan, and Iida (2010) investigated both the negative and positive strategies spouses used to urge patients with type II diabetes to improve dietary adherence. Findings showed that cautioning the patient about the consequences of eating an inadequate diet was associated with poorer adherence, and encouragement to select healthier food choices was associated with better adherence. A follow-up study of how couples managed chronic disease revealed that coordination and collaboration between the couple were necessary to carry out the work of the medical regimen (Corbin & Strauss, 1985). More recent work in the field of HIV describes the role that family caregivers provide in the complex regimen (Beals, Wight, Aneshensel, Murphy, & Miller-Martinez, 2006). Likewise, family support in adolescents suffering from asthma was positively associated with asthma control and improved quality of life (Rhee, Belyea, & Brasch, 2010). A review by Knafl and Gilliss (2002) concludes that nursing needs to be more involved with family interventions for chronic illness management. Given that shared responsibility exists, it seems reasonable to conclude that adherence-increasing strategies should be directed toward all those involved in the regimen, and that there may be a need for discussing the division of responsibility among family members.

Theoretical Underpinnings for Adherence Behavior

Theoretical frameworks and conceptual models provide direction for healthcare professionals by guiding the assessment and providing structure for the interaction between patient and provider. At this point in time, the emphasis is on translation of theories and models to effective practice interventions. Although an extensive library devoted to adherence behavior exists, few studies support strategies to improve adherence (DiMatteo & Haskard, 2006). Models for understanding individual health behavior can only be useful if they are based on empirical research and can then be used to create effective interventions. This relates to the current mandate for translational research and evidence-based practice. Brief reviews of behavioral models that are currently used are presented here.

Health Belief Model

The health belief model (HBM), developed by Hochman and colleagues (as cited in Rosenstock, 1974), was devised to explain health-related behaviors, especially preventive health behaviors, and contains a cluster of pertinent beliefs and attitudes (Becker & Maiman, 1975). The model was modified to include general health motivation (Becker, 1976) and was again modified to include sick-role behaviors. The HBM's major proposition is that the likelihood of an individual taking recommended health actions is based on 1) the perceived severity of the illness, 2) the individual's estimate of the likelihood that a specific action will reduce the threat, and 3) perceived barriers to following recommendations. The HBM is still used frequently to explain the relationships of attitudes and behaviors to adherence behavior, specifically in relation to perceived susceptibility, perceived severity, and perceived barriers (McCall & Ginis, 2004; Rodríguez-Reimann, Nicassio, Reimann, Gallegos, & Olmedo, 2004; Wutoh et al., 2005).

Health Promotion Model

A nursing model that evolved from the HBM is the health promotion model (HPM) (Pender, 1996; Pender, Murdaugh, & Parsons, 2001). Pender conceptualizes health as a goal and believes that only the desire to be healthy leads to engagement of health promotion activities. Pender organized the concepts under the framework of individual characteristics and experiences, behavior-specific cognitions and affect, and behavioral outcomes. The Health-Promoting Lifestyle Profile is an instrument that assesses health promotion behaviors, and has been translated and validated in Spanish as well as English (Walker, Sechrist, & Pender, 1987). Recent studies using this model have found that income and education negatively impact involvement in health promotion activities (Chilton, Hu, & Wallace, 2006; Lee, Santacroce, & Sadler, 2007).

Common Sense Model of Self-Regulation

The Common Sense Model of Self-Regulation was developed from two prior models. One of them, the Common Sense model, was developed by Leventhal, Meyer, and Nerenz in 1980 to explain how individuals process illness-related events and how this shapes coping and adherence. Early studies using this model were conducted primarily on individuals with asymptomatic illnesses (Baumann, Cameron, Zimmerman, & Leventhal, 1989; Meyer, Leventhal, & Gutmann, 1985).

In brief, an individual's processing of illness-related events is dependent on four dimensions: cause (what was responsible for the illness), consequences (how things will change because of the illness), identity (being able to identify the illness), and time line (the course of the illness). In 1987, Leventhal and colleagues identified a feedback mechanism to a behavioral model and called it the Self-Regulation Theory. The dimension of control–cure was examined as part of the illness representation. These two models are now combined into one model known as the Common Sense Model of Self-Regulation (Leventhal, Brisette, & Leventhal, 2003). Recent studies using this model have shown that beliefs about illness affect coping (Gould, 2011; Kelly, Sereika, Battista, & Brown, 2007; Ohm & Aaronson, 2006; Quinn, 2005; Searle, Norman, Thompson, & Vedhara, 2007).

CASE STUDY

Mr. W is a 58-year-old African American college history professor with type II diabetes. He was diagnosed with diabetes 3 years ago and had lost weight and started an exercise program. During the last year, he has gained weight back and is no longer exercising daily. He admits to you that with some changes at work, he is extremely stressed. He starts every evening with a martini, relaxes after his long day, and then has a big dinner. His blood sugars are out of control and you are concerned that he will have to start insulin injections.

Discussion Questions

1. Would you, the healthcare provider, label Mr. W as nonadherent? Why or why not?
2. Suggest several lifestyle modifications that may benefit Mr. W.
3. How might Mr. W's perspective of his illness differ from that of his provider?

The Theory of Reasoned Action and the Theories of Planned Behavior

The theory of reasoned action (Fishbein & Ajzen, 1975) and the theory of planned behavior (Ajzen, 1985) have intention as a main component. Individuals engage in health behaviors, intentionally, based on attitudes toward a behavior and social influence. The theory of planned behavior adds a component to the model, called "perceived behavioral control," which captures the extent to which a person has control over any given behavior. Both of these theories have been useful in the examination of preventive behaviors, such as engaging in exercise programs (Martin, Oliver, & McCaughtry, 2007; Norman & Connor, 2005), condom use (Gredig, Nideroest, & Parpan-Blaser, 2006), and binge drinking (Norman, Armitage, & Quigley, 2007), where intention has been found to be an important component of engaging in the desired behavior. Such theories have proven to be valuable in comprehending physical activity in chronic illness regimens (Eng & Martin Ginis, 2007).

Cognitive Social Learning Theory

Cognitive social learning theory attempts to predict behavior that is dictated by outcome and efficacy expectancies. This theory combines environment, cognition, and emotion in the understanding of health behavior change (Bandura, 2004). Three necessary prerequisites to altering health behavior are the recognition that a lifestyle component can be harmful, the recognition that a change in behavior would be beneficial, and the recognition that one has the ability to adopt a new behavior (self-efficacy) (Schwarzer, 1992). To effect any change then, each individual must be able to self-monitor and self-regulate health behavior. This aspect of self-regulation has led to a variety of self-management strategies with which to cope with illness. The additional component of self-efficacy, defined as the patient's expectations or confidence in his or her ability to perform a recommended action, has also promoted research to test efficacy-enhancing strategies important in health behavior change. Self-efficacy has been found to be an important predictor of self-management behaviors useful in the treatment of AIDS (Johnson et al., 2006), cancer (Eiser, Hill, & Blacklay, 2000), cardiac disease (Hiltunen et al., 2005), depression (Harrington et al., 2000), and diabetes (Ott, Greening, Palardy, Holderby, & DeBell, 2000).

Transtheoretical Model of Change (Stages of Change)

The stages of change, or transtheoretical model, which was developed by Prochaska and DiClemente (1983), is an eclectic model that aims to examine and predict the process of change. This model contains three constructs: the stages of change, processes of change, and levels of change. The model's underlying premise proposes that people are at different stages in their intentional desire to adopt certain health behaviors with or without assistance. It also proposes that interventions should be matched to each categorical stage of change. Although presented hierarchically, the process of change is considered to be a spiral with relapse from a healthy behavior placing an individual in a position to move backward toward contemplation of the healthy behavior. The model also incorporates self-efficacy and decision making as key factors in the process of change, but these factors have an impact at different stages of change. The stages include the following:

- Pre-contemplation: no intention of changing behavior

- Contemplation: considering future action
- Pre-action: have a timetable for action
- Action: involved in behavior change
- Maintenance: after change is adopted; relapse is a possibility

The stage model of health behavior was initially applied to the treatment of addictive behaviors. Currently, other research on behavioral change for chronic illness has embraced this model. Clinical interventions have been proposed at each stage. The use of motivational interviewing has been examined for use in moving patients to an action phase of readiness (Jackson, Asimakopoulou, & Scammell, 2007; Johnson et al., 2007), although critics warn that there is no theoretical link between motivational interviewing and the transtheoretical model.

In summary, there are many models that have been used to study adherence behavior in chronic illness. It is important to have a theoretical basis for proposed interventions; however, more work needs to be accomplished to evaluate the effectiveness of theory-based strategies.

Prevalence of Nonadherence

Individuals with chronic medical conditions face a variety of stressful life circumstances involving a range of adaptation demands. Individuals with chronic illness must deal with a loss of independence, the threat of disease progression, and the challenge of modifying their behavior to meet the demands of a prescribed regimen. Lifestyle modifications may become necessary and include, but are not limited to, dietary changes, use of medications, and change in physical activity. Adherence to these modifications has substantial implications for treatment success and decreased disease progression.

For the patient with chronic illness, failure to adhere can result in increased disease complications, increased hospitalizations, and greater treatment costs, as well as disruptions in lifestyle, family dynamics, and coping skills. Although ascertaining the true picture of nonadherence in chronic illness is difficult, the consistency with which poor adherence rates are reported indicates that nonadherence is a major problem in health care. Several studies indicate that adherence rates in chronic illness are approximately 50% (Dunbar-Jacob et al., 2000; Haynes, McDonald, Garg, & Montague, 2002; WHO, 2003), with ranges in nonadherence rates estimated to be 20–40% for acute illness, 20–60% for chronic illness, and an incredible 50–80% for preventive regimens (Bosworth, 2010). In the United States, medication adherence to antihypertensive medications is 51% (Graves, 2000). This problem is not limited to the United States. In developing countries, it is estimated that rates of adherence to antihypertensive medications are less than 50% (van der Sande et al., 2000).

Different definitions of adherence have contributed to difficulties in comparing studies of particular disease groups, and make it impossible to generalize to studies highlighting other diseases. Adherence studies are typically disease-specific; that is, the study population is defined by the presence of a specific disease. However, more recent reviews of adherence behaviors in persons with chronic illness indicate that the nature and extent of adherence problems are similar across diseases, across regimens, and across age groups (Vermeire, Hearnshaw, Van Royen, & Denekens, 2001). A review of studies examining medication adherence reported rates as low as 50%, with some differences in rates seen between settings and measurement methods (Dunbar-Jacob et al., 2000).

Medication adherence is one category of research that spans a variety of diseases. Unfortunately there is no gold standard to measure medication adherence, and current evidence suggests the use of several strategies besides disease outcomes to capture treatment adherence to medication (Krapek et al., 2004; Wagner & Rabkin, 2000; Wendel et al., 2001). Furthermore, polypharmacy in chronic disorders adds an additional variable in observing and measuring medication adherence (Vik, Maxwell, & Hogan, 2004). Despite the complex issues contributing to medication adherence, it has been posited that greater health benefits worldwide would be realized with improved adherence to existing treatments than with the development of new medical treatments (Bosworth, 2010).

Electronic monitors have been used to assess medication adherence in many recent studies. Studies of treatment adherence in HIV populations have used both self-report, diaries, and medication event monitors (MEMs). Not specific to HIV populations, electronic monitoring typically provides lower estimates of adherence than self-report data (Wagner & Rabkin, 2000). In a study of individuals with ankylosing spondylitis, only 22% adhered strictly to prescribed medication (de Klerk & van der Linden, 1996). Although adherence rates were not as low among patients with rheumatoid arthritis— consistently below 50% (Elliott, 2008), epilepsy—34% (Cramer, Vachon, Desforges, & Sussman, 1995); major depression—51% upon initiation, 42% upon continuation/follow-up (Akincigil et al., 2007), (Carney, Freedland, Eisen, Rich, & Jaffe, 1995; Demyttenaere, Van Ganse, Gregoire, Gaens, & Mesters, 1998); schizophrenia— less than 55% (Duncan &

Rogers, 1998; McCann & Lu, 2009), diabetes mellitus—47% (Mason, Matsayuma, & Jue, 1995); hypertension—30–47% (Mounier-Vehier et al., 1998; Le et al., 1996); tuberculosis—39% (Ailinger, Martyn, Lasus, & Garcia, 2010); ischemic heart disease—38–45% (Carney et al., 1998; Straka, Fish, Benson, & Suh, 1997); and use of inhaled corticosteroids in asthma— 44–72%, with only 13% continuing to fill prescriptions after 1 year (Borrelli, Reikert, Weinstein, & Rathier, 2007). These nonadherence behaviors were nonetheless significantly associated with poor control of symptoms.

Other methods for measuring medication adherence (drug-dosing recall, pill counts, self-report surveys, and pharmacy refills) have been used and have indicated similar rates of adherence (DiMatteo, 2004; Dunbar-Jacob, Schlenk, & Caruthers, 2002). In a study using subjects with chronic pain, paper diaries and electronic diaries were compared. The electronic diaries offered a time-stamped variation on the paper diary and outperformed the latter with regard to adherence of use by the subject (Stone, Shiffman, Schwartz, Broderick, & Hufford, 2003).

Forty-eight percent of patients with tuberculosis were reported as having defaulted on their recommended medication prescriptions (Pablos-Mendez, Knirsch, Barr, Lerner, & Frieden, 1997). Treatment nonadherence following renal transplantation is associated with loss of the graft. In addition, a history of poor adherence prior to transplantation has also been associated with graft loss (Butler, Roderick, Mullee, Mason, & Peveler, 2004; Marcén &Teruel Briones, 2011). Self-reported medication nonadherence among renal transplant recipients ranged between 13% and 36% (Greenstein & Siegal, 1998; Hilbrands, Hoitsma, & Koene,

1995), whereas heart transplant recipients showed nonadherence rates of up to 37% (Grady et al., 1996). Among liver transplant patients nonadherence to immunosuppressive drugs ranges between 15% and 40% while nonadherence to clinical appointments is in the range of 3–45% (Burra et al., 2011). Although persons with life-threatening disorders may adhere somewhat better than other patients, researchers suggest that even moderate alterations in their treatment have a significant clinical impact (de Geest, Abraham, & Dunbar-Jacob, 1996; Dew et al., 2007).

ISSUES RELATED TO EXAMINING ADHERENCE BEHAVIOR

Studies have demonstrated that large numbers of individuals do not follow healthcare recommendations completely. Although nonadherence is increasingly recognized as a problem, there is no consensus about appropriate or effective methods to increase adherence. Some of the difficulty lies in the inadequacies of research on adherence, some lies in differing role expectations of patients and providers, and some relates to conflict in values. As healthcare professionals prescribe, teach, and counsel patients about medical regimens, they must be cautious in making assumptions about adherence behaviors in a given situation before imposing any specific strategy on the patient.

Individual Characteristics

Several patient characteristics that influence adherence have been examined. These include demographic factors, psychological factors, social support, past health behavior, somatic

factors, and health beliefs (Dunbar-Jacob et al., 2002). Ethnicity was addressed in a review by Schlenk and Dunbar-Jacob (1996) and by Joshi (1998), indicating that more research is needed in this area. More recent literature has examined ethnicity as an influence in adherence with diagnostic testing (Cook et al., 2010; Strzelczyk & Dignan, 2002). Strzelczyk and Dignan (2002) reported that African American women were more likely to be nonadherent with mammography screening. Conversely, Cook and colleagues (2010) reported that Latino and African American women were 2 and 1.45 times more likely to receive Pap smear screening, respectively when compared to Caucasians. With respect to retention in clinical trials, African American subjects were more likely to drop out of participation in a rheumatoid arthritis treatment adherence study than Caucasians (Dunbar-Jacob et al., 2004). An interesting study by Taira and colleagues (2007) examined predictors of medication adherence among Asian American subgroups in Hawaii and found that Filipino, Korean, and Hawaiian patients were less likely to adhere than Japanese patients. More research is needed to examine strategies among various ethnic groups to increase adherence behavior.

Because of the many inconsistencies in studies that examine age and adherence behavior, no overall statement can be made. According to Barnestein-Fonseca and colleagues (2011), there may be a variety of factors that interfere with the ability of the older adult to adhere to medical instruction. It is important to rule out cognitive changes, which may occur with aging, versus the busy lifestyle barriers that pertain to the middle-aged adult. In a study by Hinkin and colleagues (2004), HIV patients who were middle aged were less adherent than older patients.

For children, there are specific issues of adherence related to age that are associated with developmental stages rather than chronologic age. However, in general, developmental issues have not been well addressed in the adherence literature (Dunbar-Jacob et al., 2000).

Psychological Factors

Intuitively, healthcare professionals believe that psychological factors may affect adherence behavior. Many studies support the premise that depression is related to poor adherence. DiMatteo, Lepper, and Croghan (2000) completed a meta-analysis examining the relationship between depression and adherence and found that depressed patients were at a threefold risk for nonadherence. Depression has also been linked to mortality in patients not following medical recommendations in acute coronary syndromes (Kronish et al., 2006), and HIV (Lima et al., 2007). It may be helpful to treat depression in patients at risk for nonadherence (Berg, Nyamathi, Christiani, Morisky, & Leake, 2005). Other psychological factors, such as ambiguity, hostility, and general emotional distress, as single factors, are not predictive of adherence behavior but may, in fact, be components of motivation (Dunbar-Jacob, Schlenk, Burke, & Mathews, 1997).

Social Support

Social support is a variable that has frequently been explored in adherence studies. However, social support has not been demonstrated to consistently have an impact on adherence behavior. In some cases social support increases adherence behavior, such as in pediatric patients with asthma who received social support from family and friends (Sin, Kang, & Weaver, 2005) and in patients with HIV (Gonzalez et al., 2004). In contrast, other studies have found that social support has no impact on adherence (Sunil & McGehee, 2007).

Prior Health Behavior

It has been suggested that adherence to a particular healthcare regimen at a single point in time may predict subsequent adherence (Dunbar-Jacob et al., 1997). In the 10-year study of the Lipid Research Clinics Coronary Primary Prevention Trial, initial medication adherence accurately predicted adherence throughout the study; however, this did not extend to other health behaviors. In general, it was found that the more similar the initial behaviors were to the behaviors that need to be predicated, the greater the likelihood of accuracy (Dunbar-Jacob et al., 1997). In a study examining HIV treatment adherence, attending clinic appointments was associated with medication treatment adherence (Wagner, 2003).

Somatic Factors

It has been postulated that the presence of symptoms may lead to greater adherence with medical recommendations. For example, hypertensive individuals who are asymptomatic indicated that they could tell when their blood pressure was high and adhered with treatment at these times because of their belief that adherence relieved the symptoms (Meyer et al., 1985). In another study, of individuals with lung disease, increased dyspnea predicted greater adherence with nebulizer therapy (Turner,

Wright, Mendella, Anthonisen, & IPPB Study Group, 1995). A more recent study found that lack of symptoms was a barrier to adherence with inhaled corticosteroids (Ulrik et al., 2006). Conversely, increased HIV symptom experience was associated with decreased medication adherence as patients' belief in the efficacy of the medication waned in the face of continued symptomatology (Cooper, 2009). Patients who are severely ill with serious illnesses have also presented with poorer treatment adherence, as relationships with care providers decline in the face of worsening health. These patients may become depressed, pessimistic, socially withdrawn, and hopeless or ambivalent about surviving, making adherence seem futile (DiMatteo, Haskard, &Williams, 2007). Illness-related symptoms may be an important cue to following treatment recommendations.

Regimen Characteristics

Regimen type and regimen complexity have been linked to adherence behavior, with complexity being a more important factor (Dunbar-Jacob, Burke, & Puczynski, 1995). Complexity includes multiple medications, frequent treatments, a variety of treatments (e.g., diet, exercise, and medications), duration of the regimen, a complicated treatment delivery system, as well as irritating side effects (Chesney, 2003; Lemanek, 1990). An early review of the literature (Wing, Epstein, Nowal, & Lamparski, 1986) substantiated that complicated regimens lead to low adherence rates. This effect has also been well documented in the HIV literature where patients have extremely complex medication regimens (Chesney, 2003; Hinkin et al.,

2002; Waldrop-Valverde, Jones, Gould, Kumar, & Ownby, 2010).

Economic Factors

Poverty, poor English-language proficiency, and limited access to health care are predictors of nonadherence (Gonzalez, 1990). The burdens of financial costs alone may serve as a barrier to obtaining healthcare services, supplies, or medications needed to manage chronic illness. Another major barrier to adherence is a lack of resources, including inadequate or difficult transportation, inadequate availability of childcare, loss of time from low-paying jobs, and little job security. Socioeconomic status has recently been associated with poor adherence in individuals using hormone-replacement therapy. This needs to be examined further with other studies of adherence (Finley, Gregg, Solomon, & Gay, 2001). Health literacy may also contribute to problems in managing chronic illness regimens. In some studies, limited health literacy has been associated with poor adherence to antiretroviral medications (Waldrop-Valverde et al., 2010;Wolf et al., 2007) and with better adherence to other HIV medications (Paasche-Orlow et al., 2006).

Some barriers to adherence are clearly related to an ineffective healthcare system for chronic disease management. For example, some individuals with chronic disease who come to emergency departments for nonurgent care have limited access to primary care services that are more appropriate for chronic disease management (Mansour, Lanphear, & DeWitt, 2000). There is decreased availability of primary care services, particularly in inner cities and rural areas, to groups such as migrant workers, new immigrants, the homeless, and those with AIDS. In addition, the maze of governmental and third-party payers' policies and regulations often deny provider reimbursement for preventive or educational services, making these services less available to patients.

Cultural Factors

More attention is being given to the ways in which culture influences health behaviors and the interactions of patients with healthcare providers. Cultural influences affect the way adults and children experience, interpret, and respond to illness and its treatment.

Because of the changing demographics and the influx of immigrants into the United States, studies examining the behaviors of different cultural groups have begun to appear in the literature. Some of these studies explore the dimension of being a minority group with a health problem. For example, minority status has been associated with lower asthma medication adherence. Minorities were found to have lower adherence and a higher prevalence of negative asthma medication beliefs than Caucasians. Tests of medication suggested that such negative medication beliefs partially mediated the relationship between minority status and adherence (Le et al., 2008). Language issues affect the utilization of health care and the ability to form relationships with healthcare professionals. Different cultural norms may also interfere with adherence behaviors. For example, in Latino families, the stigma of having tuberculosis may be a factor in poor adherence to taking medication (Cabrera, Morisky, & Chin, 2002; Hovell et al., 2003). Latinos have

also been described as seeking health care late, if at all, and then using folk healers and medications for illness (Talamantes, Lawler, & Espino, 1995; Zuckerman, Guerra, Dorssman, Foland, & Gregory, 1996). Some of the delay in healthcare utilization relates to insurance issues, language barriers, and immigration status.

Asian immigrants may have difficulty accepting and actively engaging in regimen demands. Chinese immigrants were found to have ineffective self-care and coping strategies with diabetes in a study by Jaynes and Rankin (2001). Similarly, in a study by Im and Meleis (1999), Korean women ignored the symptoms of menopause until symptoms became intolerable.

It will become increasingly important for healthcare professionals to interpret the effect of culture and ethnicity on adherence behavior. One of the issues that confounds the link between health behavior and culture is socioeconomic status. There is a need to distinguish if poor adherence is related to ethnicity, cultural, or socioeconomic factors, as opposed to the interaction of these factors.

Patient–Provider Interactions

Of all of the variables associated with nonadherence, patient–provider interactions have been highlighted as being extremely important since 2000. In 1993, in an editorial in the journal *Health Psychology*, Dunbar-Jacob asked if it was time to share the blame. Previously, the focus of adherence research and practice only examined patient characteristics. In the results from the medical outcomes study, DiMatteo and colleagues (1993) found that patient satisfaction in encounters with healthcare providers may impact health behavior. A few years later, the American Heart Association addressed the "multilevel compliance challenge" (Miller et al., 1997), referring to the contributions of the patient, provider, and the healthcare system. More recent studies have focused on the relationship between provider and patient as a way of encouraging health behavior change (Beach, Keruly, & Moore, 2006; O'Malley, Sheppard, Schwartz, & Mandelblatt, 2004). Importantly, self-management topics arise in primary care consultations infrequently, as maintaining the self-other relationship reign as a prime objective for both patients and professionals (Blakeman, Bower, Reeves, & Chew-Graham 2010). The introduction of self-management topics threaten this process, highlighting an important tension that underpins care. Strategies such as motivational interviewing have been used successfully by healthcare professionals who are advocating health behavior change (Carels et al., 2007; Cook, Emiliozzi, & McCabe, 2007). Ockene, Hayman, Pasternak, Schron, and Dunbar-Jacob (2002) detail specific strategies that healthcare providers should use in counseling patients, including:

- Simplify the regimen.
- Tailor the regimen to each individual patient.
- Ask about adherence behavior at every encounter.
- Review patient's medication containers, noting renewal dates.
- Involve the patient in designing the treatment plan.
- Provide clear instructions (written and verbal).
- Use behavioral strategies (reminder systems, cues, self-monitoring, feedback, and reinforcement).

Four phases of treatment adherence have been identified: contemplating, initiating, maintaining, and sustaining long-term behavior, with each phase having different barriers and facilitators (Bosworth, 2010). Discrepancies between a patient's stage of treatment adherence and a provider's intervention may yield nonadherence due to a patient's lack of readiness for the intervention.

Motivational interviewing is a "client-centered, directive style for enhancing intrinsic motivation to change by exploring and resolving ambivalence" (Miller & Rollnick, 2002, as cited in Lane & Rollnick, 2009, p. 154). Through the utilization of four core principles, practitioners can harness the spirit of motivational interviewing and guide patients toward greater self-motivated change: expressed empathy, rolling with resistance, supporting self-efficacy, and developing discrepancy (the latter, meaning to discover how one's personal values are at odds with current behavior through careful listening). Through the use of open-ended questions, summarizing, reflective listening directed toward empathy and eliciting "change talk," practitioners can gain an understanding of the importance of change to a patient, and the confidence the patient has in effecting such change (Rollnick, Butler, Kinnersley, Gregory, & Mash, 2010). Motivational interviewing was originally developed for the treatment of addictions (Levensky, Forcehimes, O'Donohue, & Beitz, 2007), but has been modified for use in different contexts, including adaptation to the healthcare setting, sometimes termed "behavior change counseling" (Lane & Rollnick, 2009). This technique, whether termed motivational interviewing or behavior change counseling, has been used effectively toward better treatment adherence through improving body mass index, cholesterol, and systolic blood pressure (Lane & Rollnick, 2009); hypertension, diet and exercise regimens, and smoking cessation (Anshel & Kang, 2008; Levensky et al 2007); asthma medication adherence (Borelli, Riekert, Weinstein, & Rathier, 2007); and weight loss in diabetic women (West, DiLillo, Bursac, Gore, & Greene, 2007).

Perspectives of Patients and Healthcare Professionals

Patients and providers are likely to have different perspectives on chronic illness, its treatment, and the relative merits of adherence behavior. The patient lives with the disease, and treatment is only one aspect of that individual's life. Living with treatment consequences is vastly different from offering advice, counsel, education, or exhortation about healthcare recommendations. Patients ask for help from healthcare professionals because they feel ill, they are worried, they are responding to others' recommendations, they need evidence to validate claims for entitlement benefits, and so forth. Providers, on the other hand, are concerned about adherence, which may be seen as the desired outcome of the patient–provider interaction (Anderson, 1985).

Anderson (1985) identifies two ways in which the patient's perspectives on chronic illness—in this case, diabetes mellitus—differ from those of healthcare providers. First, there is a relative difference in understanding the treatment regimen, not just on the level of specificity, rationale, and consequences, but also with respect to the sources of problems. Patients may see treatment as part of the problem of having diabetes, whereas providers see treatment as a solution. Second, patients are more concerned about the "here and now" experience, in contrast to providers' concern over a problem that

places future health at risk. For example, patients express more concerns about preventing hypoglycemic reactions than about managing higher than normal blood glucose levels. Providers, on the other hand, express more concern about the importance of achieving close to normal blood glucose levels because of their perceptions of serious long-term consequences if control of blood glucose levels is not achieved (Anderson, 1985).

Ethics and Adherence Behavior

Adherence to recommendations for health behavior is an increasingly important ethical issue in healthcare cost containment, because conflicts arise when healthcare resources are limited and decisions about the best use of time, money, and the energy of providers must be made. However, economic and ethical issues in adherence differ. Whereas economic issues are concerned with the most efficient distribution of resources, ethical issues are concerned with the most equitable distribution (Barry, 1982). Connelly (1984) believes that strategies that promote and improve a patient's active and effective self-care are both ethically and economically significant.

There is also concern about providing resources to help those with chronic disorders in developing countries, where treatment nonadherence is so high (WHO, 2003). Ethical issues center on reciprocal rights and responsibilities of caregivers and patients, use of paternalism and coercion by caregivers, autonomy of the patient, relative risks and benefits of proposed regimens, and the costs to society of nonadherence. Again, the focus upon the patients' active participation with their healthcare providers appears to also raise ethical concerns (Bernardini, 2004; Rand &

Sevick, 2000). This raises the question of whether health care directed solely by the practitioner without input by the patient is ethical and whether nonadherence should rest upon the shoulders of only the patient.

INTERVENTIONS TO ENHANCE ADHERENCE BEHAVIOR

The complexity of the variables associated with nonadherence should not deter the healthcare professional from working with the patient to achieve maximum possible integration of optimal health recommendations. To accomplish maximum adherence, those who use adherence-increasing strategies have a responsibility to ensure the patient's safety and comprehension. For the nurse, often working as liaison between patient and physician, communicating with either or both is often necessary before matters are sufficiently clear to select and begin specific adherence-increasing strategies. The WHO (2003) has suggested adopting the use of the five "As" in an effort to assist patients with self-management aspects to their chronic disease, such as treatment adherence. The five "As" include: assess, advise, agree, assist, and arrange (Locke & Latham, 2002). The interventions suggested in this chapter are adaptable within this framework. Advising the patient of the importance of treatment adherence, establishing agreement with a treatment plan, and arranging adequate follow up are necessary steps for healthcare professionals interested in providing treatment adherence interventions to their patients.

Assessment

If we are to assume that any measurement of patient adherence is an assessment of behaviors,

then we must decide how to analyze those behaviors. Adherence behaviors can be assessed in many ways. Unfortunately, there is no "gold standard" for measuring adherence, and each measurement is prone to some error, usually consisting of a bias toward an overestimation of adherence (Dunbar-Jacob et al., 2002; Burke & Dunbar-Jacob, 1995). However, using a combination of methods to measure a specific adherence behavior is recommended to increase accuracy and reliability of the results, compared with a single method of measurement (WHO, 2003). An assessment of the patient's overall well-being and psychological structure is also essential to a better understanding of his or her adherence behaviors.

A systematic assessment of the patient should include the patient's family, sociocultural and economic factors, knowledge level, beliefs, attitudes, and current understanding of the proposed regimen. Attention should also be given to the patient's perceptions of the illness threat, the efficacy of recommendations, and the patient's ability to carry these out.

Enhancing adherence behaviors is not as simple as telling patients what to do and then telling them again when the desired effect is not achieved. In studying adherence, it is necessary to understand that it is not the length of their life that is of concern to many people with chronic illness, but their perception that the recommended behavior change will be worth the effort (Rapley, 1997). Understanding and respecting the social, cultural, and psychological factors that influence adherence behaviors may enhance efforts to manage the problem of nonadherence.

There should be a determination of the "rightness" of the prescriptions for the particular patient, including an estimation of the relative harm or benefit that is expected. The assessment will allow the nurse to determine which aspects of the regimen management are most unlikely to achieve adherent behavior, are most important in attaining therapeutic goals, and require the most learning to attain the desired behavioral change. The following questions should be asked in an adherence-oriented history (Hingson, Scotch, Sorenson, & Swazey, 1981):

- Have you been taking anything for this problem already?
- Does anything worry you about the illness?
- What can happen if the recommended regimen is not followed?
- How likely is not following your recommendation regimen likely to occur?
- How effective do you feel the regimen will be in treating the disorder?
- Can you think of any problems you might have in following the regimen?
- Do you have any questions about the regimen or how to follow it?

Healthcare professionals are not infallible, and errors can occur in prescribing, in dispensing, in communicating with the patient and family caregiver, and in maintaining updated written records, especially in settings in which multiple care providers are present. A second consideration is that the patient or caregiver simply may not understand, or remember, instructions. If patients lack the knowledge or skills to undertake a recommended behavior or treatment, it is unlikely that they will do so. Instructions related to treatment regimens need to be reinforced continually over time to enhance adherence behaviors.

Enhancing a patient's motivation requires careful assessment of his or her readiness to make and maintain behavioral changes. Building skills requires that he or she be ready to learn tasks such as reading food labels, selecting appropriate foods in restaurants, and incorporating the taking of medications into his or her daily routine. In other words, patients must learn new strategies to help them adopt and maintain new behaviors, especially when daily routines are interrupted (Bandura, 1997; Barnestein-Fonseca et al., 2011; Miller et al., 1997).

It is also important to be aware of a tendency among care providers to see adherence behavior as positive, admirable, and wise (being the "good patient") and nonadherence behavior as being negative, deplorable, and unintelligible (being the "problem patient"). It seems probable that healthcare professionals who have this view would be less likely to search out barriers to nonadherence.

Assessment should also lead to a determination of the proper focus of adherence-increasing strategies. It was mentioned earlier that the notion of adherence as self-care may be too restrictive in situations where adherence with medical regimens cannot be achieved without the assistance of others. For instance, the combination of marked disability and chronic illness makes the conceptualization of adherence as self-care ability inappropriate. In such instances, social support networks may be the most important agents of adherence and, therefore, should become the focus of adherence-increasing strategies. However, the nurse should carefully assess the impact of social support on adherence. Although social support—by significant others or support networks—may help patients cope with chronic illness and reinforce adherence behavior in some populations (McWilliam, 2009; Burke & Dunbar-Jacob, 1995), this may not be true for all, because there are patients who do not always want tangible help from others.

Measuring Adherence Behaviors

There are several common methodological approaches that focus on adherence. Primary methods include self-report, practitioner report, observation, physiologic measures, medication monitoring, and electronic monitors.

Self-Report

Patient self-reports of adherence behaviors are the simplest and least expensive method of gathering nonadherence information and are feasible in virtually all care settings. Self-reports also allow the collection of more detailed information on the circumstances surrounding poor adherence than any other type of measure (Burke & Dunbar-Jacob, 1995). They may be elicited through simple questions or through a more complex, structured interview schedule. Common self-report measures include medication and symptom diaries, structured questionnaires, and interviews.

Self-reported adherence behavior has come under scrutiny because it is widely believed to be invalid and unreliable (Berg & Arnstein, 2006; Liu et al., 2006; Smith et al., 2007). There are many reasons that a patient's self-reported adherence may be inaccurate. While patients who report nonadherence tend to report their behavior accurately (Bosworth, 2010), patients may honestly not remember whether they took their medications, may be unaware that they are not following recommendations, or may have misconceptions about their dosing schedule (Barfod, Hecht, Rubow, & Gerstoft, 2006; Bosworth, 2010; Sankar, Nevedal, Neufeld, & Luborsky, 2007). There may also be other reasons for nonadherence such as economic factors, or lack of resources, or the patient's discomfort with being honest with healthcare providers. In any event, it is incumbent on the provider to be able to assess whether a patient can and is willing to follow a recommendation. Toward this end, there are studies that recommend asking questions in a nonjudgmental way to elicit valid responses about regimen adherence (Berg & Arnstein, 2006).

Several studies have attempted to evaluate and define the accuracy of self-reported adherence. Many of these have compared patient reports with pill counts, drug levels, or biological markers in body fluids. Most have found that individuals overestimate their adherence (Bender, Milgrom, Rand, & Ackerson, 1998; Dunbar-Jacob et al., 2000; Liu et al., 2006). Despite inherent problems, self-report is still the most common measure used in adherence behavior assessment, and it has the potential to be the most accurate record of what a given patient has done, as long as the patient can remember taking the medication and is motivated to be absolutely truthful about what is remembered (Morisky & DiMatteo, 2011, p. 255–257). Thus, establishing trust within the patient–provider relationship and developing strategies to enhance recall are essential to obtaining accurate information.

Practitioner Report

Reports by healthcare professionals are an indirect method of adherence assessment. However, studies indicate that this method is not accurate and often results in overestimating adherence (Bosworth, 2010). Because there are no readily observable characteristics of the patient who has trouble following a regimen, clinicians rely on intuition and presumption to gauge the adherence of a patient (Miller et al., 2002; Steele, Jackson, & Gutman, 1990). However, given that practitioner reports are fast, free, noninteractive, and consistent with the medical model, they are still used to assess adherence behavior.

Observation

Direct observation of the patient is not always possible. Therefore, observation is not a practical method of assessing adherence. Theoretically, this method would be an ideal way to provide evidence of adherence behavior; however, individuals often "play to an audience," and the knowledge that someone is watching affects behavior. An example of this behavior for the individual with asthma is the demonstration/return demonstration of the correct method of using metered-dose inhalers (MDIs). Patients with asthma are assessed on their ability to carry out the instructed regimen and adherence with teaching. Although nurses assess a patient's behavior in carrying out tasks related to healthcare management, the assumption cannot be made that this activity continues at home.

Physiologic Measures

Physiologic measures of adherence include serum drug levels, heart rate monitoring, muscle strength, urine sample analysis, cholesterol levels, and glycosylated hemoglobin levels. The advantage of physiologic methods is that these measures are not dependent on the patient's memory or veracity.

Of all of the physiologic measures, measurement of drug levels is most commonly used. Although drug-level measurements reflect a greater degree of accuracy than self-reports and practitioner reports, there are some difficulties with this type of assessment. First, these measures do not reflect the level of adherence (Dunbar-Jacob et al., 1995). They merely classify a person as having followed or not followed some of the regimen (Burke & Dunbar-Jacob, 1995). Second, although biochemical assays offer a direct and objective approach to the measurement of nonadherence, this method is neither affordable nor available for every drug, is only applicable to medications with a long half-life, and may vary from individual to individual (de Geest et al., 1996). Third, physiologic technologies are often unable to detect dosage levels. For example, many asthma medications are so rapidly absorbed systemically that it is not possible to detect them by biochemical assay (Rand & Wise, 1994). Finally, accurate detection of nonadherence through drug-level testing offers no explanation or insight into the reasons for nonadherence (Besch, 1995).

Medication Monitors

Pill counts, pharmacy-refill monitoring, and MDI canister weighing can all be used to measure medication adherence. In studies that use pill counts, the subject is given a vial each month that has a certain number of tablets, and this vial is exchanged for a new one each month. The medication left in the vial can be compared with the number that was supposed to be left if the medication were taken. Similarly, when a patient requests a refill from the pharmacy, the time of the request is compared with the expected date of refill if the medication were taken as prescribed. This does not take into account whether patients are sharing medications with others or "dumping" pills prior to refill.

MDI canister weighing is used with patients who have respiratory illnesses. The canister is weighed before it is given to the patient and then at specific times during treatment. Although medication-monitoring methods appear highly accurate, they may overestimate adherence behavior (Rand & Wise, 1994; Rudd, Ahmed, Zachary, Barton, & Bonduelle, 1990). Berg & Arnstein (2006) suggest that asking a patient to bring in the medications for a check of pill count may, in fact, be offensive and be counterproductive to the rapport building between patient and provider.

Electronic Monitoring

Electronic monitors are the newest technology for the assessment of adherence behaviors. The most common electronic monitoring device is the electronic medication monitor. Electronic monitors may also be used to capture heart rate and muscle movement with exercise adherence (Iyriboz, Powers, Morrow, Ayers, & Landry, 1991) or to document nasal continuous positive airway pressure adherence for patients with sleep apnea (Kribbs et al., 1993).

Electronic monitors that assess medication adherence are used with tablets, eye drops, and MDIs (Berg & Arnstein, 2006). These monitors function with the use of microprocessors placed in special bottle caps or blister packs and can monitor the date and time of day for each manipulation of the drug container and provide information on drug-taking behavior for days or weeks. Knowing the pattern of pill taking (or not taking) can be useful in evaluating clinical responses (or lack thereof) or side effects, and provide guidance for interventions specifically tailored for each patient (Quittner, Modi, Lemanek, Ievers-Landis, & Rapoff, 2007).

An innovative use of technology was reported in a pilot trial to monitor lung transplant recipient adherence to self-care behaviors using a Pocket Personal Assistant for Tracking Health device (Pocket PATH) (DeVito Dabbs et al., 2009). The mobile, hand-held device significantly improved self-care behaviors of monitoring vital signs, medical regimens, health habits, and communicating important changes to the transplant team between scheduled visits, as compared to standard pencil-and-paper methods.

In the end, no single measure of adherence can compete with the accuracy of a multi-method approach that combines feasible self-reporting and reasonable objective measures amidst an effective patient–provider relationship (Bosworth, 2010).

Strategies to Enhance Adherence

There is universal agreement that it is important for patients with chronic illness to follow evidence-based provider recommendations (WHO, 2003). In order to enhance adherence to treatment, there are a variety of strategies that healthcare providers can employ. Some of these strategies are educational, some are behavioral, and some are organizational.

Education

Educational interventions should include an assessment of the patient's level of knowledge, cultural background, and particular goals. Educational information should be presented in manageable segments, with additional information and reinforcement at subsequent meetings. The nurse should focus on the key issues in the management of the regimen and should select the most important aspects necessary for health maintenance. Difficult skills should be demonstrated, and then the patient should be allowed to practice and do a return demonstration. Difficult skills should also be reviewed each time the patient visits.

Written material should be geared to the patient's reading level and language. Glazer, Kirk, and Bosler (1996) evaluated printed materials to teach breast self-examination and found that, although the reading level of the materials being provided was at the ninth-grade level, the average reading level of the target population was at the sixth-grade level. Another study on health literacy found that 24% of patients could not understand even the most basic written medication instructions and that an additional 12% had very limited literacy (Gazmararian, Williams, Peel, & Baker, 2003). These findings underscore the need to prepare materials that can be used by the maximum number of patients. Other educational materials can be provided, such as videotapes, audiotapes, and computer-assisted instruction.

Often patients rely on family members to interpret regimen details at home and may feel embarrassed about their issues with health literacy (Williams et al., 2007). Therefore, when educating those with chronic illnesses, family members or significant others should be involved in the teaching session. Emphasis in teaching needs to be directed toward not only knowledge of the disease, but also the skills needed for the regimen (Morello, Chynoweth, Kim, Singh, & Hirsch, 2011; Burke & Dunbar-Jacob, 1995). In addition, the regimen should be simplified as much as possible.

Beyond Knowledge and Comprehension

Abilities beyond knowledge and comprehension are required. Therefore, educational goals must be broader than solely the acquisition of knowledge if adherence is to result. The outcome of adherence depends on participation of the learner beyond that of listening, reading, or assimilating information. Clinicians should also encourage patients' participation in their own care. Flexible self-care regimens enable people to exercise a degree of autonomy that is not an option in standard regimens, even when these are adapted to some extent for individuals. The flexibility of instructions, such as "If you have this sign or this symptom, then try this activity," allows people some freedom to make informed choices, and having choices fosters independence and a better quality of life (McWilliam, 2009; Rapley, 1997).

Behavioral Strategies to Enhance Adherence

Behavioral strategies attempt to influence specific adherence behaviors directly through the use of various techniques. These strategies may be used as a single intervention, or in combination, to achieve desired results.

It is generally believed that adherence is increased when patients actively participate in learning and deciding how to implement prescribed regimens. However, insistence by the healthcare provider on a preconceived or stereotyped notion of the most desirable level of participation may be inappropriate. A mismatch between an authoritarian provider and an assertive, active learner may influence adherence adversely. On the other hand, the provider who expects an active involvement process can overwhelm a passive and nonactive learner.

The power differential between patients and providers constitutes an important aspect of adherence behaviors. It has been posited that providers inadvertently transmit their expectations to their patients, and that this subtle projection may be even more determinative for health effects than the expectations of the patient (McWilliam, 2009; van Dulmen & Bensing, 2002). A clinician's belief in his or her own ability to enhance adherence significantly predicts actual efforts to enhance adherence, and raises expectations about adherence outcomes (Byrne, Deane, & Caputi, 2008). Interestingly, empathy for the patient on the part of the provider lowered adherence expectations, possibly indicating that understanding the difficulty in adhering to medications reduces the provider's belief in his or her ability to effect change (Byrne et al., 2008).

Tailoring

The minimal outcome of patient participation with the nurse in developing an adherence strategy should be tailoring the treatment to the patient's daily behaviors, because this process may help cue adherence (Burke & Dunbar-Jacob, 1995). Integrating treatment activities so that they coincide with routine activities, called rituals, is an important way of individualizing and enhancing the treatment plan. The daily schedule of eating, arising and retiring, hygiene, favorite television program, and so on identifies rituals that may be used to incorporate health behaviors into daily life.

Simplifying the Regimen

As a result of discussions between patient and nurse, it may become apparent that the patient is unable to manage the complexity of the prescribed regimen. Negotiation with the prescribing source may result in better adherence if this barrier is cleared and the regimen is simplified. As a general rule, the number of times medications are taken and the number of doses should be held to a minimum (Schernthaner, 2010).

Providing Reminders

Reminders or memory aids are useful when the problem is a failure of the behavior to occur because patients have forgotten to perform one or more aspects of the desired behavior. Calendars, clocks, and individually prepared posters with medication and food reminders can be very helpful. Separating a day's supply of medications can also help the person who has difficulty remembering if a particular dose was taken.

The healthcare professional can reinforce the importance of adherence at episodic visits. Such reinforcement may involve pill counting, attention to patient diaries or to other reports of behavior, and self-monitoring. These are all methods that remind the patient of the value of adherence and that elicit participation.

Telephone calls are also useful in reminding patients about healthcare recommendations; in encouraging adherence with medications in the elderly (Cargill, 1992) and low-income, minority populations with diabetes (Walker et al., 2011); and as an effective intervention in enhancing adherence with making and keeping follow-up appointments after referral from emergency (Komoroski, Graham, & Kirby, 1996). Friedman and colleagues (1996) tested a variation of telephone follow up, which demonstrated a 17.7% improvement in medication adherence among those receiving automated telephone calls. Bosworth and colleagues (2008) used a telephone intervention for patients with hypertension and found a significant change in medication-taking behavior. Telephone reminders not only provide a personal touch, but also allow individuals who wish to reschedule an appointment the opportunity to do so at that time (Crespo-Fierro, 1997). A newer strategy, the use of text messaging to adolescents with diabetes, increased disease self-efficacy and adherence to the medical regimen (Franklin, Waller, Pagliari, & Greene, 2006). SMS intervention (text messaging) in sub-Saharan Africa also improved patients' adherence to antiretroviral therapy, perhaps through an improved patient–provider relationship (Chi & Stringer, 2010; Lester et al., 2010).

Enhancing Coping

The nurse should be sensitive to cues from individual patients suggesting emotional responses that interfere with learning optimal health behaviors. Situational anxiety, marked depression, and denial are associated with low levels of adherence. These three emotional responses should be interpreted as signals that a patient's coping skills are inadequate and that a modification in approach may be more effective.

Ethnocultural Interventions

Recognition that the patient and family's patterns of communication may differ from the provider's is important for effective interactions. In addition, cultural components need to be integrated into any strategies that are proposed. There are some basics to delivering culturally competent care to enhance treatment adherence. Most of the strategies have been addressed in other documents, for example, *Healthy People 2020*. It has been acknowledged that one of providers' goals for the health of all is to eliminate the disparities that currently exist in providing care. Flaskerud (2007) acknowledges that the provision of culturally competent care rests on the shoulders of the healthcare provider. Therefore, it is up to healthcare providers, individually, to provide these key ingredients to their practices:

- Ask about health practices that may interfere with a treatment regimen.
- Seek understanding when a patient says something that you do not understand.
- Acknowledge to patients that there may be additions to recommendations that stem from culture and tradition, and inquire about these.
- Listen carefully to verbal communication and pay close attention to nonverbal communication.

For effective interaction with persons of a different culture, "cultural translation" may be needed. One requisite for a cultural translator is learning about the historical rituals and norms that relate to health of the particular group. Another requisite is evaluating health behaviors in the patient's cultural context to determine competing priorities, environmental obstacles, or degree of knowledge and skills (George, 2001). One cultural intervention study successfully improved TB medication adherence among Latino immigrants by building relationships and implementing Latino values of personal attention (seeing the same nurse during the 9-month treatment period), asking about family members, incorporating a common Latino proverb into each session (translating to "It is better to prevent than to lament"), adapting written materials to be easily understood (in Spanish at a sixth-grade level) with photos of Latino families, and use of culturally appropriate, nonverbal language of touching the arm of the woman or shoulder of the man at the end of each visit (Ailinger, Martyn, Lasus, & Lima Garcia, 2010).

Providers need to recognize that *their* belief system, values, and attitudes toward healthcare management also are culturally determined and may be responsible for ideologic or philosophic differences (McWilliam, 2009). The emphasis on self-care in Western medical systems is ideologically consistent with the value of individual enterprise in Western cultures (Anderson, Blue, & Lau, 1993). Persons of other cultures may find this value of self-care foreign.

Evidence-Based Practice Box

Purpose: The purpose of this study was to evaluate the efficacy of the telephone as a tool to improve adherence to a cholesterol-lowering diet.

Method: Subjects were randomized to a control group and to a treatment group. Usual care for the control group consisted of follow-up physician visits and/or lipid measurements every 3–6 months. Subjects assigned to the treatment group received the intervention described as follows.

Sample: The study enrolled 65 men and women diagnosed with hypercholesterolemia, who were considered nonadherent to a cholesterol-lowering diet.

Intervention: Members of the treatment group were required to participate in six intervention sessions delivered every 2 weeks via telephone. Telephone interventions were individually tailored and designed to focus on methods of managing eating behavior in difficult situations.

Results and Implications for Nursing Practice: There was a significant difference in total and saturated fat, dietary cholesterol adherence, and serum low-density lipoprotein cholesterol (LDL-C) between the control group and the intervention group. This behavioral intervention enhanced adherence to the recommended cholesterol-lowering diet. Implications are as follows: In light of the difficulties patients often face when attempting to follow a therapeutic eating plan, healthcare providers must rely on methods of improving adherence that have proved successful in similar situations.

Source: Burke, L. E., Dunbar-Jacob, J., Orchard, T.J., et al. (2005). Improving adherence to a cholesterol-lowering diet: A behavioral intervention study. *Patient Education and Counseling, 57*(1), 134–42.

There has been a blossoming interest in documenting the evidence of particular strategies to improve health outcomes. Evidence-based practice guidelines for a variety of physiologic and behavioral interventions are now readily available to all healthcare practitioners (Agency for Healthcare Research and Quality, National Guideline Clearinghouse). This means that what we recommend to patients is based on evidence of efficacy. We still, however, face the challenge of helping patients to follow recommendations. No matter the quality of our interventions, they are only beneficial if patients use them. And, it is up to healthcare professionals to better assess if patients can do what we suggest, and then to evaluate the outcomes.

This chapter has discussed hundreds of studies that have assessed adherence behavior. Ultimately, it is up to each of us to build rapport with our patients, and to simply ask the patient what they can and cannot do.

For a full suite of assignments and additional learning activities, use the access code located in the front of your book and visit this exclusive website: **http://go.jblearning.com/larsen**. If you do not have an access code, you can obtain one at the site.

STUDY QUESTIONS

Why is trying to increase adherence behaviors important for clients with chronic illness?

What factors are involved in adhering to medical regimens? Discuss them.

How prevalent is nonadherence? Can you think of examples from your own practice?

How does adherence behavior affect evidence-based practice?

What ethical issues arise when a provider tries to increase a client's adherence behavior? Discuss an ethical approach.

Using your own or a client's culture, identify how norms, rituals, and practices affect adherence with healthcare recommendations.

What are the strengths and weaknesses of education as a means of increasing adherence?

What impact does health literacy have on adherence behavior?

How can you encourage client participation to increase adherence? Discuss tailoring, simplifying the regimen, and reminders.

How can you enhance coping to increase adherence?

What are the advantages and disadvantages of support groups to aid adherence behavior?

REFERENCES

Ailinger, R. L., Martyn, D., Lasus, H., & Lima Garcia, N. (2010). Populations at risk across the lifespan: Population studies: The effect of a cultural intervention on adherence to latent tuberculosis infection therapy in Latino immigrants. *Public Health Nursing, 27*(2), 115–120.

Ajzen, L. (1985). From intention to action: A theory of planned behavior. In J. Kuhl & J. Beckman (Eds.), *Action control: From cognition to behavior*. Heidelberg: Springer.

Akincigil, A., Bowblis, J. R., Levin, C., Walkup, J. T., Jan, S., & Crystal, S. (2007). Adherence to antidepressant treatment among privately insured patients diagnosed with depression. *Medical Care, 45*(4), 363–369.

Anderson, J. M., Blue, C., & Lau, A. (1993). Women's perspectives on chronic illness: Ethnicity, ideology, and restructuring of life. *Diabetes Spectrum, 6*(2), 102–115.

Anderson, R .M. (1985). Is the problem of noncompliance all in our head? *Diabetes Educator, 11*, 31–34.

Anshel, M., & Kang, M. (2008). Effectiveness of motivational interviewing on changes in fitness, blood lipids, and exercise adherence of police officers: An outcome-based action study. *Journal of Correctional Health Care, 14*(1), 48–62.

Bandura, A. (1997). *Self-efficacy: The exercise of control*. New York: W.H. Freeman and Company.

Bandura, A. (2004). Swimming against the mainstream: The early years from chilly tributary to transformative mainstream. *Behavior Research and Therapy, 42*(6), 613–630.

Barfod, T.S., Hecht, F.M., Rubow, C., & Gerstoft, J. (2006). Physicians' communication with patients about adherence to HIV medication in San Francisco and Copenhagen: A qualitative study using grounded theory. *BMC Health Services Research, 6*, 154.

Barofsky, I. (1978). Compliance, adherence, and the therapeutic alliance: Steps in the development of self-care. *Social Science and Medicine, 12*, 369–376.

Barnestein-Fonseca, P., Leiva-Fernández, J., Vidal-España, F., García-Ruiz, A., Prados-Torres, D., & Leiva-Fernández, F. (2011). Efficacy and safety of a multifactor intervention to improve therapeutic adherence in patients with chronic obstructive pulmonary disease (COPD): Protocol for the ICEPOC study. *Trials, 14*(12), 40.

Barry, V. (1982). *Moral aspects of health care*. Belmont, CA: Wadsworth.

Baumann, L. J., Cameron, L. D., Zimmerman, R. S., & Leventhal, H. (1989). Illness representations and matching labels with symptoms. *Health Psychology, 8*(4), 449–469.

Beach, M. C., Keruly, J., & Moore, R. D. (2006). Is the quality of the patient-provider relationship associated with better adherence and health outcomes for patients with HIV? *Journal of General Internal Medicine, 21*(6), 661–665.

Beals, K. P., Wight, R. G., Aneshensel, C. S., Murphy, D. A., & Miller-Martinez, D. (2006). The role of family caregivers in HIV medication adherence, *AIDS Care, 18*(6), 589–596.

Becker, M. H. (1976). Socio-behavioral determinants of compliance. In D. L. Sackett & R. Haynes (Eds.), *Compliance with therapeutic regimens*. Baltimore: Johns Hopkins University Press.

Becker, M. H., & Maiman, L. A. (1975). Sociobehavioral determinants of compliance with health and medical care recommendations. *Medical Care, 13*, 10–24.

Bender, B., Milgrom, H., Rand, C., & Ackerson, L. (1998). Psychological factors associated with medication nonadherence in asthmatic children. *Journal of Asthma, 35*, 347–353.

Berg, J., Nyamathi, A., Christiani, A., Morisky, D., & Leake, B. (2005). Predictors of screening results for depressive symptoms among homeless adults in Los Angeles with latent tuberculosis. *Research in Nursing & Health, 28*(3), 220–229.

Berg, K. M., & Arnsten, J. H. (2006). Practical and conceptual challenges in measuring antiretroviral adherence. *Journal of Acquired Immune Deficiency Syndromes, 43*(Suppl 1), 79–87.

Bernardini, J. (2004). Ethical issues of compliance/adherence in the treatment of hypertension. *Advances in Chronic Kidney Disease, 11*(2), 222–227.

Besch, C.L. (1995). Compliance in clinical trials. *AIDS, 9*(1), 1–10.

Blakeman, T., Bower, P., Reeves, D., & Chew-Graham, C. (2010). Bringing self-management into clinical view: A qualitative study of long-term condition management in primary care consultations. *Chronic Illness, 6*(2), 136–150.

Borrelli, B., Riekert, K. A., Weinstein, A., & Rathier, L. (2007). Brief motivational interviewing as a clinical strategy to promote asthma medication adherence. *The Journal of Allergy and Clinical Immunology, 120*(5), 1023–1030.

Bosworth, H. B. (2010). *Improving patient treatment adherence: A clinician's guide*. New York: Springer.

Bosworth, H. B., Olsen, M. K., Neary, A., Orr, M., Grubber, J., Svetkey, L., et al. (2008). Take Control of Your Blood pressure (TCYB) study: A multifactorial tailored behavioral and educational intervention for achieving blood pressure control. *Patient Education and Counseling, 70*(3), 338–347.

Burke, L. E., & Dunbar-Jacob, J. (1995). Adherence to medication, diet and activity recommendations: From assessment to maintenance. *Journal of Cardiovascular Nursing, 9*(2), 62–79.

Burra, P., Germani, G., Gnoato, F., Lazzaro, S., Russo, F. P., Cillo, U., & Senzolo, M. (2011). Adherence in liver transplant recipients. *Liver Transplant, 17*(7), 760–767.

Butler, J. A., Roderick, P., Mullee, M., Mason, J. C., & Peveler, R. C. (2004). Frequency and impact of nonadherence to immunosuppressants after renal transplantation: A systematic review. *Transplantation, 77*(5), 769–776.

Byrne, M., Deane, F., & Caputi, P. (2008). Mental health clinicians' beliefs about medicines, attitudes, and expectations of improved medication adherence in patients. *Evaluation & the Health Professions, 31*(4), 390–403.

Cabrera, D. M., Morisky, D. E., & Chin, S. (2002). Development of a tuberculosis education booklet for Latino immigrant patients. *Patient Education and Counseling, 46*(2), 117–124.

Carels, R. A ., Darby, L., Cacciapaglia, H. M., Konrad, K., Coit, C., Harper, J., et al. (2007). Using motivational interviewing as a supplement to obesity treatment: A stepped-care approach. *Health Psychology, 26*(3), 369–374.

Cargill, J. M. (1992). Medication compliance in elderly people: Influencing variables and interventions. *Journal of Advanced Nursing, 17*(4), 422–426.

Carney, R. M., Freedland, K. E., Eisen, S. A., Rich, M. W., & Jaffe, A. S. (1995). Major depression and medication adherence in elderly patients with coronary artery disease. *Health Psychology, 14*(1), 88–90.

Carney, R. M., Freedland, K. E., Eisen, S. A., Rich, M. W., Skala, J. A., & Jaffe, A. S. (1998). Adherence to a prophylactic medication regimen in patients with symptomatic versus asymptomatic ischemic heart disease. *Behavioral Medicine, 24*(1), 35–39.

Chesney, M. (2003). Adherence to HAART regimens. *AIDS Patient Care and STDs, 17*(4), 169–177.

Chi, B. H., & Stringer, J. S. (2010). Mobile phones to improve HIV treatment adherence. *Lancet, 376*(9755), 1807–1808.

Chilton, L., Hu, J., & Wallace, D. C. (2006). Health-promoting lifestyle and diabetes knowledge in Hispanic American adults. *Home Health Care Management Practice, 18*, 378–385.

Connelly, C. E. (1984). Economic and ethical issues in patient compliance. *Nursing Economics, 2*, 342–347.

Conrad, P. (1985). The meaning of medications: Another look at compliance. *Social Science and Medicine, 20*, 29–37.

Cook, N., Kobetz, E., Reis, I., Fleming, L., Loer-Martin, D., & Amofah, S. A. (2010). Role of patient race/ethnicity, insurance and age on Pap smear compliance across ten community health centers in Florida. *Ethnic Disease, 20*(4), 321–326.

Cook, P. F., Emiliozzi, S., & McCabe, M. M. (2007). Telephone counseling to improve osteoporosis treatment adherence: An effectiveness study in community practice settings. *American Journal of Medical Quality, 22*(6), 445–456.

Cooper, L. (2009). A 41-year-old African American man with poorly controlled hypertension: Review of patient and physician factors related to hypertension treatment adherence. *Journal of the American Medical Association, 301*(12), 1260–1284.

Corbin, J. A., & Strauss, A. L. (1985). Managing chronic illness at home: Three lines of work. *Qualitative Sociology, 8*(3), 224–247.

Cramer, J., Vachon, L., Desforges, C., & Sussman, N. (1995). Dose frequency and dose interval compliance with multiple antiepileptic medications during a controlled clinical trial? *Epilepsia, 36*, 1111–1117.

Creer, T. L., & Levstek, D. (1996). Medication compliance and asthma: Overlooking the trees because of the forest. *Journal of Asthma, 33*, 203–211.

Crespo-Fierro, M. (1997). Compliance/adherence and care management in HIV disease. *Journal of the Association of Nurses in AIDS Care, 8*, 43–54.

Curry, S., & Fitzgibbon, M. (2009). Theories of Prevention. In S. A. Schumaker, J. K., Ockene, & K. A. Riekert (Eds.) *The handbook of health behavior change* (3rd ed., pp. 3–17). New York, NY: Springer Publishing Co.

de Geest, S., Abraham, I., & Dunbar-Jacob, J. (1996). Measuring transplant patients' compliance with immunosuppressive therapy. *Western Journal of Nursing Research, 18*(5), 595–605.

de Klerk, E., & van der Linden, S. (1996). Compliance monitoring of NSAID drug therapy in ankylosing spondylitis, experiences with an electronic monitoring device. *British Journal of Rheumatology, 35*, 60–65.

Demyttenaere, K., Van Ganse, E., Gregoire, J., Gaens, E., & Mesters, P. (1998). Compliance with depressed patients treated with fluoxetine or amitriptyline. *International Clinical Psychopharmacology, 13*(1), 11–17.

De Vito Dabbs, A., Dew, M. A., Myers, B., Begey, A., Hawkins, R., Ren, D., et al. (2009). Evaluation of a hand-held, computer-based intervention to promote early self-care behaviors after lung transplant. *Clinical Transplantation, 23*(4), 537–545.

Dew, M. A., DiMartini, A. F., DeVito Dabbs, A., Myaskovsky, L., Steel, J., Unruh, M., et al. (2007). Rates and risk factors for nonadherence to the medical regimen after adult solid organ transplantation. *Transplantation, 83*(7), 858–873.

DiMatteo, M. R. (2004). Variations in patients' adherence to medical recommendations: A quantitative review of 50 years of research. *Medical Care, 42*(3), 200–209.

DiMatteo, M. R., & Haskard, K. B. (2006). Further challenges in adherence research: Measurements, methodologies, and mental health care. *Medical Care, 44*(4), 300–303.

DiMatteo, M. R., Haskard, K. B., & Williams, S. L. (2007). Health beliefs, disease severity, and patient adherence: A meta-analysis. *Medical Care, 45*(6), 521–528.

DiMatteo, M. R., Lepper, H. S., & Croghan, T. W. (2000). Depression is a risk factor for noncompliance with medical treatment. *Archives of Internal Medicine, 160*, 2101–2107.

DiMatteo, M. R., Sherbourne, C. D., Hays, R. D., Ordway, L., Kravitz, R. L., McGlynn, E. A., et al. (1993). Physicians' characteristics influence patients' adherence to medical treatment: Results from the medical outcomes study. *Health Psychology, 12*(2), 93–102.

Dunbar, J. (1980). Adhering to medical advice: A review. *International Journal of Mental Health, 9*(1–2), 70–78.

Dunbar-Jacob, J. (1993). Contributions to patient adherence: Is it time to share the blame? *Health Psychology, 12*, 91.

Dunbar-Jacob, J., Burke, L. E., & Puczynski, S. (1995). Clinical assessment and management of adherence to medical regimens. In P. M. Nicassio & T. W. Smith (Eds.), *Managing chronic illness: A biopsychosocial perspective*. Washington, DC: American Psychological Association.

Dunbar-Jacob, J., Erlen, J. A., Schlenk, E. A., Ryan, C. M., Sereika, S. M., & Doswell, W. M. (2000). Adherence in chronic disease. *Annual Review of Nursing Research, 18*, 48–90.

Dunbar-Jacob, J., Holmes, J. L., Sereika, S., Kwoh, C. K., Burke, L. E., Starz, T. W., et al. (2004). Factors associated with attrition of African Americans during the recruitment phase of a clinical trial examining adherence among individuals with rheumatoid arthritis. *Arthritis & Rheumatology, 51*(3), 422–428.

Dunbar-Jacob, J., & Schlenk, E. (2001). Patient adherence to treatment regimen. In A. Baum & T. Revenson (Eds.), *Handbook of health psychology* (pp. 321–657). Mahwah, NJ: Lawrence Erlbaum Associates Publishers.

Dunbar-Jacob, J., Schlenk, E. A., Burke, L. E., & Mathews, J. T. (1997). Predictors of patient adherence: Patient characteristics. In S. A. Schumaker, E. B. Schron, & J. K. Ockene (Eds.), *The handbook of health behavior change* (2nd ed.). New York: Springer.

Dunbar-Jacob, J., Schlenk, E., & Caruthers, D. (2002). Adherence in the management of chronic disorders. In A. Christensen & M. Antoni (Eds.), *Chronic physical disorders: Behavioral medicine's perspective.* (pp. 69–82). Malden, MA: Blackwell Publishers.

Duncan, J., & Rogers, R. (1998). Medication compliance in patients with chronic schizophrenia: Implications for the community management of mentally disordered offenders. *Journal of Forensic Sciences, 43*, 1133–1137.

Eiser, C., Hill, J. J., & Blacklay, A. (2000). Surviving cancer: What does it mean for you? An evaluation of a clinic based intervention for survivors of childhood cancer. *Psycho-Oncology, 9*, 214–220.

Elliott, R. (2008). Poor adherence to medication in adults with rheumatoid arthritis: Reasons and solutions. *Disease Management & Health Outcomes, 16*(1), 13–29.

Eng, J. J., & Martin Ginis, K. (2007). Using the theory of planned behavior to predict leisure time physical activity among people with chronic kidney disease. *Rehabilitation Psychology, 52*(4), 435–442.

Feachem, R. G., Sekhri, N. K., & White, K. L. (2002). Getting more for their dollar: A comparison of the NHS with California's Kaiser Permanente. *British Medical Journal, 324*(7330), 135–141.

Finley, C., Gregg, E. W., Solomon, L. J., & Gay, E. (2001). Disparities in hormone replacement therapy use by socioeconomic status in a primary care population. *Journal of Community Health, 26*(1), 39–50.

Fishbein, M., & Ajzen, I. (1975). *Belief, attitude and intention: An introduction to theory and research. Reading,* MA: Addison-Wesley.

Flaskerud, J. H. (2007) Can we achieve it? *Issues in Mental Health Nursing, 28*(3), 309–311.

Franklin, V. L., Waller, A., Pagliari, C., & Greene, S. A. (2006). A randomized controlled trial of Sweet Talk, a text-messaging system to support young people with diabetes. *Diabetic Medicine, 23*(12), 1332–1338.

Friedman, R., Kazis, L. E., Jette, A., Smith, M. B., Stollerman, J., Torgeson, J., et al. (1996). A telecommunication system for monitoring and counseling patients with hypertension: Impact on medication adherence and blood pressure. *American Journal of Hypertension, 9*(1), 285–292.

Gazmararian, J. A., Williams, M. V., Peel, J., & Baker, D. W. (2003). Health literacy and knowledge of chronic disease. *Patient Education and Counseling, 51*(3), 267–275.

George, M. (2001). The challenge of culturally competent health care: Applications for asthma. *Heart and Lung, 30*(5), 392–400.

Glazer, H., Kirk, L., & Bosler, F. (1996). Patient education pamphlets about prevention, detection, and treatment of breast cancer in low literacy women. *Patient Education and Counseling, 27*, 185–189.

Golin, C. E., Smith, S. R., & Reif, S. (2004). Adherence counseling practices of generalist and specialist physicians caring for people living with HIV/AIDS in North Carolina. *Journal of General Internal Medicine, 19*(1), 16–27.

Gonzalez, J. (1990). Factors relating to frequency among low-income Mexican American women: Implications for nursing practice. *Cancer Nursing, 13*, 134–142.

Gonzalez, J. S., Penedo, F. J., Antoni, M. H., Durán, R. E., McPherson-Baker, S., Ironson, G., et al. (2004). Social support, positive states of mind, and HIV treatment adherence in men and women living with HIV/AIDS. *Health Psychology, 23*(4), 413–418.

Gould, K. A. (2011). A randomized controlled trial of a discharge nursing intervention to promote self-regulation of care for early discharge interventional cardiology patients. *Dimensions of Critical Care Nursing. 30*(2), 117–125.

Grady, K. E., Lemkau, J. P., McVay, J. M., Carlson, S., Lee, N., Minchella, M., et al. (1996). Clinical decision-making and mammography referral. *Preventive Medicine, 25*(3), 327–338.

Graves, J. W. (2000). Management of difficult-to-control hypertension. *Mayo Clinic Proceedings, 75*, 539–542

Gredig, D., Niderost S., & Parpan-Blaser, A. (2006). HIV-protection through condom use: Testing the theory of planned behaviour in a community sample of heterosexual men in a high-income country. *Psychology & Health, 21*(5), 541–555.

Greene, J. A. (2004)."Noncompliance" enters the medical literature, 1955–1975. 2002 Roy Porter Memorial Prize Essay Therapeutic Infidelities. *Social History of Medicine, 17*(3), 327–343.

Greenley, R. N., Josie, K. L., & Drotar, D. (2006). Perceived involvement in condition management among inner-city youth with asthma and their primary caregivers. *Journal of Asthma, 43*(9), 687–693.

Greenstein, S., & Siegal, B. (1998). Compliance and noncompliance in patients with a functioning renal transplant: A multicenter study. *Transplantation, 66*(12), 1718–1726.

Harrington, R., Kerfoot, M., Dyer, E., McNiven, F., Gill, J., Harrington, V., et al. (2000). Deliberate self-poisoning in adolescence: Why does a brief family intervention work in some cases and not others? *Journal of Adolescence, 23*, 13–20.

Haynes, R. B. (1979). Determinants of compliance: The disease and the mechanics of treatment. In R.B. Haynes (Ed.), *Compliance in healthcare*. Baltimore, MD: Johns Hopkins University Press.

Haynes, R. B., McDonald, H., Garg, A. X., & Montague, P. (2002). Interventions for helping patients to follow prescriptions for medications. *Cochrane Database of Systematic Reviews* (2), CD000011.

Healthy People (2020). Retrieved September 20, 2011, from www.healthypeople.gov/

Hilbrands, L., Hoitsma, A., & Koene, R. (1995). Medication compliance after renal transplantation. *Transplantation, 60*, 914–920.

Hiltunen, E. F, Winder, P. A., Rait, M. A., Buselli, E. F., Carroll, D. L., & Rankin, S.H. (2005). Implementation of efficacy enhancement nursing interventions with cardiac elders. *Rehabilitation Nursing, 30*(6), 221–229.

Hingson, R., Scotch, N., Sorenson, J., & Swazey, J. (1981). *In sickness and in health*. St. Louis: Mosby.

Hinkin, C. H., Castellon, S. A., Durvasula, R. S., Hardy, D. J., Lam, M. N., Mason, K. I., et al. (2002). Medication adherence among HIV positive adults: Effects of cognitive dysfunction and regimen complexity. *Neurology, 59*(12), 1944–1950.

Hinkin, C. H., Hardy, D. J., Mason, K. I., Castellon, S. A., Durvasula, R. S., Lam, M. N., et al. (2004). Medication adherence in HIV-infected adults: Effect of patient age, cognitive status, and substance abuse. *AIDS, 18*(1), 19–25.

Hovell, M. F., Sipan, C. L., Blumberg, E. J., Hofstetter, C. R., Slymen, D., Friedman, L., et al. (2003). Increasing Latino adolescents' adherence to treatment for latent tuberculosis infection: A controlled trial. *American Journal of Public Health, 93*(11), 1871–1877.

Im, E., & Meleis, A. (1999). A situation-specific theory of Korean immigrant women's menopausal transition. *Journal of Nursing Scholarship, 31*, 333–338.

Iyriboz, Y., Powers, S., Morrow, J., Ayers, D., & Landry, G. (1991). Accuracy of the pulse oximeters in estimating heart rate at rest and during exercise. *British Journal of Sports Medicine, 25*(3), 162–164.

Jackson, R., Asimakopoulou, K., & Scammell, A. (2007). Assessment of the transtheoretical model as used by dietitians in promoting physical activity in people with type 2 diabetes. *Journal of Human Nutrition & Dietetics, 20*(1), 27–36.

Jaynes, R., & Rankin, S. (2001). Application of Leventhal's self-regulation model to Chinese immigrants with type 2 diabetes. *Journal of Nursing Scholarship, 31*, 333–338.

Johnson, S. S., Paiva, A. L., Cummins, C. O., Johnson, J. L., Dyment, S. J., Wright, J. A., et al. (2007). Transtheoretical model-based multiple behavior intervention for weight management: Effectiveness on a population basis. *Preventive Medicine, 46*(3), 238–246.

Johnson, M. O., Chesney, M. A., Goldstein, R. B., Remien, R. H., Catz, S., Gore-Felton, C., et al. (2006). Positive provider interactions, adherence self-efficacy, and adherence to antiretroviral medications among HIV-infected adults: A mediation model. *AIDS Patient Care and STDs, 20*(4), 258–268.

Joshi, M. S. (1998). Adherence in ethnic minorities: The case of South Asians in Britain. In L. Myers & K. Midence (Eds.), *Adherence to treatment in medical conditions*. Amsterdam: Harwood.

Kelly, M. A., Sereika, S. M., Battista, D. R., & Brown, C. (2007). The relationship between beliefs about depression and coping strategies: Gender differences. *The British Journal of Clinical Psychology, 46*(3), 315–332.

Knafl, K. A., & Gilliss, C. L. (2002). Families and chronic illness: A synthesis of current research. *Journal of Family Nursing, 8*(3), 178–198.

Komoroski, E., Graham, C., & Kirby, R. (1996). A comparison of interventions to improve clinic follow-up compliance after a pediatric emergency department visit. *Pediatric Emergency Care, 12*, 87–90.

Krapek, K., King, K., Warren, S. S., George, K. G., Caputo, D. A., Mihelich, K., et al. (2004). Medication adherence and associated hemoglobin A1c in type 2 diabetes. *Annals of Pharmacotherapy, 38*(9), 1357–1362.

Kribbs, N., Pack, A., Kline, L., Smith, P., Schwartz, A. R., Schubert, N. M., et al. (1993). Objective measurement of patterns of nasal CPAP use by patients with obstructive sleep apnea. *American Review of Respiratory Disease, 147*(4), 887–895.

Kronish, I. M., Rieckmann, N., Halm, E. A., Shimbo, D., Vorchheimer, D., Haas, D. C., et al. (2006). Persistent depression affects adherence to secondary prevention behaviors after acute coronary syndromes. *Journal of General Internal Medicine, 21*(11), 1178–1183.

Lane, C., & Rollnick, S. (2009). Motivational Interviewing. In S. A. Shumaker, J. K., Ockene, & K. A. Riekert (Eds.) *The Handbook of Health Behavior Change* (3rd ed., pp. 151–167). New York, New York: Springer Publishing.

Lee, Y. L., Santacroce, S. J., & Sadler, V. (2007). Predictors of healthy behavior in long-term survivors of childhood cancer. *Journal of Clinical Nursing, 16*(11a), 285–295.

Lehane, E., & McCarthy, G. (2009). Medication non-adherence—exploring the conceptual mire. *International Journal of Nursing Practice, 15*(1), 25–31.

Le, J. Y., Kusek, J. W., Greene, P. G., Bernhard, C., Norris, K., Smith, D., et al. (1996). Assessing medication adherence by pill count and electronic monitor in the African American study of kidney disease and hypertension. *American Journal of Hypertension, 9*(8), 719–725.

Le, T. T., Bilderback, A., Bender, B., Wamboldt, F. S., Turner, C. F., Turner, C. F., Rand, C. S. et al. (2008). Do asthma medication beliefs mediate the relationship between minority status and adherence to therapy? *Journal of Asthma, 45*(1), 33–37.

Lemanek, K. (1990). Adherence issues in the medical management of asthma. *Journal of Pediatric Psychology, 15*(4), 437–458.

Lester, R. T., Ritvo, P., Mills, E. J., Kariri, A., Karanja, S., Chung, M. H., et al. (2010). Effects of a mobile phone short message service on antiretroviral treatment adherence in Kenya (WelTel Kenya1): A randomised trial. *Lancet, 376*(9755), 1838–1845.

Levensky, E. R., Forcehimes, A., O'Donohue, W. T., & Beitz, K. (2007). Motivational interviewing: An evidence-based approach to counseling helps patients follow treatment recommendations. *The American Journal of Nursing, 107*(10), 50–58.

Leventhal, H., Brisette, I., & Leventhal, E. (2003). The common-sense model of self-regulation of health and illness. In L. Cameron L. (Ed.), *The self-regulation of health and illness behaviour* (pp. 42–65). New York: Routledge.

Leventhal, H., Meyer, D., & Nerenz, D. (1980). The common sense representations of illness danger. In S. Rachman (Ed.), *Contributions to medical psychology* (pp. 27–30). Oxford: Pergamon Press.

Leventhal, H., Glynn, K., & Fleming, R. (1987). Is the smoking decision an 'informed choice'? Effect of smoking risk factors on smoking beliefs. *Journal of the American Medical Association, 257*, 3373–3377.

Lima, V. D., Geller, J., Bangsberg, D. R., Patterson, T. L., Daniel, M., Kerr, T., et al. (2007). The effect of adherence on the association between depressive symptoms and mortality among HIV-infected individuals first initiating HAART. *AIDS, 21*(9), 1175–1183.

Liu, H., Miller, L. G., Hays, R. D., Wagner, G., Golin, C., & Hu, W. (2006). A practical method to calibrate self-reported adherence to antiretroviral therapy. *Journal of Acquired Immune Deficiency Syndromes, 43*(Suppl. 1), 104–112.

Locke, E. A., & Latham, G. P. (2002). Building a practically useful theory of goal setting and task motivation. A 35-year odyssey. *American Psychologist, 57*(9), 705–717.

Mansour, M. E., Lanphear, B. P., & DeWitt, T. G. (2000). Barriers to asthma care in urban children: Parent perspectives. *Pediatrics, 106*, 512–519.

Marcén, R., & Teruel Briones, J. L. (2011). Patients with a failed renal transplant. *Minerva Urology Nefrology, 1*,35–44.

Marston, M. (1970). Compliance with medical regimens: A review of the literature. *Nursing Research, 19*, 312–323.

Martin, J., Oliver, K., & McCaughtry, N. (2007). The theory of planned behavior: Predicting physical activity in Mexican American children. *Journal of Sport & Exercise Psychology, 29*(2), 225–232.

Mason, B., Matsayuma, J., & Jue, S. (1995). Assessment of sulfonylurea adherence and metabolic control. *Diabetes Educator, 21*, 52–57.

McCall, L. A., & Ginis, K. A. (2004). The effects of message framing on exercise adherence and health beliefs among patients in a cardiac rehabilitation program. *Journal of Applied Biobehavioral Research, 9*(2), 122–135.

McCann, T. V., & Lu, S. (2009). Medication adherence and significant others' support of consumers with schizophrenia in Australia. *Nursing and Health Sciences 11*(3), 228–234.

McDonald, H. P., Garg, A. X., & Haynes, R. B. (2002). Interventions to enhance patient adherence to medication prescriptions: Scientific review. *The Journal of the American Medical Association, 288*(22), 2868–2879.

McGlynn, E., Asch, S., Adams, J., Keesey, J., Hicks, J., & DeCristofaro, A. (2003). The quality of health care delivered to adults in the United States. *New England Journal of Medicine, 348*(26), 2635–2645.

McWilliam, C. L. (2009). Patients, persons or partners? Involving those with chronic disease in their care. *Chronic Illness, 5*(4), 277–292.

Meyer, D., Leventhal, H., & Gutmann, M. (1985). Common-sense models of illness: The example of hypertension. *Health Psychology, 4*(2), 115–135.

Miller, N. H., Hill, M., Kottke, T., & Ockene, I. (1997). The multilevel compliance challenge: Recommendations for a call to action. A statement for healthcare professionals. *Circulation, 95*, 1085–1090.

Miller, L. G., Liu, H., Hays, R. D., Golin, C. E., Beck, C. K., Asch, S. M., et al. (2002). How well do clinicians estimate patients' adherence to combination antiretroviral therapy? *Journal of General Internal Medicine, 17*(1), 1–11.

Miller, W. R., & Rollnick, S. (2002). *Motivational interviewing: Preparing people for change*. New York: Guilford Press.

Misselbrook, D. (1998). Managing the change from compliance to concordance. *Prescriber, 19*, 23–33.

Morello, C. M., Chynoweth, M., Kim, H., Singh, R. F., & Hirsch, J. D. (2011) Strategies to improve medication adherence reported by diabetes patients and caregivers: Results of a taking control of your diabetes survey. *Annals of Pharmacotherapy. 45*(2), 145–153.

Morisky, D., & DiMatteo, M. (2011). Improving the measurement of self-reported medication nonadherence: Response to authors. *Journal of Clinical Epidemiology, 64*(3), 255–257.

Mounier-Vehier, C., Bernaud, C., Carre, A., Lequeuche, B., Hotton, J. M., & Charpentier, J. C. (1998). Compliance and antihypertensive efficacy of amlodipine compared with nifedipine slow-release. *American Journal of Hypertension, 11*, 478–486.

Norman, P., Armitage, C. J., & Quigley, C. (2007). The theory of planned behavior and binge drinking: Assessing the impact of binge drinker prototypes. *Addictive Behaviors, 32*(9), 1753–1768.

Norman, P., & Conner, M. (2005). The theory of planned behavior and exercise: Evidence for the mediating and moderating roles of planning on intention-behavior relations. *Journal of Sport and Exercise Psychology, 27*, 488–504.

Ockene, I. S., Hayman, L. L., Pasternak, R. C., Schron, E., & Dunbar-Jacob, J. (2002). Task force No.4: Adherence issues and behavior changes: Achieving a long-term solution. 33rd Bethesda Conference. *Journal of the American College of Cardiology, 40*(4), 630–640.

Ohm, R., & Aaronson, L.S. (2006). Symptom perception and adherence to asthma controller medications. *Journal of Nursing Scholarship, 38*(3), 292–297.

O'Malley, A. S., Sheppard, V. B., Schwartz, M., & Mandelblatt, J. (2004). The role of trust in use of preventive services among low-income African-American women. *Preventive Medicine, 38*(6), 777–785.

Ott, J., Greening, L., Palardy, N., Holderby, A., & DeBell, W. K. (2000). Self efficacy as a mediator variable for adolescents' adherence to treatment for insulin dependent diabetes mellitus. *Children's Health Care, 29*, 47–63.

Paasche-Orlow, M. K., Cheng, D. M., Palepu, A., Meli, S., Faber, V., & Samet, J. H. (2006). Health literacy, antiretroviral adherence, and HIV-RNA suppression: A longitudinal perspective. *Journal of General Internal Medicine, 21*(8), 835–840.

Pablos-Mendez, A., Knirsch, C. A., Barr, R. G., Lerner, B. H., & Frieden, T.R. (1997). Nonadherence in tuberculosis treatment: Predictors and consequences in New York City. *American Journal of Medicine, 102*(2), 164–170.

Pender, N. J. (1996). *Health promotion in nursing practice* (2nd ed.). Norwalk, CT: Appleton-Century-Crofts.

Pender, N. J., Murdaugh, C. L., & Parsons, M. A. (2001). *Health promotion in nursing practice*. Upper Saddle River, NJ: Prentice Hall.

Prochaska, J., & DiClemente, C. (1983). Stages and processes of self-change of smoking: Toward an integrative model of change. *Journal of Consulting & Clinical Psychology, 51*, 390–395.

Quinn, J. R. (2005). Delay in seeking care for symptoms of acute myocardial infarction: Applying a theoretical model. *Research in Nursing & Health, 28*(4), 283–294.

Quittner, A. L., Modi, A. C., Lemanek, K. L., Ievers-Landis, C. E., & Rapoff, M. A. (2007). Evidence-based assessment of adherence to medical treatments in pediatric psychology. *Journal of Pediatric Psychology. 33*(9), 916–936

Rand, C. S. (1993). Measuring adherence with therapy for chronic diseases: Implications for the treatment of heterozygous familial hypercholesterolemia. *American Journal of Cardiology, 72*(10), 68D–74D.

Rand, C. (2004). Non-adherence with asthma therapy: More than just forgetting. *The Journal of Pediatrics, 146*, 157–159.

Rand, C. S., & Sevick, M. A. (2000). Ethics in adherence promotion and monitoring. *Controlled Clinical Trials, 21*(Suppl. 5), 241–247.

Rand, C. S., & Wise, R. A. (1994). Measuring adherence to asthma medication regimens. *American Review of Respiratory and Critical Care Medicine, 149*, 289–290.

Rapley, P. (1997). Self-care: Re-thinking the role of compliance. *Australian Journal of Advanced Nursing, 15*, 20–25.

Rhee, H., Belyea, M. J., & Brasch, J. (2010) Family support and asthma outcomes in adolescents: Barriers to adherence as a mediator. *Journal of Adolescent Health, 47*(5), 472–478.

Rhiner, M. I., & von Gunten, C. F. (2010). Cancer breakthrough pain in the presence of cancer-related chronic pain: Fact versus perceptions of health-care providers and patients. *Journal of Supportive Oncology, 8*(6), 232–238.

Rodríguez-Reimann, D. I., Nicassio, P., Reimann, J. O., Gallegos, P. I., & Olmedo, E. L. (2004). Acculturation and health beliefs of Mexican Americans regarding tuberculosis prevention. *Journal of Immigrant Health, 6*(2), 51–62.

Rollnick, S., Butler, C. C., Kinnersley, P., Gregory, J., & Mash, B. (2010). Motivational interviewing. *British Medical Journal, 340*, 1900.

Rosenstock, I. M. (1974). Historical origins of the health belief model. *Health Education Monographs, 2*, 354–386.

Rosenstock, I. M. (1988). Enhancing patient compliance with health recommendations. *Journal of Pediatric Health Care, 2*(2), 67–72.

Rudd, P., Ahmed, S., Zachary, V., Barton, C., & Bonduelle, D. (1990). Improved compliance measures: Applications in an ambulatory hypertensive drug trial. *Clinical Pharmacology and Therapeutics, 48*(6), 676–685.

Sackett, D. L., & Haynes, R. B. (Eds.) (1976). *Compliance with therapeutic regimens*. Baltimore: Johns Hopkins University Press.

Sackett, D. L., & Snow, J. C. (1979). The magnitude of compliance and noncompliance. In R. B. Haynes, D. W. Taylor, & D. L. Sackett (Eds.), *Compliance in health care* (pp. 11–22). Baltimore: Johns Hopkins University Press.

Sankar, A. P., Nevedal, D. C., Neufeld, S., & Luborsky, M. R. (2007). What is a missed dose? Implications for construct validity and patient adherence. *AIDS Care, 19*(6), 775–780.

Schernthaner, G. (2010). Review Article: Fixed-dose combination therapies in the management of hyperglycaemia in Type 2 diabetes: An opportunity to improve adherence and patient care. *Diabetic Medicine, 27*(7), 739–743.

Schlenk E., & Dunbar-Jacob, J. (1996). *Ethnic variations in adherence: A review*. Unpublished manuscript.

Schwarzer, R. (1992). Self-efficacy in the adoption and maintenance of health behaviors: Theoretical approaches and a new model. In R. Schwarzer (Ed.), *Self-efficacy: Thought control of action* (pp. 217–243). Washington, DC: Hemisphere.

Searle, A., Norman, P., Thompson, R., & Vedhara, K. (2007). A prospective examination of illness beliefs and coping in patients with type 2 diabetes. *British Journal of Health Psychology, 12*(4), 621–638.

Smith, S. R., Wahed, A. S., Kelley, S. S., Conjeevaram, H. S., Robuck, P. R., & Fried, M. W. (2007). Assessing the validity of self-reported medication adherence in hepatitis C treatment. *The Annals of Pharmacotherapy, 41*(7), 1116–1123.

Sin, M. K., Kang, D. H., & Weaver, M. (2005). Relationships of asthma knowledge, self-management, and social support in African American adolescents with asthma. *International Journal of Nursing Studies, 42*(3), 307–313.

Steele, D. J., Jackson, T. C., & Gutmann, M. C. (1990). Have you been taking your pills? *The Journal of Family Practice, 30*(3), 294–299.

Stephens, M. A., Rook, K. S., Franks, M. M., Khan, C., & Iida, M. (2010). Spouses use of social control to improve diabetic patients' dietary adherence. *Family System Health, 28*(3),199–208.

Stone, A., Shiffman, S., Schwartz, J., Broderick, J., & Hufford. (2003). Patient compliance with paper and electronic diaries. *Controlled Clinical Trials, 24*(2), 182–199.

Straka, R., Fish, J., Benson, S., & Suh, J. (1997). Patient self-reporting of compliance does not correspond with electronic monitoring: An evaluation using isosorbide dinitrate as a model drug. *Pharmacotherapy, 17*, 126–132.

Strauss, A., Corbin, J., Fagerhaugh, S., Glaser, B., Maines, D., & Suczek, B. (1984). *Chronic illness and the quality of life* (2nd ed.). St. Louis: Mosby.

Strzelczyk, J. J., & Dignan, M. B. (2002). Disparities in adherence to recommended followup on screening mammography: Interaction of sociodemographic factors. *Ethnic Disparities, 12*(1), 77–86.

Sunil, T. S., & McGehee, M. A. (2007). Social and religious support on treatment adherence among HIV/AIDS patients by race/ethnicity. *Journal of HIV/AIDS & Social Services, 6*(1–2), 83–99.

Taira, D. A., Gelber, R. P., Davis, J., Gronley, K., Chung, R. S., & Seto, T. B. (2007). Antihypertensive adherence and drug class among Asian Pacific Americans. *Ethnicity & Health, 12*(3), 265–281.

Talamantes, M., Lawler, W., & Espino, D. (1995). Hispanic American elders: Caregiving norms surrounding dying and the use of hospice services. *The Hospice Journal, 19*, 35–49.

Trostle, J. A. (1997). The history and meaning of patient compliance as an ideology. In D. S. Gochman (Ed.), *Handbook of health behavior research II: Provider determinants*. New York: Plenum Press.

Turner, J., Wright, E., Mendella, L., Anthonisen, N., & IPPB Study Group. (1995). Predictors of patient adherence to long term home nebulizer therapy for COPD. *Chest, 108*, 394–400.

Ulrik, C. S., Backer, V., Soes-Petersen, U., Lange, P., Harving, H., & Plaschke, P. (2006). The patient's perspective: Adherence or non-adherence to asthma controller therapy. *Journal of Asthma, 43*(9), 701–704.

U.S. Department of Health and Human Services. (2010). *Healthy People 2010*. Retrieved August 7, 2011, from: http://www.healthypeople.gov

van der Sande, M. A., Milligan, P. J., Nyan, O. A., Rowley, J. T., Banya, W. A., Ceesay, S. M., et al. (2000). Blood pressure patterns and cardiovascular risk factors in rural and urban gambian communities. *Journal of Human Hypertension, 14*(8), 489–496.

Van Dulmen, A. M., & Bensing, J. M. (2002). Health promoting effects of the physician-patient encounter. *Psychology, Health and Medicine, 7*(3), 289–300.

Vermeire, E., Hearnshaw, H., Van Royen, P., & Denekens, J. (2001). Patient adherence to treatment: Three decades of research. A comprehensive review. *Journal of Clinical Pharmacological Therapy, 26*(5), 331–342.

Vik, S. A., Maxwell, C. J., & Hogan, D. B. (2004). Measurement, correlates, and health outcomes of medication adherence among seniors. *Annals of Pharmacotherapy, 38*(2), 303–312.

Wagner, G. (2003). Placebo practice trials: The best predictor of adherence readiness for HAART among drug users? *HIV Clinical Trials, 4*(4), 269–281.

Wagner, G., & Rabkin, J. G. (2000). Measuring medication adherence: Are missed doses reported more accurately then perfect adherence? *AIDS Care, 12*(4), 405–408.

Waldrop-Valverde, D., Jones, D. L., Gould, F., Kumar, M., & Ownby, R. L. (2010). Neurocognition, health-related reading literacy, and numeracy in medication management for HIV infection. *AIDS Patient Care STDS. 24*(8), 477–484.

Walker, E. A., Shmukler, C., Ullman, R., Blanco, E., Scollan-Koliopoulus, M., & Cohen, H. W. (2011). Results of a successful telephonic intervention to improve diabetes control in urban adults: A randomized trial. *Diabetes Care, 34*(1), 2–7.

Walker, S. N., Sechrist, K. R., & Pender, N. J. (1987). The health-promoting lifestyle profile: Development and psychometric characteristics. *Nursing Research, 36*, 76–80.

Wendel, C. S., Mohler, M. J., Kroesen, K., Ampel, N. M., Gifford, A. L., & Coons, S. J. (2001). Barriers to use of electronic adherence monitoring in an HIV clinic. *Annals of Pharmacotherapy, 35*(9), 1010–1015.

West, D. S., DiLillo, V., Bursac, Z., Gore, S. A., & Greene, P. G. (2007). Motivational interviewing improves weight loss in women with type 2 diabetes. *Diabetes Care, 30*(5), 1081–1087.

Williams, L. K., Joseph, C. L., Peterson, E. L., Wells, K., Wang, M., Chowdhry, V. K., et al. (2007). Patients with asthma who do not fill their inhaled corticosteroids: A study of primary nonadherence. *The Journal of Allergy & Clinical Immunology, 120*(5), 1153–1159.

Wing, R. R., Epstein, L. H., Nowal, M. P., & Lamparski, D. (1986). Behavioral self-regulation in the treatment of patients with diabetes mellitus. *Psychological Bulletin, 99*(1), 78–89.

Wolf, M. S., Williams, M. V., Parker, R. M., Parikh, N. S., Nowlan, A. W., & Baker, D. W. (2007). Patients' shame and attitudes toward discussing the results of literacy screening. *Journal of Health Communication, 12*(8), 721–732.

World Health Organization.(2003). *Adherence to long-term therapies: Evidence for action*. Geneva, Switzerland: World Health Organization.

Wutoh, A. K., Brown, C. M., Dutta, A. P., Kumoji, E. K., Clarke-Tasker, V., & Xue, Z. (2005). Treatment perceptions and attitudes of older human immunodeficiency virus-infected adults. *Research in Social and Administrative Pharmacy, 1*(1), 60–76.

Zuckerman, M., Guerra, L., Dorssman, D., Foland, J., & Gregory, G. G. (1996). Health-care-seeking behaviors related to bowel complaints: Hispanics versus non-Hispanic Whites. *Digestive Diseases and Sciences, 41*(1), 77–82.

PART II

Impact on the Client and Family

CHAPTER 10

Family Caregiving

Linda L. Pierce and Barbara J. Lutz

INTRODUCTION

Few adults receive paid homecare services. Outside support is not always welcome. Caregivers often refuse help and resources, as they may feel that professionals are prying into their private lives (Pierce, 2001).

Many adults who are in need of help receive unpaid care (Johnson & Wiener, 2006). The value of this care in the United States is estimated at $375 billion annually (National Alliance for Caregiving [NAC] & American Association of Retired Persons [AARP], 2009). The term *unpaid caregiver* refers to a range of kin and nonkin individuals who provide both functional (task-oriented) and affective (emotional) unpaid assistance to a dependent person with whom a long-term or lifelong commitment usually exists (Shirey & Summer, 2000). Family members, friends, and neighbors who provide unpaid care may also be referred to as *informal caregivers* (Pierce, Steiner, Govoni, Thompson, & Friedemann, 2007). These individuals care for spouses, other relatives, friends, and disabled children (Scott, 2006). The most common informal caregiving relationship is between an adult child and an aging parent (Scott, 2006). However, a study financed by the U.S. Administration on Aging found that more than 900,000 households include a child caregiver between the ages of 8 and 18 years who care for ill or disabled family members (Hunt, Levine, & Naiditch, 2005).

The decisions about caring for a person with chronic illness are complex and multifaceted for caregivers. Each choice an individual makes has advantages and disadvantages for the person with chronic illness, the caregiver, and the family. Healthcare professionals generally find that no two situations are alike. Each and every situation needs to be individualized to best meet the needs of everyone involved. This chapter focuses on the multiple aspects of coping and decision making that caregivers face, often on a daily basis.

Current Family Caregiving

The incidence of chronic disease in the United States is increasing. More than 133 million Americans live with chronic conditions such as diabetes, heart disease, and cancer (Bodenheimer, Chen, & Bennett, 2009). Nearly one-third of adults aged 18 to 44 years suffer from a chronic condition (Shapiro, 2002). Most important, the number of adults older than 65 years (39.6 million in 2009) will continue to rise by more than 19 million by 2020; by 2030 there will be about 72.1 million of these individuals (Administration on Aging, 2010; Moore, 2006). Medicare data document that 83% of all beneficiaries have at least one chronic condition. However, 23% of

Medicare beneficiaries with five or more conditions account for 68% of the program's funding (Anderson, 2005, p. 305). With advances in health care, the number of older adults living with debilitating and/or chronic conditions will grow (Williams, Dilworth-Anderson, & Goodwin, 2003).

At the other end of the age spectrum is the growing number of children with chronic illness, disabilities, or both. Advances in neonatal care can now save increasing numbers of preterm and low birth weight infants. According to a 2003 report from the National Center for Health Statistics, the percentage of low birth weight infants (born weighing less than 2500 grams) increased to the highest level in more than 30 years. In addition, the percentage of preterm births (infants born at less than 37 weeks of gestation) increased to 12% of live births. Low birth weight and prematurity both lead to an increased incidence of chronic health problems in the pediatric population. About 15–18% of children have a chronic disease (University of Michigan Health System, 2006) that continues into adulthood.

A 2009 study by the National Alliance for Caregiving and the American Association of Retired Persons estimated that 28.5% of the American population serves as unpaid family caregivers to an adult or child with special needs. This translates into 65.7 million caregivers in the United States (NAC & AARP, 2009). The duration of caregiving can last from a few months to decades. Caregivers report an average of 20 hours per week in caring for a person with a chronic condition (NAC & AARP, 2009).

Preferences for Family Care

It is important to clarify that some dependent individuals will always need the level of care provided in institutional settings and that not all families are willing or able to provide care over the long term. However, for all but the most severely impaired individuals, most chronically ill, dependent persons have their long-term care needs met in the home or with community-based care arrangements. Approximately two-thirds of dependent persons in the community rely solely on informal caregivers (Mittelman, 2003). For these arrangements to work, family members, friends, or neighbors must play central roles in long-term plans of care.

The decision about where and how to provide care for family members with chronic conditions is emotionally charged and multifaceted. Home-based care is financially cost effective for the healthcare system. However, the reliance on family members as care providers creates multiple stressors for the family (Hunt, 2003). When formal assistance is required, married persons prefer help in the home regardless of the level of disability of the care recipient; however, financial difficulty and the strain of extended caregiving, especially on the caregiver's health, often lead family caregivers to decisions that favor institutionalized care (Family Caregiver Alliance, 2006).

Characteristics of Family Caregivers

Today, the term *family caregiver* extends beyond the traditional family boundaries. *Caregiver* is defined as anyone who provides assistance to another in need. The *informal caregiver* is anyone who provides care without pay and who usually has personal ties to the care recipient. *Family caregiver* is a term used interchangeably with informal caregiver and can include family, friends, or neighbors. *Caregiver coalition* is a term used to describe the addition of a support person or persons in traditional relationships when the caregiver–recipient arrangement is no longer sufficient (Haigler, Bauer, & Travis, 2004).

Motivations for caregiving, such as love, duty, or obligation (often based on ethnicity and culture), strongly influence a caregiver's willingness to accept primary caregiving status (Geister, 2005). Additional reasons given by family caregivers for accepting their role are their expectations of themselves and others, religious training and spiritual experiences, and role modeling (Piercy & Chapman, 2001).

Caregiver Dyads and Caregiver Systems

Early caregiving research identified a care recipient and a caregiver as separate entities; the caregiver had primary responsibility for the care and well-being of the care recipient. These studies often did not recognize that caregiving usually occurs within the context of larger, more complex family systems (Palmer & Glass, 2003) or other social networks (Weitzner, Haley, & Chen, 2000). Furthermore, the helping networks used by widowed and never married individuals may be larger than those of married people (Barrett & Lynch, 1999).

In recent years, caregiving research has placed more emphasis on the dynamics of the family relationships (Palmer & Glass, 2003) and the dyadic relationship (Badr & Actielli, 2005; Sebern & Whitlatch, 2007). As would be expected, these studies indicate that the dynamics of the family or other close personal relationships that existed before the illness experience can influence caregiving relationships post-illness. The increasing number of stepfamilies also adds to the complexity of caregiving. Today, people of both genders and of all ages, ethnicities, and economic classes occupy positions as caregivers with varying levels and types of responsibilities, especially in long-term care arrangements. Because caregivers have varying degrees of responsibility for providing or arranging for care, the terms *care provider* and *care manager* may be used to differentiate two types of caregivers (Stoller & Cutler, 1993). This designation helps clarify the previously invisible contributions of all family caregivers. If a son is close to his dependent parents, especially if he is not married, he is likely to be accountable for seeing that things get done, even if he does not provide all of the direct care that is required (Allen, Goldscheider, & Ciambrone, 1999; Keith, 1995; Thompson, Tudiver, & Manson, 2000). Similarly, an adult grandchild may help a grandparent in the absence of a nearby adult child, or children-in-law may find their relationships to relatives with chronic illness make them better suited to caregiving roles than the biological children (Peters-Davis, Moss, & Pruchno, 1999; Pruchno, Burant, & Peters, 1997; Travis & Bethea, 2001).

Changes in the modern family social structure have resulted in more families where both parents work outside the home. This so-called sandwich generation is often not available to provide care for aging family members, which creates a new level of caregivers—children and adolescents. These young caregivers assist with or even assume care of adults with chronic illness in their homes (Hunt et al., 2005; Lackey & Gates, 2001).

Racial and Ethnic Diversity

The family caregiving experience is also shaped by race and ethnicity. These two factors influence one's life experiences in terms of socioeconomic status, education, marital status, health, living arrangements, and general lifestyle (Binstock, 1999). In chronic illness, access to programs and services and preferences for certain types of assistance are often sharply divided along racial and ethnic lines. The number of minority older adults is increasing at a faster rate than that of non-Hispanic whites, with the largest proportionate increases projected in the over-75-years group. While the number of African American older adults will increase slightly in the next 50 years, proportionately larger and more rapid increases will occur among Hispanic and Asian elders (He, Sengupta, Velkoff, & DeBarros, 2005).

Comparative research indicates that patterns of family response to a family member with a chronic illness may be significantly different across ethnic groups (Chesla & Rungreangkulkij, 2001). Gerontologic researchers are building a substantial body of literature on African American, Asian American, Native American, and Hispanic older adults and their family caregiving experiences and preferences for support. Because this literature is extensive, only one example of diversity is provided to illustrate ethnic influences.

Cultural precedence, historical events, and the needs of extended kin and family structure shape African American caregiving. Documented barriers to formal programs and services include poverty and economic disparity, lower educational levels, ageism, and racial discrimination (Jones, 1999). As a result, persistent underutilization of formal assistance programs and a reliance on family and friends are typical patterns of long-term care for dependent African American older adults (Cox, 1999).

While it is known that African American families have a strong sense of respect, duty, and obligation to elderly members of their communities, it may also be the case that generations have learned to be self- and family-reliant in the face of both overt and covert forms of racial discrimination (Binstock, 1999; Edmonds, 1999). As a result of this self-reliance, African American family caregivers, especially women, may be perceived to have a lower level of role strain than their white counterparts. Research demonstrates a large variation in the female African American caregiver's perception of role strain (Williams et al., 2003).

Gender Differences

The choice of who becomes the primary caregiver and what the family caregiving system looks like depends on many factors. In a spousal relationship, the unaffected spouse usually assumes the caregiving role. Often, both spouses are forced to cope with role renegotiation in addition to their new roles as the giver and receiver of care (Gordon & Perrone, 2004).

Among married adult children, daughters or daughters-in-law are most often the primary caregivers for aging parents (Shirey & Summer, 2000). Daughters are more likely to offer assistance to their father who is serving in a caregiving role than their mother. This may be because they are more comfortable with their mother in that role and feel that their father needs additional assistance performing the tasks required of a caregiver (Mittelman, 2003). Sarkisian and Gerstel (2004) found that much of the relationship between gender and helping parents is explained by gender differences in employment patterns. They suggest that gender differences in adult care may be fading as women's and men's work lives become more similar (Sarkisian & Gerstel, 2004). National studies in the 1980s suggested that though women predominate as caregivers, somewhere between one in five and one in three caregivers are men (Chang & White-Means, 1991; Stone, Cafferata, & Sangl, 1987). Other studies in the 1990s estimated that men constituted nearly half of in-home caregivers and of caregivers to the elderly, chronically ill, and disabled (Kramer & Thompson, 2001). Although men are just as likely as women to be involved in caring for and helping seniors, women, wives, mothers, and adult daughters spend more time as the designated primary caregiver (Stobert & Cranswick, 2004). In 2009, approximately two-thirds of family caregivers were female (NAC & AARP, 2009).

The gendered nature of caregiving is certainly one important characteristic of long-term caregiving that is likely to continue in the future. All things being equal, the person who is closest to and the most involved in the daily life of the dependent person is usually the person most accountable for either doing or seeing that care is done.

Types of Care Provided by Family Caregivers

Over the long term, a dependent person requires two types of care: social care and health-related care. Social care includes both functional and affective assistance in daily living while health-related care refers to specialized care by professionals and daily treatments performed by family caregivers, such as the administration of medication.

Functional assistance is determined by the care recipient's ability to perform various tasks of daily existence, which are categorized as either instrumental or basic activities of daily living. Instrumental activities of daily living (IADLs) are the functions an adult would be expected to perform in the process of everyday life, including cooking, cleaning, buying groceries, doing yard work, and paying bills. For a child, these tasks might include getting to school, playing, or cleaning his or her room. Basic activities of daily living (ADLs) are the tasks required for personal care and basic survival. These tasks include eating, bathing, dressing, going to the bathroom,

maintaining personal hygiene, and getting around (mobility).

Affective assistance, also called emotional support, includes behaviors that convey caring and concern to the care recipient. Affective assistance is most often linked with enhanced feelings of self-esteem, contentment, life satisfaction, hope of recovery, dignity, and general well-being (Brody & Schoonover, 1986; Horowitz, 1985).

In the past, there was a somewhat clearer division between the formal and informal care network. The informal network—family caregivers or significant others—provided both emotional and functional aspects of care and monitored the care provided by formal providers. The formal network provided specialized care that was highly task-oriented and goal-directed. Today the roles of the formal and informal network reveal a more blended approach to caregiving. Family caregivers perform highly skilled tasks formerly reserved for the professional. Professional caregivers function as a team with the family in care decisions for the client (Haigler et al., 2004).

Caregiving Histories and Maturation over Time

Longitudinal studies of family caregiving have documented the many changes that occur in the role of family caregiver and note that family caregiving is not a static event. Pearlin (1992) equated caregiving to career development. There are two factors that contribute to this notion of a caregiving career or caregiving history: maturation of the caregiver over time, and ongoing role development associated with the inevitable transitions in care over the long term.

The expectations of the family caregiver are many. They often begin their roles with little or no training or support. In addition to the psychological aspects of caregiving, they are expected to provide competent, skilled health care for their loved ones (Elliot & Shewchuk, 2003). Most caregivers begin their experiences as novices with little or no experience or knowledge of how to navigate the healthcare system (McAuley, Travis, & Safewright, 1997; Skaff, Pearlin & Mullan, 1996). Over time, mature caregivers master a new language system of entitlements (Medicare, Medicaid) and treatments (medication administration, illness symptomatology), and learn how to incorporate the needs of a dependent person into their daily lives (Leavitt et al., 1999). Some caregivers mature more quickly and with greater ease than others, and some caregivers are never able to achieve adequate skill and/or confidence in the caregiver role. Thus, tremendous variability can be found in the levels, lengths, and forms of care provided by family caregivers, which are at least partially attributed to successful mastery of their roles (Seltzer & Wailing, 2000).

Transitions in care occur at three points: entry into a caregiving relationship, institutionalization (or transitions into other formal care arrangements), and bereavement (Seltzer & Wailing, 2000). Unlike acute or episodic care that has an end point, the only natural end to long-term caregiving is the death of the care recipient. Even families that ultimately opt for institutional placement of their dependent family members do not abandon their relatives over the long term. Most caregivers stay engaged as care managers following the institutional placement decision (Seltzer & Wailing, 2000).

Montgomery and Kosloski (2000) have identified a similar concept called a caregiving trajectory. Their seven markers of caregiving are 1) performance of initial caregiving task; 2) self-definition as a caregiver; 3) provision of personal care; 4) seeking out or using assistive services; 5) consideration of institutionalization; 6) actual nursing home placement; and 7) termination of the caregiver role. In this trajectory, Montgomery and Kosloski believe that the order and timing of the markers are indicative of the individual, their culture, and the relationship of the caregiver to the care recipient.

One of the reasons that family caregiving precipitated by acute hospitalization is so stressful for new caregivers is that they have not had a period of maturation and development before the intense caregiving demands and the decision-making requirements that follow (Kane, Reinardy, & Penrod, 1999). In addition, the transitions in care occur rapidly and over a highly compressed period. In a matter of days the caregiver may transition from having no care responsibilities to being fully engaged in rehabilitation after hospitalization, or home or institutional long-term care (Kane et al., 1999).

Positive Aspects of Caregiving

In the past, research on stress, strain, burden, and burnout overshadowed the positive aspects of providing care to a dependent family member. As a result, less is understood about how and why caregivers provide care even under difficult circumstances. While not much has been published on satisfaction with caregiving, Kramer's (1997) review of research on positive aspects of caregiving noted that some caregivers gain experience when assisting others. Gain was conceptualized as "the extent to which the caregiving role is appraised to enhance an individual's life space and be enriching" (p. 219). Caregivers do report satisfaction with their role. Adults who functioned as caregivers during their childhood have reported that their participation taught them responsibility, allowed them to be "part of the family," and provided opportunities to be "appreciated" and to be "useful." They also reported pride at learning skills at an early age (Lackey & Gates, 2001). Many couples feel that caring for their partner strengthened their relationship (Gordon & Perrone, 2004). Coherence, a sense of togetherness in caring for others, was discovered by Pierce (2001) to be important for maintaining stability within the family. Through coherence, family caregivers felt connected and this helped them survive in stressful times related to caring situations (Pierce, 2001).

A number of factors have been reported since the 1980s as contributors to caregivers' satisfaction. These factors include the care recipient's levels of physical, cognitive, and social impairment (Blake & Lincoln, 2000; Deimling, & Bass, 1986; Williams, 1993); the types of care provided by the caregiver (Draper, Poulos, Cole, Poulos, & Ehrlich, 1992; Montgomery, Stull, & Borgatta, 1985); the caregiver's gender and marital status (Zarit, Todd, & Zarit, 1986); the extent to which the caregiver's personal and social life are disrupted by the demands of caregiving (George & Gwyther, 1986; Poulshock, & Deimling, 1984); the quality of the relationship between caregiver and care recipient as perceived by the caregiver (Bowdoin, 1994; Caron & Bowers, 2003); and the satisfactory assistance with caregiving perceived by the caregiver (Bowdoin, 1994; George & Gwyther, 1986). For instance, caregivers and their families may experience less satisfaction if the care recipient is severely disabled and if they perceive that needed assistance in caring is unavailable. Other

caregivers may report more satisfaction if the care recipient is only mildly disabled and if relatives, or friends, or both are able to help provide the needed assistance (Pierce, 2001). Family style, including receptivity, has been suggested as an area for future study (Gilliss, 2002). Longitudinal research and research with caregivers in diverse arrangements are needed to provide a more comprehensive view of what contributes to a positive caregiving experience.

The Future of Caregiving

Looking to the future, it is likely that the next cohort of older adults (the baby boomers) will be very different from their parents and grandparents and will further confound the current reliance on family caregivers. Declining family sizes, increasing childlessness, and rising divorce rates will limit the number of family caregivers (Johnson, Toohey, & Wiener, 2007) during the lifetimes of adult baby boomers. Parents of the baby boomer generation have several children from whom to seek assistance, while older baby boomers with smaller families will not be so fortunate. Additionally, the mobility of families often separates individuals by thousands of miles, making family assistance impossible. It remains to be seen what this societal trend will mean to this cohort.

In the future, racial caregiving trends are likely to change as well. In particular, African American and Hispanic caregivers will be more available for long-term caregiving than will Caucasian caregivers. Furthermore, Caucasian caregivers are expected to purchase more services for dependent family members (Shirey & Summer, 2000).

Most researchers agree, however, that any predictions about family caregiving in the future are tenuous because public policy is difficult to predict from one generation to the next. That policy will need to change to accommodate the caregiving needs of the aging baby boomer cohort is the only certainty.

PROBLEMS AND ISSUES

Family caregivers face multiple problems, issues, and concerns throughout their caregiving experiences. The section includes a case study on "the H. family" that is typical of the effort most family caregivers put into fulfilling their responsibilities, attending to the wants and needs of the care recipient, and continuously adjusting their lives to the physical and emotional requirements of the caregiving situation.

Family caregiving experiences incorporate societal values and are shaped by governmental policy. Policies that affect family caregiving in the United States were created with the presumption that families are responsible for caring for their disabled members and will provide the majority of the care that is needed (Montgomery, 1999). For many years, these expectations were consistent with caregivers' resources and abilities.

Since 1990, however, there has been a blurring of the lines of responsibility for long-term caregiving. Increased technology, greater acuity of those in need of assistance, and competing demands on available caregivers have created an imbalance between the demand for family care and the ability of family caregivers to provide care. Family caregivers are being asked to provide highly technical treatments; administer complex medication regimens; provide labor-intensive, hands-on care; and monitor the medical conditions of very ill family members.

The one responsibility that has remained constant over time, whether the family caregiver is a direct care provider or arranges care as a care manager, is the extensive decision-making demands placed on family caregivers. When the dependent family member cannot make decisions or has difficulty communicating choices, the responsibility for countless decisions associated with managing daily life falls to the caregiver. These decisions include the initiation, timing, and provision of assistance from informal and formal sources; integration of caregiving demands into work and family life; and planning for future long-term care needs (McAuley et al., 1997; Travis & Bethea, 2001).

The Influence of Public Policy on Family Caregiving

Containing the rising costs of healthcare services has become a national policy imperative. This goal is demonstrated through policies that promote prevention of premature or unwanted institutionalization of disabled elders in nursing homes, limit publicly funded homecare services to individuals with the lowest incomes, and curtail the Medicare home health benefit. Such policies limit the amount and scope of services that are provided to persons who need ongoing assistance by formal caregivers as well as their family caregivers. Cost-containment measures occurred precisely when the demand for help in providing long-term care at home was increasing (Riggs, 2004). These changes in government-sponsored services meant that many families, particularly low- and middle-income families, were faced with difficult choices about providing assistance while receiving minimal help from professional healthcare providers.

CASE STUDY

The H. Family

Mrs. H. had coronary artery disease and congestive heart failure that caused increasing fatigue, dyspnea, and angina over a 5-year period. Frequent upper respiratory infections exacerbated her dyspnea.

Home setting. Mrs. H. lived with her husband in a small rural town in a home they had owned since their children were small. Mr. H. was 4 years younger than his wife.

Role issues. Mr. H. assumed cooking tasks in the home and was the primary caregiver for his wife, assisting her to ambulate to the bathroom for toileting and bathing, making sure her clothes were clean and accessible, and making sure she took her medicine as prescribed.

Support. The couple's married daughter and married son lived within a 10-minute drive of their parents' house. Both had children of their own but assisted their parents at least once a week. The daughter did the major housecleaning for her parents and drove them regularly to the grocery store, to frequent doctor's visits, and to the pharmacy. The son assisted his father with lawn work and household repairs; he was also called on in cases of medical emergency to be the decision maker.

Transitions. Over several years, Mrs. H.'s health declined. Her upstairs bedroom became inaccessible because stair climbing became exhausting. The living room was converted to a bedroom. She was hospitalized for a series of short-term stays for complaints of chest pain and/or difficulty breathing over this time span. Whenever she was hospitalized, the daughter and son took turns driving their father to the hospital because he visited their mother daily. During the next 5 years, these hospitalizations increased in frequency to several times yearly. She used portable oxygen at home.

Initially oxygen was only used for brief intervals during the night, and she was able to accompany her daughter for brief shopping trips or drives "to get out of the house." As her health declined, Mrs. H. used the oxygen continuously, remaining in her room. The family got a Medi-Alert call button that Mrs. H. always wore in case she needed emergency help.

With each hospitalization, Mrs. H. returned home weaker. Mr. H. began to worry that he could no longer care for his wife at home because of her increasing weakness. He moved her commode adjacent to her wheelchair; even so, Mrs. H. had difficulty transferring from her chair to the commode. Mrs. H. was heavier than her husband; he worried about her safety, fearing that she might fall and injure herself and he would be unable to assist her. The daughter had a part-time job but visited her parents more frequently, twice weekly. She began to express concerns about both parents' health to her brother, her friends, and her husband.

Decisions. When Mrs. H. was hospitalized at the age of 78 for chest pain and difficulty breathing, the physician approached Mr. H. and his son and daughter with a request that they

(continues)

CASE STUDY   (Continued)

sign a Do Not Resuscitate (DNR) agreement. Mrs. H. had vehemently expressed, "I don't want them damn machines," so the family readily agreed to the DNR order. They were concerned for Mrs. H. because the DNR had never been brought up by the doctor before.

Mr. H. told his children that Mrs. H. would have to go to a nursing home when she was discharged from the hospital, as he could no longer care for her with her severely diminished abilities. Although the family discussed this problem, they did not resolve it. After visiting Mrs. H. one evening at the hospital, during which time she was alert and talkative, the family returned to their homes. That evening Mrs. H. died. The family expressed relief that her suffering was over, that she died the way she wanted to, without machines. They were also relieved that the whole family did not have to struggle with the nursing home decision.

Discussion Questions

1. What are the advantages and disadvantages of the client being cared for at home? For the family? For the caregiver?
2. What factors influence the cost effectiveness of home care versus institutionalization?
3. Who are the primary providers of home care? What are some of the providers' competing demands?
4. What are some of the emotional responses to family caregiving?
5. What is the financial impact of caregiving on the caregiver?
6. How does public policy affect caregiving?
7. How can health professionals assist family caregivers?
8. Where can family caregivers go for assistance and information?

Several government initiatives have attempted to address the needs of family caregivers. In 1993, the Family and Medical Leave Act (FMLA) became law. This act gives qualified caregivers the option of taking up to 12 weeks of unpaid leave from their jobs to care for a family member (U.S. Department of Labor, 1993). In 2000, approximately 24 million or 16.5% of eligible employees used family and medical leave. Of these, approximately 30% used the leave to care for an ill child, spouse, or parent. Approximately 3% of the surveyed qualified employees who needed family and medical

leave did not take it. The top barriers were not being able to afford unpaid leave (54%), being worried about losing their job (32%), or feeling that job advancement would be hurt (43%) (Workplace Flexibility 2010, 2004).

In addition to these barriers, many caregiving situations require that the caregiver be available for a longer period of time than the 12 weeks afforded by the FMLA. These barriers present difficult choices for family members of individuals in need of caregiving assistance—many are faced with leaving or reducing gainful employment to provide the necessary care because they have no other options. The Older Americans Act Amendments of 2000 established the National Family Caregiver Support Program (NFCSP) (DHHS Administration on Aging, 2011a). Federal funds are given to states based upon their proportionate share of the population age 70 years old or older. States, working in partnership with local agencies on aging and faith and community-service providers and tribes, offer five direct services to best meet the range of caregiver needs. The services include provision of the following:

- Information to caregivers about available services
- Assistance to caregivers in gaining access to supportive services
- Individual counseling, organization of support groups, and caregiver training to assist caregivers in making decisions and solving problems relating to their roles
- Respite care to enable caregivers to be temporarily relieved from their caregiving responsibilities
- Supplemental services, on a limited basis, to complement the care provided by caregivers

Family caregivers eligible for the NFCSP are those who care for adults aged 60 years or older and grandparents and relatives of children not more than 18 years of age, including grandparents who are sole caregivers of grandchildren and those individuals who are affected by mental retardation or have developmental disabilities. Priority is given to caregivers with social and economic need, particularly low-income and minority individuals, or older individuals providing care and support to persons with mental retardation and related developmental disabilities. While the NFCSP has been lauded as

an important step in recognizing the needs of family caregivers, it lacks the appropriate funding to support the needs of caregivers at any meaningful level. Furthermore, each state decides how the funds are used, resulting in inconsistencies of services across states. In addition, with the aging of the baby boomers over the next several decades, the reliance on family members and friends for the long-term care needs of those with chronic conditions is expected to increase significantly (Montgomery & Feinberg, 2003; Riggs, 2004).

The lack of adequate monetary assistance for the family unit is a complex problem. Currently, public financing of long-term care in the home setting is minimal. Medicare offers a hospice benefit with a time-limited period at the end of life and some states have limited home and community-based waiver programs that provide some home-based services for low-income residents. Often the waiting lists for these services are long, with residents never receiving the services for which they are qualified. Many private insurers offer long-term care policies through employers, fraternal organizations, retirement communities, and health management organizations. Unfortunately, in the past, most of these policies did not cover many aspects of the personal care provided by family caregivers, leaving this in-home care as out-of-pocket expenses. Long-term care policies now on the market are more comprehensive, but are expensive to purchase.

More recently, individual states were authorized to craft their own programs to provide paid leave to workers who need to care for family members. In 2001, the Clinton administration proposed relief to families in the form of a $1,000 annual tax credit for those receiving or providing long-term care in the home, but the proposal generated controversy among legisla-tors. Many believed that government interven-tion would discourage people from purchasing long-term care insurance to cover nursing home care and healthcare services in the home (DuPont, 1999). The 2010 U.S. healthcare reform legislation may provide some additional assistance for caregivers of persons with chronic illness in the United States. The legislation pro-vides new options in two areas: home and com-munity-based care and care coordination. The law establishes new options in Medicaid-funded home and community-based care that includes programs to provide attendant care services for individuals with disabilities and protection against spousal impoverishment. The law also provides incentives to physicians and healthcare organizations to improve post-discharge patient outcomes and establish care coordination ser-vices for Medi-care beneficiaries. However, this legislation is currently being contested, so the extent to which these reforms will be instituted and the involvement of the government's role in assisting caregivers remains a highly debated issue (Family Caregiver Alliance, 2010).

Emotional Effects of Being a Caregiver

Although not all persons experience stress when providing care, many do. There are a number of factors that influence caregiving and the stress it may cause. Factors include the intensity of the care provided, types of care tasks performed, gender, personal characteristics of the caregiver, the relationship between the caregiver and the person receiving care, support from other family members, and competing obligations of the caregiver. Research on caregiver stress spans more than 2 decades, and researchers have labeled caregiver stress as either strain or burden.

Strain or Burden

Caregiver strain and burden are multidimen-sional, closely related concepts that include both subjective perceptions of caregivers, such as role overload, and objective factors, such as physical care needs of the care recipient. Caregiver strain is usually related to the stress, hardship, or con-flicting feelings one has when performing the caregiving role (Hunt, 2003). For example, a caregiver may feel a high level of role strain when trying to decide between caring for an ail-ing parent and maintaining gainful employment.

One area of caregiver research that has focused heavily on caregiver strain is dementia care. In particular, caregiving is more stressful and produces more emotional and physical strain when the caregiver is caring for a person with dementia or Alzheimer's disease. Caregivers of persons with dementia are more likely than nondementia caregivers to say that they suffer mental or physical problems as a result of care-giving (Ory, Hoffman, Yee, Tennstedt, & Schulz, 1999). Caregivers also report higher levels of strain when they perceive the patient to be manipulative, unappreciative, or unreasonable (Nerenberg, 2002).

Caregiver burden is defined as "the oppres-sive or worrisome load borne by people provid-ing direct care for the chronically ill" (Hunt, 2003, p. 28). Burden is relative to the level of the care recipient's disability, including behavioral and cognitive issues; the extent of care required; and the caregiver's level of worry or feelings of being overwhelmed (Nerenberg, 2002). Fi-nancial strain also contributes to the level of caregiver burden (Evercare & NAC, 2007).

Caregiver burden has been associated with increased depressive symptoms in caregivers of patients with stroke (Chumbler, Rittman, Van Puymbroeck, Vogel, & Qin, 2004), coronary artery bypass (Halm & Bakas, 2007), and Alzheimer's disease (Mausbach et al., 2007), among others. The Family Caregiver Alliance (FCA) estimates that between 40% and 70% of caregivers have "clinically significant" depressive symptoms (FCA, 2006). Higher levels of depression have been found among dementia caregivers who cared for persons with moderate to severe functional impairment and greater amounts of behavioral disturbance (wandering and aggression) than among nondementia caregivers (Meshefedjian, McCusker, Bellavance, & Baumgarten, 1998).

In another study of caregivers and patients with dementia (n = 5627), 32% of the caregivers were classified as clinically depressed on the basis of elevated scores on the Geriatric Depression Scale (Covinsky et al., 2003). When caregivers' appraisals of the burden of caregiving are high, there is greater likelihood of caregiver depression and depressive symptoms (Clyburn, Stones, Hadjistavropoulos, & Tuokko, 2000).

Caregiving is also a risk factor for poorer health and increased mortality in caregivers versus noncaregivers (FCA, 2006). One study reported that among spousal caregivers experiencing strain, there was a 63% higher mortality risk for family caregivers during a 4-year period than among noncaregivers (Schulz & Beach, 1999).

There also appears to be a gender component associated with caregiver strain. Female caregivers experience more psychiatric disorders than do male caregivers (Yee & Schulz, 2000) and are much more likely than men to report being depressed or anxious and to experience lower levels of life satisfaction. The irony is that, while they report more caregiver burden, role conflict, or strain, women are more likely than male caregivers to continue caregiving responsibilities over the long term. Women are less likely than men to obtain assistance from others with caregiving. Finally, women are less likely than men to engage in preventative health behaviors, such as rest, exercise, and taking medications as prescribed while caregiving (Burton, Newsom, Schulz, Hirsch, & German, 1997).

Caregivers for spouses have reported a higher incidence of depression and stress than those caring for a disabled parent. The caregiving roles and responsibilities may have a major impact on the relationship itself. Healthcare professionals must realize that the relationship between the caregiver and the spouse receiving the care needs to be supported and nurtured in terms of love, affection, and intimacy (Gordon & Perrone, 2004).

Children and adolescents who have functioned in the role of caregiver report difficulty watching their loved one progress with a chronic problem. They have memories of unpleasant smells and sights. They also report feeling helpless because of their lack of knowledge and fear that they will not be able to deal with a crisis (Lackey & Gates, 2001).

Recent research has found that caregivers who have a higher sense of self-efficacy and control over their life situations (i.e., personal mastery) have less burden and fewer depressive symptoms (Chumbler et al. 2004; Chumbler, Rittman, & Wu, 2007; Mausbach et al., 2007). These studies suggest that interventions that enhance self-efficacy or personal mastery will decrease health risks and improve health-related outcomes for caregivers (Chumbler et al., 2007; Halm & Bakas, 2007; Rabinowitz, Mausbach, Thompson, Gallagher-Thompson, 2007)

Burnout

Burnout has been defined as a "state of physical, emotional, and mental exhaustion caused by long-term involvement in emotionally demanding situations" (Pines & Aronson, 1988, p. 9). For the caregiver, the term *burnout* can be used to describe this type of physical, mental, and/or emotional exhaustion (Nerenberg, 2002).

Figley (1998) developed a model of burnout for professional caregivers (e.g., nurses and social workers) that has implications for caregiver and caregiver family situations as well. In this model, burnout begins with a caregiver's stress response, that is, compassion stress, which refers to "the stress connected with exposure to a sufferer" (Figley, 1998, p. 21). In this case, the sufferer is the care recipient. When compassion stress is accompanied by prolonged exposure to the suffering and/or unresolved trauma, compassion fatigue sets in. Compassion fatigue can also be exacerbated by a substantial degree of life disruption. These factors lead to caregiver burnout, which may be dealt with by placing the care recipient in an institution, by having another family member assume primary caregiver duties, or, in some cases, by neglecting or abusing the care recipient. Parents caring for children with severe developmental disabilities or others caring for individuals with Alzheimer's disease are especially at risk for burnout due to prolonged exposure and high levels of life disruption. However, to date, little research has been done on the incidence of compassion fatigue in informal caregivers.

Family Relationships and Shifting Roles

Providing care to others, especially spouses and parents, often requires changes in the ways that family members interact with each other. For the care provider, this decision may be a lifelong commitment to another family member (Elliot & Shewchuk, 2003). These changes in family interactions have been labeled role reversal, role renegotiation, or role reconstruction. Although most family caregivers handle these role changes over time, some caregivers struggle with changes in their family relationships (Lutz, Chumbler, & Roland, 2007).

In role reversal, for example, wives providing care to husbands are often required to make financial decisions or perform tasks to maintain their homes that have always been their husbands' responsibility. Adult children often speak of becoming "parents" to their frail parents (Plowfield, Raymond, & Blevins, 2000). Some researchers view the term *role reversal* as being inadequate for describing family relationships in late life (Brody, 1990; Seltzer, 1990). They view the use of the term role reversal as a simplistic way of viewing a complex phenomenon and express concern that it reinforces negative stereotypes of dependency in general and old age in particular. If being a parent, child, or spouse is a social position in a family, these positions do not change during the lifetime of the family. A parent is always a parent. A spouse is always a spouse. Although behaviors toward each other may change as health or functioning decline, the roles remain stable. Therefore, the terms *role renegotiation* or *role reconstruction* may be more accurate to describe changes in familial relationships due to caregiving.

Support for this argument was offered in a study of adult child caregivers that found that adult child caregivers respected traditional parental autonomy for as long as possible (Piercy, 1998). The caregivers in this study described sensitivity to the parents' wishes, even when they disagreed with the parent, and well beyond the point at which the parent experienced significant cognitive or physical decline. This is particularly evident in studies of non-white cultures in which familial roles are revered and respected (Evans, Coon, & Crogan, 2007). However, Lackey and Gates (2001) found that in some cases children less than 18 years of age who provide care to their parents at times perceived a reversal of roles. When caring for a parent, children reported serving as the personal confidant of the parent. In addition to the changed family dynamics, the child caregivers reported a pronounced effect on their school life and their friendships.

Elder Abuse and Neglect

The 2000 Survey of State Adult Protective Services stated that there were 472,813 reported cases of elder or vulnerable adult abuse. For substantiated reports, the most common environment for abuse was in domestic settings. The typical abuser was a man between the ages of 26 and 50 years. Almost 62% of the perpetrators were family members (spouse, parents, children, grandchildren, siblings, and other family members). The family member or perpetrator with the highest incidence of perpetration was the spouse or intimate partner, followed by an adult child (Teaster, 2003). Even with the impact of these statistics, one must realize that it is likely that the majority of elder or vulnerable adult abuses go unreported.

The DHHS Administration on Aging (2009) defines the following types of abuse and neglect: physical abuse, sexual abuse, neglect, exploitation, emotional abuse, abandonment and self-neglect. Physical abuse is defined as the willful infliction of physical pain or injury. Examples of this are slapping, bruising, or restraining. Sexual abuse is the infliction of nonconsensual sexual contact of any kind. Neglect is failing to provide shelter, health care, or protection. Exploitation is the illegal taking, misuse, or concealment of funds, property, or assets. Emotional abuse includes inflicting pain, anguish, or distress through verbal and non-verbal acts. Abandonment is desertion of the elder by anyone who is responsible for care. Self-neglect is failure of a person to perform essential, self-care tasks and that failure creates an unsafe environment for the elder.

It is important for healthcare professionals to recognize the precipitating factors for caregiver abuse of an elder. There appears to be a strong link between the likelihood for abuse and the caregiver's perception of his or her situation. Caregivers who have had a positive relationship with care recipients are less likely to become abusive. In certain situations, the risk of abuse increased in direct relationship to the amount of care required. The personality characteristics and behaviors of the care recipient have also been indicated in relation to the caregiver's stress level. Finally, an abusive incident may be triggered by the use of alcohol, substance abuse, or psychiatric illness (Nerenberg, 2002).

Although it is more common to think about the potential abuse of a dependent person by a family caregiver, it is also possible that a caregiver may be the victim of an abusive care recipient. Patterns of dysfunctional behavior in families can extend over decades. If a wife was abused by her husband before he became ill or dependent on her for assistance, there is no reason to believe that he would suddenly discontinue all forms of abusive behavior because of illness.

Family caregivers, especially women, who have not managed the family finances and must always ask the care recipient or other family members for money or who rely solely on the care recipients' families for other types of assistance, may be very vulnerable to neglect. In addition, self-neglect, behavior that threatens a person's own health or safety, can be an adverse consequence of profound caregiving stress and associated depression. Self-neglect usually manifests as refusal to provide oneself with adequate food, water, clothing, and shelter.

Excessive Caregiving

Although a very subjective notion, providing excessive care to an impaired adult occurs in some caregiving situations. One form of excessive care is assistance that puts the caregiver's physical or emotional health at risk. Excessive care may have deleterious effects on the health of spouse caregivers (Plowfield, Raymond, & Blevins, 2000; Schultz & Beach, 1999). In the Caregiver Health Effects Study, persons who felt burdened while providing long-term care for demented spouses had a high risk of mortality over a 4-year period (Schultz & Beach, 1999).

Given and colleagues (1990) found that spousal caregivers who experienced a combination of negative care-recipient behaviors, such as cognitive impairment and antisocial behaviors, were more likely to feel higher levels of responsibility and react negatively to the caregiver role than did persons caring for spouses not exhibiting such behaviors. Despite negative responses to the caregiver role, the greater levels of responsibility felt by these spouses may contribute to the provision of excessive care and the caregivers' rejection of or failure to take advantage of respite opportunities.

A second type of excessive care occurs when caregivers assume responsibilities or perform tasks for their care recipients that they are capable of performing themselves. For example, a caregiver recently informed of her parent's heart disease may react by taking over responsibilities, such as paying bills or cooking, that her parent can still perform adequately. Such excessive care can rob parents of feelings of autonomy that may be beneficial to their health and emotional well-being. Caregiving is a delicate balance of providing for the care recipient's safety while preserving their autonomy to the fullest extent possible (Piercy, 1998). Albert and Brody (1996) found that greater feelings of burden on the part of caregivers were associated with viewing parent care as child care. These burdened caregivers were also less likely to encourage parental autonomy. Such findings suggest that promotion of care recipient autonomy to the greatest extent possible for as long as possible may be beneficial for both caregiver and care recipient.

Financial Impact of Caregiving

Caregiving has different degrees of financial impact on families, depending on their particular caregiving situations and financial resources. For elderly couples with a spouse as caregiver, the impact may range from minimal to considerable, depending on the extent to which other family help is available, formal services are used, and how they are financed. For families of frail elderly relatives, reduced employment is most likely to occur when the caregivers are of ethnic minorities and for patients with specific clinical characteristics (Covinsky et al., 2001). When adult children are the caregivers, the picture becomes murky because it is the financial resources of the care recipient that are usually considered for public assistance.

The current public financing system for in-home and community-based services targets persons with the lowest incomes. Well off family caregivers can afford to pay for home or community-based care out of pocket, regardless of the financial eligibility of the care recipient. However, families in the middle ranges of income may be unable to purchase in-home services or receive public financing for needed care. White-Means (1997) found that care recipients who were within 150–250% of established poverty levels and who were not receiving the Medicare home health benefit or state-financed programs were less likely to use in-home services than were individuals in other income ranges. In other words, these low-income care recipients were not financially eligible for assistance, nor were their family caregivers able to purchase services for them.

The cost of caregiving is associated with the level of need for the affected individual. According to the Department of Health and Human Services Administration on Aging (2001b) caregivers spend an average of 11% out of pocket for services not covered by Medicare. The Evercare and the National Alliance for Caregiving (2007) found that in a survey of 1000 caregivers the average annual costs of caregiving was $5531. However, in a smaller subsample of caregivers (n = 41), who maintained a 1-month diary of expenses, the annualized expenses were $12,348. The most common expenses were in the areas of "household goods, food, and meals" (42%), travel and transportation costs (40%), and medical care co-pays and pharmaceuticals (31%)" (Evercare & NAC, 2007, p. 7). Those in the lowest income categories provided the most

number of hours of care per week. Caregivers whose income was less than $25,000 per year provided an average of 41 hours of care each week. The estimated cost of care for these caregivers is more than $5,000 annually (or approximately 20% of their income). Forty-nine percent of the caregivers in this group also reported that their finances had gotten worse since they started providing care. Of the total sample, 43% reported that their financial worries had increased since taking on the role of caregiver.

Research shows that relatively few adult children contribute financially to parent care; only 5–10% of adult children transfer money to parents in a year's time (Boaz, Hu, & Ye, 1999). These "financial caregivers" tend to have higher levels of asset income and proportionally more women engaged in the paid labor force full time than those who do not offer any financial assistance to dependent parents. Furthermore, financial help almost always goes to single parents (usually widowed mothers) for caregiving situations that require extensive personal assistance.

Employment

In the mid-1980s, the first national study of its kind revealed the shocking effects that being a caregiver had on the nation's workforce. About 14% of caregiver wives, 12% of daughters, 11% of husbands, and 5% of sons quit their jobs to care for elderly relatives. Of employed caregivers, 29% rearranged their work schedules, 21% reduced work hours, and 19% took time off without pay (Stone et al., 1987). A 2004 national survey estimated that 44 million Americans were providing care for a friend or family member older than 18 years. Of these, 7 million were providing between 12 and 87 hours of care per week, which included personal care and other tasks such as shopping and transportation; more than 26 million had to adjust their work schedules; and almost 8 million quit working to accommodate their caregiving responsibilities (MetLife & NAC, 2004). In another survey of 1000 caregivers, of those who were employed or had been employed sometime during the caregiving experience, 37% cut back or quit working, 14% changed jobs, 48% used sick leave or vacation days, and 15% used unpaid leave (Evercare & NAC, 2007).

Employees most in need of support are those who function as primary caregivers and those who care for older adults with high care needs (Evercare & NAC, 2007; Stone & Short, 1990). Being female, Caucasian, and in fair to poor health increased the caregiver's likelihood of needing some assistance to accommodate work and caregiving demands. There is also evidence to suggest that caregivers who have lower amounts of education and those less likely to view their work as a career are more likely than others to decide to leave paid employment altogether. Dautzenberg (2000) found that the daughter living closest with the least competing demands was most vulnerable to being called upon for caregiving duties.

Clearly, there are hidden costs, both economic and noneconomic, of informal care to older adults, their caregivers, and to other family members (Evercare & NAC, 2007; Fast, Williamson, & Keating, 1999). Unfortunately, these costs are frequently ignored by policy makers focused primarily on containing costs of services. The emotional well-being of the care recipient, who struggles with conflicting issues of dependency and strain on the family, and the emotional well-being of the family caregiver, who struggles with loss of control and independence in his or her daily life, can become very tenuous in these situations (Pyke, 1999). The most dramatic economic costs to caregivers include giving up paid employment, lost income from unpaid leave or time off work,

relinquishment of career advancement opportunities, and the prospect of out-of-pocket expenses to support home care. Those in the lowest income categories have the highest economic burden. Employers need to consider flexible options to help the caregiver/employee meet the demands of their multiple roles.

INTERVENTIONS

Most interventions related to caregiving are a blend of both formal and informal networks of care. The interventions that address caregiving are unique for each person with chronic illness and cannot be generalized to others.

The Interface of Informal and Formal Caregiving Networks

The interface of a formal caregiving network with the family caregiver is important for the long-term emotional and physical health of the family caregiver. There are several diverse models currently in use to explain the ways in which informal and formal caregiving networks interact over the long term.

Dual Specialization Model

One model that is particularly useful for studying the shared care between formal and informal networks is the dual specialization or complementary model (Litwak, 1985). The model is based on the notion that formal and informal networks have certain kinds of caregiving responsibilities and abilities that are best suited to each particular network. Because of this specialized division of labor, there is the potential for friction and conflict among caregivers. Therefore, the networks work best when the amount of contact or level of involvement between them is minimized, and the groups perform only those tasks for which they are best suited.

This conceptualization of a clear division of labor worked well until the early 1990s when, as already described, highly technical aspects of care were expected of family caregivers. With a new emphasis on family caregivers receiving support and empowerment from formal providers to become competent caregivers, a somewhat less restrictive interpretation of the complementary model is required today. Still, the model is useful for thinking about potential stress and tension that family caregivers may feel toward formal caregivers.

Family Empowerment Model

A model that more appropriately reflects the current emphasis on support of the family caregiver and the inclusion of those caregivers as members of the care-planning team is the Family Empowerment Model (see **Figure 10-1**). Families with members who have chronic health conditions, especially if those members are children, often feel a sense of powerlessness in satisfying the healthcare needs of that family member and in sustaining family life (Hulme, 1999). The Family Empowerment Model depicts

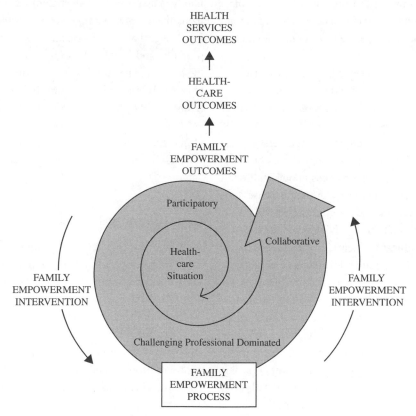

FIGURE 10-1 Family Empowerment Model.
Source: Hulme, P.A. (1999). Family empowerment: A nursing intervention with suggested outcomes for families of children with a chronic health condition. *Journal of Family Nursing*, 5(1), 33–50. Thousand Oaks, CA: Sage.

an interactive intervention process that consists of phases corresponding to the amount of trust and decision making that a family shares with health professionals: professional dominated, participatory, challenging, and collaborative (Hulme, 1999). Family members interact with each other, nurses and other healthcare professionals, the healthcare system, and their community as they participate in the family empowerment process.

In the professional-dominated phase there is a high level of trusting dependency on health professionals to direct health care while the family adjusts to the healthcare situation. This phase occurs during an initial diagnosis of the chronic illness and during a life-threatening situation or relapse (Hulme, 1999).

The participatory phase occurs as the family responds to the continuing chronic illness and its disruptive effect on family life. "Critical consciousness and action" (Hulme, 1999) become apparent and family members begin to perceive themselves as important members in the decision-making process about health care for their family member. During this phase, family members focus on learning about the care of their chronically ill family member and the rules of the healthcare system. They also seek support and try out changing roles and responsibilities to improve their family life (Hulme, 1999).

In the challenging phase the balance of power begins to shift from the healthcare professional to the family. Family members question aspects of care, sometimes triggering conflict with the healthcare professional over control of their family member's health care. Family frustration, uncertainty, disillusionment, and loss of trust in the healthcare professional are not uncommon during this phase (Hulme, 1999).

The collaborative phase is entered as the family becomes more self-confident and assertive

and less reliant on the healthcare professional. The family is now a full partner in the healthcare team (Hulme, 1999).

When using the Family Empowerment Model, it is important to remember that the phases are interdependent and overlapping, and that a family's progress through the phases may be delayed or reversed because of a prolonged or extremely challenging phase, a disruption in family life, or changes in the healthcare situation (Hulme, 1999). Healthcare professionals can help prevent these events by implementing Family Empowerment Interventions, such as guiding the family in assessing its own strengths and in mobilizing the use of those strengths for problem solving. The goal of such interventions is to recognize, promote, and enhance a family's ability to meet the healthcare needs of their family member with chronic illness and to sustain their family life (Hulme, 1999). A valuable resource for nurses as well as family caregivers is the National Organization for Empowering Caregivers (see www.nofec.org and www.care-givers.com).

Family Caregivers as Members of Care Planning Teams

Although the two terms are sometimes used interchangeably, *interdisciplinary* teams are very different from *multidisciplinary* models of care. The older concept of teaming included multidisciplinary teams. These teams typically included members from different disciplines who shared common goals but worked independently to propose and implement patient interventions. When a family caregiver interacts with a multidisciplinary team, he or she is more or less forced to compartmentalize caregiving needs, problems, or concerns into disciplines, such as a nursing problem, a therapy concern, or a social need.

In contrast, the more contemporary concept of teaming calls for interdisciplinary teams. These teams work together to identify and analyze problems, plan actions and interventions, and monitor results of the care plan. Team meetings are used to make or negotiate assignments, share information, and evaluate the team's effort toward achieving client and caregiver outcomes. Lines of communication among team members are highly visible, while disciplinary boundaries are connected on interdisciplinary teams (Travis & Duer, 2000). Family caregivers who participate as members of interdisciplinary teams need only to convey their problems, needs, issues, or concerns to activate a team effort for resolution.

Active inclusion as a member of the interdisciplinary team may help in overcoming a still common complaint of family caregivers: that of dissatisfaction with the level of their involvement in healthcare decision making. Family caregivers have identified four markers of satisfactory involvement: feeling that information is shared, feeling included in decision making, feeling that there is someone you can contact when you need to, and feeling that the service is responsive to your needs (Walker & Dewar, 2004). A goal of interdisciplinary teams should be to help family caregivers achieve these markers of involvement satisfaction. Use of the Family Empowerment Model (as previously discussed) can assist the interdisciplinary team in reaching that goal.

CASE STUDY

The C. Family

Ms. C. is a 29-year-old white woman divorced from her husband. She lives with her 2-year-old son Andrew, who has central hypoventilation syndrome (he does not breathe unassisted when asleep) and prolonged expiratory apnea (he has frequent hypoxic episodes when awake). It was Andrew's illness that led to the couple separating. After birth, Andrew was hospitalized for approximately 3 months with his mother remaining near the hospital rather than returning home, 70 miles away. Her husband saw her absence as inattentiveness and neglect. After they learned that the baby had a poor prognosis, the parents disagreed about his treatment, resulting in much conflict, domestic violence, and eventual separation.

Home setting. Ms. C. and Andrew live in a small, one-bedroom upstairs apartment on the outskirts of a small city. The living room is largely taken up with Andrew's crib and equipment: ventilator, apnea monitor, oxygen tanks, and suction equipment. Ms. C. keeps the apartment very clean to avoid respiratory irritants for her son. Toys are in every room.

Support system. Ms. C does not trust Mr. C. There is a restraining order to keep him out of the apartment, as he has stated he wishes to take Andrew off life support. Mr. C.'s mother and sister do not acknowledge Andrew as part of the family. They visited once in the hospital after Andrew was born, but tried to take out the baby's tracheostomy tube, for, in their culture only "normal" healthy babies are allowed to live.

(continues)

CASE STUDY   (Continued)

Ms. C.'s mother comes to visit her daily. Her sister visits several times a week when she is off from work. Two nephews also visit once or twice weekly. Thus, there is extended family support for her from her family and much conflict from Mr. C.'s family. The consistent emotional support provided by her family keeps Ms. C. strong in her belief that her son deserves to live as normal a life as possible. She maintains a positive, almost stoic attitude about raising him at home.

Growth and development issues. The developmental task for this family is to incorporate the child into the family unit. The family unit itself changed after Andrew's birth, given the separation of the parents due to conflicts between their beliefs about the child's right to live. Andrew is part of his mother's extended family system. Ms. C. has begun to date again, which has positive implications for her meeting her own needs as well as potential long-term implications for the family unit.

Andrew is played with in developmentally appropriate ways. He is frequently held and cuddled by his mother and her extended family. He is able to get around the apartment in his walker and is taken for age-appropriate excursions outside the home with his ventilator and the nurse.

Professional assistance for the child. Andrew has 24-hour-a-day nursing care. Importantly, Ms. C. refers to two of the nurses as part of the family, because they have cared for him for so long. In addition, he has a special education teacher once weekly, and a physical therapist and a speech therapist, who come every other week.

Assistance for the parent caregiver. The mother identified her need for support and counseling services. She was provided with the following information: The American Red Cross offers support groups for parents of children at home on high-technology care. The New York State Department of Health Council on Child and Adolescent Health offers a Directory of Self-Help/Mutual Support for Children with Special Health Needs and Their Families (Huber, 1992). The National Organization for Rare Disorders is also a reference for self-help groups. The local county Mental Health Association is an additional resource for parent caregivers. Ms. C. is fortunate that her family allows her respite from her parenting and caregiving responsibilities. She can therefore participate in such self-help and support groups.

Discussion Questions

1. What challenging behaviors do you identify in this case study?
2. What do you think is causing these behaviors? Give some examples.
3. How would you handle these behaviors?
4. What are effective ways to handle these behaviors? Please explain.
5. How might ethnicity/culture influence family caregiving?

Source: This case study was provided by Allison M. Goodell, RN, BSN, staff nurse in the Pediatric Intensive Care Unit of the Children's Hospital at Albany Medical Center, Albany, New York.

Interdisciplinary teaming works well in long-term care situations because it is virtually impossible to disentangle the ever changing social and healthcare needs of dependent individuals and their family caregivers. If an elderly diabetic client and his spousal caregiver cannot afford to purchase appropriate food and medications in the same week, the healthcare plan will fail until the social needs of the couple are met. Similarly, a wheelchair-bound adult in a potentially neglectful situation will not be able to remain in community-based care with only healthcare support. There is a need for social support and/or family involvement as well.

Transdisciplinary teams are the newest form of long-term care teams. With shrinking healthcare dollars and limited access to care, the transdisciplinary team model seeks to "maximize the strengths of team members and minimize duplication in effort" (Lutz & Davis, 2008, p. 26). In this type of team, one member is selected to direct the care on the basis of the primary needs of the family and patient. This team leader then coordinates the care with other members of the team and the family and patient. In this model, there is a blurring of disciplinary boundaries and team members may be cross-trained in the duties of other disciplines (without exceeding the standards of practice within their own discipline) to provide better continuity in care. For example, the nurse may also be cross-trained in some of the duties of the social worker or physical therapist (Lutz & Davis, 2008).

Lifespan Development and Developmentally Appropriate Care

Knowledge of growth and development helps caregivers separate normal changes from disease-related changes in the dependent family member, regardless of the client's age. This knowledge helps caregivers deal more effectively with decision-making issues, obtain appropriate available community resources, and secure emotional support for themselves. Numerous specialty organizations, such as the March of Dimes, provide this type of educational material for families of recipients of different ages (e.g., children and adolescents). The case study of the C. family with the ventilator-dependent child, Andrew, demonstrates the importance of support and education for the parent.

For families of children with chronic illness, regardless of the type of chronic illness, certain developmental changes or times of transition trigger disequilibrium and stress in the family. There are five principal periods of transition: the initial diagnosis, when symptoms increase, when the child goes to a new setting (such as the hospital), during a parent's absence, and during periods of developmental change (Meleski, 2002). Of the developmental milestones, five specific times are associated with increased stress: when most children learn to walk, when they learn to talk, when they enter school, the onset of puberty, and the child's 21st birthday. Nurses need to recognize these times of transition and teach families how to foster the healthy development of their children as well as the family. The literature reveals several types of adaptation that parents use during times of transition: support, assigning meaning to the illness, managing the condition, role reorganization, and normalization. Nursing interventions should consider the type of adaptation, the family, and the specific situation (Meleski, 2002).

Andrew's story illustrates some of the client and family needs that must be addressed. Andrew's growth, development, and social needs are addressed by his mother, her extended family, his nurses, and his therapists. As he grows older, his changing needs must be considered by individualizing the services he obtains and by treating him as normally as possible. His mother must learn about the changes he will undergo and how to interface effectively with institutions such as hospitals, clinics, and schools. To achieve this, she needs various supportive services. She also needs to have her own needs met so that she can more effectively deal with Andrew's chronic condition. Andrew's restructured family, without his father, has successfully incorporated him into a coherent unit and has not allowed his illness to be a major obstacle.

Helping Families Learn to Cope

Part of the maturation of individual family caregivers and caregiving systems involves the development of realistic expectations of the individual member's abilities and limitations, as well as an understanding of the anticipated trajectory of dependent care that lies ahead. To provide adequate care for a dependent relative and at the same time secure their own well-being, family caregivers need support, aid, and understanding from their families and friends and from the healthcare system. To get that support, it is crucial that family caregivers learn to recognize when they need help, what kind of help to ask for, how to ask for the help they need, and whom to ask (Mittelman, 2003). In doing so, caregivers may need assistance in acquiring the information, support, and services to meet those needs (Elliott & Shewshuk, 2003; Piercy & Chapman, 2001). Individual family caregivers and their caregiving systems may need assistance in learning how to cope with the positive and negative feelings and the emotional

and social impacts of caregiving. Healthcare professionals need to promote family caregivers' well-being, which is a complex, multidimensional concept that includes personal meanings (George & Gwyther, 1986).

Family caregivers need formal providers who have time and the training necessary to help them learn effective interventions. Because nurses with clinical training also understand behavioral and counseling techniques, they are often considered the most appropriate member of the team to work with family caregivers and to oversee educational programs. Stress-Point Intervention by Nurses (SPIN) (Kauffmann & Harrison, 1998) has proved useful in assisting families whose children have a chronic condition and are repeatedly hospitalized. A nurse helps the family develop a unique set of coping strategies based on the family's own concerns and resources and the nurse's expertise. The nurse helps the family explore issues together. This helps the family identify critical stress points and to design a customized family intervention. A central strategy that nurses use in the SPIN process is to express realistic confidence in the family's ability to cope (Kauffmann & Harrison, 1998). While SPIN was developed for families with children with chronic conditions, the SPIN process could be adapted for families of adult members with chronic illness.

In general, programs that build family caregiver confidence and skill and a feeling of support are more effective than those that simply impart knowledge (Piercy & Chapman, 2001). Problem-solving interventions that target the specific concerns of family caregivers are especially effective and can reduce caregiver depression and distress (Elliott & Shewshuk, 2003). Kaye and colleagues (2003) found that early intervention screening of family caregivers of older relatives resulted in caregivers accessing sources of community support before a crisis and impending burnout. In all cases, intervention programs must be developmentally appropriate and tailored to be culturally relevant and learner specific.

The types of intervention programs available range from individual or group caregiver counseling in the presence of a professional facilitator to self-paced, self-help computerized programs that can be completed in relative isolation from others. Software packages that provide caregivers with information and advice on promotion of personal psychological health, relaxation, and other coping strategies plus a caregiver self-assessment tool on coping with the caregiver role have proved useful to caregivers (Chambers & Connor, 2002). Caregivers report that the use of such software provides reassurance and emotional support and enables them to assess and enhance their own coping skills.

The time constraints of most contemporary family caregivers are now being addressed by such strategies as telephone conferencing, Internet chat rooms, and email. Link2Care (http://www.link2care.net) and Caring~Web (http://caringweb.utoledo.edu/) are examples of successful, innovative Internet-based programs that combine high technology with traditional service to increase caregiver well-being and coping skills (Pierce et al., 2004; Kelly, 2003–2004; Steiner & Pierce, 2002). Caregivers using both of these sites found features of updated news and research, information articles and fact sheets, online discussion groups, and "ask an expert" to be of value.

The Veteran's Administration (VA) is using home-telehealth technologies to link caregivers and veterans with chronic conditions to primary care providers at the VA (Lutz, Chumbler, Lyles, Hoffman, & Kobb, 2008; Lutz et al., 2007). It is no longer the case that an intervention program is only effective with direct, face-to-face contact. The key is to make the interventions relevant, multicomponent, tailored to caregivers' needs, and accessible when the caregiver needs it (Chambers & Connor, 2002; Elliott & Shewchuk, 2003; Gitlin et al., 2003; Mittelman, 2003). Many of the caregiving Internet site resources presented at the end of the chapter contain support interventions specific to caregivers.

Caregivers also need the opportunity for activities other than providing care to avoid a sense of entrapment and feelings of loss of self and burnout. Attention to self-help activities sustains one's sense of well-being and revitalizes energy that can later be used in providing care to the client, but many caregivers feel guilty about activities that focus on themselves (Medalie, 1994).

Spirituality and Caregiving

Spiritual beliefs and faith-based behaviors play multiple roles in caregivers' lives. Spirituality involves not only connectedness with a sacred other, but also with other people, perspectives, and sources of value and meaning beyond oneself (Faver, 2004). Such connectedness can produce happiness and energy to sustain a caregiver's ability to care for a chronically ill family member (Faver, 2004; Haley & Harrigan, 2004). Whether caregivers hold religious beliefs or not, they express needs for love, meaning, purpose, and, sometimes, transcendence in their lives (Murray et al., 2004). Caregivers draw strength from maintaining relationships with their families and value opportunities to give and receive love, to feel connected to their social world, and to feel useful (Murray et al., 2004).

Religious beliefs and formal religious practices are essential aspects of caregiving. Heavy reliance on prayer to cope with adversity is reported by many caregivers (Paun, 2004; Stuckey, 2001). African American women caregivers describe their prayer as an ongoing dialogue that keeps them connected with their God rather than as a formal religious ritual (Paun, 2004). Religiosity is also demonstrated by the belief that God has a plan; belief in a loving God; hope in an afterlife; and a sense of the evidence of God all around (Stuckey, 2001). Reading the bible and other religious materials and listening to music are also aspects of formal religion used by caregivers (Theis, Biordi, Coeling, Nalepka, & Miller, 2003). Churches provide an important source of encouragement and social support for caregivers (Faver, 2004; Murray et al., 2004; Theis et al., 2003). A strong connection with a caring community is what caregivers value in their church relationships. Caregivers find that the consistent presence of fellow parishioners is a powerful sustaining force (Faver, 2004). Efforts to maintain chronically ill spouses' engagement in religious practices, such as church attendance, are important for caregivers. When church attendance is no longer possible, caregivers substitute televised or recorded services and arrange for other formal religious practices like communion to be given at their home (Paun, 2004).

A spiritual or religious perspective seems to benefit caregivers in several ways. Caregivers report that attending religious services regularly is what keeps them going. Second to church attendance is prayer (Paun, 2004). Feelings of being supported and comforted by religious faith are associated with positive emotional experiences while caring for persons with Alzheimer's disease (Paun, 2004). A sense of sacred companionship with God or a sacred other acts as a sustaining force for many caregivers (Faver, 2004). Thus, a spiritual approach to caregiving may help caregivers cope with stressful situations and benefit those for whom they care. Strong faith-based beliefs, such as moral living and being of service to others, can motivate persons to become caregivers as well as to continue caregiving (Stuckey, 2001).

Although caregivers report the importance of spirituality and religion in their lives, they are often reluctant to initiate raising such issues with healthcare professionals. Murray and colleagues (2004) found that caregivers (as well as the care recipients) did not broach the subject of spiritual care need because they perceived the healthcare professionals to be busy and/or did not see spiritual care as part of healthcare professionals' role. Caregivers even actively tried to disguise their spiritual distress. Nurses need to be alert to caregivers' need for spiritual care and to create conditions where caregivers feel comfortable in discussing their spiritual needs. Giving caregivers this opportunity validates their concerns and needs and helps them feel connected and cared for. Spiritual support professionals, such as ministers and rabbis, should be included as an integral part of any interdisciplinary or transdisciplinary team.

Churches and Communities in Care Solutions

In addition to government-sponsored programs to help caregivers, churches have a potentially important role to play in caregivers' lives.

Though little research has been conducted on the role of churches in elder care, Stuckey (2001) found that churches supported caregivers by encouraging continued church participation whenever possible and by taking services to the care recipient and caregiver when needed.

An example of a church collaboration is the Interfaith CarePartners (www.interfaithcarepartners.org). This innovative church collaboration began in 1985 in the Greater Houston, Texas area. The focus of program is a care team concept of caregiving that provides in-home support to individuals with chronic health conditions and offers respite support to their caregivers. Individuals with AIDS/HIV were the first to benefit from the care team approach. Caring for those with Alzheimer's and dementia began in 1992, followed by the elderly or those with disabling conditions in 1994, and lastly families with impaired children in 2000 (Interfaith CarePartners, 2011).

Communities also have a role in providing assistance to those in need of care. An excellent example of a community partnership to accomplish this goal is the Gatekeeper Model developed in Spokane, Washington (Substance Abuse & Mental Health Administration, 2004). Employees of community businesses and corporations who work with the public (the "gatekeepers") are trained to identify and refer community-dwelling older adults who may be in need of aid. Upon referral by these gatekeepers, home-based assessments are conducted by interdisciplinary teams provided by the local mental health services, with referrals made for additional services as needed.

Another community example that benefits older adults and caregivers is the interfaith volunteer program organized by Faith in Action National Network (http://www.fianationalnetwork.org/), which administers 600 community programs across the United States. The program, originally funded by the Robert Wood Johnson Foundation, aims to connect volunteers with older and disabled people who need help and to provide a source of respite for caregivers.

Programs, Services, and Resources for Family Caregivers

A multitude of information and referral links, products and services, educational sites, and caregiver support groups are available online. There is no shortage of programs, services, and resources for family caregivers. However, one problem is finding affordable programs that are accessible and convenient for hassled family caregivers. In addition, narrowing an Internet search from a broad term like "family caregiving" to a search for agencies and organizations to assist family caregivers or books for caregivers and professionals will still yield an enormous number of results. An easy-to-use, comprehensive list of agencies and organizations with resources for family caregivers plus a list of books for caregivers and professionals can be found on the Family Caregiver Alliance website (www.caregiver.org).

Utilization of community services by family caregivers provides a range of benefits for caregivers. Unfortunately, barriers to the services continue to exist. Benefits reported by caregivers include renewal, sense of community, and knowledge and belief that their family member also benefited from the service. Barriers include care recipient resistance, reluctance of the caregiver, hassles for the caregiver, concerns about quality, and concerns about finances (Winslow, 2003). Nurses and other healthcare professionals involved in community services need to work to decrease or eliminate the barriers faced by family caregivers.

Respite Programs and Services

Respite is temporary relief from caregiving responsibilities that provides intervals of rest and relief for the caregiver. Family members may provide respite for the primary caregiver by taking over some tasks; for example, children may assist their caregiving parents by shopping, cleaning, and so forth. There are also formal sources of respite, such as adult daycare, in-home companions, and special weekend respite programs.

It is important for caregivers to recognize the warning signs that indicate that their coping skills are overwhelmed and they are in need of outside help. For many caregivers, the hardest step is acknowledging that help is needed; the next most difficult step is extending the effort to seek this help. Caregivers often feel guilty about seeking respite and delay using formal respite services until they are exhausted and debilitated. Ambivalence on the part of caregivers to make use of respite services is illustrated by a study of family caregivers' experiences with in-hospital respite care for family members with dementia (Gilmour, 2002). Caregivers' feelings varied from acceptance to qualified acceptance to marked ambivalence. Caregivers were torn between the need to have a break and the worry over the impact of the in-hospital respite care on their family member. Nurses have the interpersonal skills to help decrease tensions and anxieties that caregivers have over respite care.

Caregivers need to see respite services as a reasonable and appropriate action, not as a sign of personal failure, if they plan to continue caregiving without being overwhelmed by the physical and social demands.

When caregiving becomes too physically demanding or emotionally draining, short-term institutional placement of the client may be a care alternative. Planned short-term hospital admission provides in-facility professional care with relief for the caregiver. These programs can prevent the threshold of family tolerance from being exceeded. To enhance family caregivers' comfort with this type of respite, nurses need to put themselves in a secondary and supporting care provider role and acknowledge the family caregiver as the authority on the care required by their family member (Gilmour, 2002). Family members are more fully able to relinquish care when they are confident that their relative is receiving care comparable to what is provided at home and that the relative is not negatively affected by the hospital stay (Gilmour, 2002).

Both Medicare and many long-term care insurance policies provide a short-term nursing home placement for a dependent family member. Longer or more frequent temporary stays are also possible, if the family is able to pay the expenses out of pocket.

Adult Day Services

Adult day services (formerly known as adult daycare) are congregate programs that provide opportunities for impaired adults to socialize and participate in organized activities, and for their families to receive respite time. Use of adult daycare results in decreased caregiver worry and stress and improved psychological well-being (Ritchie, 2003). Caregivers appreciate the client socializing and improved health as well as the respite for themselves (Warren, Kerr, Smith, Godkin, & Schalm, 2003).

Great variation exists in the type and amount of services that these centers provide. In general, the centers are broadly classified as health or social models of care. Social models emphasize socialization and cognitive stimulation. Health models of care are often supported by a state's Medicaid program and include healthcare monitoring in the day program. In general, the major difference between the two types of programs is the presence or absence of a registered nurse on site. Some day health programs with advanced rehabilitation or restorative programs are certified by Medicare as day treatment hospitals and include rehabilitation specialists on staff.

Work by Campbell and Travis (1999) highlights the interesting ways in which family caregivers integrate formal programs and services into their informal caregiving routines. In their study of spousal caregivers, these researchers concluded that weekends were a time when other caregivers were not at work and were more readily available to help. Thus, better support to the primary caregiver appeared to have contributed to low interest in paying for additional adult day services during the weekend.

Social day programs have a variety of funding options, but most reimbursement sources are limited to low-income families or those with long-term care insurance (DHHS Administration on Aging, 2011b). Day health programs are primarily Medicaid programs or those skilled rehabilitation programs that are Medicare reimbursed. The out-of-pocket cost of day care to the family caregivers varies widely,

depending on the region of the country and the type of program offered. In an analysis of cost implications of adult day services for persons with dementia, Gaugler (2003) found that the daily costs to reduce caregivers' role overload and depression decreased with adult daycare utilization over 1 year. Apparently, the adult day programs are most cost effective for caregivers who use them consistently and for longer periods of time.

Home Care Programs

Home care has expanded in recent years as a result of earlier hospital discharge and the increase in technically more complex therapies. The home represents a different context for provision of care than the medical office or community clinic. Toth-Cohen and colleagues (2001) discuss four key factors that must be considered when providing care within the home setting: understand the personal meaning of the home for the family, view the caregiver as a "lay practitioner," identify the caregiver's beliefs and values, and recognize the potential impact of the interventions on caregiver well-being.

Multiple benefits as well as challenges for the caregiver and the healthcare professional are present in home care (Toth-Cohen et al., 2001). Benefits for the caregiver include: 1) saving of time and mental and physical energy, 2) remaining in control and guiding interaction with the provider, 3) being more comfortable and at ease in one's surroundings, and 4) practicing newly learned skills in the context in which they will be used.

Benefits for the healthcare professional include: 1) gaining an in-depth understanding of the client, the caregiver, and the home context; 2) designing interventions tailored to specific home situations; 3) identifying safety issues that caregivers may be unaware of; and 4) observing performance in the context in which it occurs. Toth-Cohen and colleagues (2001) provide some excellent recommendations to the challenges faced by caregivers caring for a family member with Alzheimer's disease. Nurses can work more effectively with families in their homes by being aware of the benefits, challenges, and possible solutions to those challenges. The nurse's ability to meet whatever challenges are encountered will influence a caregiver's response to interventions and recommendations.

Some home care programs provide respite services for families. Services can include homemaking, monitoring of both client and caregiver health status, and performing various skills, such as taking vital signs or changing catheters. Unfortunately, reimbursement for these programs is increasingly limited to those families with the greatest financial need. Paying out of pocket can be very expensive over the long term.

Psychotherapeutic Approaches

Individual, couple, group, or family counseling may be needed to help families respond to the demands of caregiving. Individual counseling is directed toward enhancing the caregiver's capacity to deal with the day-to-day rigors of caregiving. As described by Montcalm (1995), counseling for couples can be complex because of the multiple issues involved, such as dependency, grief over the losses in the relationship, and fear. When peer interaction and feedback seem appropriate, group therapy can be effective in steering a family caregiver toward more positive resolutions of internal conflict over the caregiving role.

Family treatment often includes a strategy called the "family meeting," at a time when all affected family members meet face to face. A family-based therapy, found effective for

caregivers of family members with dementia, is Structural Ecosystems Therapy (SET) (Mitrani & Czaja, 2000). The aim of SET is to address the entire family's needs within a "cojoint context" (p. 201). SET views the behavior of family members as interdependent and repetitive. Sometimes the repetitive patterns are maladaptive and cause symptoms such as caregiver stress. Other interaction patterns are adaptive and relieve caregiver strain. SET focuses on improving the caregiver's interactions within his or her whole social ecosystem, that is, family, community, healthcare providers, and so on, thus increasing the extent to which the caregiver's emotional, social, and instrumental needs are met. SET is particularly appropriate for minority families because it acknowledges the importance of culture as a contextual variable that can have a marked influence on family interaction (Mitrani & Czaja, 2000).

Support Groups

Also called self-help groups, these forums focus on specific client populations and related caregivers' needs. Self-help groups for caregivers have been established in many communities throughout the United States. Some are self-directed or run by volunteers; others are led by healthcare professionals who act as group facilitators. These groups provide information, emotional support, advocacy, or a combination of these services. They address such areas as skills in the care and maintenance of the disabled person and managing problems in the family; information regarding the aging process; emotional needs for recognition and support from caring people; and concrete service needs for referral and information regarding resources. Telephone support networks and Internet chat rooms are simply contemporary versions of the traditional face-to-face support group.

The Need for Culturally Sensitive Interventions

During the 20th century, the United States and Canada experienced massive waves of immigration, as well as growing populations of native-born minorities. Given the diversity of racial, ethnic, and religious groups in North America, there is a need for helping healthcare professionals learn more about the many cultural groups with which they work so that they can provide interventions that are sensitive to the client's culture. To that end, there has been a rapid rise of multicultural consciousness in the United States. However, cultural awareness among healthcare professionals continues to be inadequate to serve those of other cultures.

Awareness that the definition of family differs from one cultural group to another is important. For example, the dominant Caucasian definition focuses on the intact nuclear family. However, African Americans focus on a wider network of kin and community, and often include nonbiological family members in their family networks. The Chinese culture includes all of a person's ancestors and descendants in the definition of family and the needs of the family are valued more highly than the needs of the individual. However, these values may be changing because of globalization and the influence of Western values (Lee, 2007). Who the client considers to be family and who is providing care will influence who should be included in interventions.

Cultural groups vary greatly in how they respond to problems and their attitudes toward seeking help. For example, Hispanic families typically want to keep problems confidential and view caregiving as a responsibility of the female family members (Evans et al., 2007; Rittman, Kuzmeskus, & Flum, 1998). To assist an Hispanic family, a helping professional will have to work on *personalismo*, knowing the older adult and her caregiver as total persons, before focusing on personal matters; *dignidad*, developing a working relationship that reflects dignity and self-worth; *respeto*, respect between the helping professional and Hispanic elder; and *confianza*, trust between the two parties (Evans, Coon, & Crogan, 2007; Gallagher-Thompson, Solano, Coon, & Areán, 2003).

Ethnic differences exist in attitudes toward caregiving and caregiving responsibilities. For example, Cuban Americans often have a hierarchical relational orientation and adhere to traditional family roles. Because of this, female caregivers may have difficulty in adopting the leadership role of caregiving (Mitrani & Czaja, 2000). Other cultural characteristics of Cubans are collectivism, giving precedence to the needs of the family over the individual, and the high degree of emotional and psychological closeness or enmeshment between caregiver and the care recipient. Enmeshment, observed more frequently in Cuban families than in Caucasian American families, can produce a lack of objectivity and an unwillingness to delegate care tasks, making it difficult for the caregiver to be an effective care manager (Mitrani & Czaja, 2000). To work effectively with families from varied ethnic and cultural heritages, the nurse must tailor family interventions to be culturally congruent.

Providing assistance to family caregivers of minority elders for any number of issues is most effective when the members of the targeted minority group are represented in the provider or intervention group. For this reason, neighborhood-centered services, in which minority caregivers can interact with bilingual professionals, tend to be highly effective. These programs are well suited to respecting the values and customs of families in need of help and to offering culturally relevant solutions to the caregivers (Spector, 2000).

Evidence-Based Practice

Evidence-based practice is based on the demonstrated effectiveness of interventions tested in multiple clinical trials. Systematic reviews of the research are considered to be the highest level of evidence. As described in the previous sections, there are numerous studies testing various interventions to help improve the health and well-being of caregivers. However, there are only a few systematic reviews of the literature that focus on these widely varying interventions. Furthermore, the reviews available cite the lack of high-quality evidence and poor consistency in the clinical trials testing these interventions (Glasdam, Timm, & Vitrrup, 2010; Hempel, Norman, Golder, Aguiar-Ibánêz, & Eastwood, 2008; Smith, Forster, & Young, 2009). Therefore, it is imperative that more intervention research is conducted with a focus on replicating previous clinical trials. Researchers also suggest the inclusion of qualitative findings in the systematic reviews to better determine the specific effects of the interventions from the perspectives of caregivers (Thompson et al. 2007). **Table 10-1** includes examples of systematic reviews of the literature on caregiver interventions.

CARE RECIPIENT, CAREGIVER, AND CAREGIVING SYSTEM OUTCOMES

Providing care to another person has both positive and negative outcomes for the primary caregiver and the caregiver system. Because caregiving is a very personal journey, it is almost impossible to predict how each caregiver or care recipient will respond to the demands of

dependency and caregiving support. Therefore, all of the interventions provided by an interdisciplinary or transdisciplinary team are ultimately directed toward supporting family caregivers when the situation is going well, and to helping caregivers correct practices that will lead to potentially negative outcomes.

Much of the caregiving literature reflects a focus on the negative aspects of caregiving. Less available are the positive aspects of the caregiver role. The literature continues to need studies that identify the potential benefits of caregiving (Hudson, 2004) for the purpose of increasing our understanding of the caregiving experience (Tarlow et al., 2004) as well as preventing the likelihood of viewing caregiving only from a pathologic perspective and thus socializing caregivers to expect burden (Gaugler, Kane, & Langlois, 2000). The study of caregiver benefits can also provide data for the development of evidence-based supportive care strategies for families and family caregivers (Harding & Higginson, 2003).

Despite the paucity of information regarding the benefits derived from the caregiver role, studies available indicate that most caregivers find some element of satisfaction in the caregiving experience (Nolan, 2001; Scott, 2001). Hudson (2004) reported that 60% of caregivers readily identified positive aspects of the caregiver role. Given what is known about long-term family caregiving, there are three outcomes that are commonly monitored. Together, these outcomes form a gold standard by which caregiving experiences can be measured. Outcomes for both the family caregivers and their care recipients include improved quality of life and meaning in life, enhanced autonomy and control, and reduced family stress and enhanced coping ability.

Table 10-1 Examples of Systematic Reviews of Research on Caregiving Interventions

Authors (date)	Focus of Review and Number of Studies Reviewed	Findings	Recommendations
Selwood, Johnston, Katona, Lyketosos, & Livingston (2007)	Effectiveness of psychological interventions for family CGs of persons with dementia (n = 62 RCTs)	Individual behavioral management therapy with 6 or more sessions is effective in decreasing CG depression Group behavioral management therapy is not as effective Individual or group therapy focusing on coping strategies is also effective. Education on dementia and supportive therapy are not effective	Individual behavioral management and individual and group coping strategy therapy improves CG mental health Educational sessions should be individualized to each CG More research is needed
Thompson, Spilsbury, Hall, Birks, Barnes, & Adamson (2007)	Effectiveness of technology-, individual-, and group-based information and support interventions for CGs of persons with dementia (n = 44 RCTs)	Group-based interventions decrease depression in CGs No demonstrated effectiveness of any other type of intervention Clinical significance is uncertain. Poor quality evidence	Insufficient evidence to make a recommendation Limited evidence, more research needed Specifically, more systematic reviews of qualitative findings are needed
Hempel, Norman, Golder, Aguiar-Ibáñez, & Eastwood (2008)	Review evidence on psychosocial interventions for nonprofessional caregivers of persons with Parkinson's disease (n = 30 studies, 3 RCTs, 27 other)	Various methodological weaknesses in studies reviewed, many pilot studies Majority of caregiver interventions were embedded in patient treatment regimens Little evidence supporting effectiveness of interventions	Several interventions warrant further research Insufficient evidence to make a recommendation Need additional research with rigorous designs and more focus on the caregiver
Smith, Forster, & Young (2009)	Effectiveness of information provision on improving outcomes for patients with stroke and their CGs (n = 11 RCTs)	Providing information improves knowledge of patients and CGs, but shows no effect on CG stress.	Limited evidence. More research on information provision interventions is needed with a focus on active strategies that involve the patient and caregiver

(continues)

	Focus of Review and Number of Studies		
Authors (date)	Reviewed	Findings	Recommendations
Glasdam, Timm, & Vitrrup (2010)	Describe and critically evaluate support interventions for caregivers of chronically ill persons (n = 32 studies: 29 RCTs, 3 clinical trials published from 1997–2007)	Incomplete description of the research design in many of the studies reviewed An aim of all interventions was to improve CG knowledge and support Education and counseling were provided at individual and/or group levels Mode of delivery included in-home visits, face-to-face counseling, and telephone support	Insufficient evidence to make a recommendation Effect of support interventions for CG is inconclusive Quality of the studies questionable Future research should include interventions that go beyond knowledge transfer and cognitive behavioral therapy focusing instead on interventions that support CG relationships and activities in their home or local environments.

Table 10-1   Examples of Systematic Reviews of Research on Caregiving Interventions (continued)

CG, caregiver; RCT, randomized controlled trial.
Note: See individual citations for more details.

Quality of Life and Meaning in Life

It has been written that human beings "can be at their best when they are behaving with altruism and commitment to a person they love" (Lattanzi-Licht, Mahoney, & Miller, 1998, p. 31). Finding enhanced quality of life and meaning in life associated with the caregiving experience is one of the most positive outcomes of caregiving for the care recipient and the caregiver (Sheehan & Donorfio, 1999). Evidence of enhanced meaning of life can be seen in caregivers' comments about positive aspects of caregiving: "Love doing it—we've been given an opportunity we'd never thought we'd have" (Hudson, 2004, p. 62).

Until recently, systematic assessments of these positive outcomes of caregiving have been limited because of the difficulty clinicians have encountered in finding and accessing psychometrically sound measures of these abstract constructs (Farran, Miller, & Kaufman, 1999). The new generation of measurement tools allows interdisciplinary (or transdisciplinary) teams to tap into the day-to-day meaning and ultimate meaning of caregiving relationships so that these aspects of caregiving become a visible outcome of the experiences (Farran et al.,1999). One such measurement tool is the Positive Aspects of Caregiving (Tarlow et al., 2004).

Perceived Autonomy and Control

Autonomy, as an outcome of family caregiving, means that the choices of long-term caregivers and their care recipients are self-determined. Consistent with the principles of self-determination is the need to have some control over events and decisions. In chronic care situations, autonomy and control are interrelated and both are affected by the ability of professional providers to support family caregivers in the choices they make and the care that they give. It follows that autonomy and control may need to be renegotiated with the formal network and within the informal caregiving system as the caregiving situation changes.

Those caregivers who are able to feel most relaxed and confident in managing their caregiving situations have reported that being successful does not mean being in total control (Karp & Tanarugsachock, 2000). Learning to "go with the flow" is how caregivers frequently describe their approach to control issues (Travis, Bethea, & Winn, 2000). If interdisciplinary teams respect the values and goals of the caregivers and their care recipients and help to translate these into real-world plans of care, then perceived autonomy and control for both caregivers and care recipients are enhanced. Evidence of an enhanced sense of autonomy and control can be seen in caregivers' comments about positive aspects of caregiving: "Taking responsibility for things I had not previously been responsible for"; "I feel like I'm a stronger person now"; and "I've been able to undertake much more than I thought I could" (Hudson, 2004, p. 62).

Reduced Family Stress and Coping

As previously discussed, the many adverse effects of caregiving include an array of affective responses by caregivers to the demands of long-term caregiving. The goal of most care teams is to reduce this distress to a level that is perceived to be manageable for the caregivers. Caregivers are able to voice positive aspects in the role despite the negative aspects, such as stress and strain (Hudson, 2004; Roff et al., 2004). Perhaps caregivers use positive emotions to augment and maintain their coping strategies when faced with an ongoing stressor like caregiving (Folkman, 1997). Because family stress and coping are global, multidimensional, and multifaceted, interventions are often designed to address a specific aspect of stress and coping, such as perceived strain, depression, or fatigue (Buckwalter et al., 1999).

Societal Outcomes

A number of studies have examined the cost effectiveness of community-based home services to groups of individuals at risk for nursing home use. Even though the most consistent justification for delivering long-term care services in home- and community-based environments is cost containment, such claims have not been supported in the research (Weissert & Hedrick, 1999). Part of the problem is the way that costs of care are compared across settings. For example, while nursing home care appears to be more costly than community-based care, the calculations do not take into consideration the out-of-pocket expenses and subsidized programs and services that family caregivers must use to make community-based care a viable long-term care option for them and their dependent family members.

Delayed or Diverted Episodes of Institutional Care

Despite the fact that home- and community-based care may not be cost effective, providing such care remains a goal for many families and a priority of policy makers. This is because institutional care is perceived as more expensive by most policy makers, and as less desirable than home care by older adults and policy makers alike, who clearly prefer noninstitutional solutions to long-term care.

In their study of the influence of service use on consequences for caregivers, Bass, Noelker, and Rechlin (1996) conceptualized services as a type of social support. They found that certain services, such as health care, personal care, and homemaker services reduced the adverse effects of heavy or burdensome care on the family caregivers. These types of programs serve a clientele that may not be at imminent risk of nursing home placement, but their needs for assistance in the home or community are real (Weissert & Hedrick, 1994).

Instead of looking to home- and community-based services as a cost-effective alternative to nursing home placement, a better outcome of success may be measures of diverted hospital stays (Weissert & Hedrick, 1994). Advanced death planning and decisions about when to institutionalize, as well as working with clinicians and families as dependent persons transition from active treatment to palliation, can reduce inappropriate and expensive care (Weissert & Hedrick, 1994). This outcome requires more discussions and decision making among care recipients and their family members regarding care decisions and increased communication with their physicians to ensure that the decisions are respected and carried out. Nurses can foster this decision making by encouraging families to talk openly with one another about care and by assisting families to put the plans into place in advance of the need to make decisions about hospitalizations or other unwanted aggressive measures.

STUDY QUESTIONS

Who are the primary providers of home care? What are some of the providers' competing demands?

What are the advantages and disadvantages of the person with chronic illness or disease being cared for at home? For the family? For the caregiver?

Are there differences for caregivers in caring for children with disability versus caring for older adults? Please be specific and discuss.

How does ethnicity influence family caregiving?

In what way(s) does culture affect family caregiving?

What factors influence the cost effectiveness of home care versus institutionalization?

What is the financial impact of caregiving on the caregiver?

How does public policy affect caregiving?

How can healthcare professionals assist family caregivers?

As an advocate for family caregivers, what facts would you present to lawmakers related to supportive legislation?

What are some of the emotional responses to family caregiving? Discuss positive and negative consequences for family caregivers.

Choose a scenario that you are familiar with or use a case study from this chapter and apply the Family Empowerment Model.

How does spirituality or religious preference help family caregivers cope with their caring situation?

Where can family caregivers go for assistance and information?

Study Questions (Cont.) www

What are some of the issues with implementing evidence-based practice when working with family caregivers? How can these these issues be addressed?

What are some positive outcomes for family caregivers? What are some strategies that could be implemented to reinforce positive caregiving outcomes?

For a full suite of assignments and additional learning activities, www use the access code located in the front of your book and visit this exclusive website: **http://go.jblearning.com/larsen**. If you do not have an access code, you can obtain one at the site.

INTERNET RESOURCES www

AssistGuide Information Services: www.agis.com

Caregiver Resources. Because We Care. Administration on Aging and the U.S. Department of Health and Human Services: http://www.aasa.dshs.wa.gov/caregiving/documents/BecauseWeCare.pdf

Caregiving Resources from the American College of Physicians, Internal Medicine: http://www.acponline.org/fcgi/search?q=caregiver+site=ACP

Caring for Someone with Alzheimer's: http://nihseniorhealth.gov/alzheimerscare/toc.html

Caring from a Distance: www.cfad.org

Faith in Action National Network: http://www.fia-nationalnetwork.org

Family Caregiver Alliance: http://caregiver.org/caregiver/jsp/home.jsp

Interfaith CarePartners: www.interfaithcarepartners.org

National Alliance for Caregiving: www.caregiving.org

National Cancer Institute: Coping with Cancer: www.cancer.gov/cancertopics/coping

National Family Caregivers' Association: www.nfcacares.org

National Family Caregivers' Association and National Alliance for Caregiving: www.family-caregiving101.org

National Organization for Empowering Caregivers: www.nofec.org and www.care-givers.com

REFERENCES

Administration on Aging. (2010). *A profile of older Americans: 2009*. Washington, DC: U.S. Department of Health and Human Services.

Albert, S. M., & Brody, E. M. (1996). When elder care is viewed as child care. *American Journal of Geriatric Psychiatry, 4,* 121–130.

Allen, S. M., Goldscheider, F., & Ciambrone, D. (1999). Gender roles, marital intimacy, and nomination of spouses as primary caregivers. *The Gerontologist, 39,* 150–158.

Anderson, G. F. (2005). Medicare and chronic conditions. *New England Journal of Medicine, 343*(3), 305–309.

Badr, H., & Acitelli, L. K. (2005). Dyadic adjustment in chronic illness: Does relationship talk matter? *Journal of Family Psychiatry, 19*(2), 465–469.

Barrett, A. E., & Lynch, S. M. (1999). Caregiving networks of elderly persons: Variation by marital status. *The Gerontologist, 39,* 695–704.

Bass, D. M., Noelker, L. S., & Rechlin, L. R. (1996). The moderating influence of service use on negative caregiving consequences. *Journal of Gerontology, Social Sciences, 51B,* S121–S131.

Binstock, R. H. (1999). Public policies and minority elders. In M. L. Wykle & A. B. Ford (Eds.), *Serving minority elders in the 21st century* (pp. 5–24). New York: Springer.

Blake, H., & Lincoln, N. (2000). Factors associated with strain in co-resident spouses of patients following stroke. *Clinical Rehabilitation, 14*(3), 307–14.

Boaz, R. F., Hu, J., & Ye, Y. (1999). The transfer of resources from middle-aged children to functionally limited elderly parents: Providing time, giving money, sharing space. *The Gerontologist, 39,* 648–657.

Bodenheimer, T., Chen, E., & Bennett, H. D. (2009). Confronting the growing burden of chronic disease: Can the U.S. health care workforce do the job? *Health Affairs, 28*(1), 64–74.

Bowdoin, C. (1994). Commentary on new diagnosis: Caregiver role strain. *AACN Nursing Scan in Critical Care, 4*(1), 23.

Brody, E. M. (1990). Role reversal: An inaccurate and destructive concept. *Journal of Gerontological Social Work, 15,* 15–22.

Brody, E. M., & Schoonover, C. B. (1986). Patterns of parent-care when adult daughters work and when they do not. *The Gerontologist, 26,* 372–381.

Buckwalter, K. C., Gerdner, L., Kohout, F., Hall, G. R., et al. (1999). A nursing intervention to decrease depression in family caregivers of persons with dementia. *Archives of Psychiatric Nursing, 13,* 80–88.

Burton, L. C., Newsom, J. T., Schulz, R., Hirsch, C. H., & German, P. S. (1997). Preventative health behaviors among spousal caregivers. *Preventative Medicine, 26,* 162–169.

Campbell, D. D., & Travis, S. S. (1999). Spousal caregiving when the adult day services center is closed. *Journal of Psychosocial Nursing, 37,* 20–25.

Caron, C. D., & Bowers, B. J. (2003). Deciding whether to continue, share, or relinquish caregiving: Caregiver views. *Qualitative Health Research, 13*(9), 1252–1271.

Chambers, M., & Connor, S. L. (2002). User-friendly technology to help family carers cope. *Journal of Advanced Nursing, 40*(5), 568–577.

Chang, C., & White-Means, S. (1991). The men who care: An analysis of male primary caregivers who care for frail elderly at home. *Journal of Applied Gerontology, 10,* 343–358.

Chesla, C. A., & Rungreangkulkij, S. (2001). Nursing research on family processes in chronic illness in ethnically diverse families: A decade review. *Journal of Family Nursing, 7*(3), 230–243.

Chumbler, N. R., Rittman, M., Van Puymbroeck, M., Vogel, W. B., & Qin, H. (2004). The sense of coherence, burden, and depressive symptoms in informal caregivers during the first month after stroke. *International Journal of Geriatric Psychiatry, 19*(10), 944–953.

Chumbler, N. R., Rittman, M. R., & Wu, S. S. (2007). Associations of sense of coherence and depression in caregivers of stroke survivors across 2 years [Electronic Version]. *The Journal of Behavioral Health Services Research, 35*(2), 226–234.

Clyburn, L. D., Stones, M. J., Hadjistavropoulos, T., & Tuokko, H. (2000). Predicting caregiver burden and depression in Alzheimer's disease. *Journal of Gerontology, Social Sciences, 55B,* S2–S13.

Covinsky, K. E., Eng, C., Lui, L., Sands, L. P., Sehgal, A. R., Walter, L. C., et al. (2001). Reduced employment in caregivers of frail elders. *The Journals of Gerontology Series A: Biological Sciences and Medical Sciences, 56,* M707–M713.

Covinsky, K. E., Newcomer, R., Fox, P., Wood, J., et al. (2003). Patient and caregiver characteristics associated with depression in caregiving of patients with dementia. *Journal of General Internal Medicine, 18*(12), 1006–1014.

Cox, C. (1999). Race and caregiving: Patterns of service use by African American and white caregivers of persons with Alzheimer's disease. *Journal of Gerontological Social Work, 32,* 5–19.

Dautzenberg, M. G. H. (2000). The competing demands of paid work and parent care. *Research on Aging, 22,* 165–188.

Deimling, G., & Bass, D. (1986). Symptoms of mental impairment among elderly adults and their effects on family caregivers. *Journal of Gerontology, 41*(6), 778–84.

DHHS Administration on Aging. (2011a). National Family Caregiver Support Program (OAA Title III E). Retrieved 8/30/11, from http://www.aoa.gov/AoAroot/AoA_programs/HCLTC/Caregiver/index.aspv

DHHS Administration on Aging. (2011b). AoA Programs. Retrieved August 30, 2011, from http://aoa.gov/AoARoot/AoA_Programs/index.aspx

DHHS Administration on Aging. (2009). National Center on Elder Abuse (Title II). Retrieved August 30, 2011, from http://aoa.gov/AoARoot/AoA_programs/elder_rights/NCEA/Index.aspx

Draper, B., Poulos, C., Cole, A., Poulos, R., & Ehrlich, F. (1992). A comparison of caregivers for elderly stroke and dementia victims. *Journal of the American Geriatric Society, 40*(9), 896–901.

DuPont, P. (1999). *The short term problem facing long-term care. National Center for Policy Analysis.* Retrieved September 21, 2011 from http://www.ncpa.org/oped/dupont/dup010699.html

Edmonds, M. M. (1999). Serving minority elders: Preventing chronic illness and disability in the

African American elderly. In M. L. Wykle & A. B. Ford (Eds.), *Serving minority elders in the 21st century* (pp. 25–36). New York: Springer.

Elliot, T. R., & Shewchuk, R. M. (2003). Social problem-solving and distress among family members assuming a caregiving role. *British Journal of Health Psychology, 8,* 149–163.

Evans, B. C., Coon, D. W., & Crogan, N. L. (2007). Personalismo and breaking barriers: Accessing Hispanic populations for clinical services and research. *Geriatric Nursing 28*(5), 289–296.

Evercare & National Alliance for Caregiving. (2007). *Evercare study of family caregivers—What they spend, what they sacrifice.* Minnetonka, MN: Author. Retrieved August 8, 2011, from: http://www.caregiving.org/data/Evercare_NAC_CaregiverCostStudyFINAL20111907.pdf

Family Caregiver Alliance. (2006). *Fact sheet: Caregiver health.* San Francisco, CA: Author. Retrieved August 8, 2011, from:http://caregiver.org/caregiver/jsp/content_node.jsp?nodeid=1822

Family Caregiver Alliance. (2010). *Health care reform and family caregivers.* San Francisco, CA: Author. Retrieved August 8, 2011, from: http://www.caregiver.org/content/pdfs/HCR%20provisions%20for%20caregivers-2010.pdf

Farran, C. J., Miller, B. H., & Kaufman, J. E. (1999). Finding meaning through caregiving: Development of an instrument for family caregivers of persons with Alzheimer's disease. *Journal of Clinical Psychology, 55*(9), 1107–1125.

Fast, J. E., Williamson, D. L., & Keating, N. C. (1999). The hidden costs of informal elder care. *Journal of Family and Economic Issues, 20,* 301–326.

Faver, C. A. (2004). Relational spirituality and social caregiving. *Social Work, 49*(2), 241–249.

Figley, C. R. (1998). Burnout as systemic traumatic stress: A model for helping traumatized family members. In C. R. Figley (Ed.), *Burnout in families: The systemic costs of caring* (pp. 15–28). Boca Raton, FL: CRC Press.

Folkman, S. (1997). Positive psychological states and coping with severe stress. *Social Science & Medicine, 45*(8), 1207–1221.

Gallagher-Thompson, D., Solano, N., Coon, P., & Areán, P. (2003). Recruitment and retention of Latino dementia family caregivers in intervention research: Issues to face, lessons to learn. *The Gerontologist, 43,* 45–51.

Gaugler, J. E. (2003). Evaluating community-based programs for dementia caregivers: The cost implication of adult day services. *Journal of Applied Gerontology, 22*(1), 118–133.

Gaugler, J., Kane, R., & Langlois, J. (2000). Assessment of family caregivers of older adults. In R. Kane & R. Kane (Eds.), *Assessing older persons: Measures, meaning and practical applications* (pp. 321–359). New York: Oxford University Press.

Geister, C. (2005). The feeling of responsibility as core motivation for care giving—Why daughters care for their mothers. *Pflege, 18*(1), 5–14.

George, L. K., & Gwyther, L. P. (1986). Caregiver well-being: A multidimensional examination of family caregivers of demented adults. *The Gerontologist, 26*(3), 253–259.

Gilliss, C. L. (2002).There is science, and there is life. *Families, Systems & Health, 20*(1), 49.

Gilmour, J. A. (2002). Disintegrated care: Family caregivers and in-hospital care. *Journal of Advanced Nursing, 39*(6), 546–553.

Gitlin, L., Burgio, L., Mahoney, D., Burns, R., et al. (2003). Effect of multicomponent interventions on caregiver burden and depression: The REACH Multisite Initiative at 6-month follow-up. *Psychology and Aging, 18*(3), 361–374.

Given, B., Strommel, M., Collins, C., King, S., et al. (1990). Responses of elderly spouse caregivers. *Research in Nursing and Health, 13,* 77–85.

Glasdam, S., Timm, H., & Vitrrup, R. (2010). Support efforts for caregivers of chronically ill persons. *Clinical Nursing Research, 19*(3),233–265.

Gordon, P. A., & Perrone, K. M. (2004). When spouses become caregivers: Counseling implications for younger couples. *Journal of Rehabilitation, 70*(2), 27–32.

Haigler, D. H., Bauer, L. J., & Travis, S. S. (2004). Finding the common ground of family and professional caregiving: The education agenda at the Rosalynn Carter Institute. *Educational Gerontology, 30,* 95–105.

Haley, J., & Harrigan, R. C. (2004). Voicing the strengths of Pacific Island parent caregivers of children who are medically fragile. *Journal of Transcultural Nursing, 15*(3), 184–194.

Halm, M. A., & Bakas, T. (2007). Factors associated with depressive symptoms, outcomes, and perceived physical health after coronary bypass surgery. *Journal of Cardiovascular Nursing, 22*(6), 508–515.

Harding, R., & Higginson, I. (2003). What is the best way to help caregivers in cancer and palliative care? A systematic literature review of interventions and their effectiveness. *Palliative Medicine, 17,* 63–74.

He, W., Sengupta, M., Velkoff, V., & DeBarros, K. (2005). *65+ in the United States: 2005.* Washington, DC: U.S. Government Printing Office.

Hempel, S., Norman, G., Golder, S., Aguiar-Ibáñêz, R. & Eastwood, A. (2008). Psychosocial interventions for non-professional carers of people with Parkinson's disease: A systematic scoping review. *Journal of Advanced Nursing, 64*(3), 214–228.

Horowitz, A. (1985). Sons and daughters as caregivers to older parents: Differences in role performance and consequences. *The Gerontologist, 25,* 612–617.

Huber, M. (1992). Empowering families through self-help mutual support: Training sessions-Evaluation report. Albany, NY: Bureau of Child and Adolescent Health, New York Department of Health.

Hudson, P. (2004). Positive aspects and challenges associated with caring for a dying relative at home. *International Journal of Palliative Nursing, 10*(2), 58–64.

Hulme, P. A. (1999). Family empowerment: A nursing intervention with suggested outcomes for families of children with a chronic health condition. *Journal of Family Nursing, 5*(1), 33–50.

Hunt, C. K. (2003). Concepts in caregiver research. *Journal of Nursing Scholarship, 35*(1), 27–32.

Hunt, G., Levine, C., & Naiditch, N. (2005). *Young caregivers in the U.S.* NY: National Alliance for Caregiving and the United Hospital Fund.

Interfaith CarePartners (2011). Retrieved October 11, 2011, from http://www.interfaithcarepartners.org/index/php/home/c/home

Johnson, R., Toohey, D., & Wiener, J. (2007). *Meeting the long-term care needs of the baby boomers.* Retrieved August 8, 2011, from: http://www.urban.org/publications/311451.html

Johnson, R., & Wiener, J. (2006). *A profile of frail older Americans and their caregivers: The retirement project.* Washington, DC. The Urban Institute. Retrieved August 8, 2011, from: http://www.urban.org/UploadedPDF/311284_older_americans.pdf

Jones, S. (1999). Bridging the gap: Community solutions for black-elderly health care in the 21st century. In M. L. Wykle & A. B. Ford (Eds.), *Serving minority elders in the 21st century,* (pp. 223–234). New York: Springer.

Kane, R. A., Reinardy, J., & Penrod, J. D. (1999). After the hospitalization is over: A different perspective on family care of older people. *Journal of Gerontological Social Work, 31,* 119–141.

Karp, D. A., & Tanarugsachock, V. (2000). Mental illness, caregiving, and emotion management. *Qualitative Health Research, 10,* 6–25.

Kauffmann, E. & Harrison, M. B. (1998). Stress-point intervention for parents of children hospitalized with chronic conditions. *Pediatric Nursing, 24*(4), 362–366.

Kaye, L. W., Turner, W., Butler, S. S., Downey, R., et al. (2003). Early intervention screening for family caregivers of older relatives in primary care practices. Establishing a community health service alliance in rural America. *Family Community Health, 26*(4), 319–328.

Keith, C. (1995). Family caregiving systems: Models, resources, and values. *Journal of Marriage and the Family, 57,* 179–190.

Kelly, K. (2003–004). Link2 Care: Internet-based information and support for caregivers. *Family Caregiving,* Winter, 87–88

Kramer, B. (1997). Gain in the caregiving experience: Where are we? What next? *The Gerontologist, 37,* 218–232.

Kramer, B., & Thompson, E. (2001). *Men as caregivers: Theory, research and service implications.* New York: Springer.

Lackey, N. R., & Gates, M. F. (2001). Adults' recollections of their experiences as young caregivers of family members with chronic physical illnesses. *Journal of Advanced Nursing, 34*(3), 320–328.

Lattanzi-Licht, M., Mahoney, J. J., & Miller, G. W. (1998). *The hospice choice: In pursuit of a peaceful death.* New York: Simon & Schuster.

Leavitt, M., Martinson, I. M., Liu, C. Y., Armstrong, V., et al. (1999). Common themes and ethnic differences in family caregiving the first year after diagnosis of childhood cancer: Part II. *Journal of Pediatric Nursing, 14,* 110–122.

Lee, M. D. (2007). Correlates of consequences of intergenerational caregiving in Taiwan. *Journal of Advanced Nursing, 59*(1), 49–56.

Litwak, E. (1985). *Helping the elderly: The complementary roles of informal networks and formal systems.* New York: Guilford Press.

Lutz, B. J., Chumbler, N. R., Lyles, T., Hoffman, N, & Kobb, R. (2008). Testing a home-telehealth programme for US veterans recovering from stroke and their family caregiver. *Disability and Rehabilitation, 7,* 1–8.

Lutz, B. J., Chumbler, N. R., & Roland, K. (2007). Care coordination/home-telehealth for veterans with stroke and their caregivers: Addressing an unmet need. *Topics in Stroke Rehabilitation 14*(4), 32–42.

Lutz, B. J., & Davis, S. M. (2008). Theory and practice models for rehabilitation nursing. In S. Hoeman (Ed.) *Rehabilitation nursing: Prevention, intervention, and outcomes* (4th ed., pp. 14–29). St. Louis, MO: Mosby-Elsevier.

Mausbach, B. T., Patterson, T. L., Von Känel, R., Mills, P. J., et al. (2007). The attenuating effect of personal mastery on the relations between stress and Alzheimer caregiver health: A five-year longitudinal analysis. *Aging & Mental Health, 11*(6), 637–644.

McAuley, W. J., Travis, S. S., & Safewright, M. P. (1997). Personal accounts of the nursing home search and selection process. *Qualitative Health Research, 7,* 236–254.

Medalie, J. H. (1994). The caregiver as the hidden patient. In E. Kahana, D. E. Biegel, & M. L. Wykle (Eds.), *Family caregiving across the lifespan* (pp. 312–330). Thousand Oaks, CA: Sage.

Meleski, D. D. (2002). Families with chronically ill children. *American Journal of Nursing, 102*(5), 47–54.

Meshefedjian, G., McCusker, J., Bellavance, F., & Baumgarten, M. (1998). Factors associated with symptoms of depression among informal caregivers of demented elders in the community. *The Gerontologist, 38,* 247–253.

MetLife & National Alliance for Caregiving. (2004). *Caregiving in the U.S.* Retrieved August 8, 2011, from: http://www.caregiving.org/data/04finalreport.pdf

Mitrani, V. B. & Czaja, S. J. (2000). Family-based therapy for dementia caregivers: Clinical observations. *Aging & Mental Health, 4*(3), 200–209.

Mittelman, J. S. (2003). Community caregiving. *Alzheimer's Care Quarterly, 4*(4), 273–285.

Montcalm, D. M. (1995). Caregivers: Resources and services. In Z. Harel & R. E. Dunkle (Eds.), *Matching people with services in long term care* (pp. 159–179). New York: Springer.

Montgomery, R. J. V. (1999). The family role in the context of long-term care. *Journal of Aging and Health, 11,* 383–416.

Montgomery, A., & Feinberg, L. F. (2003). *The road to recognition: International review of public policies to support family and informal caregiving.* San Francisco: National Center on Caregiving, Family Caregiver Alliance.

Montgomery, R. J. V. & Kosloski, K. D. (n.d.). *Change, continuity and diversity among caregivers.* In P. Lawton & R. Rubenstein (Eds), *Alzheimer's disease and related dementia: Strategies in care and research.* New York: Springer.

Montgomery, R., Stull, D., & Borgatta, E. (1985). Measurement and the analysis of burden. *Research in Aging, 7*(1), 137–52.

Moore, J. (2006). *The impact of the aging population on the health workforce in the United States.* Rensselaer, NY: University at Albany. Retrieved August 8, 2011, from: http://www.albany.edu/news/pdf_files/impact_of_aging_full.pdf

Murray, S. A., Kendall, M., Boyd, K., Worth, A., Boyd K., Benton, T. F., et al. (2004). Exploring the spiritual needs of people dying of lung cancer or heart failure: A prospective qualitative interview study of patients and their carers. *Palliative Medicine, 18,* 39–45.

National Alliance for Caregiving & American Association of Retired Persons. (2009). *Caregiving in the U.S. 2009.* Retrieved August 8, 2011, from:http://www.caregiving.org/data/Caregiving_in_the_US_2009_full_report.pdf

National Center for Health Statistics. (2003). *U.S. birth rate reaches record low.* Retrieved August 8, 2011, from: http://www.cdc.gov/nchs/pressroom/03news/lowbirth.htm

Nerenberg, L. (2002). *Preventing elder abuse by family caregivers.* Washington, DC: National Center of Elder Abuse.

Nolan, M. (2001). Positive aspects of caring. In S. Payne & C. Ellis-Hill (Eds.), *Chronic and terminal illness: New perspectives on caring and carers* (pp. 22–44). Oxford: Oxford University Press.

Ory, M. G., Hoffman, R. R. III, Yee, J. L., Tennstedt, S., & Schulz, R. (1999). Prevalence and impact of caregiving: A detailed comparison between dementia and nondementia caregivers. *The Gerontologist, 39,* 177–185.

Palmer, S., & Glass, T. A. (2003). Family function and stroke recovery: A review. *Rehabilitation Psychology, 48*(4), 255–265.

Paun, O. (2004). Female Alzheimer's patient caregivers share their strength. *Holistic Nursing Practice, 18*(1), 11–17.

Pearlin, L. I. (1992). The careers of caregivers. *The Gerontologist, 32,* 647.

Peters-Davis, N. D., Moss, M. S., & Pruchno, R. A. (1999). Children-in-law in caregiving families. *The Gerontologist, 39,* 66–75.

Pierce, L. (2001). Coherence in the urban family caregiver role with African American stroke survivors. *Topics in Stroke Rehabilitation, 8*(3), 64–72.

Pierce, L., Steiner, V., Govoni, A., Hicks, B., Thompson, T., & Friedemann, M. (2004). Caring~Web: Internet-based support for rural caregivers of persons with stroke shows promise. *Rehabilitation Nursing, 29*(3), 95–99; 103.

Pierce, L., Steiner, V., Govoni, A., Thompson, T., & Friedemann, M. (2007). Two sides to the caregiving story. *Topics in Stroke Rehabilitation, 14*(2), 13–20.

Piercy, K. W. (1998). Theorizing about family caregiving: The role of responsibility. *Journal of Marriage and the Family, 60,* 109–118.

Piercy, K. W., & Chapman, J. G. (2001). Adopting the caregiver role: A family legacy. *Family Relations, 50,* 386–393.

Pines, A. M., & Aronson, E. (1988). *Career burnout: Causes and cures.* New York: The Free Press.

Plowfield, L. A., Raymond, J. E., & Blevins, C. (2000). Wholism for aging families: Meeting needs of caregivers. *Holistic Nursing Practice 14*(4), 51–59.

Poulshock, S., & Deimling, G. (1984). Families caring for elders in residence: Issues in the measurement of burden. *Journal of Gerontology, 39*(2), 230–239.

Pruchno, R. A., Burant, C. J., & Peters, N. D. (1997). Understanding the well-being of care receivers. *The Gerontologist, 37,* 102–109.

Pyke, K. (1999). The micropolitics of care in relationships between aging parents and adult children: Individualism, collectivism, and power. *The Journal of Marriage and the Family, 61,* 661–673.

Rabinowitz, Y. G., Mausbach, B. T., Thompson, L. W., & Gallagher-Thompson, D. (2007). The relationship between self-efficacy cumulative health risk associated with health behavior patterns in female

caregivers of elderly relatives with Alzheimer's dementia. *Journal of Aging and Health, 19*(6), 946–964.

Riggs, J. (2004). A family caregiver policy agenda for the twenty-first century. *Generations, 27*(4), 68–73.

Ritchie, L. (2003). Adult day care: Northern perspectives. *Public Health Nursing, 20*(2), 120–131.

Rittman, M., Kuzmeskus, L. B., & Flum, M. A. (1998). A synthesis of current knowledge on minority elder abuse. In T. Tatara (Ed.), *Understanding elder abuse in minority populations,* (pp. 221–238). Philadelphia: Brunner/Mazel.

Roff, L., Burgio, L., Gitlin, L., Nichols, L., et al. (2004). Positive aspects of Alzheimer's caregiving: The role of race. *Journals of Gerontology Series B: Psychological Sciences and Social Sciences, 59B*(4), 185–190.

Sarkisian, N., & Gerstel, N. (2004). Explaining the gender gap in help to parents: The importance of employment. *Journal of Marriage and Family, 66,* 431–451.

Schulz, R., & Beach, S. R. (1999). Caregiving as a risk factor for mortality: The caregiver health effects study. *Journal of the American Medical Association, 282,* 2215–2219.

Scott, G. (2001). A study of family carers of people with a life-threatening illness 2: The implications of the needs assessment. *International Journal of Palliative Nursing, 7*(7), 323–330.

Scott, J. (2006). *Informal caregiving.* Orono, ME: University of Maine System. Retrieved August 8, 2011, from: http://www.maine.gov/dhhs/beas/bhcoa/FinalReport-Caregiving_Family.pdf

Sebern, M. D., & Whitlatch, C. J. (2007). Dyadic relationship scale: A measure of the impact of the provision and receipt of family care. *The Gerontologist, 47*(6), 741–751.

Seltzer, M. M. (1990). Role reversal: You don't go home again. *Journal of Gerontological Social Work, 15,* 5–14.

Seltzer, M. M., & Wailing, L. (2000). The dynamics of caregiving: Transitions during a three-year prospective study. *The Gerontologist, 40,* 165–178.

Selwood, A., Johnston, K., Katona, C., Lyketsos, C., & Livingston, G. (2007). Systematic review of the effect of psychological interventions on family caregivers of people with dementia. *Journal of Affective Disorders, 101,* 75–89.

Shapiro, E. R. (2002). Chronic illness as a family process: A social-developmental approach to promoting resilience. *JCLP/in session: Psychotherapy in Practice, 58*(11), 1375–1384.

Sheehan, N. W., & Donorfio, L. M. (1999). Efforts to create meaning in the relationship between aging mothers and their caregiving daughters: A qualitative study of caregiving. *Journal of Aging Studies, 13,* 161–176.

Shirey, L., & Summer, L. (2000). *Caregiving: Helping the elderly with activity limitations.* Washington, DC: National Academy on Aging Society.

Skaff, M. M., Pearlin, L. I., & Mullan, J. T. (1996). Transitions in the caregiving career: Effects on sense of mastery. *Psychology and Aging, 11,* 247–257.

Smith, J., Forster, A., & Young, Y. (2009). Cochrane review: Information provision for stroke patients and their caregivers. *Clinical Rehabilitation, 23,* 196–206.

Spector, R. E. (2000). *Cultural diversity in health and illness* (5th ed.). Upper Saddle River, NJ: Prentice Hall Health.

Steiner, V., & Pierce, L. (2002). Building a web of support for caregivers of persons with stroke. *Topics in Stroke Rehabilitation, 9*(3), 102–111.

Stobert, S., & Cranswick, K. (2004). Looking after seniors: Who does what for whom? *Canadian Social Trends, 74,* 2–6.

Stoller, E. P., & Cutler, S. J. (1993). Predictors of use of paid help among older people living in the community. *The Gerontologist, 33*(1), 31–40.

Stone, R., Cafferata, G. L., & Sangl, J. (1987). Caregivers of the frail elderly: A national profile. *The Gerontologist, 27,* 616–626.

Stone, R. I., & Short, P. F. (1990). The competing demands of employment and informal caregiving to disabled elders. *Medical Care, 28,* 513–526.

Stuckey, J. C. (2001). Blessed assurance: The role of religion and spirituality in Alzheimer's disease caregiving and other significant life events. *Journal of Aging Studies, 15*(1), 69–84.

Substance Abuse and Mental Health Service Administration (2004). *SAMHSA model programs.* Retrieved September 21, 2011, from http://nrepp.samhsa.gov/

Tarlow, B., Wisniewski, S., Belle, S., Rubert, M., et al. (2004). Positive aspects of caregiving. *Research on Aging, 26*(4), 429–453.

Teaster, P. B. (2003). *A response to the abuse of vulnerable adults: The 2000 survey of state adult protective services.* Retrieved August 8, 2011, from: http://www.ncea.aoa.gov/ncearoot/Main_Site/pdf/research/apsreport030703.pdf

Theis, S. L., Biordi, D. L., Coeling, H., Nalepka, C., & Miller, B. (2003). Spirituality in caregiving and care receiving. *Holistic Nursing Practice, 17*(1), 48–55.

Thompson, B., Tudiver, F., & Manson, J. (2000). Sons as sole caregivers for their elderly parents. How do they cope? *Canadian Family Physician, 46,* 360–365.

Thompson, C. A., Spilsbury, K., Hall, J., Birks, Y., Barnes, C., & Adamson, J. (2007). Systematic review of information and support interventions for caregivers of people with dementia. *BMC Geriatrics, 2007,* 7–18.

Toth-Cohen, S., Gitlin, L. N., Corcoran, M. A., Eckhardt, S., et al. (2001). Providing services to family caregivers at home: Challenges and recommendations for health and human service professions. *Alzheimer's Care Quarterly, 2*(1), 23–32.

Travis, S. S., & Bethea, L. S. (2001). Medication administration by family members of elders in shared care arrangements. *Journal of Clinical Geropsychology, 7,* 231–243.

Travis, S. S., Bethea, L. S., & Winn, P. (2000). Medication administration hassles reported by family caregivers of dependent elders. *Journal of Gerontology, Medical Sciences, 55A,* M412–M417.

Travis, S. S., & Duer, B. (2000). Interdisciplinary management of the older adult with cancer. In A. S. Luggen & S. E. Meiner (Eds.), *Handbook for the care of the older adult with cancer* (pp. 25–34). Pittsburgh, PA: Oncology Nursing Press.

University of Michigan Health System. (2006). *Children with chronic conditions.* Ann Arbor, MI: Author. Retrieved August 8, 2011, from: http://www.med.umich.edu/1libr/yourchild/chronic.htm

U.S. Department of Labor. (1993). *The family and medical leave act of 1993.* Washington, DC: U.S. Department of Labor, Wage and Hour Division.

Walker, E., & Dewar, B. J. (2004). How do we facilitate carers' involvement in decision making? *Journal of Advanced Nursing, 34*(3), 329–337.

Warren, S., Kerr, J., Smith, D., Godkin, D., & Schalm, C. (2003). The impact of adult day programs on family caregivers of elderly relatives. *Journal of Community Health Nursing, 20*(4), 209–221.

Weissert, W. G., & Hedrick, S. C. (1994). Lessons learned from research on effects of community-based long-term care. *Journal of the American Geriatrics Society, 42,* 348–353.

Weissert, W. G., & Hedrick, S. C. (1999). Outcomes and costs of home and community-based long-term care: Implications for research-based practice. In E. Calkins, C. Boult, E. H. Wagner, & J. T. Pacala (Eds.), *New ways to care for older people,* (pp. 143–157). New York: Springer.

Weitzner, M. A., Haley, W. E., & Chen, H. (2000). The family caregiver of the older cancer patient. *Hematology and Oncology Clinics of North America, 14,* 269–281.

White-Means, S. L. (1997). The demands of persons with disabilities for home health care and the economic consequences for informal caregivers. *Social Science Quarterly, 78,* 955–972.

Williams, A. (1993). Caregivers of persons with stroke: Their physical and emotional well-being. *Quality of Life Resesarch, 2*(3), 213–220.

Williams, S. W., Dilworth-Anderson, P. & Goodwin, P. Y. (2003). Caregiver role strain: The contribution of multiple roles and available resources in African-American women. *Aging and Mental Health, 7*(2), 103–112.

Winslow, B. W. (2003). Family caregivers' experiences with community services: A qualitative analysis. *Public Health Nursing, 20* (5), 341–348.

Workplace Flexibility 2010. (2004). *Family and medical leave: Selective background information.* Retrieved August 8, 2011, from: http://www.law.georgetown.edu/workplaceflexibility2010/law/fmlaFiles/fmla_DataPoints.pdf

Yee, J. L., & Schulz, R. (2000). Gender differences in psychiatric morbidity among family caregivers: A review and analysis. *The Gerontologist, 40,* 147–164.

Zarit, S., Todd, P., & Zarit, J. (1986). Subjective burden of husbands and wives as caregivers: A longitudinal study. *The Gerontologist, 26*(3), 260–66.

CHAPTER 11

Sexuality

Margaret Chamberlain Wilmoth

INTRODUCTION

Humans are sexual beings from birth until death. Sexuality is an integral aspect of our personalities and is more than sexual contact and the ability to reach sexual satisfaction. Sexuality includes views of ourselves as male or female, feelings about our bodies, and the ways we communicate verbally and nonverbally our comfort about ourselves to others. It also includes the ability to engage in satisfying sexual behaviors alone or with another. Sexuality does not end when one reaches a certain age, nor does it end with the diagnosis of a chronic illness. In fact, sexuality and intimacy may become *more* important after such a diagnosis as a way of reaffirming human connection, aliveness, and continued desirability and caring. Sexuality is a critical aspect of quality of life that, unfortunately, is often ignored by healthcare professionals.

This chapter briefly reviews standards of nursing practice as they relate to sexuality, sexual physiologic functioning, alterations in sexuality caused by common chronic illnesses and their treatments, and nursing interventions. This chapter also provides nurses with suggestions for ways to incorporate discussions of sexuality into their practice.

Definitions

Sexuality is a complex construct with terminology that has yet to be defined in a manner that is accepted by all. When discussing sexuality with other professionals or with clients, it is important to be sure that everyone has the same frame of reference for the many descriptors that are used for aspects of sexuality. Nurses also are encouraged to know the more "scientific" terms, yet remember that these are not the words used by most of their clients when they talk about their sexuality. Nurses need to find out what terms their clients use, clarify the meaning to ensure understanding, then use words the client knows and understands when discussing the impact of chronic illness on sexuality. Nurses should avoid using the term *sexual dysfunction*, as this is a psychiatric diagnosis that most nurses are not qualified to make. The American Psychological Association (APA) has identified sexual dysfunctions that are a result of chronic medical conditions and that have specific diagnostic criteria. Examples of psychologically diagnosed sexual dysfunctions include hypoactive sexual desire, dyspareunia, and erectile disorder (APA, 2000). The definitions used in discussing sexuality in this chapter are in **Table 11-1.**

Table 11-1	Definitions
Sexuality	Everything that makes one a man or woman, including the need for touch, feelings about one's body, the need to connect with another human being in an intimate way, interest in engaging in sexual behaviors, communication of one's feelings and needs to one's partner, and the ability to engage in satisfying sexual behaviors
Sexual behaviors	Specific activities used to obtain release of sexual tension alone or with another in order to achieve sexual satisfaction; refers also to the multiple ways one verbally and nonverbally communicates sexual feelings and attitudes to others
Sexual functioning	The physiologic component of sexuality, including human sexual anatomy, the sexual response cycle, neuroendocrine functioning, and lifecycle changes in sexual physiology
Sexual dysfunction	Characterized by disturbances in the processes of the sexual response cycle or by pain associated with sexual intercourse; is a *DSM-IV-TR* diagnosis and should not be used by nurses unless they are specially trained in treating sexual dysfunctions

Sources: Wilmoth, M. C. (2009). Sexuality. In C. Burke (Ed.), *Psychosocial dimensions of oncology nursing care* (2nd ed., pp. 101–124). Pittsburgh: Oncology Nursing Press. American Psychological Association. (2000). *Diagnostic and statistical manual of mental disorders DSM-IV-TR* (4th ed., text revision). Washington, DC: Author.

Standards of Practice

Standards of practice confer both a legal standard of practice as well as an ethical responsibility that nurses adhere to in their practice of nursing (Andrews, Goldberg, & Kaplan, 1996). Standards of practice for the profession, published by the American Nurses Association (ANA) (2010), include six standards of care that encompass significant actions taken by nurses when providing care to their clients. These standards include the components of the nursing process. These standards also assume that all relevant healthcare needs of the client will be assessed and appropriate care provided, including needs regarding sexuality.

Specialty organizations have derived standards of nursing practice from those published by the ANA that are specific to their practice. For example, the Oncology Nursing Society (2004) published nursing practice standards that specifically identified sexuality as one potential area of client concern. These standards include both assessment criteria and outcome criteria. Nurses who care for cancer patients then are expected to follow each of these standards in the provision of patient care (**Table 11-2**).

Nurses and physicians are legally obligated to ensure that clients have the necessary information to make decisions regarding treatment. The provision of informed consent also requires that all risks, benefits, and side effects of diseases and their treatments be provided to clients as they choose treatments for any illness. This includes information about potential sexual side effects of proposed treatments. Failure to provide this information could potentially lead to legal action by the client.

The Sexual Response Cycle and Sexual Physiology

There are two frameworks commonly used to describe what is called the "sexual response

Table 11-2   Oncology Nursing Society Statement on the Scope and Standards of Oncology Nursing Practice

Standard I Assessment	**Standard III Outcome Identification**
The oncology nurse systematically and continually collects data regarding the health status of the patient.	The oncology nurse identifies expected outcomes individualized to the patient.
Measurement Criteria	**Measurement Criteria**
The oncology nurse collects data in the following 14 high-incidence problem areas that may include but are not limited to: sexuality.	The oncology nurse develops expected outcomes for each of the 14 high-incidence problem areas within a level consistent with the patient's physiology, psychosocial and spiritual capacities, cultural background, and value system. The expected outcomes include but are not limited to sexuality. The patient and/or family:
1. Past and present sexual patterns and expression 2. Effects of disease and treatment on body image. 3. Effects of disease and treatment on sexual function. 4. Psychological response of patient and partner to disease and treatment.	1. Identifies potential or actual changes in sexuality, sexual functioning, or intimacy related to disease and treatment. 2. Expresses feelings about alopecia, body image changes, and altered sexual functioning. 3. Engages in open communication with his or her partner regarding changes in sexual functioning or desire, within cultural framework. 4. Describes appropriate interventions for actual or potential changes in sexual function. 5. Identifies other satisfying methods of sexual expression that provide satisfaction to both partners, within cultural framework. 6. Identifies personal and community resources to assist with changes in body image and sexual functioning.

Source: Oncology Nursing Society. (2004). *Statement on the scope and standards of oncology nursing practice*. Pittsburgh, Author.

cycle." The first, proposed by Dr. William Masters and Virginia Johnson (1966), is a four-stage model of sexual response of the male and female. The four phases of the Masters and Johnson (1966) model are excitement, plateau, orgasm, and resolution. The excitement stage causes an increase in the heart rate and vasocongestion to the penis. This is accompanied by lengthening and widening of the vagina, elevation of the cervix and uterus, and initial swelling of the labia minora (Guyton & Hall, 2006; Masters & Johnson, 1966). These changes are caused by vasocongestion and are secondary to a parasympathetic response mediated to S2 and S4 through the pudendal nerve and sacral plexus (Guyton & Hall, 2006).

The second stage is the plateau stage, which is an increased state of arousal causing the heart rate and blood pressure to increase, with a subsequent increase in respiratory rate (Katz, 2007). The third stage is the orgasm, the phase of maximal muscular contraction (male ejaculation, and female pelvic muscle contraction), with a peak of respirations and heart rate, and a subjective feeling of intense pleasure that radiates throughout the body (Katz, 2007). Impending orgasm is determined by the presence of an intense color change in the labia minora in women and full elevation of the scrotal sac to the perineal wall in men, all a result of intense vasocongestion (Masters & Johnson, 1966). Orgasm is mediated by the sympathetic nervous system and is the physical release and peak of pleasurable expression, followed by relaxation (Guyton & Hall, 2006). The sympathetic nerves between T12 and L2 control ejaculation (Koukouras et al., 1991). The intensity of orgasm in women is dependent upon the duration and intensity of sexual stimulation.

The final stage is resolution, when vasocongestion resolves and the body returns to its normal nonaroused state (Katz, 2007). Men also have what is referred to as a "refractory period," which is the period within which the male is unable to achieve an erection satisfactory for penetration. This period of time is age and health-status dependent (Masters & Johnson, 1966).

Physical changes that occur in both men and women as a result of sexual stimulation are vasocongestion and myotonia. Vasocongestion occurs in the penis in men and in the labia in women, and is an essential requirement for orgasm and subsequent sexual satisfaction. Myotonia refers to the involuntary muscular contractions that occur throughout the body

during sexual response (Kolodny, Masters, Johnson, & Biggs, 1979).

The second framework is from Kaplan. Kaplan's (1979) modification of the sexual response cycle includes aspects of sexual physiology involving the prelude to sexual activity as well as the consequences of sexual activity. These three phases are desire, arousal, and orgasm. Desire is the prelude to engaging in satisfying sexual behaviors and is the most complex component of the sexual response cycle. Desire is often affected by factors such as anger, pain, and body image, as well as disease processes and medications (Kaplan, 1979). When sexual stimuli are perceived by women, they are processed physiologically and physically, leading to subjective feelings of arousal and a responsive feeling of desire (Katz, 2007). This may explain why psychogenic factors can be a determinant cause of male and female sexual dysfunction.

Arousal, manifested by erection in males, is mediated by the parasympathetic nervous system and is the result of either psychic or somatic sexual stimulation (Masters & Johnson, 1966). Alternately, activation of the sympathetic nervous system will lead to loss of an erection through vasoconstriction. It was previously thought that an analogous process of parasympathetic nervous system stimulation led to arousal in women. However, evidence suggests that it is stimulation of the sympathetic nervous system (SNS) that is responsible for female arousal (Meston, 2000). Data also suggest that stimulation of the SNS may enhance arousal in women with low sexual desire (Meston & Gorzalka, 1996) and that induction of relaxation may negatively affect arousal (Meston, 2000).

Although many women suggest that the Gräfenberg spot (G-spot) plays an important role in their sexuality, the existence of this sensitive area remains open for verification (Hines, 2001). The G-spot is purportedly located in the anterior wall of the vagina, about halfway between the back of the pubic bone and the cervix along the course of the urethra (Ladas, Whipple, & Perry, 1982). When stimulated, this tissue swells from the size of a bean to greater than a half dollar (Ladas et al., 1982). Stimulation of this area appears to cause a different orgasmic sensation, and it is hypothesized that this response is mediated by the pelvic nerve, causing the uterus to contract and descend against the vagina rather than elevate, as with stimulation mediated by the pudendal nerve (Ladas et al., 1982). Approximately 40% of women will experience expulsion of a fluid upon orgasm caused by G-spot stimulation (Darling, Davidson, & Conway-Welch, 1990). Research suggests that this is a prostatic-like fluid that is released during orgasm (Zaviacic & Whipple, 1993; Zaviacic & Ablin, 2000). Belief that this is not urine but a normal release of fluid that occurs during sexual response may lead to a reduction in embarrassment for many women.

The neurohormonal system influences sexual functioning through its effect on hormone production. The hypothalamic–hypophysial portal system plays an important role in sexual functioning in both genders through production of gonadotropin-releasing hormone (GnRH) and subsequent stimulation of gonadotropin production by the anterior pituitary gland. The anterior pituitary gland secretes six hormones, two of which play an essential role in sexual functioning. Follicle-stimulating hormone (FSH) and luteinizing hormone (LH) control growth of the gonads and influence sexual functioning. In men, LH influences production of testosterone by the Leydig cells in the testes through a negative feedback loop (Guyton &

Hall, 2006). Production of GnRH is reduced, once a satisfactory level of testosterone has been attained. A negative feedback loop also exists in the woman, although it is much more complex, given the concurrent production of estrogen and progesterone by the ovary and the production of androgens by the adrenal cortex.

Psychic factors appear to play a larger role in the sexual functioning in women than in men, particularly in relation to sexual desire. Multiple neuronal centers in the brain's limbic system transmit signals into the arcuate nuclei in the mediobasal hypothalamus. These signals modify the intensity of GnRH release and the frequency of the impulses (Guyton & Hall, 2006). This may explain why desire in women is more vulnerable to emotions and distractions than it is in men.

Aging affects the sexual response cycle in predictable ways, but it does not signal the end of sexuality. In fact, the old adage, "use it or lose it," is applicable to continued sexual activity throughout life (Masters & Johnson, 1981). The general impact of aging on the sexual response cycle is a slower, less intense sexual response (Lindau, Schumm, Gaumann, Levinson, O'Muircheartaigh, & Waite, 2007). The frequency of sexual activity in earlier years is predictive of frequency as one ages. The quality of the sexual relationship appears to be the greatest influence on the frequency and satisfaction of sexual activity (Masters & Johnson, 1981). As in younger adults, the quality of communication in a relationship, degree of mutual intimacy, and level of commitment to the relationship are vital to a satisfying sexual relationship and to achieving sexual satisfaction.

In clients aged 60 or older, organic factors are the most important determinant of erectile dysfunction (Corona et al., 2007). The frequent comorbidity of multiple metabolic and hemodynamic abnormalities in aging clients can substantially increase the incidence and progression of atherosclerotic lesions, leading to vascular forms of erectile dysfunction (Corona et al., 2007). Masters and Johnson (1966) found that in men between 51 and 90 years of age, the time to achieve erection was two to three times longer than in younger men. Achieving erection also required more tactile stimulation than in younger years. However, once achieved, older men can maintain a full erection for a longer period before ejaculation. Scrotal vasocongestion is reduced, with a subsequent decrease in testicular elevation. Basal and dynamic peak cavernosal velocity was shown to be reduced in older patients via Doppler ultrasound penile examination (Corona et al., 2007). The ability to attain orgasm is not impaired with aging, but there is an overall decrease in myotonia and fewer penile and rectal sphincter contractions. There is an increase in time from hours to days before older men can achieve another erection once they have ejaculated and achieved an orgasm (refractory period).

Women also experience sexual response cycle changes as they age, primarily after completing the menopausal transition. Common complaints include decreased desire, dry vagina, and difficulty attaining orgasm (Lindau et al., 2007). Vaginal changes include a thinning of the mucosa, with a decrease in vaginal lubrication. In women who abstain from sexual intercourse, narrowing and stenosis of the introitus and vaginal vault can occur (Leiblum & Segraves, 1989). Older women experience a decrease in the vasocongestion of the labia and other genitalia analogous to the decrease in penile tumescence experienced by men. Orgasm in sexually active women is not impaired; however, there is some decrease in the degree of myotonia experienced.

Intense orgasm may lead to involuntary distension of the external meatus, leading to an increase in frequency of urinary tract infections in older women.

SEXUALITY AND CHRONIC ILLNESS

The presence of a chronic illness affects all aspects of an individual's life, including their sexuality. There are numerous chronic illnesses, and discussion of the impact of each on sexuality is beyond the scope of this chapter. Therefore, this chapter is limited to a brief discussion of the effects of coronary artery disease, diabetes mellitus, cancer, and multiple sclerosis on sexuality.

Coronary Artery Disease

The heart is linked to romance and to the soul, so any threat to cardiac functioning is emotionally linked to matters of the self, sexuality, and intimacy. Cardiovascular disease, including coronary artery disease (CAD) and stroke, causes more death in both genders and all racial and ethnic groups in the United States than any other disease (Centers for Disease Control and Prevention, 2004). More men and women than ever before are living longer and continue to lead productive lives after experiencing a myocardial infarction (MI); however, recent data suggest that women experience a lower degree of quality of life than men (Agewall, Berglund, & Henareh, 2004; Svedlund & Danielson, 2004). Therefore, having adequate and accurate knowledge about sexuality post-diagnosis may have a positive impact crucial to individuals' self-concept, to their sexuality, and to their sexual relationships.

The consensus study from the Second Princeton Consensus Conference collaborates and clarifies the risk stratification algorithm that was developed by the first Princeton Consensus Panel to evaluate the degree of cardiovascular risk associated with sexual activity for men with varying degrees of cardiovascular disease (Kostis et al., 2005). The algorithm emphasizes the importance of risk factor evaluation and management for all patients with erectile dysfunction (ED). The relative safety in which clients can engage in sexual activity is dependent on their degree of cardiac disease. This panel recommended a classification system that would stratify clients into a risk category based on the

extent of their cardiac disease. These categories and management recommendations are found in **Table 11-3**. Patients with less than three major risk factors for cardiovascular disease (age, hypertension, diabetes mellitus, cigarette smoking, dyslipidemia, sedentary lifestyle, and family history of premature coronary artery disease) are generally at low risk for significant cardiac complications from sexual activity or the treatment of sexual dysfunction (Kostis et al., 2005). Clients whose cardiac conditions are uncertain, as well as those with multiple risk factors, require further testing or evaluation before

Table 11-3 Management Recommendations Based on Graded Cardiovascular (CV) Risk Assessment

Grade of Risk	Categories of CVD	Management
Low risk	Asymptomatic, 6 weeks; mild valvular disease, LVD/CHF (NYHA class I); patients with pericarditis, mitral valve prolapse, or atrial fibrillation with controlled ventricular response should be managed on an individualized basis	Primary care management; consider all first-line therapies; reassess at regular intervals
Intermediate risk	Three major risk factors for CAD; moderate, stable angina; recent MI (>2 weeks, <6 weeks); LVD/CHF (NYHA class II); noncardiac sequelae of atherosclerotic disease (e.g., CVA, PVD)	Specialized CV testing; restratification into high or low risk based on results of CV testing
High risk	Unstable or refractory angina; uncontrolled hypertension; LVD/CHF (NYHA class III/IV); recent MI (<2 weeks), CVA; high-risk arrhythmias; obstructive hypertrophic and other cardiomyopathies; moderate–severe valvular disease	Priority referral for specialized CV management; treatment for sexual dysfunction deferred until cardiac condition stabilized and dependent on specialist recommendations; sexual activity should be deferred until a patient's cardiac condition has been stabilized by treatment or a decision has been made by a specialist

CAD, coronary artery disease; CHF, congestive heart failure; CVA, cerebrovascular accident (stroke); CVD, cardiovascular disease; LVD, left ventricular dysfunction; NYHA, New York Heart Association; PVD, peripheral vascular disease.
Source: From DeBusk, R., Drory, Y., Goldstein, I., Jackson, G., Kaul, S., & Kimmel, S. E. (2000). Management of sexual dysfunction in patients with cardiovascular disease: Recommendations of the Princeton Consensus Panel. *The American Journal of Cardiology, 86* (2), 175–181.
Kostis, J. B., Jackson, G., Rosen, R., Barrett-Connor, E., Billups, K., Burnett, A. L. et al. (2005). Sexual dysfunction and cardiac risk (the second Princeton Consensus Conference). *American Journal of Cardiology, 96* (12B), 85M–93M.

resuming sexual activity (Kostis et al., 2005). Patients with a history of MI (>2 weeks and <6 weeks) may be at somewhat greater risk for coitus-induced ischemia and reinfarction, as well as malignant arrhythmias (Kostis et al., 2005). The level of risk associated within this time period post-MI can be assessed with an exercise stress test.

Counseling of all clients regarding lifestyle changes and activity restrictions should begin as soon as the client is stabilized. Discussions regarding sexual activity should be included in the counseling. Potential fear of cardiac arrest during sexual activity should be eradicated as soon as possible by assuring clients and their partners that this risk is only 1.2% and that sex accounts for only 0.5–1.0% of all acute coronary incidents (DeBusk, 2000).

Recent reports continue to validate the appropriateness of the stair-climbing tolerance test for successful return to sexual activity after 6 weeks post-MI. Sexual activity conceptualized simply as arousal is unassociated with physical exertion. It is not until exertion is coupled with arousal that energy expenditure occurs. Data indicate that the man in the top position results in greater responses of heart rate and maximum volume of oxygen (VO_2), and thus greater energy expenditure that may or may not reflect both heightened arousal and exertion. If sexual activity is conceptualized as exertion, then the capacity to climb two flights of stairs without limiting symptoms is a clinical benchmark of exercise tolerance and subsequent ability to engage in sexual activity without symptoms (DeBusk, 2000).

Depression has been indicated as a psychological cause of sexual dysfunction and may increase the risk of cardiac mortality in both genders (Roose & Seidman, 2000). A discrepancy between male and female sexual desire, which could disturb relationships, can be observed in many aging couples (Corona et al., 2007). Roose and Seidman (2000) indicate that the male client with ischemic heart disease who is depressed is also likely to have erectile difficulties. This is also a predisposing factor for other adverse cardiac events. Therefore, it appears prudent that all post-MI clients be evaluated for depression and receive appropriate therapy. A wide body of evidence supports the hypothesis of a strong association between depression and ED (Corona et al., 2007). The age-dependent increased use of psychotropic drugs such as antidepressants and antipsychotics may play an important role in ED in older clients (Corona et al., 2007).

Clients should be counseled regarding the effects of medications on sexuality. Calcium channel inhibitors, nonselective beta-blockers, angiotensin II antagonists, and diuretics may increase the risk of ED. Erectile dysfunction does not seem to be a problem in men using organic nitrates, angiotensin-converting enzyme inhibitors, selective beta-blockers, or serum lipid-lowering agents (Shril, Koskimaki, Hakkien, Auvinen, Tammela, & Hakama, 2007). Organic nitrates, including sublingual nitroglycerin, isosorbide mononitrate, isosorbide dinitrate, and other nitrate preparations used to treat angina, as well as amyl nitrite or alkyl nitrate ("poppers" used for recreation), are absolutely contraindicated in patients taking phosphodiesterase type 5 (PDE5) inhibitors (Kostis et al., 2005).

Counseling and education about return to pre-infarct activities, including sexual activities, should be a part of a comprehensive cardiac rehabilitation program. Age and marital status should not be a factor in determining who receives information about resuming sexual activity. If clients have a spouse or regular partner, they should be included in education and counseling sessions unless the clients request otherwise. Discussions about sexual activity should include talking about anxieties concerning resumption of sexual activities with one's partner, scheduling sexual encounters after periods of rest, avoiding sex after heavy meals or alcohol ingestion, and keeping nitroglycerin at the bedside as a form of reassurance (Steinke, 2000). An integral part of successful resumption of sexual activity is engaging in regular exercise based on physician recommendations. Partners of cardiac clients also experience distress because the disease may manifest as decreased intimacy and may require intervention to assist them in adjusting to disease-related stressors (O'Farrell, Murray, & Hotz, 2000).

Diabetes Mellitus

The incidence of diabetes mellitus in the United States is on the increase, with up to 1.9 million new cases in Americans aged 20 years or older in 2010 compared with 1.5 million new cases annually in 2005, according to the National Diabetes Information Clearing House (NDIC, 2011). Nurses must be prepared to assist these individuals with the multiple life changes they will experience because of this disease, including changes in sexual functioning.

It is well known that diabetes mellitus has serious effects on sexual functioning in men. Prevalence of ED in diabetic males range from 33–75% depending on age, glycemic control, and presence of other behaviors such as smoking (Jackson, 2004). There is great variability in reports on the effect of diabetes on the sexual response cycle in women (Sarkadi & Rosenquist, 2004), with one report indicating that 25% of sexually active diabetic women report low overall sexual satisfaction (Enzlin et al., 2009).

Men with diabetes typically experience minimal changes in their desire for sexual activity. Any changes in desire may be attributable to difficulties in achieving satisfactory arousal. Arousal difficulties are manifested by the lack of adequate penile erection typically referred to as ED. The term *impotence* has multiple negative psychological connotations and is no longer used by healthcare professionals (National Institutes of Health [NIH], 1992). An estimated 50–75% of diabetic men have ED to some degree, a rate about fourfold higher than in nondiabetic men (Consortium for Improvement in Erectile Dysfunction [CIEF], 2007; this organization has now merged with others to become the Collaborative for Advancement of Urologic Sexual Endocrine Education—see www.cause-education.org). Acute onset of ED may reflect poor glycemic control of the disease; however, ED may be reversible if control is regained. Acute onset of ED reflects accumulation of sorbitol and water in autonomic nerve fibers and is generally a temporary condition. Erectile dysfunction can result from vasculogenic, neurogenic, hormonal, and/or psychogenic factors as well as alterations in the nitric oxide/cyclic guanosine monophosphate pathway or other regulatory mechanisms (Qaseem et al., 2009). A more recent report from a large randomized controlled trial of 761 males with type I diabetes who were assigned to either intensive or conventional diabetic therapy reported that decreased libido was the most common form of sexual dysfunction reported (55%), rather than ED (34%) (Penson, Wessells, Cleary, Rutledge, & DCCT/EPI Group, 2009).

Treatment options for ED in diabetic men include use of sildenafil or similar medications,

Table 11-4   Treatments for Erectile Dysfunction

Treatment	Mechanism of Action	Side Effects	Pro/Con
Sildenafil citrate (Viagra), tadalafil (Cialis), vardenafil (Levitra)	Blocks enzyme phosphodiesterase type 5 and allows for persistent levels of cyclic GMP. This chemical is produced in the penis during sexual arousal and leads to smooth muscle relaxation in the penis and increases blood flow, leading to erection	Headache, flushing of face, gastrointestinal irritability, nasal congestion, muscle aches	*Pro:* Allows for some degree of spontaneity *Con:* Cannot be taken if the client also takes nitrates for cardiac disease
Intraurethral prostaglandin	Relaxes smooth muscle of ductus arteriosus. Produces vasodilation, inhibits platelet aggregation, and stimulates intestinal and uterine smooth muscle. Induces erection by relaxation of trabecular smooth muscle and by dilation of cavernosal arteries	Flushing, bradycardia, diarrhea, urethral pain, hematoma, back pain, and pelvic pain.	*Pro:* Allows for some degree of spontaneity
Intracavernosal injections	Medications act on sinusoidal smooth muscle to induce relaxation and enhance corporal filling	Penile pain during injection Priapism in 1% Hematoma in 8%	*Pro:* Allows for some degree of spontaneity *Con:* Requires office visits to ensure proper technique; can use only every other day; expensive
Vacuum extraction device (VED)	Places negative pressure on corporal bodies of the penis to allow for blood flow into the penis and to cause an erection. A constriction band is placed around the base of the penis to prevent loss of erection until the sex act is completed.	Penile hematoma; injury to erectile tissue or penile skin necrosis may lead to permanent penile deformity. Painful erections due to impairment of blood flow by the constriction band at the base of the penis.	*Pro:* Allows for penile–vaginal penetration *Con:* Loss of spontaneity; erection only involves a part of the penis
Inflatable penile prosthesis	Inflate erectile cylinders from reservoir. As fluid moves from the reservoir into corporal bodies, the penis becomes erect.	Infection in first few months after implanted; may have failure of device, requiring removal and replacement	*Pro:* Allows intercourse to continue *Con:* Reports of sexual dissatisfaction caused by loss of girth and length of erection; surgical procedure
External prosthetic penis	A strap-on dildo made of silicone rubber. Shaft of dildo is mounted at angle on flanged base, which holds it in the harness. Cleaning: soap/water	No physiologic implications; may require counseling with partner to overcome hesitancy	*Pro:* Allows intercourse to continue; enhances partner satisfaction *Con:* Personal inhibition may make this appear as a nonlegitimate option

intracavernosal injection therapy, or placement of a penile prosthesis (Jackson, 2004). Men who experience ED should be referred to a urologist for work-up before making a decision about treatment options (see **Table 11-4** for treatment options). In addition, because clients' responses to therapy vary according to risk factors, the more difficult to treat patients (e.g., those with conditions such as hypertension or diabetes) will most likely have a lower response rate and need more frequent follow-up visits than those with fewer risk factors (CIEF, 2007).

Men with diabetes are capable of experiencing orgasm and ejaculation even after developing ED, because the disease has lesser effects on the sympathetic autonomic nervous system. Men may experience a retrograde ejaculation due to autonomic system disruption of the internal vesical sphincter (Tilton, 1997). Fertility may also be impaired in diabetic men secondary to ED, low semen volume, and lowered sperm counts. Couples should be referred to a counselor to help them adjust to the relationship strains of chronic illness, and those desiring children should be referred to a fertility specialist.

Despite recent efforts in identifying and quantifying the prevalence of sexual problems in women with diabetes, data continue to be inadequate (Bhasin, Enzlin, Coviello, & Basson, 2007; Enzlin et al., 2009). What evidence is available, however, suggests that female sexual dysfunction (FSD) is an issue in about 35% of women with type I diabetes (Enzlin et al., 2009). Other prevalence data suggest that all phases of the sexual response cycle are negatively affected in women with insulin-dependent diabetes mellitus (IDDM), with diabetic women reporting 27% dysfunction as compared with 15% of those in a control group (Enzlin et al., 2002). More recent reports suggest that FSD is found in 35% of women with type I diabetes, with a greater

incidence in married women who report depression (Enzlin et al., 2009). In a sample of 424 women with type 1 diabetes, of those who met the criteria for FSD, 57% reported decreased desire, 51% reported difficulty achieving orgasm, 47% reported inadequate lubrication, 38% reported decreased arousal, and 21% reported dyspareunia (Enzlin et al., 2009). Data are scarce in comparing levels of desire between women with IDDM and non–insulin-dependent diabetes mellitus (NIDDM). Recent work suggests a correlation between sexual dysfunction and depression in women with diabetes (Bhasin et al., 2007; Enzlin et al., 2009).

Vaginal lubrication is a manifestation of sexual arousal and can be viewed as analogous to erection in men. As such, women may experience alterations in vaginal capillary dilation and loss of transudate formed in the vagina. The most common hormonally related problem associated with diminished sexual arousal is estrogen, because sexual arousal is influenced by levels of this chemical. Women experiencing estrogen deficiencies at menopause are often impacted by changes in vaginal structure and function (Grandjean & Moran, 2007). Diabetic women may be at higher risk for sexual dysfunction because of vaginal dryness, dyspareunia, decreased arousal or desire, and psychological factors. Treatment modalities are discussed for each of these specific problems (Grandjean & Moran, 2007). Women also reported that it took longer to reach a level of arousal necessary to be orgasmic, but that there were no discernible changes in their orgasms since the onset of diabetes. Other research reports varying frequencies of orgasmic difficulties. Kolodny (1971) found that 35% of his sample reported complete loss of orgasm, Jensen (1981) had 10% of his subjects report decreased or absent orgasm, and Enzlin et al. (2009) reported that 51% of women with symptoms of FSD reported difficulty with orgasm. Clearly, much more research is needed in this area.

Although the data cannot pinpoint the exact percentage of diabetic women and men with sexual difficulties or identify exactly when in the course of the disease sexual problems occur, nurses still have an obligation to address this aspect of care. Factors influencing sexual dysfunction in diabetic women include depression, marital dissatisfaction, difficulty adjusting to the diagnosis, and low satisfaction with diabetic treatment options. Sexual dysfunction in men also appears to be related to depression, as well as poor adjustment to the diagnosis and negative appraisal of the disease (Enzlin, Matieu, & Demytteanere, 2003). Nurses should assume that all clients with diabetes will experience sexual difficulty at some point in time and *routinely* assess the sexual concerns of their clients. Women who report vaginal dryness can be encouraged to use over-the-counter, water-soluble vaginal lubricants. Eating yogurt with active cultures may help in reducing the frequency of yeast infections. Maintaining close control over fluctuations in blood glucose levels will also reduce the frequency of yeast infections. Couples should be referred to counseling as issues arise related to the strains of living with a chronic illness in order that better communication may occur about these issues.

Cancer

Cancer occurs in people of all ages. Cancer happens to an individual, a couple, and to a family. A complete discussion of the multiple ways cancer can have an impact on sexuality is beyond the scope of this chapter. For more detailed information, the reader is referred to any of the major cancer nursing textbooks and publications by the Oncology Nursing Society. This discussion is limited to the general ways that cancer and cancer treatments affect sexuality.

In general, surgical treatments for cancer have an impact on body image and the ability to function sexually. Surgical procedures for cancers of the gastrointestinal system can lead to sexual difficulties secondary to damage to nerves that enervate sexual organs or cause alterations in body image that affect sexuality. Other procedures may involve removal of or alterations in organs that directly impact the ability to function sexually. Radical hysterectomy renders a woman unable to bear children and leads to a surgically induced menopause if oophorectomy is included in the procedure. Because of removal of the upper portion of the vagina, women and their partners may be concerned that having a shortened vagina will preclude satisfactory sexual intercourse. Postoperative discussions should include discussion of positions that might reduce dyspareunia.

Men also experience sexual side effects from surgical intervention. Characteristics associated with postoperative sexual recovery after radical prostatectomy include younger age, use of nerve-sparing techniques, smaller prostate at time of surgery, pretreatment erectile ability, presence of a sexually functional partner, and absence of androgen deprivation (Hollenbeck, Dunn, Wei, Sandler, & Sanda, 2004). Specific information regarding the effects of other surgical procedures on sexual functioning is included in **Table 11-5.**

Radiation therapy can cause alterations in organ functioning, primary organ failure resulting in either permanent or temporary alterations in fertility, as well as side effects that are not directly related to sexual functioning (**Table 11-6).** Fertility may be preserved by the use of modern radiation therapy techniques and the use of lead shields to protect the testes. Women diagnosed

Table 11-5   Effects of Cancer Surgery on Sexual Functioning

Type of Surgery	Effects on Sexual Functioning	Client Education
Colorectal surgery with colostomy	Varies; depends on type and extent of surgical procedure; major impact on body image and self-concept	Encourage expression of feelings and communication with partner.
Abdominoperineal resection	*Females*: shortening of vagina; vaginal scarring may cause dyspareunia; decreased lubrication if ovaries also are removed *Males*: erectile dysfunction; decrease in amount/force of ejaculate or retrograde ejaculation because of interruption of sympathetic and parasympathetic nerve supply. Amount of rectal tissue removed appears to determine degree of dysfunction. Capacity for orgasm not altered.	Use water-soluble lubricant prior to intercourse; allow more time for pleasuring before attempting penetration; with shortened vagina, use coital positions that decrease depth of penetration (e.g., side-to-side lying, man on top with legs outside the woman's, woman on top). Erectile dysfunction may be temporary or permanent; encourage use of touch, other means of communication.
Transurethral resection of bladder/partial cystectomy	Mild pain or dyspareunia	Encourage more time for pleasuring.
Radical cystectomy	*Females:* surgery usually includes removal of bladder, urethra, uterus, ovaries, fallopian tubes, and anterior portion of vagina. *Males*: surgery involves removal of bladder, prostate, seminal vesicles, pelvic lymph nodes, and possibly urethra. May cause retrograde or loss of ejaculation and decrease in or loss of erectile ability.	Vaginal reconstruction is possible; use water-soluble lubricant; encourage self-pleasuring and use of dilators; encourage use of touch and other means of sexual communication. Explore possibility for penile implant.
Radical prostatectomy	Involves removal of prostate, seminal vesicles, and vas deferens. Damage to autonomic nerves near prostate may cause loss of erectile ability; loss of emission and ejaculation.	Desire, penile sensations, and orgasmic abilities not altered. Explore possibility for penile prosthesis.
Transurethral resection of prostate	Causes retrograde ejaculation because of damage to internal bladder sphincter	Reassure that erection and orgasm will still occur but that ejaculate will be decreased or absent; urine may be cloudy.
Bilateral orchiectomy	Results in low levels of testosterone; causes sterility, decreased libido, impotence, gynecomastia, penile atrophy, and decreased growth of body hair and beard.	Discuss option of sperm banking prior to surgery; discuss optional ways of expressing sexuality with patient and partner.

(Continues)

Table 11-5	Effects of Cancer Surgery on Sexual Functioning (Continued)	
Type of Surgery	**Effects on Sexual Functioning**	**Client Education**
Retroperitoneal lymph node dissection	Damages sympathetic nerves necessary for ejaculation; results in temporary or permanent loss of ejaculation; patient maintains potency and orgasmic ability	Discuss option of sperm banking.
Total abdominal hysterectomy with bilateral salpingo-oophorectomy	Loss of circulating estrogens; decrease in vaginal elasticity, decrease in vaginal lubrication; some women report decreased desire, orgasm, and enjoyment.	Use water-soluble lubricants; intercourse may be resumed after 6-week post-op check; encourage discussion about meaning of loss of uterus to self-identity.
Mastectomy	Decrease in arousal associated with nipple stimulation; affects body image, self-concept	Encourage communication with partner.
Radical vulvectomy	Removal of labia majora, labia minora, clitoris, bilateral pelvic node dissection; loss of sexually responsive tissue with concomitant loss of vasocongestive neuromuscular response	Possibility of perineal reconstruction with split-thickness skin graft or gracilis muscle grafts. Intercourse is still possible; explore ways of achieving arousal other than genital stimulation. Preoperative and postoperative counseling are essential.
Penectomy	Degree of sexual limitation depends on length of remaining penile shaft. Glands will be removed; remainder of shaft of penile tissue will respond with tumescence and will allow ejaculation and orgasm.	Discuss possibility of artificial insemination if children are desired.

with invasive cervical cancer are frequently treated by a combination of external and internal radiation therapy. Side effects include fatigue, diarrhea, vaginal dryness, and vaginal stenosis (Maher, 2005). Vaginal dryness will definitely occur; however, vaginal stenosis can be prevented. A patent vagina is important in maintaining sexual function as well as allowing for adequate follow-up evaluations. Women must be educated about the need to either use a vaginal dilator or have vaginal intercourse on a regular basis (Wilmoth & Spinelli, 2000). In women older than 40 years, infertility may occur at lower doses of radiation. Women may undergo surgery to protect the ovaries by moving them out of the field of radiation (National Cancer Institute, 2007). Likewise, men who receive either external beam or brachytherapy for prostate cancer are at increased risk of sexual dysfunction (Hollenbeck et al., 2004). Current techniques such as conformal external-beam radiation therapy are reported to lead to ED in as many as 40–60% of men with prostate cancer (Wiegner & King, 2010). These rates of ED are also reported in newer delivery techniques of radiation therapy such as intensity-modulated radiation therapy (IMRT).

Table 11-6   Site-Specific Effects of Radiation Therapy on Sexuality

Radiated site	Effect on Sexuality	Client Education
Testes	Reduction in sperm count begins in 6 to 8 weeks and continues for 1 year. Doses of 2 Gy* will result in temporary sterility for about 12 months. Doses ≥ 5 Gy result in permanent sterility. Libido and potency will be maintained.	Discuss sperm banking prior to therapy and continued use of contraceptives.
Prostate	*External beam:* temporary or permanent erectile dysfunction because of fibrosis of pelvic vasculature or radiation damage of pelvic nerves. *Interstitial:* less incidence of impotency	Age is variable—men older than age 60 have higher incidence of impotence. Erectile dysfunction—may experience pain during ejaculation because of irritation of urethra. Potency preserved in 70–90% of men who were potent before treatment.
Cervix/vaginal canal	*External beam:* vaginal stenosis and fibrosis, fistula, cystitis *Intracavitary:* vaginal stenosis, dry, friable tissue, loss of lubrication. Both result in decreased vaginal sensation and dyspareunia.	Use of water-soluble lubricant; empty bladder before and after sex; encourage pleasuring prior to attempting penetration; use dilators or frequent intercourse to lessen amount of stenosis. Explore new positions for intercourse to allow woman control over depth of penile penetration.
Pelvic region	*Women:* temporary or permanent sterility dependent on dose of radiation, volume of tissue irradiated, and woman's age; the closer to menopause, the more likely permanent sterility will result. A single dose of 3.75 Gy will cause complete cessation of menses in women older than age 40. *Men:* temporary or permanent erectile dysfunction secondary to vascular or nerve damage	Oophoropexy and shielding may help to maintain fertility in women; continue use of contraceptives; use of water-soluble lubricant Both genders: encourage alternate means to express sexuality, such as touch.
Breast	Skin reactions, changes in breast sensations	Explore alternate pleasuring techniques and good communication techniques; breastfeeding should occur on nonradiated side.

*Gy (pronounced gray) is the international system (SI) unit of radiation dose expressed in terms of absorbed energy per unit mass of tissue (Health Physics Society, 2011). Retrieved October 11, 2011, from http://hps.org/publicinformation/radterms/radfact79.html

Source: Wilmoth, M. C. (2009). Sexuality. In C. Burke (Ed.), *Psychosocial dimensions of oncology nursing care* (2nd ed., pp. 101–124). Pittsburgh: Oncology Nursing Press.

Chemotherapy treatments frequently cause temporary or permanent infertility. These side effects are related to a number of factors, including the client's gender, age at time of treatment, the specific type and dose of radiation therapy and/or chemotherapy, the use of single therapy or multiple therapies, and the length of time since treatment (National Cancer Institute, 2007). The extent of the impact on fertility varies according to the patient's gender, type of cancer, and the type and dosage of chemotherapy. Combination chemotherapy that includes alkylating agents and being a woman older than age 35 appear to be the primary factors related to altered fertility. In addition to altered fertility, chemotherapy can lead to altered ovarian function and subsequent menopause (McInnes & Schilsky, 1996). Menopausal symptoms such as hot flashes, vaginal dryness, and skin changes in addition to chemotherapy side effects can be traumatic for women, particularly if they are not aware of the potential for menopause (Wilmoth, Coleman, Wahab, & Kneisl, 2009). The nurse could suggest use of vitamin E, use of water-soluble vaginal lubricants, and doing Kegel exercises to reduce symptoms (Wilmoth, 1996). In addition to the lubricating effect of over-the-counter water-soluble lubricants, several products have demonstrated a positive effect against HIV infection with use. Astroglide, Vagisil, and ViAmor inhibited HIV production by 0.1000-fold when mixed with cells in seminal fluid, and 0.30-fold when layered on the cells in the two experiments shown in comparison with nonoxynol-9 (Baron, Poast, Nguyen, & Cloyd, 2004).

The use of alkylating agents in men has a major impact on their sexuality and fertility. Men who receive cumulative doses greater than 400 mg are always azoospermic, as are those treated with cisplatin (Krebs, 2005). Adult men, regardless of age, are likely to experience long-term side effects of chemotherapy. However, age, total dose, and time since therapy are essential to recovery of fertility. If fertility is to recover, normal sperm counts should return to normal within 3 years after completion of treatment. As demonstrated in this section, the effects of treatment for cancer on sexual functioning may be devastating. Prior to beginning

CASE STUDY

You are an adult nurse practitioner working in the outpatient cancer clinic. Your next patient is Carol, a 43-year-old breast cancer survivor, 4 years post-diagnosis. Carol was diagnosed at age 39 with a Stage IIb, ER/PR negative tumor and had a lumpectomy followed by chemotherapy. Her chief complaint post-chemotherapy has been hot flashes.

You begin the visit asking Carol about how things are going with work and her husband. Carol noticeably tenses when she talks about her husband. You probe a little and reflect that you noticed some tension; you ask how are things between her and her husband. Have they been able to go away on any vacations? What has he said about how well she is doing after completing chemotherapy?

When Carol provides some vague responses, you talk about the menopause that chemo has caused and ask Carol if she thought that this, most likely permanent, problem was a source of stress between she and her husband. Carol begins to cry and says that she just hasn't felt like being intimate, and when she has, it has been painful.

CASE STUDY   (Continued)

You take a short sexual health history so that you have a comprehensive background on her sexual functioning, both pre- and post-diagnosis. You learn that Carol and her husband had a healthy sexual relationship prior to her diagnosis, were active three to four times weekly, and had been trying to become pregnant when Carol was diagnosed with cancer. Carol has been taking fluoxetine (Prozac), a selective serotonin re-uptake inhibitor (SSRI) since diagnosis to help cope with some mild depression. About midway during chemo, Carol began having hot flashes, mood swings, and complained of lack of interest, dyspareunia, and inability to reach orgasm whenever she and her husband were intimate.

Finally, you refer Carol and her husband to a sex therapist to help them work through some of their sexual and relationship challenges.

Discussion Questions

1. What might you include in a more focused sexual assessment? What type of chemotherapy agents cause either a temporary or permanent menopause? Is infertility an area of concern?
2. How do SSRIs affect sexuality in women? Are there any antidepressants with a lesser impact on sexuality?
3. What factors do you need to consider when recommending herbal remedies for menopausal symptoms to women with breast cancer?
4. What other specific suggestions might you make to Carol about ways to enhance her sexuality and reduce dyspareunia?

---

treatment, clear communication with the patient and family about potential effects on sexual function is needed.

Multiple Sclerosis

Multiple sclerosis (MS) has the potential to have a profound impact on the sexual relationships of couples, owing to the resulting motor, sensory, and cognitive alterations. The prevalence of sexual difficulties ranges between 60–80% in males and 20–60% in women (McCabe, 2002). Sexual difficulties in persons with MS can be classified as being primary, secondary, or tertiary in origin (Lowden, O'Leary, & Stevenson, 2005). Primary sexual problems

are those that are caused by the pathologic damage to the central nervous system and hormonal issues (Lowden et al., 2005). Secondary problems arise from symptoms including bladder dysfunction, fatigue, pain, cognitive dysfunction, and mobility issues (Lowden et al., 2005). Tertiary causes are psychological in nature, and are primarily related to attitudes and feelings about sexuality that are compounded by the interaction of the disease process and societal norms about sexuality (Lowden et al., 2005).

Neurologic changes caused by MS can affect sexual feelings as well as sexual response. There are common issues that affect both men and women in achieving sexual response—most prominent are changes in sensation that lead to sexual stimuli and the ability to achieve orgasm (Lowden et al., 2005). Counseling for underlying emotional concerns as well as depression may affect treatment of desire problems as well. Changes in genital sensations can be troubling, because something that used to feel good may now be noxious. Teaching couples to communicate about these changes and to try new techniques may be helpful (Kalb, 2008). Vaginal dryness can be improved with the use of water-soluble lubricants. Unfortunately, treatment of ED in men is not as easily remedied. Treatment options for ED in MS are the same as those for men with other chronic illnesses and can be found in Table 11-4.

Secondary sexual alterations caused by MS are a result of the physical symptoms that accompany the disease. Spasticity during sexual activity appears to affect women more than it does men and may be controlled by baclofen, chemical nerve blocks, and surgery. Bowel and bladder problems can cause significant alterations in sexuality and can severely impair spontaneity of sexual activity. Engaging in sexual activity successfully requires open communication as well as aggressive symptom management. Limiting fluid intake for several hours prior to sexual activity and urinating immediately before sexual activity can help with bladder control. Medications are available for incontinence; however, these medications may also increase vaginal dryness. Intermittent catheterization or taping a permanent catheter out of the way can allow successful activity. Bowel problems may be either ones of constipation, no control, or lack of predictability of function. A regular bowel regimen consisting of laxatives, enemas, or disimpaction can allow stress-free sexual interactions.

Fatigue is a pervasive symptom of MS as well as other chronic illnesses. In MS, fatigue can be managed with several pharmacologic agents and energy-conserving techniques. Medications include amantadine or pemoline. Use of wheelchairs or motorized carts or regular naps during the day can allow clients to conserve energy for activities they enjoy, including sexual activity. Cognitive impairment can also have a pervasive impact on a relationship. Memory loss, impaired judgment, and other problems can impair the interpersonal communication that is integral in any intimate relationship.

The psychosocial changes that accompany MS cause tertiary sexual dysfunction. Decreased self-concept, grieving for loss of self, and role changes affect both the client and the partner. Persons with MS report lower levels of sexual activity, sexual satisfaction, and relationship satisfaction than those without MS (McCabe, McKern, McDonald, & Vowels, 2003). Ongoing counseling and participation in support groups can help couples deal with these sexual and relationship issues caused by MS (McCabe, 2002). The MS Society published a pamphlet on intimacy and sexuality for persons with MS. This pamphlet provides both permission to continue being sexual and limited information for both the person with MS and their partner (Kalb, 2008).

INTERVENTIONS

Many healthcare providers are hesitant to ask patients about their sexuality, fearing privacy issues. However, sexuality is a part of one's quality of life. Assessing sexuality and responding to issues is essential in caring for the whole patient.

Sexual Assessment

Sexual assessment should be a routine part of every physician- or nurse-initiated assessment for nearly every client diagnosed with a chronic illness (Wilmoth, 2000, 2006). Assessing sexuality as routinely as other body systems serves two purposes. First, it decreases embarrassment on the part of the client and practitioner if it is accepted as a normal aspect of health care. Second, routine inclusion will give the client permission to mention sexual difficulties to the practitioner and give the practitioner permission to ask specific questions when it is suspected that the client might be experiencing a sexually related side effect of the disease or treatment.

The clinician should keep the same principles in mind when discussing sexuality with a client and/or partner, as with any other topic. The CIEF suggests that many clients have unrealistic expectations about the efficacy of not only PDE5 inhibitors but also other treatment options (CIEF, 2007). Clients need reassurance about the safety of treatments for issues with sexuality. These instances again reinforce the importance of the clinician as an educator, emphasize the professional nature of these discussions, clarify the content component of communications, and reinforce permission to include sexuality in the plan of care. An example of a bridge question is, "Has anyone talked with you about how your (injury/illness/treatments) can affect your ability to have sex?" *Unloading* a topic is another technique that is useful in discussing sexuality and can ease a client's concern once he or she learns that others have experienced this problem (Woods, 1984). An example of unloading is, "Many women who have received chemotherapy have had problems with vaginal dryness. What problems have you had with this?"

The inclusion of questions on sexuality in the admission assessment is an excellent way to legitimize the role of the nurse in addressing sexuality. Woods (1984) suggests that such questions should proceed from less intimate questions, such as role functioning, to more personal ones on sexual functioning. Closed (yes/no) questions should be avoided, as they eliminate opportunities for further discussion. Questions for an initial assessment include the following (Woods, 1984; Wilmoth, 1994a):

- How has (diagnosis/treatment) affected your role as wife/husband/partner?
- How has (diagnosis/treatment) affected the way you feel about yourself as a woman/man?
- What aspects of your sexuality do you believe have been affected by your diagnosis/treatment?
- How has your (diagnosis/treatment) affected your ability to function sexually?

A more medically focused sexual evaluation might include determination of chief complaint, sexual status, medical status, psychiatric status, family and psychosexual history, relationship assessment, and summary with recommendations (Krebs, 2007). A complete sexual history is not usually indicated unless initial assessment indicates the presence of a sexual problem. Most nurses are not adequately prepared to conduct a full sexual assessment; therefore, referral to a more appropriate practitioner is appropriate.

Including Sexuality in Practice

Four areas of competency must be achieved for nurses to successfully incorporate sexuality into practice to attain the published standards of practice: comfort with one's own sexuality and comfort in discussing sexuality with others; excellent communication skills; a knowledge base about sexuality in health and illness; and role models that demonstrate integration of sexuality into practice (Woods, 1984; Wilmoth, 1994b).

Participation in each of the aforementioned processes will add to the nurse's knowledge base about normal sexual functioning. The professional nurse should also engage in independent study within their specialty regarding the effects that the illnesses, treatments, and medications have on sexuality. Engaging in discussions with other healthcare providers, such as physicians or pharmacists, or participating in interdisciplinary journal clubs and research projects, can add depth to the nurses' knowledge. Such interdisciplinary efforts will have large payoffs for clients and their partners.

Nurses who are comfortable with their own sexuality, are proficient communicators, and have knowledge about sexuality possess the foundation necessary to incorporate sexuality into their practice. However, many are still reluctant to do so. Peers who can role model the incorporation of sexuality into nursing practice may be influential in helping others incorporate it into their practices. Role models can assist in this process by relating positive experiences with clients about discussions surrounding sexuality, by role playing ways of initiating discussions about sexuality, and by acting as a resource for staff. However, there is little research documenting the effectiveness of role models in teaching others to incorporate sexuality into practice.

Grand rounds and presentations of individual cases that exemplify typical sexual concerns associated with a particular treatment, medication, or diagnosis are other strategies for enhancing comfort in including sexual discussions in practice. Physicians and pharmacists could discuss a particular disease process and treatment options, including medications and their effect on sexual functioning. A social worker or clinical nurse specialist skilled in assessing and educating about sexual issues could lead practitioners through the sexual assessment and educational process. Finally, a clinician or sex therapist could discuss interventions that the majority of practitioners could use in their counseling of persons with sexual issues.

Comfort with sexuality and enhancement of communication skills can be attained through reading, values clarification exercises, and participation in courses on sexuality. Some options include semester-long college courses related to sexuality or shorter weekend courses, often referred to as "SARs." Sexual attitude reassessment, or SAR, programs combine explicit films with small group discussions over a 2- or 3-day period to allow for analysis of one's personal values surrounding sexuality. Knowing one's own values and attitudes toward a variety of other sexual practices and sexual orientations is the first step in becoming comfortable with sexuality (Wilmoth, 1994a). Values clarification exercises can assist in this process. The outcome of clarifying one's values about sexuality is knowing what one believes is acceptable sexual behavior. It is important to remember that there is no right or wrong set of behaviors or values, just different ones.

Comfort in discussing sexuality and enhancing the ability to communicate clearly about sexuality can be achieved through a variety of methods. One option is to form a discussion group or journal club among colleagues. This group could engage in discussion of values clarification exercises or articles related to human sexuality in general or disease-focused articles on sexuality. Sharing with a peer group, particularly an interdisciplinary peer group, is a nonthreatening way in which to become comfortable talking about sexuality. This approach also assists with increasing knowledge about a variety of illnesses, their treatments, and their effects on sexuality.

Nurses are skilled communicators, but they initially may find initiating discussions with clients about sexuality anxiety provoking. Nurses should assume that their clients have some form of sexual experience rather than none at all, and should also assume that they have questions about the impact of their disease or its treatments on their sexuality. Experience has shown that patients are most appreciative when asked about this part of life in relation to their chronic illness. Nurses should use terminology, including slang that their clients understand. Many health professionals use the PLISSIT model (Annon, 1976) to assist them in their sexual assessments. In this model, P stands for *permission;* LI, for *limited information;* SS, for *specific suggestions;* and IT, for *intensive therapy* (**Table 11-7**). All nurses should be able to intervene at all levels except for provision of intensive therapy. If assessment suggests a problem beyond the level of needing specific suggestions, the client and partner should be referred to a sex therapist.

OUTCOMES

Desired client and partner outcomes that may be anticipated after nursing intervention include the following (American Nurses Association/ Oncology Nursing Society, 2004):

- The ability to identify potential/actual changes in sexuality, sexual functioning, or intimacy related to disease and treatment
- The ability to express feelings about alopecia, body image changes, and altered sexual functioning
- The ability to engage in open communication with his or her partner regarding changes in sexual functioning or desire, within a cultural framework

Table 11-7 PLISSIT Model	
Permission (P)	(Assessment) Actions taken by the nurse to let the patient/partner know that sexual issues are a legitimate aspect in providing nursing care. This could include questions about sexuality that are incorporated into the general admission assessment or questions specifically related to their disease process or treatment.
Limited Information (LI)	(Education) Sharing of information regarding the effects of disease, treatments, and medications. Examples of limited information include discussing when sexual intercourse may be resumed after surgery, the possibility of menopause occurring in conjunction with chemotherapy, or medications leading to erectile dysfunction.
Specific Suggestions (SS)	(Counseling) This level of care requires specialized knowledge about specific conditions and their relationship to sexual functioning. Various techniques, positions, and alternate techniques useful in achieving sexual satisfaction are examples of counseling concerns.
Intensive Therapy (IT)	(Referral) Treatment of sexual dysfunction requires specialized training in psychotherapy, sex therapy techniques, crisis intervention, and behavior modification.

Source: Annon, J. S. (1976). *The behavioral treatment of sexual problems: Volume I: Brief therapy.* New York: Harper & Row.

- The ability to describe appropriate interventions for actual or potential changes in sexual function
- The ability to identify personal and community resources to assist with changes in body image and sexuality.

Evidence-Based Practice Box

The Consortium for Spinal Cord Medicine published clinical practice guidelines in 2010 drawn from a clinical and epidemiologic, evidence-based model from the Agency for Healthcare Research and Quality. The committee conducted a systematic review of the literature on the topic of spinal cord injury and sexuality and reproductive health published between 1995 and September 2007. The thorough methodology used for this review is outlined in the manuscript. Evidence-based guidelines for sexual assessment post-spinal cord injury are provided as well as education guidelines for educating the individual and their partner on ways to maintain sexual functioning post-injury. The guidelines also provide the professional with evidence-based suggestions on how to manage a variety of health problems that occur frequently in men and women with spinal cord injury that may negatively impact sexual functioning. Recommendations for further research are also provided.

Source: Consortium for Spinal Cord Medicine (2010). Sexuality and reproductive health in adults with spinal cord injury: A clinical practice guideline for health-care professionals. *The Journal of Spinal Cordedicine, 33*(3), 281–336.

STUDY QUESTIONS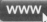

Why is it important for nurses and other healthcare professionals to include a sexual assessment and sexual education when providing care?

What are key changes in sexual response that should be expected to occur with healthy aging?

In general, what changes in sexuality are caused by chemotherapy in women? In men?

What do men and their partners need to know about the pathophysiology of diabetes mellitus on erectile ability and options to continue sexual intercourse?

What should be discussed about sexuality with a patient newly diagnosed with multiple sclerosis?

What are some methods that a nurse manager could implement with a nursing staff to increase comfort and knowledge regarding the impact of disease on sexuality?

For a full suite of assignments and additional learning activities, **WWW** use the access code located in the front of your book and visit this exclusive website: **http://go.jblearning.com/larsen**. If you do not have an access code, you can obtain one at the site.

REFERENCES

Agewall, S., Berglund, M. & Henareh, L. (2004). Reduced quality of life after myocardial infarction in women compared with men. *Clinical Cardiology, 27*(5), 271–274.

American Nurses Association. (2010). *Nursing: Scope and standards of practice.* (2nd ed.) Washington DC: Author.

American Nurses Association/Oncology Nursing Society. (2004). *Statement on scope and standards of oncology nursing practice.* Washington DC: Author.

American Psychological Association. (2000). *Diagnostic and statistical manual of mental disorders—text revision* (4th ed.). Washington DC: Author.

Andrews, M., Goldberg, K., & Kaplan, H. (Eds.). (1996). *Nurse's legal handbook* (3rd ed.). Springhouse, PA: Springhouse Corporation.

Annon, J. S. (1976). *The behavioral treatment of sexual problems: Volume I: Brief therapy.* New York: Harper & Row.

Baron, S., Poast, J., Nguyen, D., & Cloyd, M. (2004). Practical prevention of vaginal and rectal transmission of HIV by adapting the oral defense: Use of commercial lubricants. *AIDS Research and Human Retrovirus, 17*(11), 978–1002.

Bhasin, S., Enzlin, P., Coviello, A., & Basson, R. (2007). Sexual dysfunction in men and women with endocrine disorders. *Lancet, 369*(9561), 597–611.

Centers for Disease Control and Prevention, Office of Minority Health. (2004). Eliminate disparities in cardiovascular disease. Retrieved August 24, 2011, from www.cdc.gov/omhd/AMH/factsheets/cardio. htm

Consortium for Improvement in Erectile Dysfunction, (CIEF) (2007). *Collaborative for advancement of urological, sexual, and endocrine education.* Retrieved August 8, 2011, from: http://causeeducation.org/

Consortium for Spinal Cord Medicine. (2010). Sexuality and reproductive health in adults with spinal cord injury: A clinical practice guideline for health-care professionals. *The Journal of Spinal Cord Medicine, 33*(3), 281–336.

Corona, G., Mannucci, R., Mansani, R., Petrone, L., Bartolini, M., Glommi, R., et al. (2007). Aging and pathogenesis of erectile dysfunction. *International Journal of Impotence Research, 16*(5), 395–402.

Darling, C. A., Davidson, J. K., & Conway-Welch, C. (1990). Female ejaculation: Perceived origins, the Grafenberg spot/area, and sexual responsiveness. *Archives of Sexual Behavior, 19,* 29–47.

DeBusk, R. (2000). Evaluating the cardiovascular tolerance for sex. *The American Journal of Cardiology, 86*(2A), 51F–56F.

Enzlin, P., Mathieu, C., Van den Bruel, A., Bosteels, J., Vanderschueren, D., & Demyttenaere, K. (2002). Sexual dysfunction in women with Type 1 diabetes: A controlled study. *Diabetes Care, 25,* 672–677.

Enzlin, P., Matieu, C., & Demytteanere, K. (2003). Diabetes and female sexual functioning: A state-of-the-art. *Diabetes Spectrum, 16,* 256–259.

Enzlin, P., Rose, R., Wiegel, M., Brown, J., Wessells, H., Gatcomb, P., Rutledge, B., et al. (2009). Sexual dysfunction in women with Type I diabetes. *Diabetes Care, 23*(5), 780–785.

Grandjean, C., & Moran, B., (2007). The impact of diabetes mellitus on female sexual well-being. *Nursing Clinics of North America, 42*(4), 581–592.

Guyton, A. C., & Hall, J. E. (2006). *Textbook of medical physiology* (11th ed.) Philadelphia: Elsevier Saunders.

Hines, T. M. (2001). The G-spot: A modern gynecologic myth. *American Journal of Obstetrics and Gynecology, 185*(2), 359–362.

Hollenbeck, B. K., Dunn, R. L., Wei, J. T., Sandler, H. M., & Sanda, M. G. (2004). Sexual health recovery after prostatectomy, external radiation or brachytherapy for early stage prostate cancer. *Current Urology Reports, 5,* 212–219.

Jackson, G. (2004). Sexual dysfunction and diabetes. *International Journal of Clinical Practice, 58*(4), 358–362.

Jensen, S. B. (1981). Diabetic sexual dysfunction: A comparative study of 160 insulin-treated diabetic men and women and an age-matched control group. *Archives of Sexual Behavior, 10,* 493–504.

Kalb, R. C. (2008). *Intimacy and Sexuality in MS.* New York: MS Society.

Kaplan, H. S. (1979). *Disorders of sexual desire and other new concepts and techniques in sex therapy.* New York: Simon & Schuster.

Katz, A. (2007). *Breaking the silence on cancer and sexuality. A handbook for healthcare providers.* Pittsburgh: Oncology Nursing Society.

Kolodny, R. C. (1971). Sexual dysfunction in diabetic females. *Diabetes, 20,* 557–559.

Kolodny, R., Masters, W., Johnson, V., & Biggs, M. (1979). *The textbook for human sexuality for nurses.* Boston: Little, Brown.

Kostis, J. B., Jackson, G., Rosen, R., Barrett-Connor, E., Billups, K., Burnett, A. L., et al. (2005). Sexual dysfunction and cardiac risk, the second Princeton consensus conference. *American Journal of Cardiology, 96*(12B), 85M–93M.

Koukouras, D., Spiliotis, J., Scopa, C. D., Dragotis, K., Kalfarentzos, F., Tzoracoleftherakis, E., et al. (1991). Radical consequence in the sexuality of male patients operated for colorectal carcinoma. *European Journal of Surgical Oncology, 17,* 285–288.

Krebs, L. U. (2005). Sexual and reproductive dysfunction. In C. H. Yarbro, M. H. Frogge, M. Goodman, & S. L. Groenwald (Eds.), *Cancer nursing: Principles and practice* (6th ed., pp. 841–869). Sudbury, MA: Jones & Bartlett.

Krebs, L. U. (2007). Sexual assessment: Research and clinical. *Nursing Clinics of North America, 42*(4), 515–529.

Ladas, A. K., Whipple, B., & Perry, J. D. (1982). *The G-spot.* New York: Dell.

Leiblum, S. R., & Segraves, R. T. (1989). Sex therapy with aging adults. In S. R. Leiblum & R.C. Rosen (Eds.), *Principles and practice of sex therapy: Update for the 1990s* (2nd ed., pp. 352–381). New York: Guilford Press.

Lindau, S. T., Schumm, L. P., Gaumann, E. O., Levinson, W., O'Muircheartaigh, C. A. & Waite, L. J. (2007). A study of sexuality and health among older adults in the United States. *New England Journal of Medicine, 357*(8), 820–822.

Lowden, D., O'Leary, M., & Stevenson, B. (2005). Sexuality issues in patients with MS. *Multiple Sclerosis Counseling Points, 1,* 1–9.

Maher, K. (2005). Radiation therapy: Toxicities and management. In C. H.Yarbro, M. H. Frogge, & M. Goodman (Eds.). *Cancer nursing: Principles and practice* (6th ed., pp. 283–314). Sudbury, MA: Jones & Bartlett.

Masters, W. H, & Johnson, V. E. (1966). *Human sexual response.* Philadelphia: Lippincott-Raven.

Masters, W. H., & Johnson, V. E. (1981). Sex and the aging process. *Journal of the American Geriatrics Society, 24*(9), 385–390.

McCabe, M. P. (2002). Relationship functioning and sexuality among people with multiple sclerosis. *The Journal of Sex Research, 39*(4), 302–309.

McCabe, M. P., McKern, S., McDonald, E., & Vowels, L. M. (2003). Changes over time in sexual and relationship functioning of people with multiple sclerosis. *Journal of Sex & Marital Therapy, 29*(4), 305–321.

McInnes, S., & Schilsky, R. L. (1996). Infertility following cancer chemotherapy. In B. A. Chabner & D. L.

Longo (Eds.), *Cancer chemotherapy and biotherapy* (2nd ed., pp. 31–44). Philadelphia: Lippincott-Raven.

Meston, C. M. (2000). Sympathetic nervous system activity and female sexual arousal. *The American Journal of Cardiology, 86*(2) (Suppl. 1), 30–34.

Meston, C. M., & Gorzalka, B. B. (1996). The differential effects of sympathetic activation on sexual arousal in sexually functional and dysfunctional women. *Journal of Abnormal Psychology, 105,* 582–591.

National Cancer Institute (2007). Sexual and reproductive issues. Retrieved August 8, 2011, from: http://www.cancer.gov/cancertopics/pdq/supportivecare/sexuality/Patient/page1

National Institutes of Health. (1992). Impotence. *NIH Consensus Statement, 10*(4), 1–31.

National Diabetes Information Clearinghouse. (2011). Fast facts on diabetes. Retrieved August 8, 2011, from: http://diabetes.niddk.nih.gov/dm/pubs/statistics/index.htm#fast

Oncology Nursing Society. (2004). *Statement on the scope and standards of oncology nursing practice.* Pittsburgh: Author.

O'Farrell, P., Murray, J., & Hotz, S. B. (2000). Psychologic distress among spouses of patients undergoing cardiac rehabilitation. *Heart and Lung, 29*(2), 97–104.

Penson, D. F., Wessells, H., Cleary, P., Rutledge, B. N., & DCCT/EDI Group (2009). Sexual dysfunction and symptom impact in men with long-standing type I diabetes in the DCCT/EDIC study. *Journal of Sexual Medicine, 6*(7), 1969–1978.

Qaseem, A., Snow, V., Denburg, T. D., Casey, D. E., Forcica, M. A. Owens, D. K., et al. (2009). Hormonal testing and pharmalogic treatment of erectile dysfunction: A clinical practice guideline from the American College of Physicians. *Annals of Internal Medicine, 151,* 1–11.

Roose, S. P., & Seidman, S. N. (2000). Sexual activity and cardiac risk: Is depression a contributing factor? *The American Journal of Cardiology, 86*(2A), 38F–40F.

Sarkadi, A., & Rosenquist, U. (2004). Intimacy and women with type 2 diabetes: An exploratory study using focus group interviews. *The Diabetes Educator, 29*(4), 641–652.

Shril, R., Koskimaki, J., Hakkien, A., Auvinen, T., Tammela, J., & Hakama, M. (2007). Cardiovascular drug use and the incidence of erectile dysfunction. *International Journal of Impotence Research, 19*(2), 208–212.

Steinke, E. E. (2000). Sexual counseling after myocardial infarction. *American Journal of Nursing, 100*(12), 38–44.

Svedlund, M., & Danielson, E. (2004). Myocardial infarction: Narrations by afflicted women and their partners of lived experiences in daily life following an acute myocardial infarction. *Journal of Clinical Nursing, 13*(4), 438–446.

Tilton, M. C. (1997). Diabetes and amputation. In M. L. Sipski & C. J. Alexander (Eds.), *Sexual function in people with disability and chronic illness: A health professional's guide* (pp. 279–302). Rockville, MD: Aspen.

Wiegner, E. A., & King, C. R. (2010). Sexual function after stereotactic baby radiotherapy for prostate cancer: Results of a prospective clinical trial. *International Journal of Radiation Oncology, Biology, Physics, 78*(2), 442–448.

Wilmoth, M. C. (1994a, Spring). Strategies for becoming comfortable with sexual assessment. *Oncology Nursing News*, pp. 6–7.

Wilmoth, M. C. (1994b). Nurses' and patients' perspectives on sexuality: Bridging the gap. *Innovations in Oncology Nursing, 10*(2), 34–36.

Wilmoth, M. C. (1996). The middle years: Women, sexuality and the self. *Journal of Obstetric, Gynecologic, and Neonatal Nursing, 25*, 615–621.

Wilmoth, M. C. (2000). Sexuality patterns, altered. In L. J. Carpenito (Ed.), *Nursing diagnosis: Application to clinical practice* (8th ed., pp. 837–857). Philadelphia: Lippincott.

Wilmoth, M. C. (2006). Life after cancer: What does sexuality have to do with it? The 2006 Mara Mogenson Flaherty Memorial Lectureship. *Oncology Nursing Forum, 33*(5), 905–910.

Wilmoth, M. C. (2009). Sexuality. In C. Burke (Ed.), *Psychosocial dimensions of oncology nursing care* (2nd ed., pp. 101–124). Pittsburgh: Oncology Nursing Press.

Wilmoth, M. C., Coleman, E. A., Wahab, H. T., & Kneisl, J. (2009). Preliminary work in validating the symptom cluster of fatigue, weight gain, psychological distress and altered sexuality. *Southern Online Journal of Nursing Research, 9*(13), Article 13.

Wilmoth, M. C., & Spinelli, A. (2000). Sexual implications of gynecologic cancer treatments. *Journal of Obstetrics, Gynecologic and Neonatal Nursing, 29*, 413–421.

Woods, N. F. (1984). *Human sexuality in health and illness* (3rd ed.). St. Louis: Mosby.

Zaviacic, M., & Whipple, B. (1993). Update on the female prostate and the phenomena of female ejaculation. *The Journal of Sex Research, 30*, 48–151.

Zaviacic, M. & Ablin, R. J. (2000). The female prostate and prostate-specific antigen. Immunohistochemical localization, implications for this prostate marker in women, and reasons for using the term "prostate" in the human female. *Histology Histopathology, 15*, 131–142.

CHAPTER 12

Powerlessness

This was the first time . . . When I woke up the other morning I couldn't get out of bed. I couldn't believe it . . . my body, my legs, they just wouldn't move. I was terrified. I thought I'd had a stroke or something. I called for John, but he didn't hear me. I just had to lie there, staring at the ceiling, trying to calm myself. I felt so helpless, so powerless. There was nothing I could do but wait for John to come . . . he helped me into the bathtub where the warmth of the water soothed my aching body. I've always been able to handle my never ending pain . . . the stiffness and rigidity of my body, but that morning . . . that morning was different . . . and now I wonder.
—Anne, 62-year-old woman with fibromyalgia and Parkinson's disease

Faye I. Hummel

INTRODUCTION

Chronic illness changes one's sense of self and one's sense of time. Living with chronic illness requires one to adapt to a continuous changing of outlooks in which the existence of dualities, such as hope and despair, self-control and loss of power, dependence and independence, can elicit feelings of ambiguity, anxiety, and frustration (Delmar et al., 2006). Chronic illness creates threats to well-being and produces multidimensional changes and challenges for the individual and family. Whether these changes occur suddenly or over a long period, chronic illness requires that individuals and families deal with and adapt to an unrelenting altered reality. Managing real and perceived powerlessness is significant. Lack of control and the incapacity to act and change may dominate everyday life for persons with chronic illnesses. Accepting and acknowledging one's limitations as a result of chronic illness may result in a sense of helplessness and loss, as evidenced in the case of Anne:

Last week I watched John working in our garden . . . we have planted a garden for years together. I can't work outside anymore . . . I miss getting my hands in the dirt. I had to quit my job too. I was an accountant for years . . . I really miss my work, my friends; we shared so much. Now . . . now my body is just not able. I have so much pain . . . constant . . . pain is ever with me. My body seems foreign to me . . . I'm losing control of my body. It takes me the better part of the day to get around, to take care of myself . . . I try to cook for us and keep house. I try to plan ahead but I'm just not able to do what needs to be done . . . I don't have a choice. John has to do more around the house now . . . I'm not much help.

The Phenomenon of Powerlessness in Chronic Illness

At some point in the course of chronic illness, individuals experience powerlessness. Powerlessness in the absolute sense is the inability to affect an outcome; the inability to have agency in one's own life (Miller, 2000). Powerlessness may be a real loss of power or a perceived loss of power. For some persons, the feelings of powerlessness may be short lived; whereas for others, they are persistent.

What and who determines powerlessness and what factors facilitate powerlessness? The natural history of chronic illness is highly variable and does not conform to a predictable course of events. The uncertainty of chronic illness, the exacerbation of symptoms, failure of therapy, physical deterioration despite adherence to treatment regimens, side effects of drugs, iatrogenic influences, depletion of social support systems, and the disintegration of the client's psychological stamina can all contribute to powerlessness (Miller, 2000). Chronic illness results in a pronounced loss of functioning over time, disrupts social roles and activities, and limits fulfillment of role expectations (Beal, 2007). Fatigue and inability to participate and engage in social activities contribute to social withdrawal (Asbring, 2001; Beal, 2007) and loss of relationships. Loss of employment, social contacts, and physical and mental function can contribute to disempowerment of individuals with chronic illness. The quintessence of ill health is powerlessness (Strandmark, 2004).

Powerlessness occurs when an individual is controlled by the environment rather than the individual controlling the environment. Therefore, powerlessness is a situational attribute (Miller, 2000). In Anne's story, she experiences powerlessness in part because of the degenerative nature of her disease. Despite her previous life successes, Anne now feels powerless over her own circumstances. Although Anne experienced physical limitations associated with her chronic conditions for a number of years, she was able to successfully adapt and respond to the slow progressive deterioration of her physical condition. Anne maintained power and control over her daily life. When she began to experience the crushing effects of her illness symptoms and physical limitations, Anne felt a loss of control, a sense of powerlessness. No longer was Anne able to maintain her veneer of normalcy, nor was she able to sustain her work and home obligations. Anne resigned from her job, and she struggled to keep up with her household demands. When Anne begins to consider herself without worth in terms of social norms and expectations, feelings of powerlessness arise. Her autonomy and existence are threatened. Over time, Anne becomes exhausted from fatigue and grief and feels powerless over her life situation (Strandmark, 2004).

Dorothy Johnson was one of the first individuals to explore the concept of powerlessness in nursing. Johnson (1967) defined powerlessness as a "perceived lack of personal or internal control of certain events or in certain situations" (p. 40) and urged nurses to take into account the concept of powerlessness inasmuch as nursing interventions would not be effective, particularly health education, if the client felt powerless. The work of Miller (1983, 1992, 2000) has also been instrumental in the development of the concept of powerlessness in chronic illness. Miller (1983, 1992, 2000) differentiates powerlessness from similar constructs, including helplessness, learned helplessness, and locus of control. Helplessness and locus of control are based on a reinforcement paradigm; whereas powerlessness is an existential construct (Miller, 2000). Miller (2000) categorizes locus of control as a personality trait as opposed to powerlessness, which is situationally determined. Locus of control refers to the degree to which people attribute accountability to themselves (internal control) such as personal behavior or characteristics versus uncontrollable forces (external control) such as fate, chance, or luck (Rotter, 1966). The physical and psychosocial outcomes of seeking and gaining control over chronic illness have been the focus of research by social scientists for decades. Locus of control and the beliefs of individuals about whom and what controls their lives are linked to physical and psychological health (Bandura, 1989).

Chronic illness erodes individual control, and this loss of personal control results in powerlessness. Progressive physiologic changes resulting from chronic illness may limit mobility and/or diminish cognitive abilities. The progressive nature of chronic illness limits possibilities and opportunities to exert control over daily life events as well as plans for the future. Chronic illness sharply delineates the nature and quality of control, often resulting in a sense of powerlessness in individuals and their families.

Chronic illness disrupts personal control and changes life activities and expectations. Maintaining personal control is important for persons with chronic illness; lack of self-management and inability to predict the course of their disease can be distressing. Decision making to manage and control everyday life with a chronic illness is complex and bound to individually constructed lives (Thorne, Paterson, & Russell, 2003). Perceptions of control are associated with greater levels of psychosocial well-being while perceptions of powerlessness are associated with poorer health and psychosocial outcomes (Hay, 2010). Persons with inflammatory bowel disease reported personal control required maintaining a balance between what one could control versus what one needed to control for everyday life (Cooper, Collier, James, & Hawkey, 2010). Using grounded theory methodology, Pihl-Lesnovska, Hjortswang, Ek, and Frisman (2010) interviewed 11 persons with Crohn's disease. Dominant themes that emerged from their analysis of the data included quality of life, self-image, confirmatory relations, powerlessness, attitude toward life, and a sense of well-being.

Rånhein & Holand (2006) conducted a hermeneutic-phenomenologic study of women's lived experience with chronic pain and fibromyalgia. Themes of powerlessness, ambivalence, and coping emerged from interviews with 12 women with fibromyalgia. The stories of these women revealed their struggles to manage and control the severe symptoms of their disease and their efforts to reduce their feelings of powerlessness that surfaced with pain, fatigue, and immobility. Individuals with chronic illness who develop effective systems for controlling their most severe symptoms have a more positive outlook and a lessened sense of powerlessness. The main challenge of women with chronic pain is to maintain a sense of control of self and pain in order to avoid becoming discouraged. In a theory synthesis, Skuladöttir and Halldorsdóttir (2008) postulate that women with chronic pain face multiple challenges and the threat of demoralization. However, interactions with healthcare providers may be either positive or negative. Positive interactions can result in empowerment in which a sense of control is maintained. Negative interactions can disempower clients and eliminate a sense of control over self and the situation.

Persons with health failure experience increasing powerlessness (Falk, Wahn & Lidell, 2007). A systematic review of 14 qualitative research studies conducted with older adults found that living with chronic heart failure was characterized by physical limitations and stressful symptoms, feelings of powerlessness and hopelessness, and social and role interruptions (Yu, Lee, Kwong, Thompson, & Woo, 2008). Aujoulat, Luminet, and Deccache (2007) conducted interviews with 40 individuals with various chronic conditions and asked them to discuss their experiences of powerlessness. They found that powerlessness extends beyond medical and treatment issues to feelings of insecurity and threats to their social and personal identities. Desperation and powerlessness were expressed by women with long-term urinary incontinence. Women who lacked control of their urinary incontinence reported their autonomy was threatened, which promoted a sense of powerlessness to control their own bodies (Hägglund & Ahlström, 2007).

The phenomenon of powerlessness in chronic illness is a dynamic and complex issue. Powerlessness in chronic illness can be triggered by individual attributes and perceptions or stimulated by the evolving nature of the chronic disease. Powerlessness is inherent and impending in chronic illness. However, feelings of powerlessness recede and advance throughout the course of the chronic illness as individuals negotiate between control and loss and navigate the changing landscape of their daily realities. Variables such as the degree of physical limitation and ability to manage symptoms of chronic illness can also influence an individual's experience with powerlessness.

The Paradox of Powerlessness in Chronic Illness

The paradox of powerlessness in chronic illness is that power and powerlessness exist simultaneously. Power takes for granted powerlessness and vice versa (Kuokkanen & Leino-Kilpi, 2000). Power is defined as the "ability to act or produce an effect" and "possession of control, authority, or influence over others" (Merriam-Webster, 2011). Power can be enabling and enhance one's autonomous ability and capacity. Despite the limiting effects of chronic illness and feelings of powerlessness, individuals continue to exert power and control in areas of their lives through adaptation and accommodation to their evolving abilities and selves.

Power is an individual psychological characteristic (McCubbin, 2001), a personal resource inherent in all individuals, and is the ability to influence what happens to one's self (Miller, 2000). Seeking, getting, and preserving power is a dynamic process that reflects a human being's ability to achieve a desired goal in the face of personal, social, cultural, and environmental facilitators and barriers (Efraimsson, Rasmussen, Gilje, & Sandman, 2003).

In the individual-oriented society of the United States, power is associated with independence and self-determination. Although we may think of power as an individual quality, in reality, power is a relational attribute. Power has no meaning in the absence of relationships with others and the context of the interaction. Power is developed and maintained in relationships. Power can restrict self-determination with forcefulness or authority by restricting the autonomy of another in personal relationships as well as hierarchical organizations (Moden, 2004). Power is a "social, political, economic, and cultural phenomenon, since all these dimensions of human societies determine who has power and what kind" (McCubbin, 2001, p. 76).

Individual power resources include physical strength and physical reserve, psychological stamina and social support, positive self-concept, energy, knowledge, motivation, and hope (Miller, 2000, p. 8). Chronic illness can diminish these power resources. When power resources are significantly altered and affected, an individual with chronic illness may experience feelings of powerlessness. To deal with this powerlessness, persons with chronic illness should direct their energy toward their intact power resources. Power resources facilitate coping with chronic illness. Accordingly when one power resource becomes depleted, other power components may need to be developed to avert or reduce powerlessness (Miller, 2000).

Theoretical Perspectives of Powerlessness and Power

Persons with chronic illness live in a dual world, that of wellness and sickness, of control and powerlessness, and of hope and despair. The Shifting Perspectives Model of Chronic Illness (Paterson, 2001a, 2003) describes chronic illness as a complex dialectic between the individual and his or her world. This model posits that persons with chronic illness shift between the perspective of wellness in the foreground and illness in the background and vice versa. Furthermore, this model suggests that the experience of living with a chronic illness is a dynamic process that reflects the elements of both wellness and illness that comprise chronic illness. A perspective shift is a cognitive and affective strategy to negotiate the effects of chronic illness and to make sense of the experience. The perspectives of wellness and illness are not mutually exclusive, rather there is a fluctuation of the degree to which illness or wellness is in the foreground or background (Paterson, 2001a).

Rather than a static outlook, there is a continual shifting of perspectives (Paterson, 2003). Persons living with chronic illness have a preferred perspective that is assumed most frequently. Therefore, persons with an illness perspective in the foreground focus on their illness, their symptoms, and the negative impact their chronic condition has on them and others. Conversely, from a perspective of wellness in the foreground, the individual views the chronic illness at a distance and focuses on his or her abilities to navigate daily life and to perform roles and responsibilities; the negative aspects of the chronic illness recede to the background. In addition to illness and wellness, this shifting perspectives model acknowledges parallel and simultaneous contradictions in the chronic illness experience such as loss and gain, control, and powerlessness (Paterson, 2003). Hence, persons with a wellness perspective will likely exert power and control over their daily routines and social interactions.

The illness and wellness perspective is dynamic so it can be interrupted and changed at a moment's notice. Such a shift in perspective can be stimulated by physiologic changes, events, fears, and other individuals (Paterson, 2003). Social support, competent care providers, hope, and humor are factors that influence a shift from illness in the foreground to wellness in the foreground (Freeman, O'Dell, & Meola, 2003; Haluska, Jessee, & Nagy, 2002). Exacerbations of symptoms and other forms of illness intrusiveness such as pain, decreased physical function and mobility, low self-worth, and feelings of loss of life goals and aspirations (Mullins, Chaney, Balderson, & Hommel, 2000) may shift an individual's perspective to the disease state, and feelings of loss of control and powerlessness may arise. The "relative importance of the illness, physical experiences with the illness, and biomedical uncertainties" (Sutton & Treloar, 2007, p. 338) can also trigger a shift in perspective. Clinical indicators of chronic disease progression may not be congruent with individual perceptions of health and illness inasmuch as health and illness views are constructed within the individual's physical, emotional, and social spheres and may not be compatible with healthcare priorities (Sutton & Treloar, 2007). Although the focus of illness in the foreground can be self-absorbing, this perspective may provide the individual with an opportunity to learn more about his or her illness and effective strategies to treat and manage symptoms. **Figure 12-1** illustrates the shift of perspectives in chronic illness.

Self-Determination Theory (SDT)

Self-determination theory (SDT) highlights the psychological processes that promote optimal

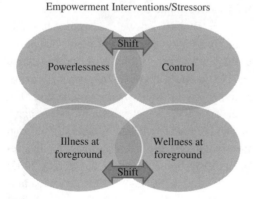

FIGURE 12-1   Shifting Perspectives in Chronic Illness.
Source: Paterson, B.L. (2001a). The shifting perspectives model of chronic illness. *Journal of Nursing Scholarship*, 33, 21–26A and Paterson, B.L. (2003). The koala has claws: Applications of the shifting perspectives model in research of chronic illness. *Qualitative Health Research*, 13(7), 987–994.

functioning and health. This theory posits three basic, innate psychological needs that are the basis for optimal functioning and personal well-being. These psychological needs—competence, relatedness, and autonomy—are universal and must be satisfied for all people to achieve optimal health. These basic psychological needs provide a framework that specifies the conditions in which people can maximize their human potential. The need for competence results in an individual's ability to adapt to new challenges in a changing context; it stimulates unique talents of individuals and produces adaptive competencies and flexible functioning in the context of changing demands. The need for relatedness is the integration of the individual into the social world in which the individual seeks attachments, security, and a sense of belonging and intimacy with others. The tendencies of relatedness are to cohere to one's group and to feel connection with and care of others. However, the need for relatedness can compete or conflict with autonomy. Autonomy, according to SDT, refers to self-organization and self-regulation, and conveys adaptive advantage. Autonomous individuals function and respond effectively within changing contexts and circumstances. When behavior is regulated by outside pressures and expectations, holistic functioning is precluded. Therefore, autonomous individuals are better able to regulate their actions in accordance with their perceived needs and available capacities as well as coordinate and prioritize courses of action that will maximize self-maintenance (Deci & Ryan, 2000; Ryan & Deci, 2000).

Self-determination theory distinguishes between autonomous and controlled behavior regulation. Behaviors are autonomous when persons experience a sense of choice to act out of personal importance of the behavior. Controlled behaviors, on the other hand, are those performed when persons feel pressured by external forces (Deci & Ryan, 1985, 1991). Autonomous regulation, or the choice to do what is important and relevant to the individual, is associated with subjective experiences of vitality and energized behavior and differentiated controlled and autonomous choice (Moller, Deci, & Ryan, 2006). Adjustment to chronic illness is influenced by the extent to which individuals believe themselves to be the source of their actions, that is, their feelings of autonomy (Igreja et al., 2000). Patient-centered care is grounded in self-determination theory. In *Crossing the Quality Chasm,* the Institute of Medicine (2001) recognizes the patient as the source of control. Patient-centered care focuses on the patient rather than the disease and gives the responsibility for disease management to the patient along with the resources and support needed to assume that responsibility.

Cognitive Adaptation Theory

Cognitive Adaptation Theory posits that an individual's attempt to maintain or regain a sense of personal control may be heightened or activated by the psychological challenge that can arise out of an unpredictable illness. The heightened sense of personal control may be used as a way to maintain positive adaptation to chronic illness. An enhanced perception of control may facilitate coping with an illness-related stressor such as exacerbation of symptoms or disease progression (Taylor, 1983), whereas absence of self-control promotes dependency, powerlessness, and erodes client autonomy (McCann & Clark, 2004).

PROBLEMS AND ISSUES ASSOCIATED WITH POWERLESSNESS

There are a number of issues associated with powerlessness. Issues discussed here are examples of what individuals and their families may experience; however, it is not an all inclusive list.

Loss

From a medical viewpoint, chronic illness is comprised of physical symptoms and limitations. From a broader perspective, chronic illness brings multiple losses for individuals and their families on the physical side, but perhaps even more so on the psychological level. The diagnosis of a chronic illness may, in and of itself, represent a loss to the individual, and for some, the diagnosis of a chronic illness may be as significant as a death. The diagnosis of the chronic illness may represent the loss of hopes and dreams, income, sexual ability, physical and mental ability, quality of life, or independence (Clarke & James, 2003). The loss of mobility and agility as a result of chronic illness affects one's ability to participate in social activities and to maintain social ties (Beal, 2007). Loss of paid employment due to chronic illness has a significant impact on one's life. Leaving work not only results in the loss of income and daily routines but triggers a loss of positive social identity (Walker, 2010).

Persons with chronic illness have restrictions in their daily lives, experience social isolation, feel they are discounted, and fear becoming a burden to others (Charmaz, 1983). Loss of self is felt by many persons with chronic illness (Charmaz, 1983), in which the serious debilitating effects of chronic illness erode the former self-image of the individual. Over time, accumulated loss of self-image can result in diminished self-concept. Loss of self is a result of chronic illness that diminishes control over lives and futures (Charmaz, 1983). Lack of self-confidence and disrupted identity are two major factors of powerlessness. In-depth interviews with clients with various chronic conditions revealed numerous losses including their loss of self-control and confidence as their environment and possibilities become diminished (Aujoulat, Luminet, & Deccache, 2007).

Uncertainty

Chronic illness generates a wide array of emotions and reactions and engenders anxiety and uncertainty. The uncertainty of chronic illness promotes feelings of loss of control and a sense of powerlessness in individuals and families (Mishel, 1999). Narratives of persons diagnosed with multiple sclerosis revealed concerns about the unpredictable progression of the disease and fear and anxiety relative to the unknown (Barker-Collo, Cartwright, & Read, 2006). Severity of the illness, the erratic nature of symptomatology, and the ambiguity of symptoms promote uncertainty in persons with chronic illness (Mishel, 1999). Anticipating and planning for the future becomes complicated. The unpredictability of physical symptoms and capabilities interferes with the individual's ability to schedule activities and events in the future and may result in an unwillingness to plan in advance. The uncertainty of the chronic illness raises salient concerns for persons about their future, about their ability to control their illness and symptoms, and their capacity to garner necessary personal and financial resources to manage their illness (see Chapter 7).

Chronic Illness Management

Chronic illness management often entails a multifaceted self-management regimen. The complexity of chronic illness has the potential to strip away a client's sense of self-worth and confidence. Clients who lack confidence often are unable to assess their needs accurately, and consequently are at risk of being manipulated or coerced by others and may capitulate to the wishes of family members or healthcare professionals. Self-management of complex chronic disease is often difficult to achieve and is reflected in low rates of adherence to treatment guidelines (Newman, Steed, & Mulligan, 2004). Although some healthcare professionals believe they can motivate persons with chronic illness to follow a treatment regimen, the impetus to follow a plan of care is internal. Healthcare professionals must acknowledge the personal context of the chronic illness and assess the individual motivators to follow a plan of care (Singleton, 2002). Persons with a chronic illness may not be willing to or capable of carrying out the complex tasks and activities to manage their chronic illness, and a simple "pep talk" from one's healthcare professional simply does not suffice. Clients' realization that their days are built around their healthcare regimen—that is, specific treatments they must perform every day, doctor visits, lab tests, body scans, consults with other healthcare providers, physical therapy, and not other aspects of their lives—can become unbearable. The power to dictate how individuals with chronic illness want to spend their day is gone. For example, Mrs. Jones, an elderly widow with end-stage renal disease must spend 3 days a week at the local dialysis unit to manage her chronic illness. Even though she has accepted the time involved to adhere to her treatment regimen and has accommodated her lifestyle accordingly, she yearns to visit her extended family that lives some distance from her. At her peril, Mrs. Jones chooses to spend time with her family, to forego prescribed treatment, and to bear the consequences of her decision. In the end, although Mrs. Jones was able to continue her dialysis treatments, her decision was motivated by her personal desire and familial priority, not the prescribed treatment.

Mr. Smith, a young man with AIDS, experiences difficulties adhering to a complex pharmacologic regimen because of financial constraints. Mr. Smith finds himself consumed with an ongoing process of seeking resources to maintain his prescribed treatment, which takes away his ability to participate in other areas of his life. The lives of the elderly woman (Mrs. Jones) and young man center around their chronic illness and treatment-regimen activities. Both experiences a loss of control over time management, personal choice, and quality of life. Their chronic illness and treatment regimens consume their daily lives to the detriment of other activities, and feelings of powerlessness arise. What was true for Mrs. Jones and Mr. Smith is also true for other persons dealing with chronic illness. The lack of self-control inherent in their disease and treatment fosters feelings of dependence and powerlessness, and undermines client autonomy (McCann & Clark, 2004).

In contrast, the ability to control one's treatment plan, choose services, and avoid coercion diminishes powerlessness (Nelson, Lord, & Ochocka, 2001). Support is essential to meet the demands and expectations of complex management regimens of chronic illness. Necessary supports include good communication with healthcare professionals, adequate financial resources, time and ability to perform care tasks, and spiritual support (Singleton, 2002).

Can we just have one day when we do not see a healthcare provider? It's a doctor appointment, re-checking lab results, radiation therapy, out-patient IV antibiotics, a port that is clogged, etc. This is a life? Where is our relationship of old when we used to talk about things other than "lab results," how much you've vomited, when the next appointment is? Why is every day of the weekend filled with an ER visit or an outpatient procedure of some type?

—*Jenny, wife of a newly diagnosed cancer patient*

Another key element to adherence to treatment regimens is meaningful participation in healthcare organizations (Nelson, Lord, & Ochocka, 2001). Choice of treatment regimen and control of that regimen are central to self-determination in persons with chronic conditions. To provide appropriate information, the nurse must listen to the needs, wants, and desires of the client. When clients feel unheard and have no voice, they feel invalidated and dismissed, and they feel powerless (Courts, Buchanan, & Werstlein, 2004). As a result of this powerlessness, the opportunity for the nurse to enhance client outcomes diminishes greatly.

Lack of Knowledge

Knowledge about chronic illness is essential for disease management and control. Lack of knowledge or skills about the disease may impact the dynamics of the disease. Often, information and education about the chronic illness occur during the acute phase of the illness or during hospitalization— overwhelming periods when the client and family may not have been able to grasp the concepts. Unfamiliar surroundings coupled with the insecurities of a new or recurrent chronic illness diagnosis impact learning. Although the client may have listened intently to the instructions and education, he or she may not have been able to internalize and actualize the content. As a result, after discharge from the acute care setting, the client may lack sufficient knowledge to effectively manage issues and problems that arise from the chronic condition. Lack of information to successfully meet the challenges of daily living further reinforces feelings of powerlessness.

Healthcare professionals frequently assume that once individuals have been provided with information about their chronic illness, they have adequate knowledge and skills to adopt necessary changes to effectively manage their chronic condition. However, Bodenheimer, Lorig, Holman, and Grumbach (2002) estimated that approximately 50% of clients leave a primary care setting with little or no understanding of what was said. Healthcare professionals must ensure that clients have a clear understanding of health information related to management of their chronic illness.

Marginalization/Vulnerability

Knowledge alone is insufficient for management and control of chronic illness. The contextual determinants of health must also be acknowledged. Social determinants of vulnerability include low income, low education, fragile social identity, and limited social networks (Crossley, 2001). Lack of resources contributes to powerlessness. Persons who experience a marginalized sociocultural status and have limited access to economic resources have a greater than average risk of developing health problems and have higher rates of morbidity and mortality associated with chronic illness (Aday, 2001).

The burden of chronic illness disproportionately affects vulnerable populations (Sullivan, Weinert, & Cudney, 2003). Vulnerable clients are the most powerless and the least able to identify and express their needs and desires beyond the completely obvious (Niven & Scott, 2003). Chronic conditions are a significant healthcare challenge, and one's vulnerability is often brought into sharp focus by a chronic disease.

Clients identify the way healthcare professionals relate to them as the cause for their vulnerability, not their chronic illness (Mitchell & Bournes, 2000). Some clients are viewed as having less social value than others (Glaser & Strauss, 1968). Social value is subjective and influenced by such factors as age, marital status, income, living conditions, hygiene, and behavior. Some clients with chronic illnesses may be perceived as having low moral worth. The nurse may believe the client's illness or condition is the result of poor or risky behaviors chosen by the client. Clients who do not behave within the prescribed norms and expectations of the institution or agency may be labeled as undesirable or noncompliant and may not have the opportunity to engage in decision making and control over their healthcare regimen.

Stigma

Persons with chronic illnesses are at risk for stigma based on the negative perceptions held by society (see Chapter 3). Stigma is a response to any physical or social attribute or characteristic that devalues a person's social identity and disqualifies him or her from full social acceptance

(Goffman, 1963). This stigma and the associated stereotypes and misconceptions about chronic illness lead to a lack of inclusion and feelings of powerlessness. Confusion and misinformation about chronic illness can lead to discrimination and stigma and result in unintended, harmful effects for persons with a chronic condition. For example, family and friends of persons with hepatitis C may be fearful and lack knowledge about the virus. For the individual with hepatitis C, the ignorance of others may stimulate feelings of helplessness and infectiousness (Zickmund, Ho, Masuda, Ippolito, & LaBrecque, 2003), or fear of judgment and stigma from those around them (Sutton & Treloar, 2007). In this way, external societal pressures can create and perpetuate feelings of powerlessness in individuals with chronic illness.

Culture

The concepts of powerlessness and power are grounded in the context of cultural values, beliefs, and practices of persons with chronic illness and their families. The traditional power and control culture in the healthcare setting may conflict with cultural customs and beliefs of an individual with a chronic illness. Many cultural groups view the individual as embedded in social relationships, thus the role of the individual in decision making is not recognized. For group-oriented persons or families, power and control may reside within the family rather than with the individual (Davis, Konishi, & Tashiro, 2003). For example, in some Native American families, healthcare decisions are made by the matriarch of the family rather than the individual with chronic illness. Failure to include the family matriarch in the decision-making process diminishes adherence to prescribed treatment regimens. In some cultures, the oldest male holds the power and control to make decisions. Cultural conflicts may arise when families are not consulted before an intervention or staff interferes with rituals deemed necessary by the client's family to promote healing.

Conversely, when a client chooses to go against his or her cultural norm or custom, the client must have the power to do so. In situations where families are in disagreement with the client about compliance with cultural customs, the nurse must support the client and give him or her the resources for self-determination (Zoucha & Husted, 2000). The desires and wishes of the individual client supersede the cultural values, beliefs, and practices of the culture in which the individual and family are in disagreement (Tang & Lee, 2004).

Culture is the context in which individuals, families, and groups make healthcare decisions. Power and control in Western society are based on the concept of individualism—a society consisting of autonomous individuals. Western societies promote the actualization of the individual self as the goal, yet other cultures do not. The Western principle of autonomy is self-determination. In other cultures, the principle of autonomy is family-determination, that is, the family is the autonomous social unit in which the entire family, not the individual, has real authority in decision making. For Chinese cancer patients living in Hong Kong, emphasizing the Chinese cultural beliefs of loyalty to family, letting go, harmony with the universe, and the cycles of life and nature was essential to the development of feelings of empowerment (Mok, Martinson, & Wong, 2004).

Values, beliefs, practices, and responses to chronic illness vary by culture and within culture. Culture impacts and dictates one's responses to normal events of everyday life and is a driving force in the decisions and choices that individuals and families make about health and care (Salas-Provance, Erickson, & Reed, 2002). Some individuals experiencing chronic illness may remain silent about their experiences and issues with chronic illness. This is not an indicator of indifference or incompetence but a reflection of cultural differences in the use of silence. Culturally appropriate care can only occur when cultural care values, expressions, or patterns are known and used appropriately (Leininger, 1995). Life experiences and situations of the past influence the present. For many African Americans, religion and spiritual values provide a method for coping with chronic conditions. Their faith and belief in God give them power to endure pain and suffering associated with their chronic conditions (Anthony, 2007). The centrality of cultural values to healthcare decisions is highlighted in the findings of a survey of 1253 African Americans in Alabama churches. This research found that 59% of the respondents reported they believed in fate or destiny in relation to healthcare decisions and health-seeking behaviors. Women who believed in fate or destiny were less likely than those who did not to have breast examinations (Green, Lewis, Wang, Person, & Rivers, 2004). Knowledge of cultural values, beliefs, and practices provides an invaluable blueprint for healthcare providers in caring for diverse clients with chronic illness. Furthermore, the promotion of cultural values can help clients with chronic illness mitigate their experiences of powerlessness.

Healthcare System

Healthcare systems are based on the assumption that patient safety and system integrity are dependent on the expertise and authority of the healthcare professional. While this type of complex process is essential for those with acute illness who lack expertise to make appropriate decisions, this system is counterproductive for those with chronic illness who develop competency and expertise with regard to management of their chronic conditions (Thorne, 2006). The healthcare system is designed for acute, episodic treatment and strives for efficient and cost-effective care. This fast-paced and impersonal care system leaves little time and individual focus for the person with a chronic condition, which requires a more long-term, illness-management approach. Thus, clients and their families are vulnerable and powerless in the healthcare power structure (Davis et al., 2003). Upon entry into the healthcare system, the client relinquishes control over his or her life, loses self-identity and initiative, and becomes distant from supportive networks. The client's voice may be ignored by healthcare professionals or quieted by dwindling energy levels that come from the disease process itself or the side effects of treatment.

Power is inherent in the healthcare system. Education and professional status are sources of power for healthcare providers in the nurse–client relationship. The procedures and language used by healthcare professionals are foreign and strange to the client and leave many persons with chronic conditions unable or unwilling to be an active participant in their health care (Anthony, 2007). The healthcare system provides fragmented care for persons with chronic illness and leaves individuals feeling isolated and left to care for themselves with inadequate knowledge and resources. Frustration and inability to overcome obstacles in accessing, receiving, and paying for services add to feelings of powerlessness.

The healthcare system perpetuates client vulnerability. It has the potential to restrict the autonomy of people and to disable and dominate them by virtue of its bureaucracy, scientific expertise, and technology. Clients surrender their independence to the healthcare system, where the physician is omniscient and clients begin the process of learned helplessness and an inability to speak for themselves (Hewitt, 2002). Today, decisions in the healthcare system are made by power brokers who are neither providers nor consumers of health care, but insurance companies, Wall Street firms, think tanks, consultants, and pharmaceutical companies (Sheridan-Gonzalez, 2000). This type of healthcare system perpetuates client powerlessness.

> Powerlessness can be seen in the context of becoming a patient, the expectations of individuals, and the ways in which they play by the rules. It is also a key to understanding the ways in which their horizons change, both as facts—the loss of mobility and contact—and as metaphor—acceptance, control, and changing outlook. It is a response to the limits of the conditions itself, and to the power which is perceived to be vested in the health care system. (Gibson & Kenrick, 1998, p. 743)

> My life is like a roller coaster . . . some days my life is full of light and joy . . . but those up days are becoming fewer and fewer now that my fibromyalgia and Parkinson's are so much a part of my life. What can I do? The uncertainty of every day makes me so angry, so confused, so sad. I want to escape from all of this but where would I go? You

> know, I really thought I could beat this. I've done it before but now . . . my pain is relentless! My body is unwilling! What choice do I have?
>
> —*Anne*

INTERVENTIONS

Persons with chronic illness feel overwhelmed, exhausted, and discouraged at times. Therefore, one of the most important challenges for nurses working with these clients is to help them overcome feelings of powerlessness. Factors that impact powerlessness in persons with chronic illness are complex and multidimensional. Nursing interventions to address powerlessness in chronic illness should be equally multifaceted and require attention to the complex nature of the healthcare situation. Appropriate and relevant nursing interventions are based on ongoing assessments and observations of the client with chronic illness in his or her environment, the context in which the person manages and copes with chronic illness. This includes not only the physical surroundings but also the psychosocial dimensions of life. Because of the dynamic nature of chronic illness, continuing evaluation of interventions with subsequent modifications to meet the current needs of the client are required. The goals of nursing interventions are to assist the client to manage the realities of one's limitations and illuminate strengths to reduce a sense of powerlessness and loss and to create new boundaries for one's changed life. Persons with chronic illness seek a sense of normalcy and a sense of dignity by focusing on personal strengths and remaining engaged in family and social activities to diminish isolation and loneliness (Skuladóttir & Halldorsdóttir, 2011).

CASE STUDY

Maria, a widowed 73-year-old Mexican American woman, lives independently in her small home in a rural community. She is a devout Catholic, attends mass daily, and is a member of the church's women's group. She works part time in the kitchen at the local nursing home to supplement her social security income. Maria attended school in Mexico and completed 8th grade. She speaks and reads limited English. Maria's only living child lives out of state and due to finances and family commitments, is able to visit infrequently. During a recent hospitalization for influenza, Maria was diagnosed with type II diabetes. When learning of her chronic illness, Maria was overcome with emotion and anxiety about what her future would hold. Would she be able to continue to work to support herself? Would she lose her legs like her mother? Would she die like her son? Maria felt overwhelmed with all of the information the nurses and doctors were telling her about her treatment plan. They used words and language she didn't understand. She was reluctant to ask questions or tell them her concerns and needs. She was silent. She prayed. Upon discharge, despite all the discharge instructions and papers she was given, Maria didn't know how to manage her care at home. She didn't feel well enough to return to work, and she stopped going to church and slept most of the day. At an office visit, the nurse practitioner noted that Maria was having difficulty managing her diabetes and ordered home health visits. During her first visit, Sara, the home health nurse, told Maria exactly what she needed to do to get her diabetes under control. Sara wrote out detailed instructions for Maria about her medications, diet, and exercise. Yet again, Maria was unable to express her fears and wishes. At each subsequent visit, Sara reinforced the treatment plan. When Maria was unsuccessful in maintaining glucose control, Maria was labeled as noncompliant. Maria became discouraged, despondent, and overcome with feelings of hopelessness and powerlessness.

Discussion Questions

1   How do the physical and psychosocial challenges experienced by Maria contribute to her feelings of lack of control and sense of powerlessness?
2. How do theoretical perspectives of power and powerlessness guide a plan of care for Maria?
3. If you were the home health nurse, what nursing interventions would you implement to restore power and control to Maria? How would you prioritize her plan of care?
4. How would you ensure culturally appropriate restoration of power and control for Maria? How would you address issues of vulnerability and power?

Nursing interventions to restore client control and increase power resources in clients with chronic illness are discussed in this section. The following are strategies and tools to strengthen the client's power base.

Empowerment

Empowerment is a health-enhancing process. The outcome of client empowerment is self-efficacy, mastery and control, and a renewed and valued sense of self. Key issues to empowerment are self-awareness and self-determination. Self-determination is the ability to make choices and accept responsibility for one's choices (Aujoulat, d'Hoore, & Deccache, 2007). Client empowerment in chronic illness is the personal transformation through a dialectic process of "holding on" to former self-representations and roles and learning to manage the disease and treatment in order to differentiate one's self from the illness and "letting go" or relinquishing control to integrate the chronic illness into a reconciled self. "Holding on" is linked to efforts to gain control and maintain a sense of mastery whereas the process of "letting go" is linked to a search for meaning and an acceptance that chronic illness is not always controllable (Aujoulat, Marcolongo, Bonadiman, & Deccache, 2008). The nurse–client relationship emphasizes the primacy of the client's own ideas, emotions, and beliefs about the chronic illness. Within this relationship, the nurse must provide information and opportunities for choice and negotiation regarding treatment-related issues. The nurse must be attentive to individual beliefs and desires with regard to choice and control. Empowerment may not be a desirable outcome or process for all clients, inasmuch as clients differ in their desire to participate in

their own healthcare decisions (Loft, McWilliam, & Ward-Griffin, 2001) and rely on others such as family members or healthcare professionals to make decisions for them.

Empowerment strategies and efforts increase power and strengthen individual life circumstances. Two dimensions of empowerment emerge from the literature. One dimension is psychological, which includes self-esteem and self-efficacy. The other dimension of empowerment is social, action oriented, and comprised of power, involvement, and control over individual life circumstances (Hansson & Bjorkman, 2005). Key features of empowering provider–client relationships include continuity of care, patient-centeredness, and mutual acknowledgement and relatedness (Aujoulat, d'Hoore, & Deccache, 2007).

Empowerment is important for clients with chronic illness because it increases perceived quality of life and promotes self-esteem. For empowerment, clients need access to information, resources, support, and opportunity (Laschinger, Gilbert, Smith, & Leslie, 2010). Empowerment results when individual perception of needs for care has been met (Roth & Crane-Ross, 2002).

Healthcare providers can promote client empowerment by providing access to relevant, timely, and appropriate information about an illness or treatment. Ongoing information can be provided through the use of information technology including email and vetted Internet sites. Client access to necessary support and resources further enhances empowerment. Nurses can assist clients with identifying sources of social support and introduce them to alternative resources within the family or community systems (Laschinger et al., 2010).

Health Coaching

Patient-centered strategies such as incorporating lifestyle changes, engaging in prevention strategies, and making decisions to promote self-management of chronic illness can be developed. Although not a new idea in the practice of nursing, the reemergence of the idea of client-centered care is reflected in health coaching. Health coaching is client centered, and clients are actively involved in determining what is important and what they want to accomplish relative to the management of their chronic illness. Health coaching motivates behavior change in clients through collaboration, open-ended inquiry, and questions and reflection (Huffman, 2007).

Discharge Planning

Effective discharge planning is another strategy of empowerment. Discharge planning strengthens the client's position and role in social and healthcare systems. A client-tailored and well orchestrated discharge plan enhances coping with relocation from one healthcare setting to another. Open and clear communication among all participants including the client, the family, and healthcare professionals is essential for mutual understanding and successful discharge. Nurses may think of discharge planning simply from the acute healthcare setting to another care setting. However, the concept of long-range discharge planning is essential when dealing with clients with chronic illness, where the client transitions from one setting to another.

Collaboration

Successful management of chronic illness and optimal wellness is based on collaboration and partnership with clients to establish mutually negotiated and established healthcare and treatment goals. Collaboration is promoted when the client is encouraged and expected to participate in his or her own care and make decisions that are based on the client's self-determined needs (Laschinger et al., 2010). Standardized approaches to empowering and improving the quality of life in persons with chronic illness are not appropriate. The lack of a match between a person's readiness and the healthcare professional's interventions may result in lack of adherence to the prescribed treatment regimen. Adherence is a dynamic process that is compromised by barriers usually related to different aspects of the chronic illness. Such barriers include social and economic factors, healthcare team and system, characteristics of the disease, therapies, and client-related factors. Solving problems related to each of these is necessary to promote client adherence (World Health Organization [WHO], 2003).

The client with a chronic illness must be a full partner with the healthcare professional in decision making. Imparting knowledge and information to clients is an exchange process and requires active client participation. However, there are times when the client may not desire information because of fear of the information, information overload, or lack of ability to understand the information. The nurse needs to assess client readiness for information by acknowledging the client's concerns, listening to their perspectives, and respecting their desire for new information. Disempowering relationships results from discounting experiential knowledge and provision of inadequate resources (Paterson, 2001b).

Self-Management

Persons with chronic illness must be empowered to be managers of their own care within their own realities and settings. The opportunities to manage self-control are dependent on the context in which the clients live their everyday lives (Delmar et al., 2006). Psychological, behavioral, environmental, social, and socioeconomic factors determine one's ability to self-manage one's chronic illness and adhere to a complex treatment regimen (Granger, Moser, Germino, Harrell, & Ekman, 2006). In an institutional setting (acute or long-term care), clients with a chronic illness may be highly motivated to manage their own care. However, the clients' environment dictates the parameters of activities of daily living and may severely limit the opportunity to fully operationalize self-management despite ability and desire. In this instance, nurses can be instrumental in altering the institutional structure to accommodate the self-control goals of clients.

Self-management is more than adherence to a treatment regimen but also takes into account the psychological and social management of living with a chronic illness. Chronic illnesses vary in how they intrude on the psychological and social worlds of individuals. The outcome of empowerment is self-management of chronic illness through the reinforcement of self-determination and control (Aujoulat, d'Hoore, & Deccache, 2007). Self-management interventions for persons with chronic conditions need to be developed to assist them to better manage their illnesses and to take increasing responsibility for their disease (see Chapter 14). Healthcare providers must take into account the shifting nature of chronic conditions and offer self-management strategies appropriate for the problems and issues that may be encountered at a particular phase of the illness. Granger and colleagues (2006) propose the use of Trajectory Theory to ensure interventions are patient-centered and

relevant to an illness phase the client is experiencing or may encounter in the future. Further, healthcare providers must be aware that some persons with chronic illness may not have the physical or mental abilities for self-management. Assess-ment of the client to determine if self-management is attainable, realistic, and desired is necessary.

The difficulty in managing complex treatment schedules of chronic illnesses has led to the development of self-management interventions (SMIs). The key feature of these SMIs is to increase clients' involvement and control in their treatment, and to improve the subsequent impact on their lives (Newman et al., 2004). The skills necessary for clients to develop a SMI are problem solving and goal setting. Even with these skills in place, most persons with chronic illnesses are likely to encounter barriers to care that create major challenges in compliance with SMIs. Those who experience increased barriers are less likely to adhere to plans of care. Barriers include time constraints, knowledge deficits, limited social support, inadequate resources, limited coping skills, poor client–provider relationship, and low self-efficacy. Patient-centered, collaborative nursing strategies reinforce client strengths and ameliorate the impact of these barriers. The nurse becomes a partner with the client to facilitate collaboration in the development of a realistic self-management program and to identify resources and support systems to reach the goal of self-management. Failure of the nurse to identify or adequately estimate barriers to and resources for self-management will negatively impact adherence to the treatment regimen (Nagelkerk, Reick, & Meengs, 2006).

Control

Aujoulat, Marcolongo, Bonadiman, and Deccache (2008) posit: "the process of relinquishing control is as central to empowerment as is the process of gaining control" (p. 1228). Perceived control is an antecedent to function, a mediator between social support and psychological well-being, and is useful for effective disease self-management (Jacelon, 2007). Perceived control is related to better adjustment to chronic illness. Nurses need to be aware of two dimensions of perceived control (Rotter, 1966). First, one can believe one is personally able to control one's outcomes and second one can believe that more powerful others control one's outcomes. The latter, vicarious control can be exerted by physicians, parents, God, or family. To assist the client in achieving optimal functioning, the nurse must assess the client's belief about the source of control, whether within self or from others.

When the professional nurse exerts too much control, the client may totally relinquish control and put his or her life in the hands of the professional to the detriment of their empowerment (Delmar et al., 2006). Client power is a fundamental element in the client–provider relationship because clients, due to their chronic illness, may become dependent and thus subordinate to healthcare professionals (Efraimsson et al., 2003). Independence, self-control, and self-responsibility are important elements for increasing patient empowerment. The ability to ask for assistance may be an indicator of self-control and self-management (Delmar et al., 2006).

Self-Determination

Self-determination is a basic human right of individual choice and control. Self-determination ensures that an individual has the autonomy and support to make decisions and to reach personal goals. Self-determination must be balanced with safety and risk of the client and family. Self-determination restores power of choice to the client.

Fostering self-control is integral to promoting wellness in persons with chronic illness, and this control is central to self-determination. To be self-determined, clients must have knowledge and resources to deal with illness-related issues as they arise (McCann & Clark, 2004). Good choices are the result of good options from which to choose. Nurses can give persons with chronic illness adequate and appropriate knowledge as a foundation for making the good choice (Delmar et al., 2006). To manage self-control and live with dignity involves support from healthcare professionals and significant others in the decision-making process. Other people can help provide knowledge and expertise as a foundation for making the right choice. Clients with significant physical or mental impairments may be unable to engage in social discourse and may require additional resources to promote self-management. The nurse should provide the client with appropriate and relevant resources and work with the client and his or her family to obtain connections and referrals to appropriate community-based services.

Establishing a Sense of Mastery

Powerlessness is reduced and empowerment is facilitated by the development of a sense of mastery. Mastery is helping clients to focus on how they can affect their chronic conditions and can foster a sense of control in an otherwise uncontrollable illness course. Intervention techniques encourage clients to identify strengths and shift the focus away from uncontrollable aspects of chronic illness, such as use of a wheelchair or dialysis treatments, to the controllable aspects, such as decision making or self-care activities, which can imbue patients with a sense of mastery over their condition (Cvengros, Christensen, & Lawton, 2005). The WHO (2003) published guidelines for healthcare professionals to facilitate client identification of strategies to reduce barriers to mastery and facilitate integration of self-care into daily activities.

Client and Family Education

Persons with chronic illnesses and their families need information, understanding, and competent interventions to help them reformulate their lives, assimilate their losses, and adjust to the changes brought about by their illnesses (Sullivan-Bolyai, Sadler, Knafl, & Gillis, 2003). Information about chronic disease management provides clients with a sense of control and thus increases empowerment (Sommerset, Campbell, Sharp, & Peters, 2001; Wollin, Dale, Spenser, & Walsh, 2000).

Over their lifetimes, persons with chronic illness and their families must shoulder the burden of coordinating medical information and treatment regimens. The need for information must be tailored to meet the needs of the individual client relative to the disease course. The client may not be able to take in information at the time of the diagnosis of a chronic illness; therefore, information should be available to the client and his or her family at a follow-up visit to ensure understanding of information and available services (Barker-Collo et al., 2006). The time of diagnosis of a chronic disease is overwhelming and confusing for clients and their families. The expectation that clients will be able to assimilate the information given to them about their chronic illness may be unrealistic.

In addition to information and knowledge about the chronic illness, the client needs information about available, accessible, appropriate, and affordable resources and services within his or her community. The nurse is the client's link to these resources (Falk-Rafael, 2001). Therefore, it is necessary for the nurse to maintain current information about community resources and services. The nurse assesses the client's needs and preferences, selects appropriate resources for the client, and evaluates the effectiveness and acceptability of the resources to the client. The nurse may also link the client and his or her family to support groups, which can promote empowerment through the expression of shared experiences.

Many clients may also seek information about their chronic illness on the Internet. The ability to obtain this information independent of a healthcare professional can give the client a sense of control and self-determination. As a result, many visit their healthcare providers with requests for specific tests or medications (Corbin & Cherry, 2001). However, this information should be evaluated by the nurse to determine the appropriateness of the suggestion. Online communication and Internet support groups have become not only sources of information for individuals with chronic illness but also sources of social support (Laschinger et al., 2010; van Uden-Kraan, Drossaert, Taal, Seydel & van de Laar, 2009). Women are more likely to use the Internet for health information and illness-related support than are their male counterparts (Pandey, Hart, & Tiwary, 2003).

Healthcare System Navigation

The concept of patient navigation first appeared in the literature in the 1990s as a means to improve access to health care for medically underserved populations. Patient navigation moves beyond advocacy to identify barriers and challenges to healthcare access and focuses on individual well-being. It is a process in which clients are guided through the bureaucracy of the healthcare system by a nurse advocate in order to complete a specific diagnostic procedure or therapeutic task. By assisting underserved individuals to "navigate" the complex healthcare system, it reduces barriers to healthcare access and treatment. Patient navigators also mobilize appropriate resources for the client. In a study of low-income women of color with breast abnormalities, patient navigation was shown to improve the timeliness of diagnosis, compliance with follow-up treatment (Psooy, Schreuer, Borgaonkar, & Caines, 2004), and diagnostic resolution follow-up by healthcare providers (Ell, Vourlekis, Lee, & Xie, 2007). Furthermore, patient navigation has been successful in reducing barriers to care and improving health outcomes in persons with HIV (Bradford, Coleman, & Cunningham, 2007).

Patient navigators promote self-determination in their clients as a means of empowering them. Although patient navigators are charged with helping clients obtain necessary healthcare services, clients must be afforded the respect to choose regarding their individual welfare. The role of patient navigators reveals the essential elements of nursing functions such as liaison and resource coordinator. Patient navigators also have potential utility for serving at-risk women with high incidences of powerlessness (Ell et al., 2007).

Advocacy

In addition to patient navigation, advocacy is an important tool for increasing empowerment in clients with chronic illness. Advocacy activities seek to redistribute power and resources to people (individuals or groups) who demonstrate a need. Although the ideal of nursing advocacy is to empower clients within the healthcare system, often institutional, social, political, economic, and cultural constraints prevent clients from accessing health care. When such constraints are present, an advocate is necessary to facilitate procurement. The manner in which the nurse advocate intercedes to increase the client's power depends on the underlying values and beliefs held by the nurse regarding the advocate role. No one wants to be dependent on others, to inconvenience others, or to be a burden to others. Dignity and respect are linked with individual independence. The nurse must take care to ensure the client is still authoritative in his or her own life and is able to maintain responsibility and self-determination. Even when these elements are present, situations may arise in which clients need help from an advocate to regain dignity and integrity.

Decision Making

When clients make their own decisions and act on them, there may be a difference between the client's choices and those that would have been made by family members or healthcare professionals. Consequently, clients may not only experience disapproval from others regarding their decisions, but also may encounter resistance when attempting to implement them. As previously discussed, Mrs. Jones made a decision to interrupt her dialysis treatments for several days to connect with her family despite protests from her primary care nurse and physician. Upon learning of Mrs. Jones's decision to discontinue treatment for a short time, the primary care nurse contacted the children of Mrs. Jones to persuade them to exert control and interrupt Mrs. Jones's plans. In the end, the sons and daughters of Mrs. Jones agreed to honor the choice and decision made by their mother. This example provides the foundation for further discussions among nurses engaged in client-empowered health care. How much control belongs to the client, the healthcare professional, or family members? How do control issues affect the nurse–client, the nurse–family, and the client–family relationships? What are the guiding principles in this approach to nursing care of clients with chronic illness?

Nurses must provide clients all information necessary to make a decision. Providing information about the illness and the services that are available will facilitate informed decisions (Aylett & Fawcett, 2003). As clients come to know the nature and meaning of their illnesses, their power tends to be restored and their vulnerability is reduced.

Anticipatory Guidance

Anxiety is triggered by an uncertain future. Uncertainty of the illness trajectory suggests the need for the nurse to offer anticipatory guidance to persons with chronic illnesses. Anticipatory guidance is based on identifying expected future needs and can begin weeks, months, or years before any actual help is required. Future needs can have a profound effect on clients' lives because major life decisions can be influenced by them. Clients need a coach to help them chart an anticipated course throughout their chronic illness (Courts et al., 2004). Anticipating future dependency needs allows clients with progressive chronic illnesses to express their own wishes and preferences for care options. Informed anticipation lacks certainty, but it facilitates greater rational future planning for clients and their families, minimizing potentially difficult decisions made during a time of crisis.

Cultural Competence

Cultural competence is a process in which the nurse integrates cultural awareness, cultural knowledge, cultural skills, cultural encounters, and cultural desire to provide care (Campinha-Bacote, 2002). This model assumes variation among persons of different ethnic and cultural groups. For example, in collectivist culture, people may resonate to group norms to experience relatedness and autonomy. In individualist cultures, acting in accordance to the group norm may be viewed as lack of individuality and a threat to autonomy (Ryan & Deci, 2000). It is imperative for nurses to explore potential differences and similarities among clients and their beliefs to ensure culturally competent care (Leininger & McFarland, 2002). Leininger (1995) asserts, "clients who experience nursing care that fails to be reasonably congruent with the client's beliefs, values, and care life ways will show signs of cultural conflicts, noncompliance, stresses, and ethical or moral concerns" (p. 45). When nurses acknowledge and incorporate the client's cultural perspective, an environment of communication and understanding increases feelings of power and control in the client and family.

OUTCOMES

Outcomes associated with powerlessness in clients with chronic conditions can be measured from three perspectives: self, relationships with others, and client behaviors. From the first perspective, changes in self are evaluated by measures such as increased self-confidence and self-esteem, which facilitate coping with and management of chronic illness. The best outcomes for persons with chronic illness occur when clients learn to self-manage their chronic illness. The client must monitor and make adjustments in the management of the chronic illness, just as a driver of a car turns the wheel, monitors speed, and applies the brakes while driving a car. Self-management presumes the client is given the opportunity to communicate effectively, seek information, collect data, analyze options, and make decisions. Clients need to have information and resources available to them when the need arises, as opposed to when it may be convenient for the healthcare provider to give the information to the client. Healthcare providers must recognize the limits of science for self-management of chronic illness and respect the inherent expertise and primary authority of the client in matters pertaining to living with a chronic illness. In doing so, healthcare providers become consultants and resource brokers within the context of shared care (Thorne, 2006).

Evidence-Based Practice Box

As chronic illness moves from a medical model of treatment and cure to one of self-management of illness with or without professional health care, the literature reveals a variety of strategies designed to enhance and promote patient empowerment. One such approach, face-to-face support groups, is an effective resource for information and support for persons with chronic illness. However, barriers such as geography, distance, time, and physical limitations can exclude persons with chronic conditions from participating in these support groups. As the Internet has become accessible and available to more and more people, online support groups have become a viable alternative to in-person support groups. Research suggests that persons with chronic conditions who participate in online support groups are empowered and report a sense of well-being. Van Uden-Kraan, Drossaert, Taal,

Seydel, and van de Laar (2009) conducted a quantitative research project with 528 individuals who were active in online support groups for persons with breast cancer, fibromyalgia, and arthritis. Results of the online questionnaire found respondents were empowered in several ways by their participation in online support groups. The most significant empowering outcomes were "being better informed" and "enhanced social well-being" (p. 64). Participants had a better understanding of their illness from the personal experience of others and more information about what to expect in the future as a result of peer support. Study participants indicated that the online support group provided more social contacts for them and decreased their loneliness. Further, this research did not note any differences between the diagnostic groups with regard to empowering processes and outcomes. The authors concluded that empowerment is a generic mechanism among persons with chronic illness. Online patient support groups enhance empowerment in persons with chronic conditions. Healthcare providers need to become aware of online support groups as a resource for information and empowerment for their healthcare clients.

Source: van Uden-Kraan, C. F., Drossaert, C. H. C., Taal, E., Seydel, D. R., and van de Laar, M. A. F. J. (2009). Participation in online patient support groups endorses patients' empowerment. *Patient Education and Counseling, 74,* 61–69.

The second outcome of measured change of powerlessness is relationships with others. Changes in relationships include improved relationships with family, friends, and healthcare professionals. Relationships are reciprocal in nature. That is, family, friends, and healthcare professionals must play an active role in providing social support and positive interaction with the client with chronic illness. Positive relationships have a powerful impact on the health and well-being of healthcare clients.

The last measurable outcome of reduced powerlessness is behavior. Changes in behavior include healthcare and goal-oriented decisions, which promote personal responsibility for health (Falk-Rafael, 2001). Positive changes in behavior can result in increased treatment-regimen adherence, better management of symptoms, and decreases in feelings of powerlessness.

Recommendations for Further Conceptual and Data-Based Work

Chronic illness research with a focus on empowerment interventions is essential not only at the micro-level but at the macro-level. Continued development of knowledge and understanding of the experiences and needs of individuals with serious, chronic, progressive, and largely uncontrollable illnesses is essential to the development of effective strategies for greater perception of power and control. As we move away from the medical model to a sociological model of care, client and family empowerment are essential. The process of empowerment interventions at the social level would benefit clients with chronic illness, their families, and healthcare professionals.

STUDY QUESTIONS   www

Using the theoretical perspectives presented, design nursing interventions to reduce powerlessness in persons with chronic illness.

Critique the potential strengths and limitations of nursing interventions to reduce powerlessness.

Discuss the relationship between chronic illness and powerlessness.

Compare and contrast the concepts of power and powerlessness.

Discuss the factors that promote powerlessness in clients with chronic illness.

Examine the association between physiologic and psychosocial factors and powerlessness.

For a full suite of assignments and additional learning activities, **www** use the access code located in the front of your book and visit this exclusive website: **http://go.jblearning.com/larsen**. If you do not have an access code, you can obtain one at the site.

REFERENCES

Aday, L. (2001). *At risk in America*. San Francisco, CA: Jossey-Bass.

Anthony, J. S. (2007). Self-advocacy in health care decision-making among elderly African Americans. *Journal of Cultural Diversity, 14*(2), 88–94.

Asbring, P. (2001). Chronic illness: A disruption of life – identity-transformation among women with chronic fatigue syndrome and fibromyalgia. *Journal of Advanced Nursing, 34*, 312–319.

Aujoulat, I., Luminet, O., & Deccache, A. (2007). The perspective of patients on their experience of powerlessness. *Qualitative Health Research, 17*, 772–785.

Aujoulat, I., d'Hoore, W., & Deccache, A. (2007). Patient empowerment in theory and practice: Polysemy or cacophony? *Patient Education and Counseling, 66*(1), 13–20.

Aujoulat, I., Marcolongo, R., Bonadiman, L., & Deccache, A. (2008). Reconsidering patient empowerment in chronic illness: A critique of models of self-efficacy and bodily control. *Social Science & Medicine, 66*(5), 1228–1239.

Aylett, E., & Fawcett, T. N. (2003). Chronic fatigue syndrome: The nurse's role. *Nursing Standard, 17*(35), 33–37.

Bandura, A. (1989). Human agency in social cognitive theory. *American Psychologist, 44*, 1175–1184.

Barker-Collo, S., Cartwright, C., & Read, J. (2006). Into the unknown: The experiences of individuals living with multiple sclerosis. *Journal of Neuroscience Nursing, 38*(6), 435–446.

Beal, C. C. (2007). Loneliness in women with multiple sclerosis. *Rehabilitation Nursing, 32*(4), 165–171.

Bodenheimer, T., Lorig, K., Holman, H., & Grumbach, K. (2002). Patient self-management of chronic disease in primary care. *Journal of the American Medical Association, 288*(19), 2469–2475.

Bradford, J. B., Coleman, S., & Cunningham, W. (2007). HIV system navigation: An emerging model to improve HIV care access. *AIDS Patient Care and STDs, 21*, S49–S58.

Campinha-Bacote, J. (2002). The process of cultural competence in the delivery of health care services: A model of care. *Journal of Transcultural Nursing, 13*(3), 180–184.

Charmaz, K. (1983). Loss of self: A fundamental form of suffering in the chronically ill. *Sociology of Health & Illness, 83*(2), 168–195.

Clarke, J. N., & James, S. (2003). The radicalized self: The impact on the self of the contested nature of the diagnosis of chronic fatigue syndrome. *Social Science and Medicine, 57*(8), 1387–1395.

Cooper, J. M., Collier, J., James, V., & Hawkey, C. J. (2010). Beliefs about personal control and self-management in 30–40 year olds living with inflammatory bowel disease: A qualitative study. *International Journal of Nursing Studies, 47*, 1500–1509.

Corbin, J. M., & Cherry, J. C. (2001). Epilogue: A proactive model of health care. In R. B. Hyman & J. M. Corbin (Eds.), *Chronic illness research and theory for nursing practice.* New York: Springer.

Courts, J. F., Buchanan, E. M., & Werstlein, P. O. (2004). Focus groups: The lived experience of participants with multiple sclerosis. *Journal of Neuroscience Nursing, 36*(1), 42–47.

Crossley, M. (2001). The "Armistead" project: An exploration of gay men, sexual practices, community health promotion and issues of empowerment. *Journal of Community and Applied Social Psychology, 11*, 111–123.

Cvengros, J. A., Christensen, A. J., & Lawton, W. J. (2005). Health locus of control and depression in chronic kidney disease: A dynamic perspective. *Journal of Health Psychology, 10*(5), 677–686.

Davis, A. J., Konishi, E., & Tashiro, M. (2003). A pilot study of selected Japanese nurses' ideas on patient advocacy. *Nursing Ethics, 10*(4), 404–413.

Deci, E. L., & Ryan, R. M. (1991). A motivational approach to self: Integration in personality. In R. Dienstbier (Ed.), *Nebraska symposium on motivation: Perspectives on motivation, 38* (pp. 237–288). Lincoln, NE: University of Nebraska Press.

Deci, E. L., & Ryan, R. M. (1985). *Intrinsic motivation and self-determination in human behavior.* New York: Plenum Publishing Co.

Deci, E. L., & Ryan, R. M. (2000). The 'what' and 'why' of goal pursuits: Human needs and the self-determination of behavior. *Psychological Inquiry, 11*(4), 227–268.

Delmar, C., Bøje, T., Dylmer, D., Forup, L., Jakobsen, C., Møller, et al. (2006). Independence/dependence–a contradictory relationship? Life with a chronic illness. *Scandinavian Journal of Caring Sciences, 20*(3), 261–268.

Efraimsson, E., Rasmussen, B. H., Gilje, F., & Sandman, P. (2003). Expressions of power and powerlessness in discharge planning: A case study of an older woman on her way home. *Journal of Clinical Nursing, 12*, 707–716.

Ell, K., Vourlekis, B., Lee, P-J., & Xie, B. (2007). Patient navigation and case management following an abnormal mammogram: A randomized clinical trial. *Preventive Medicine, 44*, 26–33.

Falk, S., Wahn, A. K., & Lidell, E. (2007). Keeping the maintenance of daily life in spite of chronic heart failure. A qualitative study. *European Journal of Cardiovascular Nursing, 6,* 192–199.

Falk-Rafael, A. (2001). Empowerment as a process of evolving consciousness: A model of empowered caring. *Advances in Nursing Science, 24*(1), 1–16.

Freeman, K., O'Dell, C., & Meola, C. (2003). Childhood brain tumors: Children's and siblings' concerns regarding the diagnosis and phase of illness. *Journal of Pediatric Oncology Nursing, 20*(3), 133–140.

Gibson, J. M. E., & Kenrick, M. (1998). Pain and powerlessness: The experience of living with peripheral vascular disease. *Journal of Advanced Nursing, 27*(4), 737–745.

Glaser, B. G., & Strauss, A. L. (1968). *Time for dying.* Chicago: Aldine.

Goffman, E. (1963). *Notes on management of spoiled identity.* Englewood Cliffs, NJ: Prentice-Hall.

Granger, B. B., Moser, D., Germino, B., Harrell, J., & Ekman, I. (2006). Caring for patients with chronic heart failure: The trajectory model. *European Journal of Cardiovascular Nursing, 5,* 222–227.

Green, B. L., Lewis, R. K., Wang, M. Q., Person, S., & Rivers, B. (2004). Powerlessness, destiny, and control: The influence on health behaviors of African Americans. *Journal of Community Health, 29*(1), 15–27.

Hägglund, D., & Ahlström, G. (2007). The meaning of women's experience of living with long-term urinary incontinence is powerlessness. *Journal of Clinical Nursing, 16*(10), 1946–1954.

Haluska, H. B., Jessee, P. O., & Nagy, M. C. (2002). Sources of social support: Adolescents with cancer. *Oncology Nursing Forum, 29,* 1317–1324.

Hansson, L., & Bjorkman, T. (2005). Empowerment in people with a mental illness: Reliability and validity of the Swedish version of an empowerment scale. *Scandinavian Journal of Caring Sciences, 19,* 3 2–38.

Hay, M. C. (2010). Suffering in a productive world: Chronic illness, visibility, and the space beyond agency. *American Ethnologist, 37*(2), 259–274.

Hewitt, J. (2002). A critical review of the arguments debating the role of the nurse advocate. *Journal of Advanced Nursing, 37*(5), 439–445.

Huffman, M. (2007). Health coaching: A new and exciting technique to enhance patient self-management and improve outcomes. *Home Healthcare Nurse, 25*(4), 271–275.

Igreja, I., Zuroff, D. C., Koestner, R., Saltaris, C., Bropuillette, M. J., & LaLonde, R. (2000). Applying self-determination to the prediction and well-being in gay men with HIV and AIDS. *Journal of Applied Psychology, 30*(4), 686–706.

Institute of Medicine. (2001). *Crossing the quality chasm. A new health system for the 21st century.* Washington, DC: National Academies Press.

Jacelon, C. S. (2007). Theoretical perspectives of perceived control in older adults: A selective review of the literature. *Journal of Advanced Nursing, 59*(1), 1–10.

Johnson, D. (1967). Powerlessness: A significant determinant in patient behavior? *Journal of Nursing Education, 6*(2), 39–44.

Kuokkanen, L., & Leino-Kilpi, H. (2000). Power and empowerment in nursing: Three theoretical approaches. *Journal of Advanced Nursing, 31*(1), 235–241.

Laschinger, H. K. S., Gilbert, S., Smith, L. M., & Leslie, K. (2010). Towards a comprehensive theory of nurse/patient empowerment: Applying Kanter's empowerment theory to patient care. *Journal of Nursing Management, 18,* 4–13.

Leininger, M. L. (1995). *Transcultural nursing: Concepts, theories, research and practice.* Columbus, OH: McGraw-Hill College Custom Series.

Leininger, M. L., & McFarland, M. R. (2002). *Transcultural nursing: Concepts, theories, research and practices* (2nd ed.). New York: McGraw-Hill.

Loft, M., McWilliam, C., & Ward-Griffin, C. (2003). Patient empowerment after total hip and knee replacement. *Orthopedic Nursing, 22*(1), 42–47.

McCann, T., & Clark, E. (2004). Advancing self-determination with young adults who have schizophrenia. *Journal of Psychiatric and Mental Health Nursing, 11,* 12–20.

McCubbin, M. (2001). Pathways to health, illness and well-being: From the perspective of power and control. *Journal of Community and Applied Social Psychology, 11,* 75–81.

Merriam-Webster. (2011) Power. Retrieved December 30, 2010, from: www.merriam-webster.com/dictionary/power

Miller, J. F. (Ed.). (1983). *Coping with chronic illness: Overcoming powerlessness.* Philadelphia: F.A. Davis

Miller, J. F. (Ed.). (1992). *Coping with chronic illness: Overcoming powerlessness* (2nd ed.). Philadelphia: F. A. Davis.

Miller, J. F. (Ed). (2000). *Coping with chronic illness: Overcoming powerlessness* (3rd ed.). Philadelphia: F.A. Davis.

Mishel, M. H. (1999). Uncertainty in illness. *Annual Review of Nursing Research, 19*, 269–294.

Mitchell, G.J., & Bournes, D. A. (2000). Nurse as patient advocate? In search of straight thinking. *Nursing Science Quarterly, 13*(3), 204–209.

Moden, L. (2004). Power in care homes. *Nursing Older People, 16*(6), 24–26.

Mok, E., Martinson, I., & Wong, T. K. (2004). Individual empowerment among Chinese cancer patients in Hong Kong. *Western Journal of Nursing Research, 26*(1), 59–75.

Moller, A. C., Deci, E. L., & Ryan, R. M. (2006). Choice and ego-depletion: The moderating role of autonomy. *Personality and Social Psychology Bulletin, 32*(8), 1024–1036.

Mullins, L., Chaney, J., Balderson, B., & Hommel, K., (2000). The relationship of illness uncertainty, illness intrusiveness and asthma severity to depression in young adults with long-standing asthma. *International Journal of Rehabilitation and Health, 5*, 177–186.

Nagelkerk, J., Reick, K., & Meengs, L. (2006). Perceived barriers and effective strategies to diabetes self-management. *Journal of Advanced Nursing, 54*(2), 151–158.

Nelson, G., Lord, J., & Ochocka, J. (2001). Empowerment and mental health in community: Narratives of psychiatric consumer/survivors. *Journal of Community and Applied Social Psychology, 11*, 125–142.

Newman, S., Steed, L., & Mulligan, K. (2004). Self-management interventions for chronic illness. *Lancet, 364*(9444), 1523–1537.

Niven, C. A., & Scott, P.A. (2003). The need for accurate perception and informed judgment in determining the appropriate use of the nursing resource: Hearing the patient's voice. *Nursing Philosophy, 4*, 201–210.

Pandey, S. K., Hart, J. J., & Tiwary, S. (2003). Women's health and Internet: Understanding emerging trends and implications. *Social Science and Medicine, 56*, 179–191.

Paterson, B. L. (2001a). The shifting perspectives model of chronic illness. *Journal of Nursing Scholarship, 33*, 21–26.

Paterson, B. L. (2001b). Myth of empowerment in chronic illness. *Journal of Advanced Nursing, 34*(5), 574–581.

Paterson, B. L. (2003). The koala has claws: Applications of the shifting perspectives model in research of chronic illness. *Qualitative Health Research, 13*(7), 987–994.

Pihl-Lesnovska, K., Hjortswang, H., Ek, A. C., & Frisman, G. H. (2010). Patients' perspective of factors: Influencing quality of life while living with Crohn's disease. *Gastroenterology Nursing, 33*(1), 37–44.

Psooy, B. J., Schreuer, D., Borgaonkar, J., & Caines, J. S. (2004). Patient navigation: Improving timeliness in the diagnosis of breast abnormalities. *Canadian Association of Radiologists Journal, 55*(3), 145–150.

Rånhein, M., & Holand, W. (2006). Lived experience of chronic pain and fibromyalgia: Women's stories from daily life. *Qualitative Health Research, 16*(6), 741–761.

Roth, D., & Crane-Ross, D. (2002). Impact of services, met needs and service empowerment on consumer outcomes. *Mental Health & Mental Health Services Research, 4*, 43–56.

Rotter, J. P. (1966). Generalized expectancies for internal versus external control of reinforcement. *Psychological Monographs, 80*, 1–28.

Ryan, R. M., & Deci, E. L. (2000). Self-determination theory and the facilitation of intrinsic motivation, social development, and well-being. *American Psychologist, 55*(1), 68–78.

Salas-Provance, M., Erickson, J. G., & Reed, J. (2002). Disability as viewed by four generations on one Hispanic family. *American Journal of Speech-Language Pathology, 11*, 151–162.

Sheridan-Gonzalez, J. (2000). It's not my patient. *American Journal of Nursing, 100*(1), 13.

Singleton, J. K. (2002). Caring for themselves: Facilitators and barriers to women home care workers who are chronically ill following their care plan. *Health Care for Women International, 23*, 692–702.

Skuladöttir, H., & Halldorsdöttir, W. (2011). The quest for well-being: Self-identified needs of women in chronic pain. *Scandinavian Journal of Caring Science, 25*(1), 81–91.

Skuladöttir, H., & Halldorsdöttir, S. (2008). Women in chronic pain: Sense of control and encounters with health professionals. *Qualitative Health Research, 18*, 891–901.

Sommerset, M., Campbell, R., Sharp, D. J., & Peters, T. J. (2001). What do people with MS want and expect from health care services? *Health Expectations, 4,* 29–37.

Strandmark, M. K. (2004). Ill health is powerlessness: A phenomenological study about worthlessness, limitations and suffering. *Scandinavian Journal of Caring Science, 18,* 135–144.

Sullivan, T., Weinert, C., & Cudney, S. (2003). Management of chronic illness: Voices of rural women. *Journal of Advanced Nursing, 44*(6), 566–574.

Sullivan-Bolyai, S., Sadler, L., Knafl, K. A., & Gillis, C. L. (2003). Great expectations: A position description for parents as caregivers: Part 1. *Pediatric Nursing, 29*(6), 457–461.

Sutton, R., & Treloar, C. (2007). Chronic illness experiences, clinical markers and living with Hepatitis C. *Journal of Health Psychology, 12*(2), 330–340.

Tang, S. T., & Lee, S. C. (2004). Cancer diagnosis and prognosis in Taiwan: Patient preferences versus experiences. *Psycho-Oncology, 13,* 1–13.

Taylor, S. E. (1983). Adjustment to threatening events: A theory of cognitive adaptation. *American Psychologist, 38,* 1161–1173.

Thorne, S. (2006). Patient-provider communication in chronic illness: A health promotion window of opportunity. *Family and Community Health, 29*(1S), 4S–11S.

Thorne, S., Paterson, B., & Russell, C. (2003). The structure of everyday self-care decision making in chronic illness. *Qualitative Health Research, 13*(10), 1337–1352.

Van Uden-Kraan, C. F., Drossaert, C. H. C., Taal, E., Seydel, D. R., & van de Laar, M. A. F. J. (2009). Participation in online patient support groups endorses patients' empowerment. *Patient Education and Counseling, 74,* 61–69.

Walker, C. (2010). Ruptured identities: Leaving work because of chronic illness. *International Journal of Health Services, 40*(4), 629–643.

Wollin, J., Dale, H., Spenser, N., & Walsh, A. (2000). What people with newly diagnosed MS (and their families and friends) need to know. *International Journal of MS Care, 2,* 4–14.

World Health Organization (WHO). (2003). *Adherence to long-term therapies: Evidence for action.* Geneva, Switzerland: Author. Retrieved January 21, 2011, from: www.who.int/chp/knowledge/publications/adherence_report/en/

Yu, D. S. F., Lee, D. T. F., Kwong, A. N. T., Thompson, D. R., & Woo, J. (2008). Living with chronic heart failure: A review of qualitative studies of older people. *Journal of Advanced Nursing, 61*(5), 474–483.

Zickmund, S., Ho, E., Masuda, M., Ippolito, L., & LaBrecque, D. (2003). "They treated me like a leper": Stigmatization and the quality of life of patients with hepatitis C. *Journal of General Internal Medicine, 18,* 835–844.

Zoucha, R., & Husted, G. L. (2000). The ethical dimensions of delivering culturally congruent nursing and health care. *Issues in Mental Health Nursing, 21,* 325–340.

CHAPTER 13

Culture and Cultural Competence

Pamala D. Larsen and Sonya R. Hardin

INTRODUCTION

Concepts of health and illness are deeply rooted in culture, race, and ethnicity and influence an individual's perceptions and behavior. Additionally cultures are never homogeneous (Helman, 2007), as there are variations and subcultures within culture, affecting health and illness perceptions differently. So, although, one may know the "norms" of Chinese culture, Puerto Rican culture, or Indian culture, for instance, there will always be unique differences in each individual from that culture.

According to the Office of Minority Health (2005), culture (and language) influences:

- Health, healing, and wellness belief systems
- How illness, disease, and their causes are perceived; both by the patient/consumer and the provider
- The behaviors of patients/consumers who are seeking health care and their attitudes toward providers compromising access and care for those of other cultures
- The delivery of services by the provider who looks at the world through his or her own limited set of values, which can compromise access for patients from other cultures

There are factors other than culture that influence health and illness. Factors include,

but are not limited to, environment, economics, genetics, age, previous and current health status, personality, social support, and psychosocial factors. Caring for the individual, family, and community is therefore influenced by numerous factors of which culture is only one. In Canada, culture is identified as one of the 12 determinants of health (Racher & Annis, 2007).

Currently in the United States there are continuing disparities in health care among those of different cultures, races, ethnicities, and socioeconomic status (Agency for Healthcare Research and Quality [AHRQ], 2010). Throughout the literature, becoming culturally competent is seen as the first step in decreasing and eventually eliminating those disparities. Although being culturally competent is important on an individual basis, becoming so as an organization is just as important. The National Center for Cultural Competence has identified six reasons that organizations should incorporate cultural competence into policy:

1. To respond to the current and projected demographic changes in the United States
2. To eliminate long-standing disparities in the health status of people of diverse racial, ethnic, and cultural backgrounds
3. To improve the quality of services and health outcomes

4. To meet legislative, regulatory, and accreditation mandates
5. To gain a competitive edge in the market place
6. To decrease the likelihood of liability/malpractice claims (Cohen & Goode, 2003)

Defining Terms

Culture

The literature provides many definitions of culture. Within the nursing literature, each individual with his or her model/theory of transcultural nursing has a different definition. Although there is value in those definitions, perhaps one from medical anthropology offers a broader perspective. Helman (2007) defines culture as "a set of guidelines (both explicit and implicit) that individuals use to view the world and tell them what behaviors are appropriate" (p. 2). Culture is shared, learned, dynamic, and evolutionary (Schim, Doorenbos, Benkert, & Miller, 2007). This evolution is described by Dreher and MacNaughton (2002): "People live out their lives in communities, where circumstances generate conflict, where people do not always follow the rules, and where cultural norms and institutions are massaged and modified in the exigencies of daily life" (p. 184).

Typically one thinks of culture as associated with race and ethnicity. However, other cultures exist if a broader definition of culture is used. Examples include the culture of poverty, the culture of cancer survivors, the culture of rurality, and the culture of chronic illness (see Chapter 2), to name a few. Each of these cultures has explicit and implicit guidelines that determine how their members view the world, decide upon appropriate behaviors, and perform those behaviors.

Cultural Competency

Many definitions of culture mandate that there are many definitions of cultural competence. **Table 13-1** lists some of the more common definitions found in the literature. The National Prevention Information Network (2011) lists eight principles of cultural competence:

1. Define culture broadly.
2. Value clients' cultural beliefs.
3. Recognize complexity in language interpretation.
4. Facilitate learning between providers and communities.
5. Involve the community in defining and addressing service needs.
6. Collaborate with other agencies.
7. Professionalize staff hiring and training.
8. Institutionalize cultural competence.

Cultural competence for systems and organizations may be seen on a continuum (Racher & Annis, 2007; Srivastava, 2007). The Cultural Competence Continuum was developed by the National Center for Cultural Competence (NCCC) at Georgetown University, in Washington, DC. There are six levels on the continuum, spanning from cultural destructiveness at level 1 to cultural proficiency at level 6, the highest level. When an organization is culturally proficient, it holds culture in high esteem and uses this perspective to guide its work (Racher & Annis, 2007, p. 263).

Cultural Awareness and Sensitivity

Often times we hear the terms *cultural awareness* and *cultural sensitivity*. What is their relationship with cultural competency? Purnell (2008a, p. 6) explains awareness as an appreciation of the external signs of culture, whereas

Table 13-1   Cultural Competency Definitions

Author	Definition
National Prevention Information Network, 2011	Having the capacity to function effectively as an individual and an organization within the context of the cultural beliefs, behaviors, and needs presented by consumers and their communities
Spector, 2009	A provider understands and attends to the total context of the patient's situation, and it is a complex combination of knowledge, attitudes, and skills
Mutha, Allen, & Welch, 2002, p. 25	A set of skills, knowledge, and attitudes that enhance 1) your understanding of and respect for patients' values, beliefs, and expectations; 2) awareness of your own assumptions and value system in addition to those of the U.S. medical system; and 3) your ability to adapt care to fit with the patient's expectations and preferences
Campinha-Bacote, 2002	A process that consists of 5 interrelated constructs: cultural desire, cultural awareness, cultural knowledge, cultural skill, and cultural encounters
Office of Minority Health, 2005	A set of congruent behaviors, attitudes, and policies that come together in a system, agency, or among professionals that enables effective work in cross-cultural situations
Giger & Davidhizar, 2004, p. 8	A dynamic, fluid, continuous process whereby an individual, system or healthcare agency finds meaningful and useful care-delivery strategies based on knowledge of the cultural heritage, beliefs, attitudes, and behaviors of those to whom they render care

sensitivity is one's personal attitude toward others of different cultures. Although awareness and sensitivity are part of cultural competence, competency implies that awareness and sensitivity have been operationalized (Schim et al., 2007).

Myths of Culture and Diversity

Myths of culture and diversity must be challenged. Masi (1996) and Srivastava (2007) discuss six myths that can influence caring for culturally diverse clients.

The Myth of Equality

This myth describes that fairness means equal treatment for all (Srivastava, 2007, p. 42). Proponents of this myth cite success stories of individuals of varying ethnic, racial, and gender backgrounds who have overcome great obstacles and "made it" as individuals. However, this view reflects a lack of awareness of systemic barriers and institutional racism. It is a narrow view that places all responsibility on the individual without acknowledging systemic inequities.

The Myth of Sameness

The assumption of this myth is that someone who shares the client's ethnicity and language will be able to more effectively provide health care and thus eliminate miscommunication (Masi, 1996; Srivastava, 2007). However this "sameness" may be only on the surface, as there may be many other differences that affect the client and healthcare professional relationship. This also presumes a narrow definition of culture (race and ethnicity) as opposed to a broader view.

The Myth That Cultural Differences Are a Problem

Health care has often viewed issues of culture and diversity from a negative perspective, that there are problems or barriers to overcome. Srivastava (2007, p. 46) suggests that culture should not viewed as a problem, but as a leverage point, a point that can affect the health outcome of the client if energy is focused on it.

The Myth That Everything Must Be Acceptable

There is a perception that if something is a cultural value that it must be "accepted." Masi (1996) suggests that respecting an individual's cultural value not be confused with acceptance. He describes that although society states that child abuse is unacceptable, the definition of child abuse may vary among individuals from different cultures. A practice known as "scratching the wind," where bruises are caused by cupping and scratches are created by running a coin on the skin, is used to relieve fevers and illness in some cultures. Respecting this cultural value does not mean acceptance of this practice.

The Myth That Generalizations Are Unacceptable

Masi (1996) and Srivastava (2007) suggest that there is a large difference between generalizations and stereotypes. Generalizations are a necessary starting point to understand groups of individuals as they indicate trends and patterns. These generalizations may help a healthcare professional initiate a conversation with a client. In contrast, stereotypes close conversation and knowledge development (Srivastava, 2007, p. 47).

The Myth That Familiarity Equals Competence

Familiarity with cultural differences may make the difference invisible (Srivastava, 2007, p. 48). This myth dovetails with the one about generalizations, and means that being familiar with a certain culture does not make one competent, as familiarity may not allow for individual differences.

Transcultural Nursing

Transcultural nursing had its beginnings in the 1950s with Madeleine Leininger. With her work over more than 50 years, in addition to other theorists, transcultural nursing has evolved as a specific and unique specialty. Transcultural nursing is defined as "as a formal area of study and practice focused on comparative human-care (caring) differences and similarities of the beliefs, values and patterned lifeways of cultures to provide culturally congruent, meaningful, and beneficial health care to people" (Leininger & McFarland, 2002, p. 6).

Leininger and McFarland (2002) summarize eight factors that led to the development of and need for transcultural nursing:

1. Increase in immigration and migration of people across the world
2. Implicit expectation that nurses and other healthcare providers need to know, understand, respect, and respond appropriately to care for others of diverse cultures
3. Increase in the use of technologies in caring or curing, with different responses and effects on clients of diverse cultures
4. Increased signs of cultural conflicts, cultural clashes, and cultural imposition practices between nurses and those from diverse cultures
5. Increase in number of nurses who travel and work in different places in the world
6. Anticipated legal defense suits against nurses resulting from cultural negligence, cultural ignorance, and cultural imposition practices in working with diverse cultures
7. Rise in gender and the issues and rights of special groups
8. Growing trend to care with and for people, whether well or ill, in their familiar or particular living and working environments (Leininger & McFarland, 2002, pp. 13–18)

The Transcultural Nursing Society, founded in 1974 by Leininger, is a worldwide organization for nurses and others interested in and prepared to advance transcultural nursing. The society provides a forum to bring nurses together worldwide with common and diverse interests to improve the care for culturally diverse people. The goals of the society include:

• To advance cultural competencies for nurses worldwide

• To advance the scholarship (substantive knowledge) of the discipline
• To develop strategies for advocating social change for cultural competent care
• To promote a sound financial non-profit corporation (www.tcns.org)

IMPACT

Changing Demographics

According to the 2010 U.S. Census, approximately 35% of the U.S. population is defined as racial and ethnic minorities. Currently four states—Hawaii, New Mexico, California, and Texas—as well as the District of Columbia have minority populations that exceed 50%. Texas is the newest addition to this short list. In 2050, 20% of the population aged 65 and older is projected to be Latino. (U.S. Census Bureau, 2010a)

The North American healthcare system(s) is based on Western culture, and that includes using a biomedical model. With an increasingly diverse society, this narrow view continues to create a mismatch with clients and their healthcare needs and services.

As we age, the potential for having one or more chronic diseases increases significantly, thus the need to look at demographics of aging Americans is paramount. Currently non-Latino older adults account for approximately 83.5% of the older adult population. Projections for 2050 indicate that this percentage will decrease significantly. Given these projections, a culturally competent workforce will be needed to meet the needs of individuals from many cultural and ethnic groups (see **Table 13-2**).

Table 13-2 Projected Distribution of the Population, Age 65 and Older, by Race and Hispanic Origin: 2010, 2030, and 2050			
	2010	**2030**	**2050**
Total	100.0	100.0	100.0
White	14.2	20.7	21.0
Non-Hispanic White	16.1	24.8	25.5
Black	8.6	15.2	18.5
American Indian and Alaska Native	7.4	14.5	16.8
Asian	9.3	16.5	21.9
Native Hawaiian and Other Pacific Islander	6.5	13.2	17.9
Two or More Races	5.1	7.2	7.8
Hispanic	5.7	10.0	13.2

Note: Data are middle-series projections of the population. Hispanics may be of any race. Reference population: These data refer to the resident population. *Source:* U.S. Census Bureau. (2010a). The next four decades: The older population in the United States: 2010 to 2050. Retrieved August 22, 2011, from: http://www.census.gov/prod/2010pubs/p25-1138.pdf

Health Disparities

Although the focus of this chapter is culture and its influence on individuals with chronic illness, health disparities that occur with individuals from different cultures must be noted as well. Race, ethnicity, and culture sharply divide the health and health care of the population in the United States. Although such disparities have been noted for some time, the Institute of Medicine report, *Unequal Treatment* (Smedley, Stith, & Nelson, 2003), was a landmark publication that put these disparities in the forefront. This report demonstrated that racial and ethnic disparities in health care, with a few exceptions, are consistent across a range of illnesses and healthcare services.

The same year that *Unequal Treatment* was published, the AHRQ released the first annual *National Healthcare Disparities Report*.

Their seventh report was released in March of 2010. Overall, three themes emerged from that report:

- Disparities are common and uninsurance is an important contributor.
- Many disparities are not decreasing.
- Some disparities merit particular attention, especially care for cancer, heart failure, and pneumonia. (AHRQ, 2010, p. 1)

Some of the biggest disparities noted in this latest report include:

- Blacks had a rate of new AIDS cases 10 times higher than Whites, for Latinos more than 3 times as high, and for American Indians/Alaska Natives 1.4 times as high.
- Black older adults and older adults of multiple races were more likely than White older adults to delay care due to cost.

- In small metropolitan areas, the heart attack death rate was higher for Latinos than for Whites: 97.2 per 1,000 admissions compared with 70.8 per 1,000 admissions. (AHRQ, 2010)

Another national document that addresses health disparities is *Healthy People 2020*. The document has four overarching goals, two of which address health disparities: 1) achieve health equity, eliminate disparities, and improve the health of all groups; and 2) promote quality of life, healthy development, and healthy behaviors across all life stages. As healthcare professionals, the need is paramount to incorporate appropriate strategies into clinical practice with an awareness of different cultures to allocate resources fairly within society. Efforts to address racial, ethnic, and other disparities in health care requires nurses to employ creative interventions to assure culturally competent care for these populations.

Beidler (2005) states that health disparities occur in vulnerable patients who are uninsured, racially and ethnically diverse, and frequently speak languages other than English. Maze (2005) refers to health disparities existing among individuals who are disenfranchised, living in poverty, stigmatized, homeless, immigrants, victims of crimes, children, women, prisoners, persons with AIDS, persons with mental illness, and those who have little social support or education. These individuals make up a vulnerable population and may present with a variety of ethical issues for the healthcare professional. For example, illegal immigrants may be hesitant to provide a name, address, and phone number for follow-up care. Should the healthcare provider try to obtain this information from the illegal immigrant? Remember, the client may be fearful that you will "turn them in" to the authorities.

In 2009, the number of people without health insurance decreased overall and for most racial and ethnic groups, but Asian Americans experienced an increase in uninsurance. Overall out-of-pocket healthcare costs increased by 4.3%, which resulted in the rate of delaying medical care increasing by 5.4% (The Opportunity Agenda, 2009).

Racial and Ethnicity Classification

In 1997 the Office of Management and Budget (OMB) identified the following categories to be used by federal programs when reporting data: American Indian or Alaska Native; Asian; Black or African American; Hispanic or Latino; Native Hawaiian or other Pacific Islander; and White. American Indian or Alaska Native refers to people of North and South America and those who maintain tribal affiliations (Wallman, 1998). An Asian is a person with origins in the Far East, Southeast Asia, or the Indian subcontinent. Black or African American refers to individuals with origins from any Black racial groups of Africa. Hispanic or Latino is an individual of Cuban, Mexican, Puerto Rican, South or Central American, or other Spanish culture or origin. Native Hawaiians or other Pacific Islanders have origins in Hawaii, Guam, Samoa, or other Pacific Islands. White is a person having origins in any of the original people of Europe, the Middle East, or North Africa. However, with individuals from mixed origins, it may be difficult to assign an individual to one specific ethnic group. In 2007, the Department of Education added a seventh category of "two or more races" for the purpose of collecting and maintaining racial and ethnic data from students and staff, which was to be used starting in 2010 (Department of Education, 2007).

Examples of Different Cultures

The following examples of the Haitian culture, Mexican culture, and Japanese culture are brief overviews and generalizations of what is known about each culture. Disease labels in each of these cultures have different influences and meanings among clients (Turner, 1996).

In addition, the longer that one is a resident in this country (or other countries), subcultures of the original culture evolve, with each one being more unique.

Haitians

Haitians are from Haiti, an island between Cuba and Puerto Rico about the size of the state of Maryland. The Haitian population in the United States is approximately 830,000 (U.S. Census Bureau, 2010b), or approximately 0.3% of the total population.

The influence of France's rule of Haiti from 1697 to 1804 identified two distinct categories of Haitians. Members of the upper class used the marker of *mulatto* (color), the French culture, and the French language to differentiate themselves from the lower class. Those speaking French rose within the social system. The lower class was mostly black and spoke the Haitian Creole language, which is a combination language of multitribe slaves of Africa. Today, Creole is the official language of Haiti (Colin & Paperwalla, 2008).

Traditionally, the man has been considered the head of the household, the primary income provider, the decision maker, and the sexual initiator, whereas women are to be faithful, honest, respectful, and oversee the house (Dash, 2001). However, this may be changing, as a number of families are becoming matriarchal today (Colin & Paperwalla, 2008). The family unit remains an important concept of Haitian culture.

Haitian people are openly demonstrative in their emotions and typically speak loudly. They have a close personal space and may ignore territorial space. Many may pretend to understand, when in reality they are nodding to be nice and to avoid showing a lack of understanding. The use of simple and clear instructions is needed when providing education to enhance the health of the individual. Haitians are private, and if they do not understanding something, will more than likely choose to use a professional interpreter over a family member (Colin & Paperwalla, 2008).

Drinking alcohol and cigarette smoking is culturally approved for men and is the norm. The Haitian diet is high in carbohydrates and fat, with weight loss being a sign of illness. Lifestyle changes needed when faced with a chronic illness will be a challenge for the provider when trying to help clients understand the impact of alcohol, smoking, and diet on chronic illness (Colin & Paperwalla, 2008).

Even though Haitians are deeply religious, they also have many superstitions. These beliefs include the fear of a loved one not actually dying, but becoming a zombie. If it is believed that an individual is not really dead, they may ask for an autopsy to ensure death. Beliefs of *voodooism,* with its roots in Africa, are often co-aligned with their other religious beliefs. Voodoo occurs when an individual has the power to communicate by trance with ancestors, saints, or animistic deities. This can have an influence on the psychological status of the client. Hence, illness can be perceived as punishment for being evil or occurring from evil spirits (Corrine, Bailey, Valentin, Mortantus, & Shirley, 1992). Given that voodoo and folk remedies are used among this group, providers should always ask what prior home interventions have been tried before prescribing (Galembo & Fleurant, 2005).

Mexicans

Hispanic is a term that is commonly used in the United States to designate all those who speak Spanish. This cultural group includes those from Puerto Rico, Cuba, Mexico, Latin America, and other countries as well. Typically many Hispanic people wish to be described by terms that are specific to their culture; thus using the term *Mexican American* is more appropriate (Zoucha & Zamarripa, 2008). Because of the poor economy in Mexico, there has been a constant influx of immigrants from Mexico to the United States during most of the 20th century and into the 21st century. The media consistently report stories of undocumented aliens who continue to cross the border into the United States to earn money for their families left behind in Mexico.

Religious beliefs are very important to Mexican Americans, who believe that there is a divine power that has ultimate control of their lives and that one must accept what God gives (Berry, 2002, p. 365). The majority of Mexican Americans are Roman Catholics, and although they may not all attend formal church regularly, pictures and statues with a religious theme are evident in many of their homes.

Family and kinship are important social structures to Mexican Americans. In addition, this group is collectively oriented versus the individual orientation so common in North America. Mexican Americans may prefer to live close to their family and extended family, but not necessarily in the same household, as has been seen in the past. Family extends beyond the immediate circle to include fictive kin or *compadres*, friends who are chosen for special occasions (Berry, 2002). The elderly are valued and respected, and their knowledge about health information often takes precedence over that of professional healthcare providers (Berry, 2002; Zoucha & Zamarripa, 2008). Younger generations have the obligation to care for the older generations. Typical families are viewed as patriarchal, with males being dominant and females being passive. *Machismo* in the Mexican culture views men as having strength, valor, and self-confidence (Zoucha & Zamarripa, 2008).

Because family is a priority for Mexican Americans, it takes precedence over work issues. Many are sensitive to confrontation and difference of opinion, and will shun those challenges, especially in the workplace. Truth is often tempered with diplomacy and tact (Zoucha & Zamarripa, 2008). As an example, in the workplace when a service is promised for tomorrow even though it cannot be completed by then, that promise is made to please the customer, not to deceive. For some Mexican Americans, truth is a relative concept; whereby for most European Americans, it is an absolute value (p. 314).

Mexican American concepts of health and illness are a combination of Aztec and Spanish beliefs (Berry, 2002). Within the culture there is a folk belief system, based in part on religion, regarding cause and cure of illnesses. This system stresses the omnipotence of God, the inevitability of suffering, and the lack of personal control (p. 367). Mexican Americans have a fatalistic worldview and an external locus of control. Thus, if someone becomes ill, "that's just the way things are." With preventive health care in short supply in Mexico, many Mexican Americans believe that what happens to them is God's will.

A health belief still prevalent today is that illness is caused by a hot and cold imbalance (Gonzalez & Kuipers, 2004). To cure the illness, the opposite quality of the causative agent must be applied (p. 234). Cold diseases or conditions include menstrual cramps, pneumonia, cancer, earaches, and arthritis. Hot diseases include pregnancy, diabetes, hypertension, infection, and kidney and liver conditions. Mexicans regard pain as a part of life and part of the inevitable suffering (Zoucha & Zamarripa, 2008, p. 321).

Generally, Mexican Americans respect healthcare professionals because of their training and expertise (Zoucha & Zamarripa, 2008). If healthcare professionals demonstrate respect with their clients, incorporate folk practitioners as necessary and appropriate, and incorporate the concept of *personalismo* into their care, they will gain the Mexican American client's confidence and trust.

Japanese

In Japan today, physicians are clearly in charge of the healthcare team, and are held in high esteem. The majority of hospitals in Japan are managed by physicians as opposed to individuals with a healthcare management background. Because self-care is not highly regarded in Japan, and physicians are held in high regard, being told what to do by the physician is expected (Turale & Ito, 2008).

Education is highly valued in Japan, and the illiteracy rate is only 1%. Nearly 95% of students in Japan complete the 12th grade, and the standards for this accomplishment are high. As an example, calculus is part of the mandatory junior high school curriculum (Turale & Ito, 2008).

Japanese American immigrants are the only group to refer to themselves by the generation in which they were born. For instance, *issei* refers to first-generation immigrants; *nisei*, to second-generation immigrants; *sansei*, to third-generation immigrants; *yonsei*, the fourth generation;

gosei, the fifth generation; and *rokusei*, the sixth generation. These generational categories provide a framework for understanding their cultural values (Ishida & Inouye, 2004, p. 335).

Japanese society is both structured and traditional. Politeness, personal responsibility, loyalty, and working together for the greater good are important concepts. Group harmony is stressed above all else. Japan is a collectivist society, where group needs and wants take precedence over individuals. Japanese culture discourages individualism. There is much sensitivity to social status and one's relative position in life (Brightman, 2005; Turale & Ito, 2008).

The culture is also a relatively non–eye-contact culture when communicating. For some it is considered disrespectful to look someone directly in the eye, particularly if that individual is in a superior position (Galanti, 2004). Japanese culture is also seen as a nontouch culture (Ishida & Inouye, 2004). Although there is touch and close contact with infants, there is much less touch and physical contact between adults. Lastly, the ideal pattern of communication in Japanese society is silent communication. Japanese do not appreciate aggressive conversation and prefer to remain silent.

The family is important to Japanese Americans. There is a phrase, *kodomo no tame ni* (for the sake of the children), that reflects the sacrifices that parents and adults make for the success of the next generation (Ishida & Inouye, 2004, p. 342).

Pain is a concept that should not be expressed verbally. Bearing pain is seen as a virtue and one of family honor (Turale & Ito, 2008). In fact in Japan, medications to relieve pain are used much less than in the United States. Furthermore, narcotic use, in particular, is restricted.

CASE STUDY

An older Chinese patient refused pain medication following cataract surgery. When asked, he replied his discomfort was bearable and he could survive without any medication. Later the nurse found him restless and uncomfortable. Again the nurse offered pain medication. Again he refused, explaining that her responsibilities at the hospital were far more important than his comfort and he did not want to impose.

Discussion Questions

1. How would you, as the nurse, interpret this man's behavior?
2. What belief of this man's heritage has the nurse in this situation offended?
3. How can you avoid offending someone in a similar situation?

Asians

A common stereotype is to categorize those from the Far East and Southeast Asia broadly as Asians, versus Japanese, Chinese, Korean, Malaysian, Vietnamese, Thai, and so forth. In fact, using the U.S. Census as an example, Asians include individuals from 28 Asian countries (Itano, 2005).

The Chinese culture has influenced the health care of many Asian groups, including the Japanese. For instance, there must be a balance between hot (*yang*) and cold (*yin*). *Yin* and *yang* are life forces, and it is believed that illness occurs when there is an imbalance between the two forces (Itano, 2005). The approach to care is to restore harmony, order, and control through one's environment. Harmony is highly valued as a healing mode and to control one's emotions (Leininger, 2002, p. 459).

Culture of Poverty

The culture of poverty impacts the health care of a socioeconomic group, which is often faced with numerous barriers such as access, cost of care, health literacy, and a focus on surviving from one day to the next. Individuals living in poverty may place health lower on their list of priorities as they attempt to live day to day without financial resources. The lack of financial resources often results in less diagnostic tests, use of generic drugs, goal setting that is short term, and the challenge of ensuring compliance (Benson, 2000).

Poverty is synonymous with a present-moment orientation, a lack of planning ahead, and a fatalistic future. Generation after generation can perpetuate poverty by basing decisions on previous decisions that have been made by family members, parental employment and earnings, family structure, and parent education. With poverty, chronic health issues such as substance abuse, smoking, obesity, and incarceration (which may result in diseases such as HIV, hepatitis, or tuberculosis) may emerge (Pearson, 2003).

Poverty impacts migrants such as Mexicans; North American Indians; and immigrants from the Middle East, India, and China. Providing care to migrants and immigrants poses an added challenge as these individuals are notonly impoverished but also from a different cultural orientation. Healthcare professionals need to consider the cultural and social complexities that increase the challenges of managing chronic illnesses. Being uninsured, having a lower income, and lower educational levels have been associated with a decrease in hypertension and cholesterol screening (Stewart & Silverstein, 2002).

INTERVENTIONS

Key to providing culturally competent interventions are the CLAS standards. These standards form the basis for nursing frameworks and communication used with clients of different cultures.

CLAS Standards

In 2000, the U.S. Department of Health and Human Services (USDHHS) Office of Minority Health (OMH, 2007) released 14 national standards for culturally and linguistically appropriate services (CLAS) as a means to address and correct inequities in the provision of health care to culturally and ethnically diverse groups. These standards are available at the OMH website (www.omhrc.gov/CLAS). These standards are organized by themes: culturally competent care (standards 1–3), language access services (standards 4–7), and organizational supports for cultural competence (standards 8–14). Some of these standards are mandates, such as 4, 5, 6, and 7, whereas others are guidelines that should be adopted by federal, state, and national accrediting agencies. Standard 14 is suggested as voluntary.

Standard 4 mandates that healthcare organizations must offer and provide language assistance at no cost to clients during all hours of operation. Standard 5 mandates that healthcare organizations must have a mechanism to provide clients, in their language, information on their rights to receive language assistance. Standard 6 mandates that the language assistance be competent, and that families and friends should not be utilized unless requested by the client. Standard 7 mandates that signs should be posted in a facility that reflect the most commonly encountered language in the service area. These signs and patient materials should be easily understood. The remaining standards are guidelines and recommendations (**Table 13-3** includes all of the mandated guidelines and recommendations).

To help implement the standards on an organizational level, the Alliance of Community Health Plans Foundation, with funding from the Merck Company Foundation, developed 13 case studies and a final report about making a "business case" for projects addressing the CLAS Standards. Each of these case studies covers the business benefits from addressing the cultural and linguistic needs of clients (Alliance of Community Health Plans Foundation, 2007).

Nursing Frameworks for Practice

Currently a variety of models, theories, and frameworks are available to assist nurses in providing appropriate care for diverse populations. The website of the Transcultural Nursing Society (www.tcns.org) provides information about six transcultural nursing theories and models. Models include those by Margaret Andrews and Joyceen Boyle; Josepha Campinha-Bacote; Joyce Giger and Ruth Davidhizar; Madeline

Table 13-3	CLAS Standards
Standard 1	Healthcare organizations should ensure that patients/consumers receive from all staff members effective, understandable, and respectful care that is provided in a manner compatible with their cultural health beliefs and practices and preferred language.
Standard 2	Healthcare organizations should implement strategies to recruit, retain, and promote at all levels of the organization a diverse staff and leadership that are representative of the demographic characteristics of the service area.
Standard 3	Healthcare organizations should ensure that staff at all levels and across all disciplines receive ongoing education and training in culturally and linguistically appropriate service delivery.
Standard 4	Healthcare organizations must offer and provide language assistance services, including bilingual staff and interpreter services, at no cost to each patient/consumer with limited English proficiency, at all points of contact, in a timely manner during all hours of operation.
Standard 5	Healthcare organizations must provide to patients/consumers in their preferred language both verbal offers and written notices informing them of their right to receive language assistance services.
Standard 6	Healthcare organizations must ensure the competence of language assistance provided to limited English proficient patients/consumers by interpreters and bilingual staff. Family and friends should not be used to provide interpretation services (except on request by the patient/consumer).
Standard 7	Healthcare organizations must make available easily understood patient-related materials and post signage in the languages of the commonly encountered groups and/or groups represented in the service area.
Standard 8	Healthcare organizations should develop, implement, and promote a written strategic plan that outlines clear goals, policies, operational plans, and management accountability/oversight mechanisms to provide culturally and linguistically appropriate services.
Standard 9	Healthcare organizations should conduct initial and ongoing organizational self-assessments of CLAS-related activities and are encouraged to integrate cultural and linguistic competence-related measures into their internal audits, performance improvement programs, patient satisfaction assessments, and outcomes-based evaluations.
Standard 10	Healthcare organizations should ensure that data on the individual patient's/consumer's race, ethnicity, and spoken and written language are collected in health records, integrated into the organization's management information systems, and periodically updated.
Standard 11	Healthcare organizations should maintain a current demographic, cultural, and epidemiologic profile of the community as well as a needs assessment to accurately plan for and implement services that respond to the cultural and linguistic characteristics of the service area.
Standard 12	Healthcare organizations should develop participatory, collaborative partnerships with communities and utilize a variety of formal and informal mechanisms to facilitate community and patient/consumer involvement in designing and implementing CLAS-related activities.
Standard 13	Healthcare organizations should ensure that conflict and grievance resolution processes are culturally and linguistically sensitive and capable of identifying, preventing, and resolving cross-cultural conflicts or complaints by patients/consumers.
Standard 14	Healthcare organizations are encouraged to regularly make available to the public information about their progress and successful innovations in implementing the CLAS standards and to provide public notice in their communities about the availability of this information.

Source: Office of Minority Health. (2008). National standards on culturally and linguistically appropriate services (CLAS). Retrieved August 22, 2011, from: www.omhrc.gov/templates/browse.aspx?lvl=2&lvlID=15

Leininger; Larry Purnell; and Rachel Spector. Three of those models are discussed here.

Leininger's Cultural Care Theory of Diversity and Universality

Cultural values, beliefs, and practices impact health and illness and inform and guide the client and the client's family in the choices and patterns of health care. Care is universal; however, patterns of care vary among and between cultural groups with regard to healthcare beliefs and behaviors (Leininger, 2002; Leininger & McFarland, 2002, 2006). Leininger's Culture Care Theory provides a theoretical framework for healthcare professionals to discover the differences and similarities between and among cultural groups related to their cultural values, beliefs, and practices. The meanings and uses of these diversities and universalities among the cultures of the world need to be uncovered and understood (Leininger & McFarland, 2002, p. 78).

The social structure of the client and his or her family such as economics, religion, and worldview influence cultural care meanings, expressions, and patterns in different cultures (Leininger & McFarland, 2002, p. 78). Embedded within these structures are generic (folk) care practices, which are separate and distinct from professional care practices (Leininger, 1997; Leininger & McFarland, 2002). This theoretical tenet is particularly instructive for healthcare providers. For example, an individual with chronic pain may rely on the home remedies taught by an elder in the family or use a variety of herbs and compounds that have been obtained from a traditional healer to manage pain. The healthcare provider must be vigilant in the belief and use of generic care practices, and incorporate those into the plan of care. The last theoretical tenet of Leininger's theory provides three modes

of nursing decisions and actions for culturally congruent care: 1) culture care preservation and maintenance, 2) culture care accommodation and/or negotiation, and 3) culture care restructuring and/or repatterning (Leininger, 2002; Leininger & McFarland, 2002, 2006).

For example, Mrs. Huerta has degenerative arthritis. Her mother was a traditional healer in the village where she grew up. As a young child, Mrs. Huerta learned the healing ways and practices from her mother. As an elderly woman, Mrs. Huerta continues to use these traditional methods to manage her chronic pain. When Mrs. Huerta was admitted to the acute care setting, she brought with her remedies that have brought her comfort and relief in the past. Leininger's three modes of nursing decisions and action are informative and directive for the nurse to provide culturally competent care for Mrs. Huerta. The nurse can incorporate these home remedies into the care within the acute setting, the nurse can talk with Mrs. Huerta, or, in the event the home remedies Mrs. Huerta is taking are known to be unsafe or contraindicated with her present care regime, the nurse can explore alternative comfort and pain relief strategies with Mrs. Huerta. The cultural care values, beliefs, and practices are honored and maintained. Therefore, Leininger advocates cultural holding knowledge by healthcare providers in order to provide culturally competent care and, further, to minimize the potential for culturally inappropriate care that has the potential for harm and pain to the healthcare client and his or her family.

Giger-Davidhizar Transcultural Assessment Model

The Giger-Davidhizar Model was developed initially in 1991. The model is built upon concentric concepts with the client—a unique cultural being—in the center. The next circle contains concepts of religion, culture, and ethnicity (Giger & Davidhizar, 2004). The last circle focuses on six cultural concepts: 1) communication, 2) space, 3) social organization, 4) time, 5) environmental control, and 6) biological variation.

Communication refers to all human interaction and behavior, both verbal and nonverbal. Space refers to the distance between individuals when they interact, communicate, or reside together. Time can be past, present, or future oriented. How individuals view this concept is often uncovered through their style of communication. Individuals who focus on the past attempt to maintain tradition, whereas those focused on the present do not formulate goals. Environmental control refers to the ability of the individual to control nature and to plan and direct factors in the environment that affect them. If persons come from cultural groups where there is external control, there may be a fatalistic view ultimately resulting in the belief that seeking health care is useless. Biological differences, especially genetic variations, exist between individuals. These biologic differences among various racial groups are often less understood (Giger & Davidhizar, 2004)

The Purnell Model for Cultural Competence

Purnell's Model for Cultural Competence is graphically represented in a model that includes both the macro and micro concepts. The model is depicted by four concentric circles, each depicting a macro concept. The outer circle represents global society, and is defined as:

world communications and politics; conflicts and warfare; natural disasters and famines; international exchanges in business, commerce, and information technology; advances in the health sciences; space exploration; and the increased ability for

people to travel around the world and to interact with diverse societies. (Purnell, 2008b, p. 20)

The second circle is the community, and it is defined as a group of people who have common interests, but not necessarily living in the same geographic area. It is the physical, social, and symbolic characteristics of the community that enable it to feel connected, not common geography (p. 21). The third circle represents the family that is made up of two or more individuals who are emotionally connected, and who or may not live together. The fourth circle represents the individual who is continually adapting to his or her community (p. 22).

The model's organizing framework comprises 12 micro concepts, or domains, that are interconnected and common to all cultures with implications for health and health care. To assess the ethnocultural attributes of the community, family, or person, each of the following domains needs to be addressed:

- Overview, inhabited localities, and topography
- Communication
- Family roles and organization
- Workforce issues
- Biocultural ecology
- High-risk behaviors
- Nutrition
- Pregnancy and childbearing practices
- Death rituals
- Spirituality
- Healthcare practices
- Healthcare practitioners (Purnell, 2008b, p. 22)

Purnell (2008b) has identified barriers that individuals, families and communities may face in securing health care. Healthcare professionals

Table 13-4   Communication Guidelines

Assess your personal beliefs surrounding persons from different cultures.
 Review your personal beliefs and past experiences.
 Set aside any values, biases, ideas, and attitudes that are judgmental and may negatively affect care.

Assess communication variables from a cultural perspective.
 Determine the ethnic identity of the patient, including generation in America.
 Use the patient as a source of information when possible.
 Assess cultural factors that may affect your relationship with the patient and respond appropriately.

Plan care based on the communicated needs and cultural background.
 Learn as much as possible about the patient's cultural customs and beliefs.
 Encourage the patient to reveal cultural interpretation of health, illness, and health care.
 Be sensitive to the uniqueness of the patient.
 Identify sources of discrepancy between the patient's and your own concepts of health and illness.
 Communicate at the patient's personal level of functioning.
 Evaluate effectiveness of nursing actions and modify nursing care plan when necessary.

Modify communication approaches to meet cultural needs.
 Be attentive to signs of fear, anxiety, and confusion in the patient.
 Respond in a reassuring manner in keeping with the patient's cultural orientation.
 Be aware that in some cultural groups discussion with others concerning the patient may be offensive and
  impede the nursing process.

Understand that respect for the patient and communicated needs are central to the therapeutic
relationship.
 Communicate respect by using a kind and attentive approach.
 Learn how listening is communicated in the patient's culture.
 Use appropriate active listening techniques.
 Adopt an attitude of flexibility, respect, and interest to help bridge barriers imposed by culture.

Communicate in a nonthreatening manner.
 Conduct the interview in an unhurried manner.
 Follow acceptable social and cultural amenities.
 Ask general questions during the information-gathering stage.
 Be patient with a respondent who gives information that may seem unrelated to the patient's health
  problem.
 Develop a trusting relationship by listening carefully, allowing time, and giving the patient your full
  attention.

Use validating techniques in communication.
 Be alert for feedback that the patient is not understanding.
 Do not assume meaning is interpreted without distortion.

Be considerate of reluctance to talk when the subject involves sexual matters.
 Be aware that in some cultures sexual matters are not discussed freely with members of the
  opposite sex.

Table 13-4   Communication Guidelines (Continued)

Adopt special approaches when the patient speaks a different language.
  Use a caring tone of voice and facial expression to help alleviate the patient's fears.
  Speak slowly and distinctly, but not loudly.
  Use gestures, pictures, and play acting to help the patient understand.
  Repeat the message in different ways if necessary.
  Be alert to words the patient seems to understand and use them frequently.
  Keep messages simple and repeat them frequently.
  Avoid using medical terms and abbreviations that the patient may not understand.
  Use an appropriate language dictionary.

Use interpreters to improve communication.
  Ask the interpreter to translate the message, not just the individual words.
  Obtain feedback to confirm understanding.
  Use an interpreter who is culturally sensitive.

Source: Giger, J., & Davidhizar, R. (2004). *Transcultural nursing: Assessment and intervention* (4th ed., p. 35). St. Louis: Mosby.

need to be aware of these 12 barriers. Barriers include availability, accessibility, affordability, appropriateness, accountability, adaptability, acceptability, awareness, attitudes, approachability, alternative practices, and additional services available.

Communication

Communication is the crux of cultural care. It is important for nurses to be aware of appropriate body stance and proximities, gestures, languages, listening styles, and eye contact when communicating with clients, as different cultural groups, nearly 3000 worldwide, vary widely in their ideas regarding these (Narayanasamy, 2003). Differences in language between the client and healthcare professional impede detection of health needs, treatment, and patient care. For nursing interventions to be effective, it is imperative that nurses give attention to all aspects of the client's care as well as the communication process involving them.

The practice of cultural care requires negotiations and compromise as well as an understanding of how the patient views his health problem. Clients cared for by a nurse who has developed an awareness of cultural care practice have the opportunity to be fully acknowledged. Nurses who have an awareness of appropriate cultural care practice need to encourage their peers and promote the delivery of cultural care nursing by utilizing it in their everyday nursing practice.

Giger and Davidhizar (2004) have developed guidelines for communication (see **Table 13-4**). Although these are general guidelines, they provide a basis or a starting point. Although all of the guidelines are important, perhaps the most important one is to assess your own personal beliefs about persons from different cultures. It is difficult to understand others' beliefs if you do not have an awareness of your own, and how they may influence your attitudes toward others.

The use of symbols to facilitate communication in healthcare facilities can serve as a means to represent a world object, place, or concept. Unfortunately in hospitals, universal symbols on signs are rare; instead text in another language is more often found. The idea of symbols for healthcare signage originated from the subway system in Mexico City, which uses cultural icons to identify destinations. In 2003, Hablamos Juntos utilized a consultant to explore the use of healthcare symbols for wayfinding, including recommendations for future steps (Hablamos Juntos, 2008). The conclusion of the white paper was that symbols were a viable option for wayfinding in health care, that a set of tested symbols, publicly available, would help designers of health facilities increase communication and understanding. A total of 28 symbols were developed, with 17 of them being understood by at least 87% of a subject group of 300 participants from four language groups: English, Spanish, Indo-European, and Asian languages. This information is readily available, so why haven't facilities implemented these symbols?

Communication can be difficult between different cultures because of misunderstandings, inability to speak a language, or the use of technical terminology. Each culture has patterns for word choice, inflection, gestures and facial expressions, eye movement and eye contact, volume and speed of speech, use of silence, directness, and the degree of emotion. Nonverbal cues also impact communication. The amount of personal space, social space, and public space often differ between cultures, and one should always note another person's comfort zone.

Health Assessment

As the initial step in the nursing process, it is critical that healthcare professionals understand certain cultural behaviors related to their physical assessment. Simple things like eye contact and touch can affect an individual's response to the healthcare professional and determine what can and cannot be done regarding the individual's health care. Giger and Davidhizar (2004) have provided a table with some basic cultural variations that may be seen in health assessment (see **Table 13-5**). Again, as with all cultures, there is uniqueness in each individual, and these behaviors should be seen as general guidelines only.

Professional Education

The need for education about different cultures to progress toward cultural competency is evident. There are an increasing number of resources available online that may provide assistance. For instance, the National Technical Assistance Center at the University of Hawaii provides information about Asian Americans and Pacific Islanders to increase the potential of individuals with disabilities in these groups to gain employment. Their website contains overviews of each culture, newsletters, success stories, and training (http://www.ntac.hawaii.edu).

The USDHHS OMB has developed culturally competent nursing modules for nurses to increase awareness, knowledge, and skills in caring for those from diverse populations (Scott, 2008). The content of those modules is focused on the themes of the CLAS Standards. There is no cost for the modules, and continuing education credit is offered.

The National Center for Cultural Competence based at the Georgetown University Center for Child and Human Development has multiple resources available on its website

Table 13-5 Behaviors Related to Health Assessment

Cultural Group	Belief/Practice	Nursing Implication
African Americans	Dialect and slang terms require careful communication to prevent error.	Question the client's meaning.
Mexican Americans	Eye behavior is important. An individual who looks at and admires a child without touching the child has given the child the "evil eye."	Always touch the child you are examining.
American Indians	Eye contact is considered a sign of disrespect.	Recognize that the client may be attentive and interested even though eye contact is avoided.
Appalachians	Eye contact is considered impolite or a sign of hostility. Verbal patter may be confusing.	Avoid excessive eye contact.
American Eskimos	Body language is very important. Individual seldom disagrees publicly with others. May nod yes to be polite, even if not in agreement.	Monitor own body language.
Jewish Americans	Orthodox Jews consider excess touching offensive, particularly from members of the opposite sex.	Establish whether client is an Orthodox Jew and avoid excessive touch.
Chinese Americans	Individual may nod head to indicate yes or shake head to indicate no. Excessive eye contact indicates rudeness. Excessive touch is offensive.	Ask questions carefully and clarify responses. Avoid excessive eye contact and touch.
Filipino Americans	Offending people is to be avoided at all cost; nonverbal behavior is very important.	Monitor nonverbal behaviors.
Haitian Americans	Touch is used in conversation. Direct eye contact is used to gain attention and respect.	Use direct eye contact when communicating.
East Indian Hindu Americans	Women avoid eye contact as a sign of respect.	Be aware that men may view eye contact by women as offensive. Avoid eye contact.
Vietnamese Americans	Avoidance of eye contact is a sign of respect. The head is considered sacred; it is not polite to pat the head. An upturned palm is offensive in communication.	Limit eye contact. Touch the head only when mandated and explain clearly before proceeding to do so. Avoid hand gesturing.

Source: Giger, J., & Davidhizar, R. (2004). *Transcultural nursing: Assessment and intervention* (4th ed., p. 15). St. Louis: Mosby.

(http://www11.georgetown.edu/research/gucchd/nccc). The center also has a curricula-enhancement module series.

The Commonwealth Fund with their work in cultural competency provides papers, a video, and presentations on their website (http://www.commonwealthfund.org). This fund has supported significant research in the area of cultural competency.

Measuring Cultural Competence from the Patient's Perspective

As health care tries to identify best practices in providing culturally competent care, who better to ask than the patient? The Commonwealth Fund's division of health policy, health reform, and performance improvement has identified five domains of culturally competent care that can best be assessed from the patient perspective. The five components include: 1) patient–provider communication, 2) respect for patient preferences and shared decision making, 3) experiences leading to trust or distrust, 4) experiences of discrimination, and 5) linguistic competency (Ngo-Metzger et al., 2006). The five components have been incorporated into a conceptual framework as well.

Putting the Pieces of the Puzzle Together

Schim, Doorenbos, Benkert, and Miller (2007) view the bigger picture as culturally congruent care versus culturally competent care. Leininger was the first to use the term *culturally congruent care*, and Schim and colleagues' model builds on Leininger's work

and definition. Culturally congruent care is defined as:

> Those cognitively based assistive, supportive, facilitative, or enabling acts or decisions that are tailor made to fit with individual, group, or institution cultural values, beliefs, and lifeways in order to provide or support meaningful beneficial and satisfying health care or well-being services (Leininger, 1991, p. 49).

Schim and colleagues apply the puzzle metaphor to this care and see the finished puzzle with four constructs (2007, p. 105). These constructs include cultural diversity, cultural awareness, cultural sensitivity, and cultural competence.

1. **Cultural Diversity:** varies in quality and quantity across place and time; is dynamic, ever changing
2. **Cultural Awareness:** cognitive construct; a reality to be contemplated and a corresponding capacity for processing knowledge
3. **Cultural Sensitivity:** affective or attitudinal construct; attitude about their own person and others
4. **Cultural Competence:** behavioral construct; is the action that is taken in response to diversity, awareness, and sensitivity

Schim and colleagues suggest that there is one piece missing from their puzzle model and that is the client, whether it be an individual, family, or community. The client "layer" of the puzzle, although essential, is not visualized in the current model (p. 106).

Evidence-Based Practice Box

There is consensus that older Hispanic American women have a high rate of invasive cervical cancer due to lack of insurance, limited health care access, language barriers, and under utilization of screening. This study identified the association between economic factors and acculturation levels with Pap smear and mammography among Mexican American women aged 75 years and older. A total of 1272 older Mexican American women were included in the study. A major finding of the study was that cancer screening practices among older Mexican American women were associated with a number of socioeconomic factors:

Mammography use. The factors associated with mammography use included age, education, income, health insurance, functional status, depressive symptoms, cognitive status, and perceived healthcare needs.

Pap smear factors. The factors associated with Pap smear use included age education, financial strain, and health insurance.

Higher mammography use was associated with a cancer history and higher depression. Neither immigration status nor language was associated with either form of cancer screening.

Nursing implications. This study underlined the value of nurses being aware of older Latinas' healthcare practices and how factors influence the decisions for cancer screening. The myth that acculturation influences healthcare practices was not supported with older Mexican American women in decisions regarding cancer screening. Cultural competence is key to ensure optimal outcomes and improved health.

Source: Reyes-Ortiz, C. A., & Markides, K. S. (2010). Socioeconomic factors, immigration status, and cancer screening among Mexican American women aged 75 and older. *Health Care for Women International, 31*(12), 1068–1081.

In addition, as suggested by the Commonwealth Fund, giving credence to patients' perceptions of cultural competence makes sense. Healthcare professionals may think they are culturally competent, but do their patients agree? Ngo-Metzger and colleagues (2006) suggest monitoring patient populations through both quantitative and qualitative methods.

OUTCOMES

The literature is clear that providing culturally competent (or congruent) care is a primary strategy in reducing or eliminating racial and ethnic health disparities in the United States. Thus, outcome measures such as the annual National Health Disparities Report produced by the AHRQ and *Healthy People 2020* would provide evidence of decreasing health disparities that examine health literacy, English proficiency, language spoken at home, and the use of complementary and alternative medical practices (AHRQ, 2010, p. 26).

The Commonwealth Fund suggests giving credence to patients' perceptions of cultural competence. Healthcare professionals may think they are culturally competent, but do their patients agree? Ngo-Metzger and colleagues (2006) suggest monitoring patient populations through both quantitative and qualitative methods.

STUDY QUESTIONS

Evaluate the barriers to health care in a culturally diverse client you have recently seen using Purnell's identified barriers of availability, accessibility, affordability, appropriateness, accountability, adaptability, acceptability, awareness, attitudes, approachability, alternative practices, and additional services available.

How do the different transcultural nursing theories view cultural competence?

How are the different cultures (Haitian, Japanese, and Mexican) similar and different in their views of health and illness?

Explain how becoming culturally competent might decrease health disparities.

Why does culture matter in the care of an individual, family, or community?

How does one become culturally competent?

Distinguish between being culturally sensitive, aware, and competent.

Standard 12 of CLAS states: "Healthcare organizations should develop participatory, collaborative partnerships with communities and utilize a variety of formal and informal mechanisms to facilitate community and patient/consumer involvement in designing and implementing CLAS-related activities." What strategies would facilitate standard 12?

INTERNET RESOURCES

Association of Asian Pacific Community Health Organizations: www.aapcho.org

Centers for Disease Control and Prevention National Prevention Information Network: www.cdcnpin.org

EthnoMed: www.ethnomed.org

Hablamos Juntos: www.hablamosjuntos.org/signage/symbols/default.symbols.asp

Healthcare Communities: http://www.healthcarecommunities.org/

Initiative to Eliminate Racial and Ethnic Disparities in Health: raceandhealth.hhs.gov

Minority Health Program University of North Carolina at Chapel Hill: www.minority.unc.edu

Multicultural Health Communication Service: www.mhcs.health.nsw.gov.au

Multilingual Health Education Net: http://www.healthliteracy.worlded.org/docs/culture/materials/websites_009.html

National Center for Cultural Competence: www11.georgetown.edu/research/gucchd/nccc/

National Multicultural Institute: www.nmci.org

National Standards for Culturally and Linguistically Appropriate Services: http://minorityhealth.hhs.gov/templates/browse.aspx?lvl=2&lvlID=15

Office of Minority Health Resource Center Health Resources and Services Administration: http://www2.niddk.nih.gov/OMHRC/OMHRCAbout/AboutOMHRC.htm

Provider's Guide to Quality and Culture: erc.msh.org/quality&culture

Resources for cross-cultural health care: www.diversityrx.org

For a full suite of assignments and additional learning activities, use the access code located in the front of your book and visit this exclusive website: **http://go.jblearning.com/larsen**. If you do not have an access code, you can obtain one at the site.

REFERENCES

Agency for Healthcare Research and Quality. (2010). *National healthcare disparities report 2009* (AHRQ Pub. No. 08-0004). Rockville, MD: U.S. Department of Health and Human Services.

Alliance of Community Health Plans Foundation. (2007). *Making the business case for culturally and linguistically appropriate services in health care: Case Studies from the field*. Retrieved on May 31, 2008, from www.achp.org/page.asp?page_id=1059

Beidler, S. M. (2005). Ethical issues experienced by community-based nurse practitioners addressing health disparities among vulnerable populations. *International Journal for Human Caring, 9*(3), 43–50.

Benson, D. S. (2000). Providing health care to human beings trapped in the poverty culture. *Physician Executive, 26*(2), 28–32.

Berry, A. (2002). Culture care of the Mexican American family. In M. Leininger & M. R. McFarland (Eds.), *Transcultural nursing: Concepts, theories, research and practice* (3rd ed., pp. 363–373). New York: McGraw Hill.

Brightman, J. D. (2005). *Asian culture brief: Japan*. Retrieved August 22, 2011, from: http://www.ntac.hawaii.edu/downloads/products/briefs/culture/pdf/ACB-Vol2-Iss6-Japan.pdf

Campinha-Bacote, J. (2002). The process of cultural competence in the delivery of health care services: A model of care. *Journal of Transcultural Nursing, 13*(3), 181–184.

Cohen, E., & Goode, T. D. (2003). *Policy Brief 1: Rationale for cultural competence in primary care*. Washington, DC: National Center for Cultural Competence, Georgetown University Center for Child and Human Development.

Colin, J. M., & Paperwalla, G. (2008). People of Haitian heritage. In L. Purnell & B. Paulanka (Eds.), *Transcultural health care: A culturally competent approach* (3rd ed., pp. 231–247). Philadelphia: F.A. Davis.

Corrine, L., Bailey, V., Valentin, M., Mortantus, E., & Shirley, L. (1992). The unheard voices of women: Spiritual interventions in maternal-child health. *Maternal Child Nursing, 17*, 141–145.

Dash, J. M. (2001). *Culture and customs of Haiti (culture and customs of Latin America and the Caribbean)*. Westport, CT: Greenwood Press.

Department of Education. (2007). Final guidance on maintaining, collecting, and reporting racial and ethnic data to the U.S. Department of Education. Retrieved August 22, 2011, from: http://www2.ed.gov/legislation/FedRegister/other/2007-4/101907c.html

Dreher, M., & MacNaughton, N. (2002). Cultural competence in nursing: Foundation or fallacy? *Nursing Outlook, 50*, 181–186.

Galanti, G. A. (2004). *Caring for patients from different cultures: Case studies from American hospitals* (3rd ed.). Philadelphia: University of Pennsylvania.

Galembo, P., & Fleurant, G. (2005). *Vodou: Visions and voices of Haiti*. Berkley, CA: Ten Speed Press.

Giger, J., & Davidhizar, R. (Eds.). (2004). *Transcultural nursing: Assessment and intervention* (4th ed.). St. Louis: Mosby.

Gonzalez, T., & Kuipers, J. (2004). Mexican Americans. In J. Giger & R. Davidhizar (Eds.). *Transcultural nursing: Assessment and intervention* (4th ed., pp. 221–253). St. Louis: Mosby.

Hablamos Juntos (2008). Language policy and practice in health care. Retrieved February 15, 2008, from: www.hablamosjuntos.org

Healthy People 2020. (2010). Retrieved August 22, 2011, from: http://www.healthypeople.gov/2020/about/default.aspx

Helman, C. G. (2007) *Culture, health and illness* (5th ed.). London: Hodder Arnold.

Ishida, D., & Inouye, J. (2004). Japanese Americans. In J. Giger & R. Davidizar (Eds.), *Transcultural nursing: Assessment and intervention* (4th ed., pp. 332–361). St. Louis: Mosby.

Itano, J. K. (2005). Cultural diversity among individuals with cancer. In C. H. Yarbro, M. H. Frogge, & M. Goodman (Eds.), *Cancer nursing: Principles and practice* (6th ed., pp.69–94). Sudbury, MA: Jones and Bartlett.

Leininger, M. (Ed.). (1991). *Culture care diversity and universality: A theory of nursing*. New York: National League of Nursing.

Leininger, M. (1997). Overview of the theory of culture care with the ethnonursing research method. *Journal of Transcultural Nursing, 8*(2), 32–53.

Leininger, M. (2002). Culture care theory: A major contribution to advance transcultural nursing knowledge and practices. *Journal of Transcultural Nursing, 13*, 189–192.

Leininger, M. M., & McFarland, M. R. (2002). *Transcultural nursing: Concepts, theories, research & practice* (2nd ed.). New York: McGraw-Hill.

Leininger, M. M., & McFarland, M. R. (2006). *Culture care diversity and universality: A worldwide nursing theory* (3rd ed.). Sudbury, MA: Jones & Bartlett.

Masi, R. (1996). Inclusion: How can a health system respond to diversity. In A. S. Zieberth (Ed.), *Pinched: A management guide to the Canadian health care archipelago* (pp. 147–157). Nepean, ON: Pinched Press.

Maze, C. D. (2005). Registered nurses' personal rights vs. professional responsibility in caring for members of underserved and disenfranchised populations. *Journal of Clinical Nursing, 14*(5), 546–554.

Mutha, S., Allen, C., & Welch, M. (2002). *Toward culturally competent care: A toolbox for teaching communication strategies*. San Francisco: Regents of the University of California.

Narayanasamy, A. (2003). Transcultural nursing: How do nurses respond to cultural needs? *British Journal of Nursing, 12*(3), 185–194.

National Prevention Information Network. (2011). *What is cultural competency?* Retrieved October 18, 2011, from http://www.cdcnpin.org/scripts/population/culture.asp#what

Ngo-Metzger, Q., Telfair, J., Sorkin, D. H., Weidmer, B., Weech-Maldonado, R., Hurtado, M., et al. (2006). Cultural competency and quality of care: Obtaining the patient's perspective. The Commonwealth Fund. Retrieved August 22, 2011, from: http://www.commonwealthfund.org/Publications/Fund-Reports/2006/Oct/Cultural-Competency-and-Quality-of-Care--Obtaining-the-Patients-Perspective.aspx

Office of Minority Health. (2007). National standards on culturally and linguistically appropriate services (CLAS). Retrieved August 22, 2011, from: www.omhrc.gov/CLAS

Office of Minority Health. (2008). National standards on culturally and linguistically appropriate services (CLAS). Retrieved August 22, 2011, from: www.omhrc.gov/templates/browse.aspx?lvl=2&lvlID=15

Office of Minority Health. (2005). What is cultural competency? Retrieved August 22, 2011, from: www.omhrc.gov/templates/browse.aspx?lvl=2&lvlID=11

The Opportunity Agenda. (2009). *The state of opportunity in America, 2009: Key findings and recommendations.* Retrieved August 22, 2011, from: http://opportunityagenda.org/files/field_file/State%20of%20Opportunity%202009%20Key%20Findings%20Recommendations_0.pdf

Pearson, L. (2003). Understanding the culture of poverty. *The Nurse Practitioner, 28*, 4–6.

Purnell, L. (2008a). Transcultural diversity and healthcare. In L. Purnell & B. Paulanka (Eds.), *Transcultural health care: A culturally competent approach* (3rd ed., pp. 1–18). Philadelphia: F.A. Davis.

Purnell, L. (2008b). The Purnell model for cultural competence. In L. Purnell & B. Paulanka (Eds.), *Transcultural health care: A culturally competent approach* (3rd ed., pp. 19–55). Philadelphia: F.A. Davis.

Racher, F. E., & Annis, R. C. (2007). Respecting culture and honoring diversity in community practice [Electronic version]. *Research and Theory for Nursing Practice: An International Journal, 21*(4), 255–270.

Reyes-Ortiz, C. A., & Markides, K. S. (2010). Socioeconomic factors, immigration status, and cancer screening among Mexican American women aged 75 and older. Health Care for Women International, 31(12), 1068–1081.

Schim, S., Doorenbos, A., Benkert, R., & Miller, J. (2007). Culturally congruent care: Putting the puzzle together [Electronic version]. *Journal of Transcultural Nursing, 18*(2), 103–110.

Scott, D. E. (2008, January/February). The multicultural health care work environment [Electronic version]. *The American Nurse, 40*(1), 7.

Smedley, B. D., Stith, A. Y., & Nelson, A. R. (2003). *Unequal treatment: Confronting racial and ethnic disparities in health care*. Washington, DC: National Academies Press.

Spector, R. (2009). *Cultural diversity in health and illness* (6th ed.). Upper Saddle River, NJ: Pearson Prentice Hall.

Srivastava, R. H. (2007). Understanding cultural competence in health care. In R. H. Srivastava (Ed.), *The healthcare professional's guide to clinical cultural competence* (pp. 3–27). Toronto: Mosby Elsevier.

Stewart, S. H., & Silverstein, M. D. (2002). Racial and ethnic disparity in blood pressure and cholesterol measurement. *Journal of General Internal Medicine, 17,* 458–464.

Turale, S., & Ito, M. (2008). People of Japanese heritage. In L. Purnell & B. Paulanka (Eds.), *Transcultural health care: A culturally competent approach* (3rd ed., pp. 260–277). Philadelphia: F.A. Davis.

Turner, D. W. (1996). The role of culture in chronic illness [Electronic version]. *American Behavioral Scientist, 39(*6), 717–728.

U.S. Census Bureau. (2010a). The next four decades: the older population in the United States: 2010 to 2050 Retrieved January 5, 2011, from: http://www.census.gov/prod/2010pubs/p25-1138.pdf

U.S. Census Bureau. (2010b). The Population with Haitian ancestry in the United States: 2009. Retrieved January 5, 2011, from: http://www.census.gov/prod/2010pubs/acsbr09-18.pdf

Wallman, K. K. (1998). Data on race and ethnicity: Revising the federal standard. *The American Statistician, 52,* 1, 31–33.

Zoucha, R., & Zamarripa, C. A. (2008). People of Mexican heritage. In L. Purnell & B. Paulanka (Eds.), *Transcultural health care: A culturally competent approach* (3rd ed., pp. 309–324). Philadelphia: F.A. Davis.

CHAPTER 14

Self-Care

Judith E. Hertz

INTRODUCTION

On the surface, self-care is simply taking care of one's self to remain healthy. However, self-care within the context of living with a chronic illness is more complex. Self-care is required for successful management and control of chronic illnesses such as arthritis (McDonald-Miszczak & Wister, 2005; Yip, Sit, & Wong, 2004), heart disease (Burnette, Mui, & Zodikoff, 2004; Chriss, Sheposh, Carlson, & Riegel, 2004; Inglis, Pearson, Treen, Gallasch, Horowitz, & Stewart, 2006; Washburn, Hornberger, Klutman, & Skinner, 2005), diabetes (Berg & Wadhwa, 2007), HIV/AIDS (Mendias & Paar, 2007), asthma (Cortes, Lee, Boal, Mion, & Butler, 2004), and fecal incontinence (Bliss, Fischer, & Savik, 2005).

Self-care is also viewed as a pivotal concept in health promotion, disease prevention, and disease-screening programs (Haber, 2002; Potempa, Butterworth, Flaherty-Robb & Gaynor, 2010; Resnick, 2001, 2003). Furthermore, self-care has been viewed as essential to health in persons with chronic illnesses who receive care in nursing homes (Bickerstaff, Grasser & McCabe, 2003), home care (Sharkey, Ory, & Browne, 2005), and rehabilitation (Singleton, 2000), and during transitions from one healthcare setting to another (Coleman,

Smith, Frank, Min, Parry, & Kramer, 2004). Finally, self-care is applicable globally and transculturally when discussing health status in persons with chronic illnesses (Borg, Hallberg, & Blomqvist, 2006; Cortes et al., 2004; Inglis et al., 2006; Leenerts, Teel, & Pendelton, 2002; McDonald-Miszczak & Wister, 2005; Wang, Hsu, & Want, 2001; Yip et al., 2004).

Despite the widespread belief that self-care is integral to persons living with chronic illness, there is little agreement about the meaning of self-care. Sometimes self-care is defined as adherence/compliance with treatment regimens (Chriss et al., 2004), whereas other times it is referred to as having the functional ability to carry out activities of daily living (ADLs) and instrumental activities of daily living (IADLs) (Burnette et al., 2004). Other definitions imply that self-care is the belief that one can implement disease-treatment regimens (i.e., self-efficacy) (McDonald-Miszczak & Wister, 2005; Yip et al., 2004) or that one can manage and report symptoms associated with an illness (Chriss et al., 2004; Edwardson & Dean, 1999; Musil, Morris, Haug, Warner & Whelan, 2001). The ability to meet basic holistic human needs and achieve self-actualization provides yet another perspective (Hertz & Rossetti, 2006; Mendias & Paar, 2007; Potempa et al., 2010). The meaning of self-care becomes even more complex, because often it is equated solely to independent behaviors to care for self (Borg et al., 2006; Burnette et al., 2004); therefore, if one is dependent on others for assistance, as often happens when living with chronic illnesses, then it is implied that self-care cannot exist. However, Naik and colleagues recognize this situation in their analyses and recommendations for assessing two aspects of autonomy related to self-care (Naik, Dyer, Kunik, & McCullough, 2009a, 2009b; Naik, Teal, Pavlik, Dyer, & McCullough, 2008).

Although there is lack of agreement about the definition of self-care, there is implicit and explicit agreement that self-care is vital to individual health maintenance, disease prevention, and health promotion. When persons are living with chronic illnesses, the importance and need to care for self is further underscored.

KEY ISSUES AND FRAMEWORKS FOR VIEWING SELF-CARE WITHIN CHRONIC ILLNESS

The focus of this section is to compare and contrast the many definitions of self-care (or lack of self-care) with evidence to support each view, followed by a working definition of self-care. A self-care framework is presented, and key issues related to self-care in persons living with chronic illnesses are illustrated by reviewing the *Healthy People 2020* objectives. The framework and key issues set the stage for application of the nursing process by highlighting important considerations for nurses to address when promoting self-care in clients.

Perspectives on Self-Care

Diverse perspectives of self-care are provided via research on self-care in various populations living with chronic illnesses. These include the idea that self-care means: 1) to comply or adhere to prescribed medical treatments for chronic illnesses; 2) to have a personal belief that one is capable of following disease treatment regimens; 3) to have the functional abilities to carry out daily activities including ADLs and IADLS independently; and 4) to self-determine how to meet one's unique, personal basic human and self-actualization needs. Still others have addressed self-care as being multidimensional. Each perspective will be discussed.

Self-Care as Adherence with Medical Treatments

Haber's (2002) critical analysis of federal initiatives regarding health promotion and aging emphasizes physical aspects and a medical orientation toward self-care and health promotion. Self-care is implied as adherence to recommended secondary prevention interventions through disease risk reduction (e.g., smoking cessation) and screening practices (e.g., mammograms).

Edwardson and Dean (1999) explored how selected demographic, social, situational, and symptom-experience factors influence the "appropriateness" of self-care responses to symptoms. In other words, the way persons manage symptoms is influenced by many factors. In this study, self-care was equated to medical management of symptoms. Healthcare professionals judged clients' responses to symptoms as either "appropriate" or "inappropriate," using an evidence-based algorithm. If persons did not seek professional care, used "unsafe" remedies, or did not follow guidelines from professionals, their response was considered "inappropriate."

Sharkey, Ory, and Browne (2005) studied homebound older persons receiving meal delivery in North Carolina to identify the extent that older persons use strategies to reduce out-of-pocket medication expenses when self-managing their medications. From this perspective, lack of self-care was assumed to include noncompliance with medical treatment regimens. Twenty percent admitted to using one or more of the following behaviors to restrict medication use and costs: 1) taking less medicine than the prescribed amount, 2) going without the medication because of cost, 3) getting free drug samples from physicians, 4) obtaining a partial refill of a prescription, 5) taking the drug only when "needed," or 6) buying only the most important medications. Although these results seem to be "anti-self-management" or "anti-self-care," they highlight the need to address the concerns and perceptions of patients when trying to promote self-care. Sometimes caring for one's self conflicts with recommended treatment regimens.

In reviewing the literature regarding health outcomes in persons living with chronic illnesses (diabetes, chronic obstructive pulmonary disease, or chronic heart disease), self-care was equated to self-management of the person's disease state as well as adherence to medical treatment (Scollan-Koliopoulos & Walker, 2009; Sutherland & Hayter, 2009). The purposes of these reviews differed. Scollan-Koliopoulos and Walker were examining studies on the effects of previous exposure to diabetes in family members on self-care, referred to as a multigenerational timeline. Sutherland and Hayter's review was focused on self-care as an outcome of nurse-managed care. Nonetheless, both review teams limited their perspective on self-care to self-management of a disease process according to recommended medical treatments.

Others differentiate self-care from self-management (Ryan & Sawin, 2009). Self-care was linked primarily to carrying out ADLs without the advice of healthcare providers. Barlow, Sturt, and Hearnshaw (2002) also identified tasks performed by healthy people at home, including preventative strategies, as self-care. Self-management was viewed as daily tasks carried out at home by individuals to control or reduce the impact of disease on physical health. According to Ryan and Sawin, these behaviors must be learned and require assistance from health providers. After reviewing the literature on self-management programs for arthritis, asthma, and diabetes, Barlow and colleagues made recommendations for development of programs to promote self-management of other chronic health conditions.

In summary, self-care has been linked to compliance with recommended medical treatment. However, sometimes self-initiated behaviors may be in conflict with those recommendations. Learning to live with chronic illness most certainly involves following medical recommendations to reduce exacerbations. However, in some situations self-care is not the same as self-management of an illness or compliance with medical recommendations.

Self-Care as Belief in Being Able to Self-Manage

Typical disease self-management programs for arthritis, chronic heart disease, HIV/AIDS, diabetes mellitus, and asthma focus on monitoring and reporting symptoms as well as monitoring adherence to medical regimens. Research on self-management programs often attempts to identify how self-efficacy beliefs (i.e., belief that one is capable of self-managing one's treatment regimen) along with other psychological characteristics such as locus of control, perceived threat, or a sense of well-being and situational variables such as demographics, living arrangements, and overall health influence the ability to self-manage a health condition. Outcomes from these studies often look at symptom relief, functional ability status, changes in self-efficacy beliefs, and laboratory values indicative of "disease control."

An arthritis self-management program with older persons in Hong Kong introduced Tai Chi as a self-management technique. In this study, self-efficacy was greater, pain decreased, and motor strength increased in the intervention group (Yip et al., 2004) when compared with the control group receiving "usual care." Self-efficacy beliefs were linked to self-care approaches in disease self-management and to positive health outcomes.

A longitudinal study (McDonald-Miszczak & Wister, 2005) with a national Canadian sample also linked self-efficacy to the 11 arthritis self-management "self-care" behaviors of diet, exercise, sleep, self-help group participation, use of alternative remedies, modifications of environment, reading, stress reduction, meditation/prayer, consulting family/friends, and consulting others with the same condition. Self-efficacy beliefs did not predict the use of these 11 behaviors to manage arthritis. However, previous use of these behaviors (i.e., past experience) was a strong predictor of these prescribed self-care behaviors and supplemented self-efficacy beliefs.

Similarly, at the end of 3 months, previous use of self-care behaviors was a significant predictor of self-care in monitoring symptoms, following medical guidelines, reporting symptoms, and seeking help in a self-management program designed for persons with heart failure in a study conducted in the southwestern United States (Chriss et al., 2004). Other characteristics such as social support, education, gender, age, income, comorbidities, and symptom severity were not predictive of this type of self-care.

A descriptive correlational study was conducted with persons living with heart failure (Britz & Dunn, 2010). The relationship between self-care abilities (maintenance, management, and confidence) and multiple dimensions of quality of life was explored. Self-care confidence, similar to the concept of self-efficacy, was significantly related to physical, emotional, and overall quality of life.

These studies illustrate that previous lifestyle and experiences are predictive of how persons will manage chronic illnesses in terms of adhering to prescribed behaviors. Although some personal demographic characteristics, emotional state, and personal beliefs about being able to take control and manage a disease on a daily basis had some effect on following the prescribed behaviors, the strongest predictor was previous experience in using the behaviors. This leads one to believe that life experiences and personal values may be very important in determining each individual's self-care behaviors.

Self-Care as Functional Abilities and Independence

Burnette and colleagues (2004) used functional abilities as an indicator of self-care in their study with a national sample of 597 persons diagnosed with coronary heart disease (CHD) compared to those without CHD. These researchers proposed that most of the everyday work of managing CHD relied upon self-care as opposed to professional care. They defined self-care as the active role persons play in determining outcomes resulting from professional care. The coping strategies of behavioral change, environmental adaptations, and medical equipment use represented self-care strategies in their study. These strategies were also linked to functional abilities related to ADLs, IADLs, and mobility. Impaired functional abilities indicated a lack of self-care.

Borg and colleagues (2006) proposed that "older persons who are not able to manage daily life by themselves may have a different view of life satisfaction than those with preserved self-care capacity" (p. 608). Self-care capacity was defined as having functional abilities to carry out activities independently. This study's findings imply that functional limitations are linked to self-care and that those limitations, more so than the presence of a chronic illness, can affect holistic health outcomes. Persons with functional limitations might need special assistance and attention to support their self-care practices to promote health.

The impact of functional abilities on self-care and making autonomous decisions was also identified by Naik and colleagues (2009a, 2009b). They noted that some persons, particularly older adults, might have decisional autonomy capabilities in determining self-care, but lack the executional autonomy capabilities and functional abilities to actually follow through in carrying out self-care. Naik and colleagues (2008) proposed methods to assess these two dimensions of autonomy and self-care.

Self-neglect is inability to meet basic needs and is viewed as the opposite of self-care (Dyer, Goodwin, Pickens-Pace, Burnett, & Kelly, 2007). In older clients receiving adult protective services in the United States, the prevalence of self-neglect is 50.3% nationally. Dyer and colleagues developed a case definition of self-neglect based on characteristics of 538 cases. The mean age of these clients was 75.6 years, and 70% were women. Executive dysfunction, or the inability to execute specific complex tasks such as ADLs and IADLs independently, was at the root of self-neglect. Executive dysfunction was also associated with several chronic illnesses, including dementia, depression, diabetes, psychiatric illness, cardiovascular disease, and nutritional deficiency. Self-neglect—seemingly the converse of the definition of self-care—links self-care to the functional ability of acting independently.

CASE STUDY

You are employed in an ambulatory healthcare clinic in a rural healthcare system. One of your clients is Mrs. Smith, an 82-year-old widow who lives alone in a mobile home. Mrs. Smith was diagnosed with osteoarthritis more than 10 years ago and recently was diagnosed as being in the early stages of congestive heart failure. Mrs. Smith's 55-year-old daughter and family live 50 miles from her home, and her 45-year-old son lives with his wife and four teenage children 10 miles away. Mrs. Smith recently fell on the steps leading into her home. She was transported by ambulance to the closest emergency department located within the healthcare system at which you are employed, about 40 miles from Mrs. Smith's home. Luckily, Mrs. Smith did not fracture any bones when she fell. She was discharged but is now unable to drive a car and must use a walker because of severe leg pain. She has been taking five medications

(continues)

CASE STUDY   (Continued)

for her arthritis and heart condition but her current pain is unrelieved. She has an appointment at your clinic 2 days after her discharge from the emergency department.

Discussion Questions

1. How do you begin your assessment of Mrs. Smith? Why?
2. Identify at least one self-care goal related to each of Mrs. Smith's diagnosed chronic illnesses.
3. What intervention strategies should be used to help Mrs. Smith achieve each self-care goal? Why did you choose these strategies?
4. List at least three self-care outcomes related to the identified self-care intervention strategies.

Self-Care as Self-Determined Behaviors That Meet the Individual's Unique Needs

Singleton (2000) traced the history of self-care from Florence Nightingale to the present in an eloquent analysis of self-care. The analysis provided a framework for her study on how nurses encourage rehabilitation clients to care for themselves. She emphasized that self-care should be defined by how clients actually care for themselves, and that greater understanding is needed regarding the methods used by nurses to encourage clients to care for themselves in ways that meet their unique needs.

In a nurse-led, home-based multidisciplinary intervention with older persons after hospitalization for heart failure in South Australia, Inglis and colleagues (2006) incorporated unique self-determined behaviors in their definition of self-care. Although interventions were aimed at promoting adherence to medical treatments as a means of promoting self-care, the researchers also included special interventions to empower older persons to facilitate their self-determination. Thus, self-determination of self-care was emphasized.

The self-care practices of older persons who had fecal incontinence and who were enrolled in one health maintenance organization were investigated by Bliss and colleagues (2005). On average, these persons reported 2.3 chronic conditions with a range from 0–10, and 1.9 specific self-care practices with a range from 0–7. Self-care activities included diet modifications, use of panty liners, reduction in activities, and use of medications to stop diarrhea. Only 43% reported discussing this problem and their self-care practices with their healthcare providers. Only the self-care practice of diet changes was routinely discussed with providers. This emphasizes that sometimes the self-care carried out by persons with chronic illnesses truly is unique to meet personal needs, and that often these self-care practices are not discussed with healthcare providers.

In a 27-month longitudinal study with 387 randomly selected older community-dwelling adults (Musil et al., 2001), arthritis and cardio-pulmonary symptoms were assessed for consistent recurrence and their effects on well-being and symptom management with self-care. Self-care was defined as the use of home remedies, over-the-counter medications, or changes in lifestyle, but did not include deciding when to seek professional help. There were differences in the use of self-care for persons with each diagnosis. Persons with arthritis and chronic pain complaints across time used self-care, whereas those with cardiopulmonary symptoms did not. It was concluded that patterns differ by the type of symptom and illness and that managing chronic illness is a complex phenomenon.

Essential dimensions of self-care and an integrated model were proposed after reviewing research on self-care conducted in Sweden and Finland (Leenerts et al., 2002). In the model, it was emphasized that self-care activities were related to the individual person's unique view of health and the individual's self-concept. The authors recommended that nurses incorporate the client's personal beliefs about health into their teaching about self-care activities, and that nurses partner with clients to support meeting their personal needs. They also identified evidence-based outcomes of health promotion in aging individuals as connectedness to others, resource use, transcendence, and well-being. Self-care activities or skills were classified as communication, healthy lifestyle, building meaning in life, and socializing. They added that self-care takes place within the context of internal and external human environments.

In another study (Bickerstaff et al., 2003), activities that help nursing home residents transcend difficulties and live with contentment and satisfaction in life were identified. In this study, self-care meant activities that promoted holistic health. The 95 respondents, with an average age of 82.2 years, had lived in the nursing home from 3–177 months ($M = 35.6$ months) and reported a variety of self-care activities. They included 1) generativity activities through helping or reaching out to others and involving family; 2) introjectivity activities such as hobbies, travel, and lifelong learning; (3) temporal integration activities which were past-, present-, and future-based behaviors; 4) body-transcendence activities that incorporated flexibility and making changes in life; and 5) spirituality activities to develop relationships with self, others, and a higher being. These self-care activities encompassed more than a physical orientation to health and well-being and were based on the individual's perception of needs.

Likewise, Wang and colleagues (2001) used focus groups to explore the perceptions of health-promoting self-care in community-dwelling, Taiwanese older adults. All but 4 of the 21 men and women participants were living with some type of chronic illness. The investigators identified five types of self-care activities that these older persons employed in caring for themselves. They included: 1) balancing or adjusting one's health; 2) initiating or purposefully using self-care activities; 3) regularizing or maintaining a daily rhythm over time; 4) socializing or involving and connecting with society; and 5) sublimating or seeing the positive side and transcending their situations. They concluded that older adults in Taiwan viewed health and self-care activities as mind–body connections with holistic harmony rather than merely as physical health.

Maddox (1999) conducted a 3-year qualitative study of older women in three different age groups to identify their self-care activities and the meaning they assigned to health. The groups were comprised of: 1) 12 nuns ages 72 to 104; 2) eight 55- to 76-year-old women who lived in single-family dwellings and worked in blue-collar occupations; and 3) five 55- to 86-year-old residents of an urban retirement community who were previously employed as domestic help or worked on farms or in factories. Their reported self-care activities included: 1) interactions with a being greater than one's self; 2) acceptance of self; 3) humor; 4) flexibility; and 5) quality of being other-centered. It was pointed out that these self-care activities incorporated more than the traditional physical self-care activities of nutrition, exercise, and relaxation but also included holistic, spiritual, social, and emotional behaviors.

Hertz and Rossetti (2006) also found that self-care actions or activities were unique for older persons with chronic illness who lived independently in apartments. Common themes and patterns were identified from the activities reported by the 14 male and female respondents. These themes represent types of self-care activities including: 1) adapting to life as an older adult by using coping strategies, assistive devices, and avoiding hassles; 2) meeting needs for affiliated individuation by balancing activities that meet needs for independence and time alone with those that meet needs for dependence and socialization; (3) using self-care knowledge to promote and strive for holistic health by using personal beliefs and values to promote quality of life and self-actualization; 4) self-managing health problems through seeking medical and alternative treatments and by sometimes avoiding medical intervention or treatment; and 5) preventing health problems and issues by following recommendations for screenings and health promotion and by taking safety precautions. The diversity of these individually determined self-care activities also reflect the multidimensionality of self-care.

Self-Care as a Multidimensional Concept

Beattie, Whitelaw, Mettler, and Turner (2003) proposed a model that uses community-based organizations such as area agencies on aging, faith-based organizations, and public health departments to promote health. The dimensions of self-care were implied to include reducing risks to illnesses, managing illnesses, and coping with functional limits.

Lubben and Damron-Rodriguez (2003) analyzed the World Health Organization's Kobe Centre model for organizing health care at the community level for the older adult population. Within this model, self-care was differentiated from professional care (i.e., disease management) and social network care. The authors viewed self-care as multiple activities that prolonged active life and prevented functional declines. Recommendations were made initially to foster the individual's self-care capacity by encouraging productive roles and self-direction, followed by building social network support that accommodates the diverse needs of older adults, and finally engaging community professional services for health care of older adults. Enhancing home and community environments is important because those environments are the contexts in which persons live.

Summary and Working Definition of Self-Care

In summary, there are diverse perspectives about what self-care means and evidence exists to support each perspective. Therefore, the working definition of self-care for this chapter incorporates these diverse perspectives.

Self-care has multiple dimensions, is self-determined, and is unique to each individual based on that person's life experiences, values, beliefs, and personal characteristics and abilities, including biopsychosocial-spiritual and functional abilities. Self-care influences each individual's holistic health. Self-care includes a variety of activities such as following prescribed medical treatments and lifestyle recommendations for chronic illnesses (e.g., take medications, monitor and report symptoms, smoking cessation, diet modifications); carrying out daily activities including ADLs, IADLS, and mobility (e.g., hygiene, dressing, toileting); adhering to recommended guidelines for disease prevention and health promotion (regular screenings, dietary guidelines, exercise); meeting basic needs (e.g., food, shelter, safety, socializing, individuation); and pursuing personal interests that promote spiritual well-being and self-actualization (e.g., meditation, prayer, hobbies, learning).

Self-care includes performing activities both independently and dependently. Furthermore, self-care can be supported and nurtured by nurses and other healthcare professionals. The following framework provides guidelines for promoting self-care in persons living with chronic illnesses.

Self-Care: A Framework for Assessment and Intervention

In nursing, Orem's (2001) theory and perspective on self-care is frequently cited. The original focus of this theory was on patients' self-care deficits or the inability to carry out self-care tasks required for physical health. Conversely, self-care agency is the capability to care for one's self and emphasizes physical abilities. It is implied that healthcare professionals, including nurses, define for clients what self-care is needed and then carry out those activities for the client if the client lacks the capability to do so. Within this definition, there is logical incongruence. If self-care is caring for one's self, then it makes sense that the client, rather than the nurse or other healthcare provider, should be the expert regarding what is needed. Therefore, a theory that is more congruent with the working definition of self-care is presented.

The self-care model (Hertz & Baas, 2006) from modeling and role-modeling (MRM) nursing theory (Erickson, Tomlin, & Swain, 1988; Erickson, 2006) provides a more congruent framework for addressing assessment, interventions, and outcome evaluations of self-care in persons living with chronic illnesses. This perspective takes into account the unique, self-determined, multidimensional nature of self-care based on individual biology, values, and life experiences. It also recognizes that self-care is possible when persons are living with chronic illnesses and when they might be dependent on others for assistance. Finally, the overriding framework of MRM theory provides a focus for interventions that are self-care supportive via the five aims of intervention.

Figure 14-1 illustrates the MRM self-care model. In this model, self-care has three components: self-care knowledge, self-care resources, and self-care actions. Self-care knowledge is the individual's personal knowledge regarding their personal needs and goals. Those personal needs can include basic and higher level human needs as described by Maslow and others (see Erickson et al., 1988; Erickson, 2006) as well as the need for affiliated individuation, a concept unique to MRM theory and representing the need for persons to sense a separateness and independence

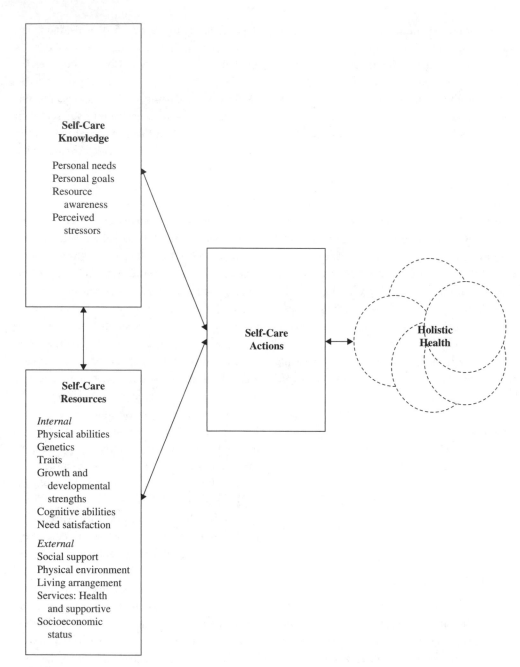

FIGURE 14-1   Framework for Self-Care in Persons Living with Chronic Illnesses.

from others while at the same time needing to feel connected to and being able to rely on others. Self-care knowledge also incorporates knowledge, either at a conscious or subconscious level, regarding what may have caused a health problem/issue and what will help resolve that issue. This personal knowledge includes perceptions of availability of resources and stressors in the individual's life. Self-care knowledge is the foundation for each individual's unique "model" or view of one's own world or life situation. Self-care knowledge is interrelated to self-care resources.

Self-care resources are internal and external to the individual. Internal resources include genetic makeup; physical, mental, and cognitive functioning; as well as psychosocial and spiritual characteristics and traits developed over the person's lifetime and as a result of need satisfaction. External resources include persons who provide social support, the physical environment (e.g., geography, urban versus rural, climate, community design), living arrangements (e.g., type of housing, accessibility, safety, neighbors, living alone), service availability (e.g., health care, transportation, social services), and socioeconomic status. These self-care resources are interdependent on self-care knowledge. For example, each person must recognize social support as such; an outsider's view of the presence of social support is less valid than the individual's view of the support. Although support may be available, the client may perceive the behaviors of those support persons as not helpful. Both self-care knowledge and resources are interrelated with self-care actions.

Self-care actions are those activities undertaken by persons to influence health status. Self-care actions require using one's personal self-care knowledge and mobilizing self-care resources to do what is best for one's self. Therefore, self-care actions require that each person perceive a sense of autonomy (Hertz, 1996). To some extent, self-care actions are unique for each individual.

For example, all persons have a need for love and belonging and to affiliate with others. One person might meet this need by purposefully participating in social activities such as a family reunion where one feels they belong and are loved as a member of a family unit; likely, this approach is based on life experiences within the family unit when that person previously felt love and belonging. Another person with different experiences and who has not experienced those feelings within the family unit might have their personal needs for love and belonging met through the caring behaviors of a nurse. For that person, self-neglect of a health problem might lead to reestablishment of a relationship with a nurse, which, in turn, could meet that person's need for love and belonging. In both instances, persons are meeting needs for love and belonging and, therefore, are influencing their holistic health status. Obviously, the person who acted in a self-neglectful mode to meet those needs might eventually deplete their resources (physical and other coping resources). Therefore, the nurse can use nursing knowledge of health processes to assist this person to find other means for meeting those needs that will build up rather than deplete resources over the long-term.

According to this model of self-care, health is holistic, meaning that it is more than the absence of physical and mental illness. It incorporates aspects of biopsychosocial-spiritual well-being, quality of life, and self-actualization in addition to addressing and reducing the harmful effects of illnesses. This definition of health is applicable to persons living with chronic illnesses. A high level of health and chronic illness can coexist. Nurses can facilitate and nurture self-care through unconditionally accepting the person and that person's unique view or "model" of the world and then by "role-modeling" interventions that fit with that person's model.

There are five aims of interventions in MRM that guide the nurse with each person. They include:

- Build trust with each client in the nurse–client relationship so that the client trusts others.
- Promote a positive orientation to one's self as a person of worth and to foster hope for the future.
- Facilitate client control so that each person feels and perceives a sense of control over the environment (internal and external) and the person's life situation.
- Build on strengths in terms of building on the person's capabilities and life experiences even in the presence of an illness
- Set mutual health-directed goals based on the client's model of the world.

Structuring interventions around these aims is supportive of self-care.

KEY ISSUES IN PROMOTING SELF-CARE IN PERSONS WITH CHRONIC ILLNESS

According to *Healthy People 2020* (U.S. Department of Health and Human Services [USDHHS], 2010), health outcomes are determined by biology and genetics (e.g., diseases, body functioning), individual behavior (e.g., exercise, smoking, sleep, diet, etc.), social environment (e.g., resources to meet needs such as education and jobs, social support, transportation, public safety), physical environment (e.g., weather, exposure to toxic substances, aesthetics, physical barriers for persons with disabilities), and health services (e.g., access, quality,

costs; see *Healthy People 2020* Framework [USDHHS, n.d.b]). This perspective on health is also congruent with the MRM self-care framework. Many of the behaviors, objectives, and goals referred to in the *Healthy People* document are integral to self-care.

In **Table 14-1**, relevant national objectives and goals from the *Healthy People 2020* (USDHHS, 2010) highlight the key issues to be addressed when supporting the self-care of persons with one or more chronic illnesses. Self-care requires taking actions on one's own behalf to influence health. Self-care goals and objectives found in *Healthy People* are focused on the following key issues: 1) *health education* about key aspects of living with chronic illness (e.g., knowledge about disease processes and management of disease, treatments, monitoring for symptoms); 2) adjustment to or *coping* with the illness (e.g., living with loss of function associated with illness, adaptive equipment, maintaining/improving psychosocial health while living with illness, adjusting to activity limitations); 3) *health promotion* and prevention of other related physical and psychosocial problems (e.g., health promotion, counseling for healthy behaviors); and 4) development of *support and assistance* from family/friends and others (e.g., support groups, caregiver support and education, ensuring ADLs and IADLs are met).

Healthcare Reform and Self-Care

On March 23, 2010, President Obama signed into law the Affordable Care Act, commonly referred to as the healthcare reform act, for persons living in the United States (USDHHS, n.d.b). Several provisions in this comprehensive law can facilitate self-care in persons living with chronic diseases.

Table 14-1   Examples of Relevant Healthy People 2020 Goals and Objectives Highlighting Key Issues Regarding Self-Care in Persons Living with Chronic Illnesses

Healthy People 2020 Goals and Objectives	Key Self-Care Issues
1. Access to quality health services *Goal:* Improve access to quality healthcare services *Objectives:* AHS-2: Health insurance coverage for clinical preventive services AHS-3: Persons with usual primary care provider AHS-5: Source of ongoing care AHS-7: Receipt of evidence-based clinical preventive services	Health promotion
2. Arthritis, osteoporosis, and chronic back conditions *Goal:* Prevent illness and disability related to arthritis and other rheumatic conditions, osteoporosis, and chronic back conditions *Objectives:* AOCBC-4: Reduce the proportion of adults with doctor-diagnosed arthritis who have difficulty in performing two or more personal care activities, thereby preserving independence AOCBC-5: Reduce the proportion of adults with doctor-diagnosed arthritis who report serious psychological distress AOCBC-7: Increase the proportion of adults with doctor-diagnosed arthritis who receive healthcare provider counseling AOCBC-8: Increase the proportion of adults with doctor-diagnosed arthritis who have had effective, evidence-based arthritis education as an integral part of the management of their condition	Health promotion; support and assistance; coping; health education
8. Diabetes *Goal:* Reduce the disease and economic burden of diabetes mellitus (DM) and improve the quality of life for all persons who have, or are at risk for, DM *Objectives:* D-13: Increase the proportion of adults with diabetes who perform self-blood glucose-monitoring at least once daily D-14: Increase the proportion of persons with diagnosed diabetes who receive formal diabetes education	Health education

U.S. Department of Health and Human Services (USDHHS). (2010). *Healthy People 2020.* Retrieved August 23, 2011, from: http://www.healthypeople.gov/2020/default.aspx

First, the preexisting insurance plan program (HealthCare.gov, n.d.f) ensures that those persons who have preexisting conditions, such as chronic illnesses, will not be denied insurance coverage. This will also be true for children younger than age 19 who are living with preexisting conditions (HealthCare.gov, n.d.c). In addition, children up to the age of 26 can be included on their parents' healthcare insurance plan (HealthCare.gov, n.d.j). The law also stops insurance companies from placing lifetime and annual limits on spending (HealthCare.gov, n.d.a). These mandates are intended to facilitate the ability of persons to pay for health care.

For those with Medicare prescription plans, two aspects of the law influence the ability of persons to afford their prescribed drugs. The provision for a one-time rebate of $250 will help those persons who are in the "donut hole"—that is having to pay out of pocket for drugs after a certain amount has been spent (HealthCare.gov, n.d.b). Provisions are in place to also offer 50% discounts on drugs after spending certain amounts (HealthCare.gov, n.d.d). This helps persons having to choose between prescription drugs and paying for food, housing, etc. (Sharkey et al., 2005).

Wellness services will be covered for those receiving Medicare and other healthcare insurance plans (HealthCare.gov, n.d.i; HealthCare.gov, n.d.h). This includes wellness examinations, some screening procedures, vaccinations, and counseling services to aid persons in making decisions about how to care for self, including how to self-manage their chronic illnesses.

The Patient's Bill of Rights (HealthCare.gov, n.d.e) is aimed at putting the client in charge of their health care in collaboration with the healthcare provider. Persons will be encouraged to seek the health care that best meets their needs, that is, to pursue self-care. This includes provisions that mandate the ability to choose a primary care provider within the insurance plan's network of providers (HealthCare.gov, n.d.g).

Overall, these provisions should facilitate the abilities of persons to obtain effective interventions that promote their abilities to care for themselves.

INTERVENTIONS

There is a lack of evidence-based clinical practice guidelines focused specifically on supporting self-care in persons living with chronic illnesses. However, on the National Guideline Clearinghouse website (www.guideline.gov), multiple tangentially related guidelines are identified (see **Table 14-2**). Examples include ones that focus on "counseling" or "management," contain a patient resource for implementation, include patients as intended users, address the care needs of "living with illness" or "staying healthy," and focus on the domain of patient-centeredness. In particular, there is a guideline to promote self-management in persons living with chronic illnesses. Oddly, this guideline does not contain a client resource. However, its focus is on children living with chronic illnesses and their families. Likewise, several guidelines address the key issues and health problems found in *Healthy People 2020* (USDHHS, 2010) and listed in Table 14-1. These guidelines address specific assessment, medical management, intervention strategies, and outcome evaluation.

In addition to these guidelines, programs that support self-care have been studied empirically. What follows are guidelines for assessment and intervention. All are based on the MRM self-care model, results of empirical studies, and comprehensive literature reviews.

Assessment

Based on the MRM self-care framework (Erickson et al., 1988; Erickson, 2006; Hertz & Baas, 2006) and because the client's model of the world is most important in setting priorities and planning interventions, the client should be the

Table 14-2   Relevant Clinical Practice Guidelines to Support Self-Care Through Health Education, Coping, Health Promotion, and Support and Assistance

Chronic Care Self-Management

Chronic Care Self-management Guideline Team, Cincinnati Children's Hospital Medical Center. (2007, March). *Evidence-based care guideline for chronic care: Self-management* (Guideline no. 30). Cincinnati OH: Cincinnati Children's Hospital Medical Center.
http://guidelines.gov/content.aspx?id=10593&search=evidence-based+guideline+for+chronic+care%3a+self-management

Arthritis

National Collaborating Centre for Chronic Conditions. (2008, February). *The care and management of osteoarthritis in adults* (Clinical guideline no. 59). London UK: National Institute for Health and Clinical Excellence (NICE).
http://guidelines.gov/content.aspx?id=14322&search=osteoarthritis#Section434

Asthma

Global Initiative for Asthma (GINA). (2009). *Global strategy for asthma management and prevention*. Bethesda, MD: Author.
http://guidelines.gov/content.aspx?id=15556&search=global+strategy+for+asthma

Depression in Persons with Chronic Illness

National Collaborating Centre for Mental Health. (2009, October). *Depression in adults with a chronic physical health problem. Treatment and management* (Clinical guideline no. 91). London, UK: National Institute for Health and Clinical Excellence (NICE).
http://guidelines.gov/content.aspx?id=15522&search=depression+in+adults

Hypertension

Medical Services Commission. (2008, February). *Hypertension-detection, diagnosis and management*. Victoria, BC: British Columbia Medical Association.
http://guidelines.gov/content.aspx?id=14257&search=hypertension

Chronic Obstructive Pulmonary Disease

Institute for Clinical Systems Improvement (ICSI). (2009, January). *Diagnosis and management of chronic obstructive pulmonary disease* (COPD). Bloomington, MN: Author.
http://guidelines.gov/content.aspx?id=14439&search=diagnosis+and+management+of+chronic+obstructive

Medication Adherence

National Collaborating Centre for Primary Care. (2009, January). *Medicines adherence. Involving patients in decisions about prescribed medicines and supporting adherence* (Clinical guideline no. 76). London, UK: National Institute for Health and Clinical Excellence (NICE).
http://guidelines.gov/content.aspx?id=14342&search=medicines+adherence

Diabetes

American Association of Diabetes Educators (AADE). (2009). *Guidelines for the practice of diabetes education*. Chicago, IL: Author.
http://guidelines.gov/content.aspx?id=14696&search=diabetes+education

Stroke

Lindsay, P., Bayley, M., Hellings, C., Hill, M., Woodbury, E., & Phillips, S. (2008). Public awareness and patient education. Patient and family education. Canadian best practice recommendations for stroke care. *Canadian Medical Association Journal, 179*(12 Suppl), E13–E15.
http://guidelines.gov/content.aspx?id=14183&search=patient+and+family+education#top

primary source of information when doing an assessment. The initial assessment questions should focus on identifying the person's perceived needs and understanding of the health issue for which nursing care is sought or recommended. For example, at the beginning of each encounter, the nurse should ask, "What is your biggest concern right now?" This immediately identifies the client's primary concern(s). Appropriate prompts include: "Tell me why you came to the [clinic, hospital, nursing home, rehabilitation setting]," "Tell me why home healthcare nurses were asked to visit you," and "Tell me what has been happening to you." These questions help the nurse comprehend the client's view of the health problem. Conversely, questions such as "How can I help you?" focus on the nurse by using the word "I" rather than the client. Furthermore, when asking for the client's perspective, the nurse should be prepared for an unexpected response.

Many times the responses from clients will be surprising. For instance, a client might believe that hospitalization occurred so that the client can get some sleep, whereas the healthcare professional's reason is to ensure close monitoring of a chronic illness. The nurse must accept the client's response rather than try to explain that the response is "wrong." Indeed, research studies have found that identifying personal needs is a key to promoting and supporting self-care (Leenerts et al., 2002) along with the perception of overall health (Borg et al., 2006; Resnick, 2001, 2003). Those with higher perceived health are more likely to also pursue recommended self-care healthy behaviors (e.g., exercise program, eating a healthy diet, regular health screenings).

After the problem or needs are identified, the next focus of assessment is to gain an understanding of the client's self-care knowledge regarding what might help relieve this problem. Simply asking, "What do you think will help you?" will provide a picture of the client's model of the world. Again, it is important for the nurse to accept the client's response as accurate and realize that it is important to understand the client's views. Often the perceptions between providers and clients differ regarding self-care (Cortes et al., 2004). Assessing preferences and satisfaction with services leads to successful self-care supportive interventions (Matsui & Capezuti, 2008; Mendias & Paar, 2007; see Evidence-Based Practice Box) and can facilitate self-care actions.

After asking these essential questions, data should be gathered regarding the client's health-related goals, personal values, and internal and external self-care resources. According to research exploring predictors of self-care, information could be asked of the client's family members as well as the client, which provides a secondary source of information. As noted by Naik and colleagues (2008), not only should the client's desires and goals in the form of decisions be addressed but also the client's ability to follow through and carry out their decisions.

Internal resources should be assessed. Age has been found to influence self-care actions. Older community-residing adults participated in more self-care activities that focused on health promotion such as exercise programs, eating a healthy diet, and getting adequate sleep (Resnick, 2001, 2003). The belief that one can carry out self-care actions, in other words, self-efficacy, required for disease management is also important to assess (Callaghan, 2005). Self-efficacy may vary according to ethnicity. Callaghan found that blacks and Latinos had lower levels of self-efficacy than did white non-Latinos. Cognitive ability should also be assessed, as those with lower cognitive abilities may not be able to carry out self-care actions or to direct others to assist them (Cortes et al., 2004; Resnick, 2003). Functional abilities to carry out self-care tasks should be assessed as well. Studies have found that individuals who lack functional abilities predicted the number of recommended health-promoting self-care behaviors (e.g., healthy diet, exercise program) more than the presence of chronic illness (Borg et al., 2006; Callaghan, 2005). The presence of medical problems and disabilities can also influence self-care (Callaghan, 2005; Cortes et al., 2004; Resnick, 2001).

External resources found to predict self-care actions include perceived adequacy of income and insurance to pay for health care (Borg et al., 2006; Callaghan, 2005; Cortes et al., 2004). Persons with income levels of between $750 and $1000 per month in the United States at the time of this study were more likely to choose between buying food and medications, were less likely to have supplemental drug coverage, and were more likely to restrict medication use through various means such as taking less than prescribed, taking the drug only in response to symptoms, prioritizing the drugs that were most important, or obtaining a partial refill on prescriptions (Sharkey et al., 2005). Likewise, it is important to find out what services the client is using and how satisfied the client is with those services (Matsui & Capezuti, 2008).

Perceived social support should be assessed (Callaghan, 2005; Matsui & Capezuti, 2008). It is not the number of persons who are available to give support but rather the clients' perceptions of who is supportive in helping them get what is needed that is critical. Perception of social support should include the assessment of the quality of the relationship with a primary care provider, because a poor relationship might provide a barrier to self-care (Cortes et al., 2004). Finally, transportation is an important resource to assess whether recommended self-care includes traveling to support group meetings, formal classes, or clinics (Cortes et al., 2004; Mendias & Paar, 2007).

Nursing Interventions

Diverse approaches to supporting and promoting self-care have been studied. Interventions discussed here are based on individual reports of nursing interventions but share some commonalities. Self-management programs for discrete chronic illnesses will be addressed, followed by comprehensive programs for individuals with multiple chronic illnesses.

Singleton's (2000) ethnographic study identified methods used by nurses to encourage clients to care for themselves in rehabilitation. Nurses reported that they focused on the individual person and included coordinating care, talking to clients, and teaching. In addition, the investigator observed the nurses taking time with clients, using presence, and building trust to promote the client's control over their own self-care. Oddly, the nurses themselves did not verbally report these activities, but the investigator observed them. Nonetheless, they are congruent with the MRM self-care framework and aims of interventions.

Washburn, Hornberger, Klutman, and Skinner (2005) examined nurses' knowledge of six key topic areas for educating patients about heart failure management and key self-management principles in a Midwestern U.S. healthcare system. Topic areas and principles were derived from evidence-based practice guidelines. Nurses ($N = 51$) were mostly registered nurses (RNs) employed in the intensive care unit or general medical unit of the hospital. Only 2 of the 20 questions were answered correctly by 100% of the nurses. Percentages of nurses answering the other questions correctly ranged from 40% for 5 questions to 90% for 6 questions. These findings emphasize the importance of ensuring that the nurse's knowledge base is accurate before teaching clients about self-management of specific chronic illnesses.

Research of self-care globally has pointed out some commonalities regarding self-care supportive interventions. Studies have been conducted in Taiwan (Wang et al., 2001), in the United States (Callaghan, 2006; Sharkey et al., 2005; Sullivan, Weinert, & Cudney, 2003), sometimes with minority groups (Cortes et al., 2004), and in Sweden and Finland (Borg et al., 2006; Leenerts et al., 2002). Specific self-care interventions with an emphasis on follow-up after hospitalization have also been assessed globally. These include a nurse-led, multidisciplinary post-hospitalization follow-up program for persons with heart failure in South Australia (Inglis et al., 2006), a post-hospitalization intervention in the United States for persons with nonspecific illnesses (Coleman et al., 2004), and a nurse-led customized program for persons with diabetes, also in the United States (Berg & Wadhwa, 2007).

Within the past several years, several clinicians and research teams have proposed a variety of other theory- and evidence-based interventions to support and facilitate self-care and self-management. McCarley (2009) recommends using motivational interviewing techniques. Weinert, Cudney and Kinion (2010) propose a simple, evidence-based personal health record for managing and organizing personal health information so persons can make the most of short interactions with providers. This promotes active care of self and management of chronic illnesses. Potempa and colleagues (2010) delineate a comprehensive model for promoting self-care in primary care settings. Parker, Teel, Leenerts, and Macan (2011) describe a standardized comprehensive, theory-based approach that can be tailored to meet individual client needs and that helps clients build self-care skills. All of these proposals merit validation through research.

One of the most striking aspects of the studies and proposed interventions is that they all recommend basing interventions on the client's model of the world. Assessing the perceived needs of clients is essential and can overcome barriers to "nonadherence." Integrating special self-care activities to manage a chronic illness must fit within the context of the client's day-to-day lifestyle. Another common aspect of these interventions is that they address the holistic health needs of clients, including spiritual and socialization needs, and are not limited solely to adherence to medical treatments or focused on living with a specific chronic illness.

Another commonality is that the programs embrace a multipronged approach to supporting and promoting self-care. For example, teaching is a major component of these interventions but comprehensive skilled assessments, coaching, empowerment, referral, and intermittent follow-up contact are also part of the recommended interventions. Finally, the interventions are based on the philosophy that promoting a positive orientation of self-worth fosters hope for the future. This philosophy is operationalized by pointing out the positive rather than negative or problematic aspects of the person's situation.

Self-Management Programs

Lorig (2001), a nursing leader in self-management program development and testing, comprehensively summarized findings from more than 20 years of research studies testing self-management programs for arthritis. Charac-teristics of the programs tested in sequential studies were analyzed to isolate the most important factors when designing programs to support self-care in terms of disease self-management, one aspect of self-care. First, programs must be focused on the problems and concerns of clients. In other words, modeling the client's world is a key factor. Programs should also be designed for a particular target population. The process of implementing the program is as important as the content to be addressed. Written materials must be included as a reference and for additional reading. Programs should promote self-efficacy by building on the client's strengths; congruent with the self-care model, positive aspects of abilities should be recognized and nurtured. Problem solving and decision making by the client should be emphasized rather than relying solely on professional judgment. Skills for communicating with healthcare professionals should be incorporated. Other important aspects include providing a structure for the program that is adhered to during each of its segments, encouraging sharing of ideas and feelings among group members attending the program, employing lay instructors, and recognizing that other education and health teaching are valuable as well.

Chodosh and colleagues (2005) identified similar characteristics through a meta-analysis of 53 randomized trials testing chronic disease self-management programs for older adults with diabetes, osteoarthritis, and hypertension. Although they did not find statistically significant elements

of these programs, they extrapolated that self-care, in the form of self-management, requires active participation in decision making and self-monitoring. In addition, programs should be tailored to meet needs, be offered in group settings, provide feedback to participants, and emphasize psychological aspects of self-management in addition to medical management.

Rogers, Kennedy, Nelson, and Robinson (2005) identified the importance of the physician–patient relationship style in promoting self-management. Physicians and the health systems in which they practice need to be responsive to patient needs and preferences, and decision making must be shared with the patient. Indeed, the idea of responsiveness to client needs is essential to MRM interventions that promote self-care.

Likewise, the notion of active involvement and participation is also compatible with the self-care model. However, for some clients, active participation might take the form of dependence on others as a self-care action. For example, the person with limited self-care resources might need to depend on others for aspects of self-care to preserve, rather than deplete, their limited resources.

Comprehensive Self-Care Programs

Lynch, Estes, and Hernandez (2005) compared three types of chronic care initiatives for older adults. These comprehensive programs are viewed as alternatives to the traditional medical model of care. The first is the integrated medical, home, and community-based services model, which focuses on providing holistic, integrated health services to persons with complex, chronic care needs in their homes. An example is the Program for All-Inclusive Care for the Elderly (PACE) that has been in place for more than 20 years and has produced many positive health outcomes, despite demanding a high level of ambulatory services.

The second type of chronic care initiatives are the disease management programs offered by a variety of providers. An example is the Kaiser Permanente Best Practice Collaborative approach with group clinics and education on disease self-care in primary care settings. The Kaiser programs are interdisciplinary and incorporate motivational interviewing to promote self-care. The benefit is a focus on active participation. But, as previously noted, demanding active, independent participation can be detrimental to some clients' health.

A third and newer model is that of high-risk care management developed by managed care insurers to control costs and to improve the care management of persons living with multiple chronic illnesses. The Guided Care Nurse model represents this approach (Boyd et al., 2007). This model emphasizes coordination and nonduplication of services that are individualized to meet clients' unique needs. A specially educated nurse works in a primary care practice with two to five physicians, and manages care for 50 to 60 older clients. An electronic health record is used to communicate among team members. The focus of guided care nursing interventions is on comprehensive assessment and monitoring of chronic conditions, coaching to aid in self-management of diseases, referral and coordination of services to secure needed resources and to facilitate transitions between healthcare settings, and provision of caregiver education and support. A key component of this model is that the client's highest priority needs for health must be addressed by the nurse. This is a multipronged

approach with many client-centered aspects. Research on this model of care indicates that clients rate the quality of healthcare services highly (Boyd et al., 2010).

Evidence-Based Practice Box

Purpose: Examined relationship between perceived autonomy, representing the potential for self-care action, and internal and external self-care resources from the perspective of the MRM self-care model.

Research design: Descriptive, correlational study

Sample: The study used a convenience sample of 120 older adults aged 60 to 101 years old who resided in the community and who attended a senior center. All could read and write English. Most were women, Caucasian, not currently married, and lived alone. More than 80% had Medicare insurance, with 79% also insured by another health insurance policy. More than 62% used 2 or more community care services and on average they used 2.1 services; the most frequent services were meals, health screenings, housing, and information and referral.

Setting: Six senior centers in Manhattan, New York City.

Findings: Participants demonstrated relatively high scores on perceived autonomy. They also scored highly on functional ability, indicating that the group was independent. The internal self-care resources of white race and functional status were significantly correlated to perceived autonomy. Social support, overall and that from family, friends, and significant others, separately, and satisfaction with service utilization were the only external self-care resources significantly linked to perceived autonomy. Using a multiple linear regression model, perceived autonomy was predicted by race, service satisfaction, and social support.

Implications: In this relatively independent sample of older persons, functional status was linked to perceived autonomy. Thus, those who have declining functional abilities need to be given support to care for self. Furthermore, social support was also related to perceived autonomy, indicating that self-care can be facilitated through social support. It is unclear why being white was related to self-care, represented by perceived autonomy. However, the sample was predominantly Caucasian. Further study is warranted. The finding regarding satisfaction with services and its linkage to perceived autonomy is important. This may reflect that these services were a good match and met the participants' unique needs. In practice, it is important to ask clients to evaluate service satisfaction as an indicator of meeting self-care needs.

Source: Matsui, M., & Capezuti, E. (2008). Perceived autonomy and self-care resources among senior center users. *Geriatric Nursing, 29*(2), 141–147.

There are other types of programs such as case management programs led by social workers, state-funded programs for low-income persons with chronic illnesses, and wellness management programs in senior centers (Lynch et al., 2005). All of these promote self-care in

some fashion. However, a limitation is that most of these programs have a very narrow focus. Therefore, the clients' holistic health needs are not always addressed. There is a need for more innovative, comprehensive programs to be developed in the future to help promote self-care in persons living with chronic illnesses. These could be located in housing units or community-based sites where persons with chronic illnesses congregate—for example, churches, shopping centers, and grocery stores. Future models should incorporate the recommended multipronged approaches and address needs related to multiple chronic illnesses. All models need to adopt a client-centered and holistic perspective so that interventions can be tailored to meet clients' unique needs, values, and lifestyles.

OUTCOMES

Grey, Knafl, and McCorkle (2006) developed a framework for describing and organizing outcomes of self-management programs. The categories of outcomes also apply to programs other than ones that promote self-care. The categories are condition outcomes, individual outcomes, family outcomes, and environmental outcomes. Positive outcomes in each category would be optimal.

Condition Outcomes

These outcomes indicate the individual's adherence and responsiveness to treatment regimens. For example, in persons with diabetes, hypertension, and osteoarthritis, outcomes include reduced levels of hemoglobin A1c; decreased systolic blood pressure by 5 mm Hg and decreased diastolic by 4.3 mm Hg; as well as pain reduction, respectively (Chodosh et al., 2005). Following recommended screening procedures (Berg & Wadhwa, 2007) would also be a condition outcome. Other outcomes might include morbidity, mortality, and improved or stable functional status (Burnette et al., 2004; Grey et al., 2006; Lynch et al., 2005).

Individual Outcomes

Any outcomes that reflect clients' perceptions regarding health status, quality of life, and well-being are included in this category. Connectedness to others, transcendence, a sense of well-being (Leenerts et al., 2002), life satisfaction (Borg et al., 2006), satisfaction with health care (Matsui & Capezuti, 2008), and reports of needs being met (Inglis et al., 2006) are examples. Quality of life and physical, mental, and spiritual health ratings (Boyd et al., 2007; Campbell & Aday, 2001); increased health-related knowledge; and a greater sense of being in control of one's situation or sense of autonomy are other individual outcomes (Campbell & Aday, 2001).

Family Outcomes

Outcomes that indicate an effect on the family of the person receiving the promotion intervention are included in this group. Depression in caregivers, improved family functioning, and degree of caregiver burden (Grey et al., 2006) are examples of family outcomes.

Environmental Outcomes

Outcomes that reflect the costs of health care or influence the healthcare system are considered environmental outcomes. For example, cost reductions, unplanned hospital admission rates, lengths of stay, and frequencies of healthcare utilization (Inglis et al., 2006) fall into this category. In addition, nonduplication of services

(Boyd et al., 2007), decreased nursing home admissions, and use of ambulatory services may be included in this category (Berg & Wadhwa, 2007; Lynch et al., 2005).

STUDY QUESTIONS

Define self-care as it relates to persons living with one or more chronic illnesses.

Identify the relationship between self-care and health outcomes. Why is self-care a key concept to positive health outcomes?

How can nurses promote self-care in the clients they care for? Identify the key elements of a self-care supportive intervention.

Delineate at least one positive outcome for the individual client, family, and healthcare system as a result of the individual client demonstrating self-care in relation to his or her chronic illness.

INTERNET RESOURCES

Center for Self and Family Management of Vulnerable Populations, Yale University School of Nursing: nursing.yale.edu/Centers/ECSMI/

Communities Putting Prevention to Work: Chronic Disease Self-Management Program: http://www.aoa.gov/AoAroot/PRESS_Room/News/2009/03_18_09.aspx

Internet Resources (Cont.)

Expert Patients Programme Community Interest Company (EPP CIC) in the UK: http://www.selfcareconnect.co.uk/

Family Caregiver Alliance, Taking Care of YOU: Self-Care for Family Caregivers: www.caregiver.org/caregiver/jsp/content_node.jsp?nodeid=847

Guided Care; www.guidedcare.org/index.asp

International Orem Society for Nursing Science and Scholarship: http://www.orem-society.com/

The Society for the Advancement of Modeling and Role-Modeling: mrmnursingtheory.org/index.html

Self-Management Science Center, University of Wisconsin–Milwaukee, College of Nursing: http://www4.uwm.edu/smsc/

Stanford Self-Management Programs: http://patienteducation.stanford.edu/programs/

Supporting Self Care in Primary Care—The Book, Chapter 14 has many suggestions for promoting self-care in clients (and self): http://www.selfcareconnect.co.uk/167

Understanding the Affordable Care Act: http://www.healthcare.gov/law/introduction/index.html

For a full suite of assignments and additional learning activities, use the access code located in the front of your book and visit this exclusive website: **http://go.jblearning.com/larsen**. If you do not have an access code, you can obtain one at the site.

REFERENCES

Barlow, J. H., Sturt, J., & Hearnshaw, H. (2002). Self-management interventions for people with chronic conditions in primary care: Examples from arthritis, asthma and diabetes. *Health Education Journal, 61*(4), 365–378.

Beattie, B. L., Whitelaw, N., Mettler, M., & Turner, D. (2003). A vision for older adults and health promotion. *American Journal of Health Promotion, 18*(2), 200–204.

Berg, G. D., & Wadhwa, S. (2007). Health services outcomes for a diabetes disease management program for the elderly. *Disease Management, 10*, 226–234.

Bickerstaff, K. A., Grasser, C. M., & McCabe, B. (2003). How elderly nursing home residents transcend losses of later life. *Holistic Nursing Practice, 17*(3), 159–165.

Bliss, D. Z., Fischer, L. R., & Savik, K. (2005). Managing fecal incontinence: Self-care practices of older adults. *Journal of Gerontological Nursing, 31*(7), 35–44.

Borg, C., Hallberg, I., & Blomqvist, K. (2006). Life satisfaction among older people (65+) with reduced self-care capacity: The relationship to social, health and financial aspects [Electronic version]. *Journal of Clinical Nursing, 15*(5), 607–618.

Boyd, C. M., Boult, C., Shadmi, E., Leff, B., Brager, R., Dunbar, L., et al. (2007). Guided care for multimorbid older adults. *The Gerontologist, 47*, 679–704.

Boyd, C. M., Reider, L., Frey, K., Scharfstein, D., Leff, B., Wolff, J., et al. (2010). The effects of guided care on the perceived quality of health care for multi-morbid older persons: 18-month outcomes from a cluster-randomized controlled trial. *Journal of General Internal Medicine, 25*(3), 235–242.

Britz, J., & Dunn, K. (2010). Self-care and quality of life among patients with heart failure. *Journal of the American Academy of Nurse Practitioners, 22*(9), 480–487.

Burnette, D., Mui, A. C., & Zodikoff, B. D. (2004). Gender, self-care and functional status among older persons with coronary heart disease: A national perspective. *Women & Health, 39*(1), 65–84.

Callaghan, D. (2005). Healthy behaviors, self-efficacy, self-care, and basic conditioning factors in older adults [Electronic version]. *Journal of Community Health Nursing, 22*(3), 169–178.

Callaghan, D. (2006). The influence of growth on spiritual self-care agency in an older adult population. *Journal of Gerontological Nursing, 32*(9), 43–51.

Campbell, J., & Aday, R. H. (2001). Benefits of a nurse-managed wellness program: A senior center model.

Using community-based sites for older adult intervention and self-care activities may promote an ability to maintain an independent lifestyle. *Journal of Gerontological Nursing, 27*(3), 34–43.

Chodosh, J., Morton, S. C., Mojica, W., Maglione, M., Suttorp, M. J., Hilton, L., et al. (2005). Meta-analysis: Chronic disease self-management programs for older adults. *Annals of Internal Medicine, 143,* 427–438.

Chriss, P. M., Sheposh, J., Carlson, B., & Riegel, B. (2004). Predictors of successful heart failure self-care maintenance in the first three months after hospitalization. *Heart & Lung, 33,* 345–353.

Coleman, E. A., Smith, J. D., Frank, J. C., Min, S-J., Parry, C., & Kramer, A. M. (2004). Preparing patients and caregivers to participate in care delivered across settings: The care transitions intervention. *Journal of the American Geriatrics Society, 52,* 1817–1825.

Cortes, T., Lee, A., Boal, J., Mion, L., & Butler, A. (2004). Using focus groups to identify asthma care and education issues for elderly urban-dwelling minority individuals. *Applied Nursing Research, 17*(3), 207–212.

Dyer, C. B., Goodwin, J. S., Pickens-Pace, S., Burnett, J., & Kelly, P. A. (2007). Self-neglect among the elderly: A model based on more than 500 patients seen by a geriatric medicine team. *American Journal of Public Health, 97,* 1671–1676.

Edwardson, S. R., & Dean, K. J. (1999). Appropriateness of self-care responses to symptoms among elders: Identifying pathways of influence. *Research in Nursing & Health, 22,* 329–339.

Erickson, H. C., Tomlin, E., & Swain, M. A. (1988). *Modeling and role-modeling: A theory and paradigm for nursing* (2nd ed.). Lexington, SC: Pine Press.

Erickson, H. L. (2006). *Modeling and role-modeling: A view from the client's world.* Cedar Park, TX: Unicorns Unlimited.

Grey, M., Knafl, K., & McCorkle, R. (2006). A framework for the study of self- and family management of chronic conditions. *Nursing Outlook, 54,* 278–286.

Haber, D. (2002). Health promotion and aging: Educational and clinical initiatives by the federal government. *Educational Gerontology, 28,* 253–262.

HealthCare.gov. (n.d.a). Eliminating lifetime and annual limits on your benefits. Retrieved August 23, 2011, from: http://www.healthcare.gov/law/provisions/limits/limits.html

HealthCare.gov. (n.d.b). Filling medicine part D "donut hole." Retrieved August 23, 2011, from: http://www.healthcare.gov/law/provisions/donuthole/donuthole.html

HealthCare.gov. (n.d.c). Insurance protections for children in the Affordable Care Act. Retrieved August 23, 2011, from: http://www.healthcare.gov/law/provisions/ChildrensPCIP/childrenspcip.html

HealthCare.gov. (n.d.d). Making Medicare prescription drug costs more affordable. Retrieved August 23, 2011, from: http://www.healthcare.gov/law/provisions/prescription/drugdiscounts.html

HealthCare.gov. (n.d.e). Patient's bill of rights. Retrieved August 23, 2011, from: http://www.healthcare.gov/law/provisions/billofright/patient_bill_of_rights.html

HealthCare.gov. (n.d.f). Pre-existing condition insurance plan. Retrieved August 23, 2011, from: http://www.healthcare.gov/law/provisions/preexisting/index.html

HealthCare.gov. (n.d.g). Preserving doctor choice and ensuring emergency care. Retrieved August 23, 2011, from: http://www.healthcare.gov/law/provisions/choice_access/index.html

HealthCare.gov. (n.d.h). Preventive care and services. Retrieved August 23, 2011, from: http://www.healthcare.gov/law/provisions/preventive/index.html

HealthCare.gov. (n.d.i). Preventive services under Medicare. Retrieved August 23, 2011, from: http://www.healthcare.gov/law/provisions/medicare/preventiveservices.html

HealthCare.gov. (n.d.j). Young adult coverage until age 26. Retrieved August 23, 2011, from: http://www.healthcare.gov/law/provisions/youngadult/index.html

Hertz, J. E. (1996). Conceptualization of perceived enactment of autonomy in the elderly. *Issues in Mental Health Nursing, 17*(3), 261–273.

Hertz, J. E., & Baas, L. (2006). Self-care: Knowledge, resources, and actions. In H. L. Erickson (Ed.), *Modeling and role-modeling: A view from the client's world* (pp. 97–120). Cedar Park, TX: Unicorns Unlimited.

Hertz, J. E., & Rossetti, J. (2006, March). *Senior apartment residents' reported self-care activities.* Paper presented at the 2006 Midwest Nursing Research Society Conference, Milwaukee, WI.

Inglis, S. C., Pearson, S., Treen, S., Gallasch, T., Horowitz, J. D., & Stewart, S. (2006). Extending the horizon in chronic heart failure: Effects of multidisciplinary, home-based intervention relative to usual care. *Circulation, 114*, 2466–2473.

Leenerts, M. H., Teel, C. S., & Pendleton, M. K. (2002). Building a model of self-care for health promotion in aging. *Journal of Nursing Scholarship, 34*(4), 355–361.

Lorig, K. (2001). Arthritis self-management. In E. A. Swanson, T. Tripp-Reimer, & K. Buckwalter (Eds.), *Health promotion and disease prevention in the older adult: Interventions and recommendations* (pp. 56–80). New York: Springer.

Lubben, J. E., & Damron-Rodriguez, J. A. (2003). An international approach to community health care for older adults. *Family and Community Health, 26*(4), 338–349.

Lynch, M., Estes, C. L., & Hernandez, M. (2005). Chronic care initiatives for the elderly: Can they bridge the gerontology-medicine gap? *Journal of Applied Gerontology, 24*, 108–124.

Maddox, M. (1999). Older women and the meaning of health. *Journal of Gerontological Nursing, 25*(12), 26–33.

Matsui, M., & Capezuti, E. (2008). Perceived autonomy and self-care resources among senior center users. *Geriatric Nursing, 29*(2), 141–147.

Maslow, A. H. (1962). *Toward a psychology of being.* New York: John Wiley & Sons.

McCarley, P. (2009). Patient empowerment and motivational interviewing: Engaging patients to self-manage their own care. *Nephrology Nursing Journal, 36*(4), 409–413.

McDonald-Miszczak, L., & Wister, A. V. (2005). Predicting self-care behaviors among older adults coping with arthritis: A cross-sectional and 1-year longitudinal comparative analysis. *Journal of Ageing and Health, 17*, 836–857.

Mendias, E. P., & Paar, D. P. (2007). Perceptions of health and self-care learning needs of outpatients with HIV/AIDS. *Journal of Community Health Nursing, 24*(1), 49–64.

Musil, C. M., Morris, D. L., Haug, M. R., Warner, C. B., & Whelan, A. T. (2001). Recurrent symptoms: Well-being and management. *Social Science & Medicine, 52*, 1729–1740.

Naik, A., Dyer, C., Kunik, M., & McCullough, L. (2009a). Patient autonomy for the management of chronic conditions: A two-component reconceptualization. *American Journal of Bioethics, 9*(2), 23–30.

Naik, A., Dyer, C., Kunik, M., & McCullough, L. (2009b). Response to commentaries on "Patient autonomy for the management of chronic conditions: A two-component re-conceptualization." *American Journal of Bioethics, 9*(2), W3–W5.

Naik, A., Teal, C., Pavlik, V., Dyer, C., & McCullough, L. (2008). Conceptual challenges and practical approaches to screening capacity for self-care and protection in vulnerable older adults. *Journal of the American Geriatrics Society, 56*, S266–S270.

Orem, D. (2001). *Nursing: Concepts of practice* (6th ed.). St. Louis, MO: Mosby.

Parker, C., Teel, C., Leenerts, M. H., & Macan, A. (2011). A theory-based self-care TALK intervention for family caregiver-nurse partnerships. *Journal of Gerontological Nursing, 37*(1), 30–35.

Potempa, K., Butterworth, S., Flaherty Robb, M., & Gaynor, W. (2010). The healthy ageing model: Health behaviour change for older adults. *Collegian, 17*(2), 51–55.

Resnick, B. (2001). Promoting health in older adults: A four-year analysis. *Journal of the American Academy of Nurse Practitioners, 13*(1), 23–33.

Resnick, B. (2003). Health promotion practices of older adults: Model testing. *Public Health Nursing, 20*(1), 2–12.

Rogers, A., Kennedy, A., Nelson, E., & Robinson, A. (2005). Uncovering the limits of patient-centeredness: Implementing a self-management trial for chronic illness. *Qualitative Health Research, 15*, 224–239.

Ryan, P., & Sawin, K. (2009). The individual and family self-management theory: Background and perspectives on context, process, and outcomes. *Nursing Outlook, 57*(4), 217–225.

Scollan-Koliopoulos, M., & Walker, E. (2009). Multigenerational timeline and understanding of diabetes and self-care. *Research & Theory for Nursing Practice, 23*(1), 62–77.

Sharkey, J., Ory, M., & Browne, B. (2005, April). Determinants of self-management strategies to reduce out-of-pocket prescription medication expense in homebound older people [Electronic version].

Journal of the American Geriatrics Society, 53(4), 666–674.

Singleton, J. K. (2000). Nurses' perspectives of encouraging clients' care-of-self in a short-term rehabilitation unit within a long-term care facility. *Rehabilitation Nursing, 25*(1), 23–35.

Sullivan, T., Weinert, C., & Cudney, S. (2003). Management of chronic illness: Voices of rural women. *Journal of Advanced Nursing, 44*(6), 566–574.

Sutherland, D., & Hayter, M. (2009). Structured review: Evaluating the effectiveness of nurse case managers in improving health outcomes in three major chronic diseases. *Journal of Clinical Nursing, 18*(21), 2978–2992.

U.S. Department of Health and Human Services (DHHS). (2010). *Healthy People 2020. Retrieved August 23, 2011, from:* http://www.healthypeople.gov/2020/default.aspx

U.S. Department of Health and Human Services (DHHS). (n.d.a) *Affordable care act.* Retrieved August 23, 2011, from: http://www.healthcare.gov/law/introduction/index.html

U.S. Department of Health and Human Services (DHHS). (n.d.b). Framework: The vision, mission, and goals of *Healthy People 2020.* Retrieved August 23, 2011, http://www.healthypeople.gov/2020/Consortium/HP2020Framework.pdf

Wang, H. H., Hsu, M. T., & Want, R. H. (2001). Using a focus group study to explore perceptions of health-promoting self-care in community-dwelling older adults. *Journal of Nursing Research, 9*(4), 95–104.

Washburn, S., Hornberger, C., Klutman, A., & Skinner, L. (2005, May). Nurses' knowledge of heart failure education topics as reported in a small Midwestern community hospital [Electronic version]. *Journal of Cardiovascular Nursing, 20*(3), 215–220.

Weinert, C., Cudney, S., & Kinion, E. (2010). Development of My Health Companion to enhance self-care management of chronic health conditions in rural dwellers. *Public Health Nursing, 27*(3), 263–269.

Yip, Y. B., Sit, J. W. H., & Wong, D. Y. S. (2004). A quasi-experimental study on improving arthritis self-management for residents of an aged people's home in Hong Kong. *Psychology, Health & Medicine, 9,* 235–246.

CHAPTER 15

Client and Family Education

Elaine T. Miller

INTRODUCTION

For the majority of clients and their families, a chronic illness constitutes a life-changing event uniquely affecting them as they deal with the added demands and long-term nature of the particular disease. Perhaps more importantly, chronic illnesses do not always have a similar trajectory of presentation and management (e.g., asthma, heart disease, depression, cancer, stroke, arthritis, diabetes, and hypertension), and they do not discriminate according to age, race, gender, socioeconomic status, culture or ethnicity, or learning capability. Furthermore, the client and family's response and resources to cope with chronic illnesses may vary tremendously, requiring healthcare professionals (HCPs) to be attuned to each client and family's particular needs, expectations, resources, and personal goals.

Data further indicate that treating clients with chronic diseases accounts for 75% of U.S. healthcare spending and two-thirds of our current increase in healthcare spending is related to the expanded prevalence of treating chronic disease (Centers for Disease Control and Prevention, Chronic Disease Prevention and Health Promotion, 2010). The vast majority of chronic diseases (e.g., pulmonary, hypertension, heart disease) could be prevented or better managed by adopting a more client-centered,

multidisciplinary approach that fosters client and family involvement, client self-management, and continuous quality im-provement (Partnership to Fight Chronic Disease, 2010). For example, Woodhouse, Peterson, Campbell, and Gathercoal (2010) found a significant reduction in the costly use of emergency room visits by high user clients with chronic pain who received targeted educational/behavioral interventions to better manage their condition. Thus, maximizing the client and family's coping with chronic illness and improving their knowledge, attitudes, and behaviors in conjunction with HCPs providing a more unified approach and subsequent monitoring, management, and evaluation of care outcomes are central aspects of the care-delivery process. Given that many clients and their families are likely to experience more than one chronic illness in a lifetime, it is critical for HCPs to be cognizant of the potential interplay of diverse chronic illnesses that may influence the client and family's responses to further losses such as incontinence, fatigue, diminishing cognitive function, or mobility.

It is also well documented that educating clients and their families is critical to successful coping with chronic illnesses and overall long-term quality of life. Plus, the family frequently serves as the client's primary support system affecting the client's decision making about health, seeking health care, and adherence to recommended healthcare recommendations (e.g., taking prescribed medication, following a diet, having a recommended procedure or test) (Falvo, 2011). Although there are often some commonalities, each client and family situation has its distinctive characteristics that require HCPs to approach every situation carefully and systematically without making assumptions as to the client and family's resources, capability to learn, and ability to achieve educational outcomes. Moreover, HCPs must continually assess the factors influencing the client and family's educational needs, the teaching and learning approach, and evaluation of short- and long-term outcomes. Another central element in this educational process is identifying what clients and their families want to learn, their priorities in terms of their educational needs, and having mutual goal setting, so that clients, families, and HCPs are working together to achieve common goals.

Because numerous factors contribute to the success or failure of client and family education pertaining to chronic illness, this chapter presents an overview of the fundamental elements that should be considered and clarifies the state of evidence-based knowledge pertaining to client and family education related to chronic illnesses. Even though much is known regarding client and family education, the literature and research do not suggest simple solutions or approaches that will optimize this educational process in all situations. In addition, the nature of the chronic disease(s) as well as the specific attributes of the learner(s) such as age, gender, race/ethnicity, culture, socioeconomic status, motivation, self-efficacy, psychological conditions (depression,

bipolar disorder), sensory deficits (low-level vision, hearing impairment, literacy, learning capability), and/or learning disabilities will significantly influence how the HCP approaches and evaluates the success of each client and family educational encounter. The primary focus of this chapter is the adult learner. However, a basic distinction is described regarding key learning differences between adults and children. Finally, because this chapter only purports to present a broad overview of key issues affecting client and family educational processes regarding chronic illnesses, it is highly recommended that additional evidence-based resources be obtained to more specifically target the chronic illness and client population of concern, recognizing that research and the associated findings continue to expand the science of what is known.

The Teaching–Learning Process

The teaching–learning process is characterized by multifaceted, dynamic, and interactive exchanges that are fundamental to client–family education and nursing practice. Teaching involves a deliberative, intentional act of communicating information to individuals in response to their identified educational needs and with the objective of achieving a desired outcome (Falvo, 2011; Bastable, 2006). Learning, on the other hand, assists the individual to acquire new knowledge, skills, and/or attitudes that can be measured (Bastable, 2006). A review of the literature reveals that there are more than 50 major teaching–learning theories that can shape an educational intervention (Learning Theories Knowledge Base, 2011).

Although many theories and frameworks are applicable to client and family education, behaviorist theory, social–cognitive learning theory, humanistic learning theory, and constructionist theory have been identified as particularly helpful in shaping educational interventions. Each offers a different orientation of what is most important and what should be the HCP's focus of attention when educating individuals with chronic illness and their families. In addition, each has a particular perspective in terms of how teaching and learning are defined, measured, and structured, as well as the phases of learning.

For example, the behaviorist framework states that learning is the result of connections between the stimuli in the environment and the individual's responses (Skinner, 1974). So if an educator wants a client and/or family to learn new information or alter their attitudes and responses, such as the new need for a client to receive a subcutaneous insulin injection twice daily, the educator would alter the conditions in the environment (e.g., information available on the hospital educational cable system) and reinforce positive new behaviors when they occur (e.g., praise when the injection is given correctly).

On the other hand, social–cognitive theory includes role modeling as a central concept and offers a different approach to teaching clients and their families to perform the same task (Bandura, 1986). In this identical situation, using the social–cognitive theory, the nurse educator would demonstrate how to perform the insulin injection and then have the client, if capable, perform the insulin injection when next scheduled.

Meanwhile, if Maslow's Hierarchy of Needs, one of the best known humanistic frameworks, was applied to this identical scenario, the educator would first need to fulfill lower level needs such as physiologic needs and safety before being concerned about teaching the client how to perform the insulin injection.

Finally, the constructionistic learning theory offers an additional alternative theoretical perspective to guide the HCP's educational encounter, asserting that learners are actively creating meaning as they learn. When viewed from this constructionist orientation, learning is perceived as contextual, requiring not only time, social contact, and motivation, but also creating meanings that foster learning over time and its application (Hein, 1991). In the case of learning how to properly give an insulin injection, the constructionist theory provides a framework to connect the client's understanding/meaning of how the insulin injection should be correctly given, the client's motivation to learn this activity, the time required to correctly perform this task, and the contribution of the HCP who is teaching this skill.

In summary, theoretical frameworks offer alternative ways to approach a teaching–learning situation involving clients and their families. Because there are a myriad theoretical frameworks, it is important that HCPs determine what is most relevant to their situations, examine available evidence-based research pertaining to that framework (preferably evidence published in the last 5 years), and then translate that framework to their particular client–family interactions, and systematically evaluate the efficacy of using that perspective to direct their educational interventions.

In conjunction with the numerous teaching–learning theories that guide the HCP's client–family educational encounters, it is valuable to contemplate several basic assumptions underpinning these interactions. According to Petty (2006), learning involves "an active process of making sense and creating a personal interpretation of what has been learned" (p. 8), rather than simply an exact interpretation of what has been taught. What occurs is more than just a storing of personal interpretations of facts and ideas, it is "also linking them in a way that relates ideas to other ideas, and to prior learning, and so creates meaning and understanding" (p. 8). When viewed from this perspective, learners construct meaning that is more easily applied to solve problems, make judgments, and assist clients and their families to perform the numerous tasks associated with living with one or more chronic illnesses. Evidence is steadily expanding to support the constructivism perspective and its positive outcomes (Muijs & Reynolds, 2005). In addition, results from multiple meta-analyses of educational research reinforce the pivotal influence that feedback and reinforcement exert on individual as well as group learning (Petty, 2006).

CASE STUDY

Mrs. McGill is a 63-year-old African American grandmother with a history of chronic obstructive pulmonary disease and obesity (BMI > 30) as well as 2 falls in the last 4 months resulting in bruises, but no fractures. About 6 months ago, she was also diagnosed as a type 2 diabetic and is receiving medication, but getting her blood sugars under control and adhering to her diet restrictions has been somewhat of a challenge.

Mrs. McGill lives with her husband of 34 years and is currently raising 2 grandsons ages 6 and 10. Although she loved being a substitute English teacher in the high school where she taught, Mrs. McGill has been unable to do so since obtaining custody of her 2 grandsons 9 months ago. Her husband, who is a pharmacist, still works part-time and is very supportive of his wife. The couple live with their grandsons in a comfortable duplex.

Discussion Questions

1. What appear to be the primary educational objectives for Mrs. McGill?
2. What additional assessment data would be helpful in identifying your educational objectives and structuring your related interventions?
3. What teaching method(s) would be most appropriate and what is your rationale for this decision?
4. What websites or national practice standards may be of assistance in helping to develop your teaching plan?
5. Briefly describe what your teaching plan would consist of in terms of objective(s), content, timeline, and teaching strategies?

Significance of Client and Family Teaching to Practice and Healthcare Costs

Practice standards from the American Nurses Association (ANA), the American Association of Colleges of Nursing (AACN), the National League for Nursing (NLN), specialty nursing practice standards, and other national documents consistently identify health teaching as a fundamental component of nursing practice (ANA, 2004; Lindell et al., 2005). Even in the early writings of Florence Nightingale, teaching was recognized as a prominent nursing activity (Nightingale, 1992). In addition, all state nurse practice acts include teaching within the scope of nursing practice responsibilities and essential to promoting optimal health and disease management of clients and their families.

The underlying premise of *Healthy People 2010* and *Healthy People 2020* (U.S. Department of Health and Human Services, 2010) is that an individual's health is almost inseparable from the health of the larger community and is profoundly influenced by the collective beliefs, attitudes, and behaviors of this community. Throughout this comprehensive national health promotion and disease prevention roadmap, there is a recurrent theme emphasizing the improvement of "the availability and dissemination of health related information" (*Healthy People 2010,* p. 17) pertaining to the leading health indicators of our society. Central to accomplishing these health objectives is education of all stakeholders (i.e., clients, families, HCPs, the overall community). *Healthy People 2020* further emphasizes how disparities in income and education are associated with higher levels of occurrence of illness and death and place greater importance on targeting community-based health educational programming. For instance, *Healthy People 2020* focuses on the systematic and targeted health promotion education and preventative actions for adults who are most at risk for long-term health problems/diseases. Plus, the 2020 edition emphasizes the coordination and targeting of health promotion education and other activities beginning in preschool and continuing through high school. *Healthy People 2020* concentrates on health problems such as unintentional injury, violence, dental caries, unhealthy dietary patterns, tobacco use and addiction, and alcohol and drug use—all having ramifications for long-term chronic health issues.

In addition to *Healthy People 2020* emphasizing the importance of evidence-based, coordinated, targeted, and individualized client and family education, the Joint Commission (JC, 2010) *2011 Hospital Accreditation Standards* identify specific critical educational standards that must be achieved by organizations seeking accreditation. The JC (2010) standards include:

PC.02.03.01 The hospital provides client education and training on each client's needs and abilities.

1. The hospital performs a learning needs assessment for each client, which includes the client's culture and religious beliefs, emotional barriers, desire and motivation to learn, physical or cognitive limitations and barriers to communication.

4. The hospital provides education and training to the client based on his or her assessed needs.

5. The hospital coordinates the client education and training provided by all disciplines involved in the patient's care, treatment, and services.

10. Based on the client's condition and assessed needs, the education and training provided to the client by the hospital include any of the following: An explanation of the plan of care, treatment, and services. Plus, basic health and safety information need to be included with a special emphasis on the safe and effective use of medication....Discussion of pain, risk for pain, the importance of effective pain management, the pain assessment process, and methods for pain management, information on oral health, safe and effective use of medical equipment, supplies provided by the hospital, also what rehabilitation techniques need to be in place to help the client reach maximum independence, strategies to reduce falls.

25. The hospital evaluates the client's understanding of the education and training it provided.

27. The hospital provides the client education and how to communicate concerns about the client's safety issues that occur before, during, and after care is provided.

The Joint Commission patient education standards further specify that clients and families assume an active role in this process and have responsibilities just as the educator does. In instances where they do not understand the information, they are to indicate this and must take responsibility for self-management of their needs when capable (e.g., medication, safety, nutrition, pain). Moreover, the educator is expected to consistently and comprehensively assess the client and family's learning needs and barriers affecting the educational outcomes. In addition, the Joint Commission expects that educational activities be coordinated, tailored according to the clients and families needs/abilities, and evaluated to determine if learning has occurred.

During the 2002 Summit on the Education of Health Care Professionals (Institute of Medicine [IOM], 2003), it was emphasized that the education of all HCPs is in serious need of a "major overall" (p. 1) to be better prepared to fulfill the needs of clients and the changing healthcare system. Current nursing graduates must engage in evidence-based practice and integrate research findings pertaining to client and family teaching (IOM, 2003). Building upon this trend of expanding nursing roles, the National League for Nursing Task Group on Nurse Educator Competencies identified core competencies of nurse educators, underscoring their need to engage in scholarly activity pertaining to teaching and learning.

Data from the Centers for Disease Control and Prevention (CDC) highlight the pivotal role that education has in clients' self-management of chronic illness. For instance, the CDC reports that for each dollar invested in diabetic education to assist clients to self-manage their diabetes and prevent hospitalizations, healthcare costs are reduced by $8.76 (CDC, 2005). With regard to heart disease and stroke, they further emphasize that much of the burden associated with these two diseases can be eliminated by reduction of major risk factors such as high blood pressure, high cholesterol, tobacco use, limited physical activity, and poor nutrition. By targeting client and family education on those modifiable risk factors, the likelihood of heart disease and stroke can be significantly diminished and personal and financial costs reduced. The 2010 passage of the

Patient Protection and Affordable Care Act into law is estimated to reduce the number of uninsured by 31 million in 2019 at a net cost of $938 billion over 10 years while reducing the deficit emerging from escalating healthcare costs by $124 billion during that same time period (Kaiser Foundation, 2010). Several of the benefits of this law are as follows:

- Insurance for people with pre-existing conditions
- Coverage for preventive care and screenings such as immunizations and screening for conditions such as cancer and diabetes
- More spending on care—at least 80% of a customer's premium dollars need to be for direct medical care and efforts to improve quality care
- All insurance plans must include mental health and substance abuse services by 2014
- Starting in 2011 persons with Medicare will have an annual wellness visit that includes a personalized prevention plan that identifies health risk factors and treatment options

A main feature of these changes and others included within this legislation is the focus on prevention and management of chronic healthcare conditions. As a result, identifying evidence-based effective, timely, and targeted educational interventions will be pivotal to achievement of short- and long-term health outcomes in settings spanning from acute to long-term care. In addition, with the passage of this legislation, there is a growing demand to perform research focusing on the expansion of the evidence that underpins our educational interventions and attainment of the preferred client and family outcomes. When contemplating how to choose and develop written educational materials, Pierce (2010) provides valuable recommendations that should be considered.

Basic Differences Between Child and Adult Learners

The term *pedagogy* is defined as the art and science of teaching children, while *andragogy* refers to adult learning (Bastable, 2006, p. 451, 466). When teaching children versus adults, the key principles operating during the teachable moment are distinctly different, as indicated in **Table 15-1.**

Quality of Research and Evidence

When developing educational interventions for clients and their families, it is important to first determine the quality of the evidence forming the basis for the planned actions. Evidence-based practice (EBP) refers to a problem-solving approach used in practice that combines the following three components: the best available evidence; the HCP's clinical expertise; and the client's values and preferences (Melnyk & Fineout-Overhold, 2010). The highest level of evidence is a well conducted meta-analysis and systematic review of randomized control trials (RCTs) (Craig & Smyth, 2002; Melynk & Fineout-Overhold, 2010). However, a review of the literature reveals that a sizable portion of present knowledge directing our educational interventions is of a lower level of evidence quality than preferred such as single randomized trials, nonrandomized studies, consensus opinion of experts, and case studies. Results of a systematic review of 139 educational RCTs involving more than 22,000 clients with diabetes, asthma, or congestive heart failure (CHF) reveal that many of these RCTs draw inappropriate conclusions, with researchers frequently tending to overgeneralize their findings and include their opinions that are

Table 15-1   Comparison of Assumptions Pertaining to Teaching and Learning for Children and Adults

Pedagogy (children)	Andragogy (adults)
Rely on others to decide what is important to learn. Teacher is dominant. Learning is teacher led.	Decide for themselves what is important to learn (self-directive).
Expect what they learn will be helpful in the future.	Expect what they are learning to be immediately useful/applicable.
Have little or no experience on which to build knowledge/skill.	Have abundant experience.
Possess little ability to serve as a resource to teacher or classmates.	Possess great ability to serve as a resource to teacher and other learners (active student role).
Expect to be taught and take no responsibility.	Like to take control of the situation.
Not necessarily ready to learn.	Imply their motivation to learn, because they are present in the learning situation.
View learning as a process of acquiring information to be used at a later time.	View learning as a process of increasing competence to achieve a fuller life potential.

Sources: Bastable, S. B. (2006). *Essentials of patient education.* Sudbury, MA: Jones andBartlett; Conner, M. L. (2005). Andragogy and pedagogy. *Ageless Learner, 1997–2004.* Retrieved August 24, 2011, from:http://agelesslearner.com/intros/andragogy.html; Knowles, M. (1998). *The adult learner: The definitive classic in adult education and human resource development.* Houston, TX: Gulf Publishing; Mihall, J., & Belletti, J. (1999). Adult learning styles and training methods. *FDIC ADR Presentation Handouts.* Retrieved September 6, 2011 from http://www.justice.gov/adr/workplace/pdf/learstyl.pdf

not based on research evidence (Boren, Balas, & Mustafa, 2003). Therefore, educators need to carefully scrutinize the level of available evidence that underpins their practice, determine whether stated implications in research studies extend beyond the documented evidence, and recognize the tentative nature of our knowledge.

An excellent illustration of how knowledge evolves is demonstrated by the Internet and the increasing prevalence of online learning that has reshaped, in many instances, the education of clients, families, and HCPs worldwide. In a study investigating clients' seeking trends for additional health information regarding their disease/health problem, Rahmqvist and Bara (2007) identified from a sample of 24,800 respondents that young and middle-aged clients primarily use the Internet to expand their knowledge. Despite

this Internet access facilitating clients becoming more informed, they stress the inherent quality issues associated with public access to a blend of poor as well as high-quality, evidence-based online health information. Their findings were reaffirmed by Gremeaux and Coudeyre (2010), who performed a systematic review of the Internet and therapeutic education of patients and found that HCPs must work to create quality sites that provide accurate evidence-based data and best practices pertaining to chronic disease management for clients and their families.

Assessment of the Learner

A critical aspect of the client and family educational process is the assessment phase that shapes the other steps in the process, such as planning the educational event/program, its implementation, and evaluating outcomes. However, just as vital signs are obtained to determine the client's physiologic state, so too must certain essential information be obtained in this initial assessment that will affect how the education is structured, delivered, and evaluated. Because it is assumed that the client and family dealing with the chronic illness are equal partners with the HCP, the following are critical questions to ask the client and family:

- What information do you want provided? Recognize that the client and family may identify different needs. If so, make sure each of their needs is addressed.
- Are there any new skills that you want to learn or ones you want to review?
- What are your specific educational goals for the client and family? You may need to give an example (e.g., correctly identify signs/symptoms of hypoglycemic reactions; know what to do when an insulin reaction occurs and how to correctly give an insulin injection). The HCP must recognize that client and family goals can focus on knowledge, attitude (i.e., self-efficacy), and/or skill acquisition.
- Of the goals identified, what is most important? Once again, the client and family may differ markedly in specific goals and priorities. Listen carefully to both of them.
- What do you perceive as factors that affect your ability to achieve these educational goals? How will barriers be overcome?
- Do you feel confident using the information provided to you? If not, how may I assist you in increasing your confidence and ability to use this information?

When clients and family members are providing answers, the HCP must always be an astute listener, nonjudgmental, capable of developing individualized and attainable client and/or family goals, and reflect back to the client and family their understanding of what has been heard (Miller, 2003). While collecting the relevant client and family data, the HCP needs to be organized, perform the assessment in a timely manner, and be aware of readability of assessment materials. In addition, the client with chronic illness often has associated limitations that affect the assessment (e.g., easily fatigued and diminished hearing and/or vision and/or comprehension).

INFLUENCES ON TEACHING AND LEARNING

This section identifies a variety of factors that may influence the teaching–learning process; however, the list is not all inclusive as each individual with chronic illness is unique and their teaching–learning may be influenced by other factors.

Family Structure and Function

Families can vary significantly in structure and function. The chronic illness of a family member can precipitate changes in the family structure and function, as do changes associated with marriage, raising children, or death of a family member. When a family has a member with a chronic illness, the family's response to this change and its capability to adapt and make decisions can influence their receptiveness to education. When the client and family experience high anxiety, it can markedly interfere with their ability to receive and comprehend information, maintain normal patterns of family functioning, and use appropriate coping skills. Because culture and lifestyle affect the development of family norms and beliefs, differences in these client/family and

HCP factors can affect the dynamics of the educational process (Rankin, Stallings, & London, 2005). Once these beliefs and values are identified, they can be addressed through individualized teaching. It is imperative, therefore, that the family structure, function (i.e., roles, resources, strengths, and weaknesses), and norms be considered in the assessment and educational planning process.

According to the 2010 Joint Commission standards, the family is to be included in client teaching (e.g., fall-reduction strategies, reporting concerns related to care and safety). Because the client's family may be large with varying functions, the HCP must determine the primary family member who should receive the relevant education. Just as in the case of the client, the HCP needs to assess the primary family caregiver's role, expectations, learning needs/goals, learning style, fears, concerns, cognitive and physical abilities, and present knowledge pertaining to the client's healthcare needs (Bastable, 2006). Moreover, the client and the family member may need to receive similar information, reinforcement, and feedback related to their knowledge and/or skill performance. In many instances, the family member is the single most important factor in determining the success or failure of the teaching plan (Haggard, 1989).

Culture

When working with clients and their families, culture can dramatically affect how educational activities are structured, delivered, and evaluated. The client and family's culture comprise "an integral part of each person's life and includes knowledge, beliefs, values, morals, customs, traditions, communication patterns, and habits acquired by members of a society" (Bastable, 2006, p. 455).

When educating clients and families, an important initial step is becoming culturally sensitive. This refers to the process of becoming aware of one's own biases and prejudices about another culture or ethnic group. Cultural competence, a higher level, denotes educational interventions reflecting knowledge, understanding, respect, and acceptance of the clients and/or family's culture (Bastable, 2006).

For a successful educational encounter to occur, HCPs and clients and their families must bridge these cultural differences through the use of effective interpersonal communication. This establishment of common understanding between HCPs and clients and their families is facilitated by the HCP performing the following:

- Explore and respect the client's/family's beliefs, values, meaning of the chronic illness, preferences, and needs.
- Identify what will build rapport and trust. Potential sources of information to assist in this process are other colleagues, family members of the client, community groups, and reputable websites.
- Determine if there are any common views or interests.
- Identify own biases and assumptions.
- Maintain and convey an unconditional positive regard. Be an excellent listener, be open and nonjudgmental, and use consistent perception checks to assess comprehension of what has been communicated.
- Become knowledgeable of the culture and health disparities/discrimination of the particular client/family's culture. Review some of the websites listed at the end of this chapter that provide a starting point for resources from reputable sources.
- Use interpreter services when needed.

Cultural differences make each client and family situation unique, but there are also essential considerations in communication, interactions, and the ultimate delivery of any educational activity. Because culture has been linked to cancer-related beliefs and practices, Kreuter and associates (2003) examined the effects of culture on responses to cancer education materials. With a convenience sample of 1227 African American women, it was determined that responses to culturally tailored materials were no different than to other materials, regardless of the women's cultural characteristics. However, for all types of educational materials, women with higher religiosity and racial pride paid more attention to the educational materials. In this study, it appeared that select cultural attributes (e.g., religiosity and racial pride) moderated responses to tailored health education materials.

A number of other contextual factors have been demonstrated to influence health-related attitudes and beliefs of the cancer information–seeking behavior of African American men. For example, living in the South where the Tuskegee Syphilis Study took place has resulted in distrust of the healthcare delivery system among many African Americans (Freimuth et al., 2001; Green et al., 2000). In a study investigating factors predicting prostate cancer information seeking by 52 African American men, it was discovered that the men increased their awareness by obtaining accurate information regarding the disease, early detection and screening, and treatment. However, negative beliefs such as fear, distrust, and inconvenience of the symptoms and treatment were identified. It was further revealed that peers, siblings, and religious leaders had a significant influence on the study subjects' behaviors.

Viswanathan and Lambert (2005), in a study with 20 adult African Americans with cardiovascular disease, ranging in age from 45 to 64 years, discovered that the subjects expressed fear. Subjects' fears were related to side effects from their medication, fear of dependence, and worry about forgetting to take their medication correctly. Despite the fears identified, these subjects perceived their medications to be lifesaving, an important part of life, and recognized the necessity to take medication properly to prevent the complications associated with hypertension. In Hatcher and Wittemore's study (2007), the subjects also experienced fear, but the stated reasons were distinctly different. This finding emphasizes that not all African Americans experience situations in the same manner, and that individualized assessment and planning needs to occur without making assumptions and applying them to all members of that cultural group.

In an integrative review that focused on Hispanic adults and their beliefs about type II diabetes, Hatcher and Wittemore (2007) identified several valuable findings that should be considered when developing educational interventions for this population. After reviewing 15 research studies, they identified that generally Hispanic adults' understanding of the etiology of diabetes was an integration of biomedical causes (e.g., heredity) and traditional folk beliefs. With knowledge of the importance of heredity and folk beliefs in how Hispanics view diabetes, Hatcher and Wittemore (2007) recommend this as a starting point to clarify misconceptions and develop individualized plans of teaching and care. Results from this synthesis of the research literature highlight the necessity of obtaining specific knowledge of how race and culture can affect the structure, implementation, and evaluation of educational outcomes.

Determination of the family's sense of burden, ability to cope, and the role of culture is another aspect of the client and family assessment that needs to be taken into consideration when planning individualized educational activities. Cain and Wicke (2000), in a study involving 138 family caregivers of clients with chronic obstructive pulmonary disease (COPD), discovered that African American caregivers experienced less burden than their Caucasian counterparts. Similar levels of burden occurred in men compared with women and spouse caregivers compared with nonspouse caregivers. In addition, younger caregivers indicated more burden than those age 55 and older. Although these findings are not generalizable beyond this study, the researchers acknowledge the importance of educators being cognizant of contextual factors such as caregiver burden and age, and how these factors may affect other activities such as client and family teaching. **Table 15-2** provides additional resources to facilitate cultural competence with diverse client and family populations.

Gender and Learning Styles

In addition to cultural background, gender and learning styles have a significant influence on the learner's willingness and ability to respond

---

Table 15-2   Cultural Competence Resources for Client–Family Education

Center for Human Diversity; provides consulting and training in cultural competence, diversity, and customer service: www.centerforhumandiversity.org

Joint Commission- Advancing effective communication, cultural competence, and patient-and-family-centered care: A roadmap for hospitals. Retrieved September 6, 2011, from http://www.jointcommission.org/Advancing_Effective_Communication

Kaiser's monthly update on health disparities (2011). Retrieved September 9, 2011, from http://www.kff.org/minorityhealth/report.cfm

Knowledge Path; electronic resource guide to racial and ethnic disparities in health that includes information on (and links to) websites, electronic and print publications, webcasts, and databases: www.mchlibrary.info/KnowledgePaths/kp_race.html

National Center for Cultural Competence; increase the capacity of health and mental health programs to design, implement, and evaluate culturally and linguistically competent service delivery systems (there is also a Spanish version): www11.georgetown.edu/research/gucchd/nccc/

National Mental Health Information Center; U.S. Dept. of Health and Human Services Substance Abuse and Mental Health Services Administration (SAMHSA): http://promoteacceptance.samhsa.gov/topic/SubstanceUseDisorders.organizations.aspx

Network for Multicultural Health Research on Health and Healthcare. Retrieved September 9, 2011, fromhttp://www.multiculturalhealthcare.net/

Office of Minority Health: www.omhrc.gov/templates/browse.aspx?lvl=2&lvlID=15

Rural Assistance Center for Minority Health; U.S. Department of Health and Human Services Rural Initiative Center's resource on issues of minority health in rural communities: www.raconline.org/info_guides/minority_health/

Working Together to End Racial and Ethnic Disparities: One Physician at a Time; AMA toolkit designed to help physicians eliminate health care disparities: www.ama-assn.org/ama1/pub/upload/mm/433/health_disp_kit.pdf

Table 15-3	Comparison of Brain-Based Learning Differences According to Gender	
	Males	**Females**
Deductive and inductive reasoning	Are more inclined to use deductive thinking	Prefer inductive thinking
Abstract and concrete reasoning	Gravitate to abstract arguments	Perform better with concrete analysis
Language usage	Write, read, and speak but usually less than females; in a group of males, one or two tend to dominate	Usually prefer writing, reading, and speaking more words than males
Logic and evidence	Tend to ask for more evidence to support a claim	Tend to be better listeners, more secure in conversation, and require less control of discussion compared with males
Symbolism usage	Respond to pictures with males; more dependent on pictures, diagrams, and graphs in their learning process	Respond to pictures, but not as dependent on pictures, diagrams, and graphs as males to learn

Source: Gurian, M., & Ballew, A. C. (2003). *The boys and girls learn differently: Action guide for teachers.* San Francisco: Jossey-Bass; Sax, L., Bryant, A., & Harper, C. (2005). The differential effects of student-faculty interaction on college outcomes for women and men. *Journal of College Student Development, 46*(6), 642–657; Connell, D. & Gunzelmann, B. (2004). The new gender gap: Why are so many boys floundering while so many girls are soaring? Retrieved August 24, 2011, from: http://www.teacher.scholastic.com/products/Instructor/Mar04_gendergap.htm

to and apply educational content. Numerous studies have identified gender differences in the structure of the brain and how it functions (Gur et al., 1999; Luders et al., 2008; Witelson, Beresh, & Kigar, 2006). **Table 15-3** provides an overview of basic gender differences that have been identified, but educators are strongly encouraged to individually determine the applicability of these differences to a particular client and family population (Gurian & Ballew, 2003; Sax, 2005; Connell & Gunzelmann, 2004).

With the increased usage of online courses and Web-based educational materials, research is revealing that there is a variation in learning styles of online students and students in face-to-face courses (Garland & Martin, 2005). Moreover, these researchers determined that gender is related to learning style and engagement. In their study involving 7 online courses and 168 students (102 female and 66 male), there was a significant relationship with regard to male students who favored an abstract conceptualization mode of learning and how many times they accessed the communication area of Blackboard, an online course management system. Female students, meanwhile, were more highly motivated to perform required class activities than male students. The researchers emphasize that faculty constructing online courses need to be aware of how discussions, chats, and groups are influenced by gender, while keeping in mind that postings may be intimidating to some female students. Garland and Martin (2005) further stress the need for additional studies that investigate the relationship between online learning, learning style, and gender, but also the importance of considering gender equity in building and designing online courses and educational programs.

In another study involving an online health-education program, Women-to-Women (WTW), Cudney, Sullivan, Winters, Paul, and Orient (2005) were interested in determining issues and solutions in a sample of 50 middle-aged women with cancer, diabetes, multiple sclerosis, or rheumatoid arthritis who lived in rural communities. The problems identified included difficulties carrying out self-management programs, negative fears/feelings, poor communication with HCPs, and disturbed relationships with family and friends. Self-identified solutions pertained to problem-solving techniques that were tailored to their rural lifestyle. Although most women indicated that their health promotion problems were not easily solvable, they continued to identify feasible ways to self-manage their chronic illnesses (e.g., small achievable goals, taking one day at a time, taking responsibility for being informed, improving communication with HCPs, being proactive in family relationships, being able to say "no"). Results from this study affirm the importance of performing research to expand the best available evidence to guide our practice.

Just as gender differences need to be assessed, many educators indicate that determination of the individual's learning style is equally important. The presumed method by which an individual learns best is defined as one's learning style. The difficulty is that there are more than 80 learning style models and limited scientific evidence to support any of them (Coffield, Moseley, Hall, & Ecclestone, 2004; Stahl, 2002). Despite the controversy over the presence and quality of the evidence, it is still worthwhile to ask clients and families what approach to learning they prefer (e.g., spoken word, reading, writing, doing, or interacting). With this information the HCP can then more effectively plan the teaching interventions. Moreover, age, intelligence, motor skills, degree of impairment, anxiety, and past experiences can significantly affect an individual's ability to learn (Rankin et al., 2005). Along with the aforementioned factors, educational activities must be adapted to clients' and families' style of learning and preferences regarding what they need to learn.

Readiness to Learn, Self-Efficacy, and Readiness to Change

Once the learning needs of the client and family are identified, determination of their readiness to learn and self-efficacy are important next steps. Readiness to learn refers to the time when learners are receptive to learning, whereas self-efficacy indicates that they have confidence in their capability of attaining a particular goal (Bastable, 2006). In order for learning to occur, clients and family members must be ready to learn and possess average to high self-efficacy.

Readiness to learn manifests in a variety of areas such as physical readiness, emotional readiness, experiential readiness, and knowledge readiness (Lichtenthal, 1990). More specifically, physical readiness can be affected by the client's ability to perform the task, the task's complexity, environmental conditions that keep the client's attention and interest, the client's health status, and gender (Lichtenthal, 1990; Bastable, 2006). Research supports that women are more receptive to medical care and less likely to take risks associated with their health compared with men (Bertakis, Rahman, Helms, Callahan, & Robbins, 2000). Emotional readiness to learn, on the other hand, has been demonstrated to be affected by anxiety level, strength of one's support system, motivation, state of mind, and developmental stage (Bastable, 2006). Previous positive as well as negative learning experiences can dramatically affect experiential readiness of clients and family members. Therefore, HCPs planning an educational activity should identify any previous learning successes and failures and prior ways of coping with similar situations, and understand the potential influence of culture and human motivation. Finally, readiness to learn new knowledge can be influenced by what the client or family member already knows, their cognitive ability, any learning disabilities, and general learning style (Bastable, 2006; Muijs & Reynolds, 2005; Rankin et al., 2005).

While assessing clients and family members for readiness to learn, self-efficacy must also be determined. In the research literature, a strong sense of self-efficacy, confidence in one's ability to achieve a behavior, has repeatedly been demonstrated to have significant positive influence on accomplishing a health-promoting behavior change in individuals with chronic illness (Coleman & Newton, 2005; Osborne, Wilson, Lorig, & McColl, 2007; Tung & Lee, 2006).

Readiness to change is another increasingly familiar term applied to chronic illness and reducing unhealthy behaviors. Although readiness to change has varied definitions, the best known emerges from the Transtheoretical Model of Change (TTM), which involves intentional decision making and was developed to promote effective interventions to facilitate positive behavioral change. TTM is a model that reflects an integration of constructs from other theories and describes how individuals modify problem behaviors such as smoking, limited exercise, and overeating to acquire a more positive behavior (Prochaska & DiClemente, 1983; Prochaska,

DiClemente, & Norcross, 1992; Prochaska & Velicer, 1997). The central organizing construct is Stages of Change, but the model also includes other variables (e.g., self-efficacy, processes of change, decisional balance, and temptation). TTM focuses on stage-focused interventions pertaining to the individual's readiness to change an unhealthy behavior (e.g., smoking, limited exercise). Within TTM, there are five stages of readiness to change (i.e., pre-contemplation, contemplation, preparation, action, and maintenance). Measurement instruments with demonstrated reliability and validity can be obtained at the Cancer Prevention Research Center website (CPRC, 2008).

Developmental Stage

Chronologic age provides a basic indication of clients' and family members' projected physical, cognitive, and psychological state of development. When planning a teaching–learning activity for a client and family member, consideration of the clients' or family members' developmental stage is pivotal, along with past learning experiences, stress level, physical and emotional health, personal motivation, environmental conditions, and available support systems (Bastable, 2006).

Within the literature, there are several prominent developmental theorists who have shaped how HCPs view life stages (Erikson, 1968; Piaget, 1951, 1976). In contrast with childhood where learning is student centered, adult learning tends to be more problem centered, with the primary emphasis on how to apply new knowledge and skills to immediate problems (Bastable, 2006). Adults tend to be more resistant to change, which is why establishing mutual goals and an action plan with HCPs markedly improves the

Table 15-4   Linking Developmental Stage with Learner Characteristics and Teaching Strategies

Developmental Stage	Learner Characteristics	Recommended Teaching Strategies
Young adulthood (18–39.9 years)	Peak body function	Immediate application
	Self-directive	Active participation
	Independent in learning	Learning needs to be convenient, self-paced, and blend of visual and written
	Making decisions about career, education, social roles	Tend to like group interaction
	Competency-based learner	Organized materials and presentation
	If has a chronic illness, tends to want to learn as much as possible to remain independent and lead as normal a life as possible	Use past experiences as a resource for learning
		Provide practical answers to their problems
		Give opportunity for immediate application of teaching
		Seek credible/evidence-based information
Middle age (40–64.9 years)	Well developed sense of self	Maintain independence and perhaps reestablish what constitutes normal life patterns
	Usually at career peak	Assess prior positive and negative learning experiences
	Concerned about physical changes	Identify potential stressors
	Reexamines goals and values	Provide information that fits to life problems and/or concerns; use past experiences as a resource for learning
	Confident in abilities	
	Tends to want to reduce unsatisfying aspects in life	Provide practical answers to their problems
	May be experiencing midlife crises	Give opportunity for immediate application of teaching
Older adult (65 years and older)	Cognitive changes	Use concrete examples
	Decreased ability to think abstractly	Build on past experiences
	Reduced short-term memory	Make information relevant
	Increased reaction time	Allow time for processing and responses
	Focus on past life experiences	Use verbal interactions and coaching
	Motor and sensory losses	Encourage active involvement
	Auditory and visual changes	Keep explanations brief (20–40 minutes)
	Hearing loss especially with high-pitched tones, consonants, and rapid speech	Speak distinctly and slowly
		Minimize distractions while teaching
		Avoid shouting—if large group, microphone may be needed
	Decreased peripheral vision	Use large font in handouts
	Decreased risk taking	Avoid glares
		Provide a safe environment
		Keep teaching sessions short
		Provide rest periods
		Rooms where conducted should be neutral temperature (not too hot or cold)

Sources: Bastable, S. B. (2006). *Essentials of patient education.* Sudbury, MA: Jones and Bartlett; Mauk, K. L. (Ed.). (2006). *Gerontological nursing: Competencies for care.* Sudbury, MA: Jones and Bartlett; Rankin, S. H., Stallings, K. D., & London, F. (2005). *Patient education in health and illness* (5th ed.). Philadelphia: Lippincott.

achievement of educational outcomes (Miller, 2003; Rankin, Stallings, & London, 2005).

Table 15-4 provides a brief overview of the developmental stages of adults, the major attributes of the learner, and the most applicable teaching strategies. A common misconception is that older adults cannot learn. When older adults are provided information at a slower rate, material being taught is relevant, and positive feedback is received, they are very capable of learning new knowledge and skills (Bastable, 2006; Mauk, 2010). Because depression, grief, and loneliness are not restricted to older adults, these factors can markedly affect any client or family members' ability to concentrate on content being presented. HCPs, moreover, must be continually aware of other potential cognitive as well as physical limitations (i.e., pain, fatigue, diminished vision, reduced hearing) that can affect the ability of clients and family members to learn. **Table 15-5**

Table 15-5 Helpful Resources to Facilitate Teaching and Learning of Older Adults

Organization	Website
American Society on Aging	www.asaging.org
Association for Gerontology in Higher Education	www.aghe.org
The John A. Hartford Foundation Institute for Geriatric Nursing	www.hartfordign.org
National Center for Education Statistics	www.nces.ed.gov
National Institute on Aging	www.nia.nih.gov
National Council on Aging	www.ncoa.org
Osher Lifelong Learning Institute	www.olli.gmu.edu

provides a listing of recommended resources for HCPs to identify how to optimally structure and evaluate educational activities involving older adults.

Literacy

Health literacy or the ability to understand and apply information to care for one's self is a challenge for approximately one in two adults in the United States, who cannot read above the 5th-grade level (Nielson-Bohlman, Panzer, & Kindig, 2004; Mayer & Vallaire, 2007). Throughout the entire healthcare delivery process, low literacy levels can affect the ability of clients and family members to read and comprehend health information (e.g., discharge instructions, labels on prescription bottles), which serves as an important prerequisite to compliance and overall successful client outcomes (Bastable, 2006; Lasater & Mehler, 1998; Nielson-Bohlman, Panzer, & Kindig, 2004). A variety of measurement tools are available to HCPs to assess the readability of written educational materials as well as reading capability of clients and family members. Refer to **Table 15-6** for a brief description of several tools that have proved useful.

System Factors That Influence the Teaching and Learning Process

To ensure an optimal client, family, and HCP educational situation, certain elements need to be in place. System factors that can significantly contribute to positive educational outcomes include (Edwardson, 2007; Nobel, 2006; Rankin et al., 2005):

- Preparation of the HCP in terms of knowledge of the educational content and teaching capabilities

Table 15-6   Tools to Assess Readability of Educational Materials and Individuals' Reading Comprehension

Measurement Tools to Assess Readability of Educational Materials	**Measurement Tools to Assess an Individual's Reading Comprehension**
Flesch Formula	*Wide Range Achievement Test (WRAT)*
In use more than 70 years to assess news reports, adult educational materials, and government publications. Based on a count of two basic language components: average sentence length in words and average word length measured in syllables per word of selected samples of text (Flesch, 1948; Spadero, 1983). Helpful Web source to assist with these calculations is:	WRAT is a word-recognition screening test that typically takes about 5 minutes to complete. It assesses the client's ability to recognize and pronounce a list of words out of context to determine reading skills. It has two levels of testing: Level 1 is for children 5–12 years; Level 2 is for individuals older than 12 years of age (Doak, Doak, & Root, 1996). Helpful Web source is:
http://www.readabilityformulas.com/flesch-reading-ease-readability-formula.php and www.csun.edu/~vcecn006/read1.html	http://www4.parinc.com/Products/Product.aspx?ProductID=WRAT4
Fog Formula	*Rapid Estimate of Adult Literacy in Medicine (REALM)*
Assesses the reading level of materials from 4th grade to college level. One of the easier tools to use with the calculation based on the average sentence length and percentage of multisyllabic words based on a sample of 100 words (Bastable, 2006; Spadero, 1983). Helpful Web sources are:	The REALM tests the client's ability to read medical and health-related vocabulary (advantage over the WRAT), takes less time, and has easy scoring (Duffy & Synder, 1999). Although the test has validity, it offers less precision and reliability than other word tests (Hayes, 2000). Sixty-six medical and health-related words are placed in three columns ranging from short and easy to more difficult. Clients are to begin reading the words from the top and go down. The total number of correctly pronounced words is the raw score that is then converted to a grade range (Doak et al., 1996). Helpful Web source is:
http://www.readabilityformulas.com/gunning-fog-readability-formula.php	Faculty-Development/MediaLibraries/Faculty-Development/Media/PDF/The-REALM-Test-(Hazen-3-07-07).pdf
www.thelearningweb.net/fogindex.html	
SMOG Formula	*Test of Functional Health Literacy in Adults (TOFHL)*
This formula has been used primarily to evaluate the grade-level readability of patient educational materials (PEMs) and can measure reading level with as little content as 10 sentences. This formula determines readability from grades 4 to college level, and is based on number of multisyllable words (3 or more) within a set number of sentences (McLaughlin, 1969). Helpful Web source is:	TOFHL is a newer measurement tool to assess clients' literacy skills and actually uses hospital materials (i.e., appointment slips, informed consent documents, and prescription labels). The test consists of two parts: reading comprehension and numeracy (Bastable, 2006). It has demonstrated validity and reliability, takes approximately 20 minutes to administer, and has an English and Spanish version (Quirk, 2000). Helpful Web source is:
http://www.readabilityformulas.com/smog-readability-formula.php	http://education.gsu.edu/csal/TOFHLA.htm

- Cultural competence and knowledge related to all of the other factors that help to personalize the educational approach (i.e., age, developmental stage, and cognitive and physical status related to the chronic illness)
- Required resources for effective teaching (e.g., equipment/technology, materials—booklets, figures).
- Time limitations that permit updating teaching plans, evaluation tools, and developing/updating educational protocols
- Coordinating educational activities that are consistent with discharge plans and other important client and family information that needs to be communicated
- Succinct and timely documentation of what was taught, when, and the outcome, so others can build on and reinforce prior teaching
- If client and family education is not valued by the system and rewards are not given for educational excellence and positive outcomes
- If there is inadequate record-keeping and reimbursement policies that reimburse fully for direct, hands-on illness interventions, but poorly for client/family education and interventions via telephone and computer

The following strategies (Mayer & Vallaire, 2007; Bastable, 2006; Petty, 2006; Falvo, 2011) may serve as a starting point when assessing and educating clients and families with low literacy:

- Materials should not be above 5th-grade level and should be culturally appropriate.
- Keep sentences short and limited to 20 words or fewer if possible.
- Speak and write using short words with only one or two syllables whenever possible. Rely on common words that are easily recognized by most individuals.
- Put the most important information first and limit focus on what the client and family member need to know.
- Clearly and simply define technical words or ones that are unfamiliar (e.g., fasting blood glucose, hypertension), or replace with simpler words (high blood pressure for hypertension).
- Remember that those with low literacy skills may require more time to read and absorb the materials.
- Visual presentation (a picture is worth a thousand words) can be especially helpful to someone with low literacy skills.
- Avoid abbreviations (e.g., MI, FBS, I, and O).
- Use consistent words throughout the presentation (e.g., don't switch from "diet" to "menu" to "dietary prescription").
- Organize information into "chunks" that facilitate recall. Use numbers only when necessary and realize that statistics are usually confusing and meaningless for the low-literate client and family member.
- Keep the number of items in a list at no more than seven.
- Keep teaching sessions short and preferably no longer than 10–15 minutes.
- Use the teach-back method with clients to ensure that they understand their care routine and warning signs if there is a problem (i.e., signs of a wound infection or urinary tract infection, signs of a stroke or heart attack—not myocardial infarction). Never ask, "Do you understand?" Ask the patient to explain the processes or state the signs of an infection, stroke, or heart attack. These perception checks are an important part of

the teaching–learning process and enable the HCP to assess whether learning is occurring as planned. Plus, these perception checks allow the HCP to redirect their activities if the client and/or family educational outcomes are not being achieved as planned.

- Have your written materials reviewed by a literacy expert to determine the grade reading level. Also, ask the client and family member a question to determine their specific ability to read and comprehend what is described. In addition, do not assume that the teaching materials address all of the client and/or family concerns. Ask if there is something missing or whether they have questions about anything that is not included in the materials provided. Remember too that blending written materials combined with auditory interactions enhances learning and retention of information.

- Present information one step at a time to pace instruction and allow clients and family members to understand each step and ask questions before moving on to the next step.

In conjunction with the system challenges just identified, HCPs must also consider other diverse attributes (i.e., age, gender, culture, developmental stage, literacy, and functional status) that make each client and family educational encounter unique. In addition, what is the best available evidence that will help shape these interventions? Townsend, Bruce, Hooten and Rome (2006) also assert that HCPs do not always recognize the tensions and ambiguities permeating clients' experiences, particularly those who have multiple chronic illnesses. Results of this research revealed that clients with chronic illness utilize multiple techniques

to manage their symptoms, and frequently felt pressure to manage "well" and have a "normal life" for both their families and HCPs.

Despite the limited strong evidence to support all aspects of HCPs' educational interventions, the research continues to expand as do the meta-analyses and systematic reviews that synthesize the evidence and identify additional areas to be explored. In order to more comprehensively document the specific contribution of nursing to the education and self-care of clients with chronic illness, Edwardson (2007) recommends two focus areas for research. The first is to measure the outcomes of client and family education and have this information included in both the clinical and administrative databases. Whenever possible, the client and family educational process and outcomes should be separated according to type of education, objectives, timing, dose (i.e., strategies, length), and so forth. In addition, systematic reviews and meta-analysis suggest that inpatient education followed by some form of post-discharge intervention may be the most promising approach to reduce hospitalizations (Gonseth, Castillion, Banegas, & Artalejo, 2004). However, for this care system to succeed, databases from ambulatory care, acute care, and after-care services need to be linked to monitor symptoms, monitor adherence to treatment prescription, and to modify treatment plans as needed (Edwardson, 2007).

EDUCATIONAL INTERVENTIONS FOR THE CLIENT AND FAMILY

As indicated in previous sections of this chapter, there are multiple factors to be carefully assessed and considered in the development of an educational plan for clients with chronic illness and their families. Because of the variance in how these elements manifest, the mutually established goals by the client, family, and HCP; associated interventions; and outcomes will need to be uniquely planned, implemented, and evaluated. In most instances, nurses will be the principal HCP who participates in this ongoing educational process and provides the continuity of care for clients with chronic illness and their families.

Development of the Teaching Plan

The teaching plan provides the overall blueprint or outline for instruction that clearly defines the relationship among the behavioral objectives, instructional content, teaching strategies, timeframe for teaching, and methods of evaluation (Bastable, 2006). All aspects work together to achieve a predetermined goal that should be mutually agreed upon by the client and family and HCP. The domains of learning that are to be accomplished divide into one of three domains: cognitive (knowledge), psychomotor (physical activities), and affective (attitudes or emotions). When constructing teaching plans to address these learning domains for specific chronic illnesses, HCPs should also refer to published practice standards such as those from the Agency for Healthcare Research and Quality (AHRQ), specialty nursing groups, and the American Heart Association, which present evidence-based guidelines. The specific teaching plan includes the following aspects: purpose of the teaching plan; goal(s), broad statement of what is to be achieved; objective(s) that need to be specific and measurable; content covered to achieve each objective; teaching strategies; time required; and evaluation methods to determine if the learning has occurred. Key aspects of the teaching plan are described, followed by a specific example.

Teaching Strategies

Knowing how to use varied teaching strategies to achieve educational objectives can make client and family education more interesting, challenging, and effective for HCPs and learners (Rankin et al., 2005). A general overview of common teaching strategies and their predominant characteristics is presented in **Table 15-7**. For the client with chronic illness, the research strongly supports that combining multiple teaching methods during several educational sessions consistently produces more positive client outcomes than single teaching methods and events (Bastable, 2006; Beranova & Sykes, 2007; Edwardson, 2007; The Joanna Briggs Institute, 2006). However, the HCP must also remain cognizant of the system factors contributing to the success and/or failure of the teaching and learning process.

A pivotal aspect of any client and family teaching event is preparing measurable objectives that can be achieved in the timeframe specified. For example, the client with diabetes may need to learn the signs and symptoms of a hypoglycemic reaction. An appropriate measurable objective could be "Ms. Jones will state four signs/symptoms of a hypoglycemic reaction by the end of this 12-hour shift."

Increasingly, more clients with chronic illness and their family members are receiving education regarding disease management from Web-based sources, with the young to middle aged being the biggest consumers (Beranova & Sykes, 2007; Lee, Yeh, Liu, & Chen, 2007). Research from a new survey published by the Pew Research Center's Internet and American Life Project and the California Healthcare Foundation (2011) found that 80% of Internet users look online for health information, making it the third most popular online pursuit following email and

Table 15-7   General Overview of Common Teaching Strategies

Teaching Strategy	Learning Domain	Learner Role	Teacher Role	Strength	Weakness
Lecture	Cognitive	Passive	Presents information	Cost effective; targeted to larger groups	Not individualized
Group discussion	Cognitive; affective	Active, if learner participates	Directs and focuses discussion	Share emotions and ideas	Shy or dominant members affect participation; may lose focus
One-to-one teaching	Cognitive; affective psychomotor	Active	Presents information and encourages individualized learning	Tailored to client or family member's needs and goals	Great diversity; labor intensive; learner isolated
Demonstration	Cognitive	Passive	Modeling of skill or behavior	Preview of skill or behavior, can ask questions	Need individual or small group to visualize
Return demonstration	Psychomotor	Active	Individualized feedback to refine skill performance	Immediate feedback	Labor intensive; anxiety may affect actions
Gaming	Cognitive; affective	Active if client–family participates	Oversees pacing; debriefs	Stimulates learners' enthusiasm and participation	May be too competitive; over-stimulating
Simulation	Cognitive; psychomotor	Active	Designs situation; facilitates learning; debriefs	Practice a reality situation in a safe setting	Labor intensive; equipment costs/access; scheduling issues
Online learning	Cognitive; affective	Passive, but can be active if participates in group discussions, problem solving, group projects	Usually designs program/class; presents information; provides active learning exercises, discussions, case studies, and group projects	Learners usually at a distance; flexibility when access learning content and activities; learners need to be motivated; feedback provided is usually individualized and immediate	Need equipment to access; lack of personal contact; accessibility; all feedback may not be instantaneous
Computer-assisted instruction	Cognitive; affective	Active	Purchases or designs program; expected to provide feedback to student	Individualized instruction; learner controls pace of the learning; can program to receive feedback; valuable modality if hearing impaired, learning disability, or aphasic	Must have equipment and software

Sources: Bastable, S. B. (2006). *Essentials of patient education.* Sudbury, MA: Jones & Bartlett; Miller, E. (2010). Scientific basis for clinical reasoning I (29NURS840), Online Course Manual. Cincinnati, OH: University of Cincinnati, College of Nursing; Wantland, D. J., Portillo, C. J., Holzemer, W. L., & Slaughter, R. (2004). The effectiveness of Web-based vs. non-Web-based interventions: A meta-analysis of behavioral change outcomes. *Journal of Medical Internet Research, 6*(4), 40–71.

using a search engine (Fox, 2011). For clients with chronic illness, the use of the Internet provides a means to encourage behavior change necessitating knowledge sharing, education, and greater understanding of their condition. Results of a meta-analysis comparing Web-based and non–Web-based education of chronically ill adults (mean age 41.2 years) from 1996 to 2003 revealed that there was substantial evidence that Web-based interventions improved behavioral change outcomes (Wantland, Portillo, Holzemer, & Slaughter, 2004). The specific positive outcomes identified were increased knowledge of nutritional status, increased knowledge of asthma treatment, increased exercise time, slower health decline, and 18-month weight-loss maintenance. Web-based interventions that were relevant and individually tailored had more and longer website visits. Wantland and associates further discovered that sites with chat rooms increased social support scores of the users. They caution, however, that the long-term effects on individual persistence with the chosen therapies and the cost effectiveness of the Web-based therapies and hardware and software development demand ongoing evaluation.

Learning Curve

Whenever a learner is acquiring knowledge, an attitudinal change, or motor skill, there is a learning curve (Bastable, 2006). Typically individual learning curves are irregular, with fluctuations attributed to changes in the learner such as attention, energy, ability, or situational factors (Gage & Berliner, 1998). In the case of clients with chronic illness, learning to walk again following a stroke may take time and create frustration, as expectations do not match physical capability. Because learning may not always occur in a linear fashion, HCPs must recognize

this and assist clients and their families when they experience anger, discouragement, or depression associated with achievement not progressing as anticipated. In addition, research supports that retention of learning is enhanced when there are opportunities to see, hear, observe demonstrations, discuss, and practice as well as teach others (Bastable, 2006; Muijs & Reynolds, 2005; Petty, 2006).

Evaluation

Evaluation of educational outcomes is a critical step in the teaching and learning process. It encompasses a systematic and continuous activity that involves collecting and using information to determine whether the educational objectives have been achieved. This outcome evaluation is labeled summative evaluation, but there can also be formative evaluation. Formative evaluation occurs during the actual teaching process when the implementation is still in process. Formative evaluation permits the HCP to adjust or change aspects of the implementation process that may improve the quality or delivery of the educational program or session. For instance, the HCP may decide to use a Web-based program and face-to-face demonstration of a task to clients and their families. On the basis of immediate negative feedback received regarding a client's unfamiliarity with computers and reluctance to use such a program, the HCP may decide to replace the Web-based education with a small group discussion involving the client and his family.

When performing any type of evaluation, it is also important to identify what outcome is being measured, how and when the data will be collected, and then how it will be interpreted. For example, assume the HCP and client have established the following outcome objective: "Client will state three signs/symptoms of hypoglycemia

Table 15-8 Sample Teaching Plan

Objectives	Content (topics)	Time Frame	Teaching Strategy	Evaluation Method
The client will be able to: 1. Distinguish the signs and symptoms of hypoglycemia from hyperglycemia. *Cognitive domain of learning*	a. Definition of hypoglycemia compared to hyperglycemia b. Signs of hypoglycemia c. Signs of hyperglycemia d. Actions to take when each are present	5 minutes	One-to-one teaching presentation Visual materials: poster listing signs and symptoms of hypoglycemia and hyperglycemia, booklet to keep If client has difficulty getting the content correct, repeat teaching as well as discuss other strategies that may facilitate retention of the information.	Use several vignettes and then ask client to identify signs and symptoms of each from a list. Need 100% correct response. Ask immediate action when each is present. Must get all correct.
2. Demonstrate ability to correctly perform a finger stick and reading of glucose level. *Psychomotor domain of learning*	a. Purpose of client glucose self-monitoring b. Key aspects in the correct performance of a finger stick and accurate reading of the results	20 minutes	One-to-one teaching presentation Provide a demonstration of the correct technique Then have client perform the finger stick and interpretation of results Nurse provides feedback, reinforcement of behaviors, and may have client do this again if needed. May have online or hospital TV channel available so that client can review this again	Client correctly performs the finger stick and glucose interpretation Have a video of incorrect performance of this skill or nurse incorrectly do and client identify incorrect elements performed
3. Verbalize confidence in performing key elements in glucose monitoring. *Affective domain of learning*	Importance of daily monitoring of blood glucose in the continued management of diabetes Accountability and self-monitoring associated with a chronic disease	2 minutes	One-to-one teaching and blend brief discussion, reinforcement, and feedback	Have rate on a scale of 0 = no confidence to 10 = complete confidence in performing daily glucose monitoring

| | | Time | | Evaluation |
Objectives	Content (topics)	Frame	Teaching Strategy	Method
4. State purpose, dose, time to take, and side effects of single medications prescribed at discharge. *Cognitive domain of learning* During the second interaction when this fourth objective is the focus, assess the client's retention of the correct information associated with objectives 1–3.	Medication prescribed— including purpose, dose, time to take, side effects, and other considerations	10 minutes	One-to-one teaching, poster, or other written materials to provide a blend of visual and auditory information is advisable Determine if the client has any questions since receiving instruction pertaining to objectives 1–3	Orally and/or on paper list the medication's purpose, dose, time to take, prominent side effects, and other considerations Assess knowledge, actions, and attitudes pertaining to objectives 1–3 with the same evaluation standard as in the first encounter

Table 15-8   Sample Teaching Plan (Continued)

by the end of a 12-hour shift." Determination of achievement for this objective is straightforward. Yet, sometimes barriers occur that hinder the evaluation process. Several barriers that can be particularly problematic are: lack of clarity regarding what is being evaluated, lack of ability to perform the evaluation, and, finally, fear of punishment or low self-esteem (Bastable, 2006). With regard to lack of ability, the HCP may not know how to construct a short test to determine if the client and family have a basic understanding of diabetes or feel comfortable orally quizzing them to assess their learning. In other situations, clients may be too ill to learn the information, how to perform a new task, or respond as they anticipate the HCP wants them to.

In many settings, practice guidelines or protocols identify how formative and summative evaluations are to be conducted and what information needs to be documented. Data from the evaluation process, especially as it applies to the teaching and learning process for the client and family, can be extremely valuable as the chronic illness progresses and additional knowledge, attitudinal, and psychomotor skills need to be developed.

Example of a Teaching Plan

This teaching plan was developed in accordance with the following case situation (see **Table 15-8**): You have a newly diagnosed client with diabetes who is going to be discharged in the next 48 hours. The client is a 24-year-old Caucasian male who is single and lives alone. He is currently working as a cashier at a grocery store, but wants to go to college. He also tells you that his parents live about 2 hours away and are concerned about him, but they work full-time and called once while he was in the hospital. Given that you are his primary care nurse, you need to make sure that these four objectives are accomplished.

The specific approach to this client will consider such elements as gender, culture, learning curve, importance of feedback, and reinforcement, as were already described. Given the content and objectives of this specific teaching plan, it is recommended that *not all* of this teaching occur at the same time. The teaching plan pertaining to the first three objectives could be performed, and then teaching of the fourth objective occurs later in the day. During this second educational session, review the key points associated with the first teaching episode. Furthermore, make sure that each teaching session is not interrupted and that there is adequate time to permit questions from the client and family, who should also be present if at all possible.

SUMMARY AND CONCLUSIONS

Education serves as an essential vehicle to provide the client and family with the knowledge, skills, and confidence to address the many facets associated with living with a chronic illness. Although numerous factors contribute to the success or failure of this educational process, HCPs and nurses in particular play a fundamental role as part of their scope of practice and other national standards such as *Healthy People 2020* and Joint Commission benchmarks.

Research evidence continues to expand and guides the assessment of all learners, teaching plan development, and ultimate educational outcomes. Teaching and learning is a complex process and requires consideration of many elements such as family structure and function, culture, gender, learning styles, readiness to learn/change, self-efficacy,

developmental stage, literacy, socioeconomic status, resources, and learning capability. In addition, as HCPs partner with clients and their families during this educational process, it is critical that the HCPs assess their educational objectives and redirect their actions when needed. Because well over 50% of the U.S. population has at least one chronic illness, the teaching and learning process is paramount to attaining greater quality of life and adapting to the frequently dynamic nature of most chronic diseases.

Another central ingredient that is sometimes overlooked is the mutual goal setting that occurs among the client, family, and HCP. Working together, clients are much more inclined to achieve the planned educational objectives whether targeted at knowledge, attitudes, and/or behaviors pertaining to the chronic health problem.

EVIDENCE-BASED PRACTICE BOX

Purpose and background: Client education is an important intervention in the management of heart disease. This article is a systematic review of the literature that examined the educational interventions implemented for clients with heart failure that assessed their related outcomes.

Methods: Randomized control trials from 1998–2008 in CINAHL, MEDLINE, EMBASE, PsychINFO, and the Cochrane Library were reviewed with the search terms: *patient education, educational intervention, self-care* in combination with *heart failure*. Two reviewers independently examined 1515 abstracts.

Results: A total of 2686 patients in 19 studies met the inclusion criteria for this literature review. The initial intervention for all reported studies was typically a one-to-one educational intervention. Seven of these studies had a theoretical framework for their educational intervention. Of the studies reviewed, 15 revealed that the educational intervention had a significant positive outcome on at least one of the desired outcomes.

Conclusions: Even though there were improvements in educational outcomes, the study samples varied considerably. As a result, it was difficult in this systematic review to determine the most effective educational strategy because of the variance in delivery methods, duration of the interventions, and the outcomes evaluated. A client-centered approach to education based on an educational theory and evaluated consistently with that framework is recommended.

Source: Boyde, M., Turner, D., Thompson, D. R., & Stewart, S. (2010). Educational interventions for patients with heart failure: A systematic review of randomized controlled trials. *Journal of Cardiovascular Nursing, 26*(4), E27–E35.

Study Questions (Cont.)

What are the pros and cons of three teaching strategies that can be used to educate an individual with a chronic illness?

What is the difference between pedagogy and andragogy and what affect does it have on your approach to teaching?

What are major factors that should be considered when planning an educational session for a client with chronic illness?

How may the approach of an educational intervention differ if the client is a male compared to a female?

How may cultural and ethnic/race differences specifically affect how you structure and evaluate the outcomes of a specific educational intervention?

How would you specifically assess the literacy of a client and his/her family?

What is the difference between a formative and summative evaluation?

Describe how *Healthy People 2020* and/or Joint Commission standards affect the importance of educational interventions in your practice.

STUDY QUESTIONS

What level of evidence provides the greatest confidence in the applicability of research findings to practice?

For a full suite of assignments and additional learning activities, use the access code located in the front of your book and visit this exclusive website: **http://go.jblearning.com/larsen**. If you do not have an access code, you can obtain one at the site.

REFERENCES

American Nurses Association (2004). *Nursing: Scope and standards of practice* (5th ed.). Washington, DC: Author.

Bandura, A. (1986). *Social foundations of thought and action: A social cognitive theory.* Englewood Cliffs, NJ: Prentice Hall.

Bastable, S. B. (2006). *Essentials of patient education.* Sudbury, MA: Jones and Bartlett.

Beranova, E., & Sykes, C. (2007). A systematic review of computer based software for educating patients with coronary heart disease. *Patient Education and Counseling, 66*(1), 21–28.

Bertakis, K., Rahman, A., Helms, L. J., Callaham, E., & Robbins, J. (2000). Gender differences in the utilization of health care services. *Journal of Family Practice, 49*(2), 147–152.

Boren, S., Balas, E., & Mustafa, Z. (2003). Evidence-based patient education for chronic care. *Abstract Academy Health Meeting, 20*(788). Retrieved August 24, 2011, from: http://gateway.nlm.nih.gov/MeetingAbstracts/102275756.html

Boyde, M., Turner, D., Thompson, D. R., & Stewart, S. (2010). Educational interventions for patients with heart failure: A systematic review of randomized controlled trials. *Journal of Cardiovascular Nursing, 26*(4), E27–E35.

Cain, C. J., & Wicke, M. N. (2000). Caregiving attributes as correlates of burden in family caregivers coping with chronic obstructive pulmonary disease. *Journal of Family Nursing, 6*(1), 46–68.

Cancer Prevention Research Center. (2008). *Measures.* Retrieved August 24, 2011, from: www.uri.edu/research/cprc/measures.htm

Centers for Disease Control and Prevention. (2005). *Preventing diabetes and its complications.* Retrieved August 24, 2011, from: www.cdc.gov/nccdphp/publications/factsheets/prevention/pdf/diabetes.pdf

Centers for Disease Control and Prevention, *Chronic Disease Prevention and Health Promotion* (2010). Retrieved October 18, 2011, from http://www.cdc.gov/chronicdisease/overview/index.htm

Coffield, F., Moseley, D., Hall, E., & Ecclestone, K. (2004). *Learning styles and pedagogy in post-16 learning: A systematic and critical review.* Retrieved August 24, 2011, from: http://www.pedagogy.ir/images/pdf/learning-styles-pedagogy.pdf

Coleman, M., & Newton, K. (2005). Supporting self-management in patients with chronic illness. *American Family Physician, 72*(8), 1503–1510.

Connell, D., & Guzelman, B. (2004). *The new gender gap: Why are so many boys floundering while so many girls are soaring?* Retrieved September 15, 2011, from http://teacher.scholastic.com/products/instructor/Mar04_gendergap.htm#bio

Conner, M. L. (2005). Andragogy and pedagogy. *Ageless Learner, 1997–2004.* Retrieved August 24, 2011, from: http://agelesslearner.com/intros/andragogy.html

Craig, J. V., & Smyth, R. L. (2002). *The evidence-based practice manual for nurses.* New York: Churchill Livingstone.

Cudney, S., Sullivan, T., Winters, C., Paul, L., & Orient, P. (2005). Chronically ill rural women: Self-identified management problems and solutions. *Chronic Illness, 1,* 49–60.

Doak, C, C., Doak, L. G., & Root, J. H. (1996). *Teaching patients with low literacy skills* (2nd ed.). Philadelphia: Lippincott.

Duffy, M. M., & Snyder, K. (1999). Can ED patients read your patient education materials? *Journal of Emergency Nursing, 25*(25),294–297.

Edwardson, S. (2007). Patient education in heart failure. *Heart and Lung: The Journal of Critical Care, 36*(4), 244–252.

Erikson, E. H. (1968). *Identity: Youth and crisis.* New York: Norton.

Falvo, D. R., (2011). Effective patient education: A guide to increased adherence (2nd ed.). Sudbury, MA; Jones and Bartlett Publishers.

Flesch, R. (1948). A new readability yardstick. *Journal of Applied Psychology, 32*(3), 221–233.

Fox, S. (Pew Internet project and California Healthcare Foundation) (2011). *Health topics.* Retrieved September 15, 2011, from http://www.pewinternet.org/Reports/2011/HealthTopics.aspx

Freimuth, V. S., Quinn, S. C., Thomas, S. B., Cole, G., Zook, E., & Duncan, T. (2001). African Americans' view on research and the Tuskegee Syphilis Study. *Social Science and Medicine, 52*(2), 797–808.

Gage, N. L., & Berliner, D. C. (1998). *Educational psychology* (6th ed.). Boston: Houghton Mifflin.

Garland, D., & Martin, B. (2005). Do gender and learning style play a role in how online courses should be designed? *Journal of Interactive Online Learning, 4*(2), 67–81.

Gonseth, J., Castillion, G. P., Banegas, J. R., & Artalejo, F. R., (2004). The effectiveness of disease management programmes in reducing hospital re-admission in older adults with heart failure: A systematic review and meta-analysis of published reports. *European Heart Journal, 25*(18), 1570–1590.

Green, B., Partridge, E., Fouad, M., Kohler, C., Crayton, E., & Alexander, L. (2000). African American attitudes regarding cancer clinical trials and research studies: Results from focus group methodology. *Ethics and Disease, 10*(1), 76–86.

Gremeaux, V., & Coudeyre, E. (2010). The Internet and therapeutic education in patients: A systematic review of the literature. *Annals of Physical and Rehabilitation Medicine, 53*(10), 669–692.

Gur, R., Turetsky, B., Matsui, M., Yan, M., Bilker, W., Hughett, P., et al. (1999). Sex differences in brain gray and white matter in healthy young adults: Correlations with cognitive performance. *The Journal of Neuroscience, 19*(10), 4065–4075.

Gurian, M., & Ballew, A. C. (2003). *The boys and girls learn differently: Action guide for teachers.* San Francisco: Jossey-Bass.

Haggard, A. (1989). *Handbook of patient education.* Rockville, MD: Aspen.

Hatcher, E., & Whittemore, R. (2007). Hispanic adults' beliefs about type 2 diabetes: Clinical implications. *Journal of the American Academy of Nurse Practitioners, 19*(10), 536–545.

Hayes, K. S. (2000). Literacy for health information of adult patients and caregivers in a rural emergency department. *Clinical Excellence for Nurse Practitioners, 4*, 35–40.

Healthy People 2010: Understanding and improving health (2nd ed.). Washington, DC: U.S. Government Printing Office.

Hein, G. E. (1991). *Constructivist learning theory. Institute of inquiry.* Retrieved October 18, 2011, from http://www.exploratorium.edu/ifi/resources/constructivistlearning.html

Institute of Medicine, Committee on Health Professions Education Summit (2003). *Health professions education: A bridge to quality (Quality Chasm Series).* Washington, DC: National Academies Press.

The Joanna Briggs Institute. (2006). Educational interventions for mental health consumers receiving psychotropic medication. *Best Practice, 10*(4), 1–4.

The Joint Commission. (2010). 2011 *Hospital accreditation standards.* Oakbrook, Terrace, IL: Author.

Kaiser Foundation. (2010). *Focus on health reform.* Menlo Park, CA: Author.

Knowles, M. (1998). *The adult learner: The definitive classic in adult education and human resource development.* Houston, TX: Gulf Publishing.

Kreuter, M., Steger-May, K., Bobra, S., Booker, A., Holt, C., Lukwago, S., et al., (2003). Sociocultural characteristics and responses to cancer education materials among African American women. *Cancer Control: Journal of the Moffitt Cancer Center, 10*(5), 69–80.

Lasater, L., & Mehler, P. S. (1998). The literate patient: Screening and management. *Hospital Practice, 33*(4), 163–165, 169–170.

Learning Theories Knowledge Base (2011). *Constructivism at learning-theories.com.* Retrieved September 6, 2011 from www.learning-theories/constructivism.com

Lee, T., Yeh, Y., Liu, C., & Chen, P., (2007). Development and evaluation of a patient-oriented education system for diabetes management. *International Journal of Medical Informatics, 76*, 655–663.

Lichtenthal, C. (1990). *A self-study model of readiness to learn.* Unpublished manuscript.

Lindell, D., Aucoin, J. W. Adams, C. E., Connolly, M. A., Devaney, S., Love, A., et al. (2005). *The scope of practice for academic nurse educators.* New York: National League for Nursing.

Luders, E., Narr, K., Bilder, R., Szeszko, P., Gurbani, M., Hamilton, A., et al. (2008). Mapping the relationship between cortical convolution and intelligence: Effects of gender. *Cerebral Cortex, 18*(9), 2019–2026.

Maslow, A. H. (1962). *Towards of psychology of being.* New York: John Wiley and Sons.

Mauk, K. E. (Ed.) (2006). *Gerontological nursing: Competencies for care.* Sudbury, MA: Jones & Bartlett.

Mauk, K. L. (Ed.). (2010). *Gerontological nursing: Competencies for care (2nd ed.).* Sudbury, MA: Jones & Bartlett.

Mayer, G. G., & Vallaire, M. (2007). *Health literacy in primary care: A clinician's guide.* New York: Springer.

McLaughlin, G. H. (1969). SMOG-grading: A new readability formula. *Journal of Reading, 12*, 639–646.

Melnyk, B. M., & Finehold-Iverholt, E. (2010). *Evidence-based practice in nursing and healthcare (2nd ed.).* Philadelphia: Lippincott.

Mihall, J., & Belletti, J. (1999). Adult learning styles and training methods. *FDIC ADR Presentation Handouts,* Retrieved September 6, 2011, from: http://justice.gov/adr/workplace/pdf/learstyl.pdf

Miller, E. (2010). Scientific basis for clinical decision making (29NURS84). *Online Course Manual. Cincinnati, OH:* University of Cincinnati, College of Nursing.

Miller, E. (2003). Readiness to change and brief educational interventions: Successful strategies to reduce stroke risk. *Journal of Neuroscience Nursing, 35*(4), 215–222.

Muijs, D., & Reynolds, D. (2005). *Effective teaching: Evidence and practice* (2nd ed.). Thousand Oaks: Sage Publications.

National League for Nursing. (2003). *Innovation in nursing education: A call to reform* (Position statement). Retrieved September 6, 2011 from http://www.nln.org/aboutnln/PositionStatements/innovation082203.pdf

Nielson-Bohlman, L., Panzer, A. M., & Kindig, D. A. (2004). *Health Literacy: A prescription to end confusion.* Institute of Medicine, Washington DC: National Academies Press.

Nightingale, F. (1992). *Notes on nursing: What it is and what it is not.* Philadelphia: Lippincott.

Nobel, J. (2006). Bridging the knowledge-action gap in diabetes: Information technologies, physician incentives and consumer incentives converge. *Chronic Illness, 2,* 59–69.

Osborne, R., Wilson, T., Lorig, K., & McColl, G. (2007). Does self-management lead to sustainable health benefits in people with arthritis? A 2-year transition study with 452 Australians. *The Journal of Rheumatology, 34*(5), 1112–1117.

Partnership to Fight Chronic Disease. (2010). *An unhealthy truth: Rising rates of chronic disease and the future of health care in America.* Retrieved August 24, 2011, from: http://www.caaccess.org/pdf/6_unhealthy_truths.pdf

Petty, G. (2006). *Evidence based teaching: A practical approach.* United Kingdom: Nelson Thornes.

Piaget, J. (1951). *The origin of intelligence in children.* New York: International Universities Press.

Piaget, J. (1976). *Behavior and evolution.* Richmond, CA: McCutchen Publishing.

Pierce, L. L. (2010). How to choose and develop written educational materials. *Rehabilitation Nursing, 35*(3), 99–105.

Prochaska, J. O., & DiClemente, C. C. (1983). Stages and processes of self-change of smoking: Toward an integrative model of change. *Journal of Consulting and Clinical Psychology, 51,* 390–395.

Prochaska, J. O., & DiClemente, C. C., & Norcross, J. C. (1992). In search of how people change: Applications to addictive behavior. *American Psychology, 47*(9), 1102–1114.

Prochaska, J. O., & Velicer, W. F. (1997). The Transtheoretical Model of health behavior change. *American Journal of Health Promotion, 12,* 38–48.

Quirk, P. A. (2000). Screening for literacy and readability: Implications for the advanced practice nurse. *Clinical Nurse Specialist, 14*(1), 26–32.

Rankin, S. H., Stallings, K. D., & London, F. (2005). *Patient education in health and illness* (5th ed.). Philadelphia: Lippincott.

Rahmqvist, M., & Bara, A. (2007). Patients retrieving additional information via the Internet: A trend analysis in a Swedish population, 2000–2005. *Scandinavian Journal of Public Health, 35*(2), 533–539.

Sax, L., Bryant, A., & Harper, C. (2005). The differential effects of student-faculty interaction on college outcomes for women and men. *Journal of College Student Development, 46*(6), 642–657.

Skinner, B. F. (1974). *About behaviorism.* New York: Merrill.

Spadero, D. C. (1983). Assessing readability of patient information materials. *Pediatric Nursing, 4,* 274–278.

Stahl, S. A. (2002). Different strokes for different folks? In L. Abbeduto (Ed.), *Taking sides: Clashing on controversial issues in educational psychology* (pp. 98–107). Guilford, CT: McGraw Hill.

Townsend, C., Bruce, B., Hooten, M., & Rome, J. (2006). The role of mental health professionals in multidisciplinary pain rehabilitation programs. *Journal of Clinical Psychology, 62*(11), 1433–1443.

Tung, W. C., & Lee, I. F. (2006). Effects of an osteoporosis educational programme for men. *Journal of Advances in Nursing, 56*(1), 26–34.

U.S. Department of Health and Human Services (DHHS). (2010). *Healthy People 2020.* Retrieved August 23, 2011, from: http://www.healthypeople.gov/2020/default.aspx

Viswanathan, H., Lambert, B. L. (2005). An inquiry into medication meanings, illness, medication use, and the transformative potential of chronic illness among African Americans with hypertension. *Research in Social and Administrative Pharmacy, 1*(1), 21–39.

Wantland, D. J., Portillo, C. J., Holzemer, W. L., & Slaughter, R. (2004). The effectiveness of Web-based vs. non-Web-based interventions: A meta-analysis of behavioral change outcomes. *Journal of Medical Internet Research, 6*(4), 40–71.

Witelson, S., Beresh, H., & Kigar, D. L. (2006). Intelligence and brain size in 100 postmortem brains: Sex lateralization and age factors. *Brain, 129*(2) 386–398.

Woodhouse, J., Peterson, M., Campbell, C., & Gathercoal, K. (2010). The efficacy of a brief behavioral intervention for managing high utilization of ED services by chronic pain patients. *Journal of Emergency Nurses, 36* (5), 399–403.

PART III

Impact of the Healthcare Professional

CHAPTER 16

Health Promotion

Alicia Huckstadt

INTRODUCTION

Health-promoting behaviors strongly influence whether one prematurely succumbs to disease or whether one postpones and possibly avoids many major diseases. Yet, health promotion is often viewed as insignificant as healthcare systems scramble to treat heart disease, cancer, and other diseases that are often in advanced stages. Only recently has national attention been directed toward understanding the underlying cause of disease and how health promotion may have changed the course of the disease. The once believed single causation theory of morbidity has now been largely replaced by multifactorial causation theories and chronicity of conditions. Improved recognition and management of disease processes, better sanitation, immunizations, and other health measures have increased the longevity of Americans. The life expectancy in the early 1900s was the late 40s; it has now increased to the upper 70s for both genders. Diseases that once brought sudden death have been surpassed by chronic disease. Americans are living longer but not necessarily healthier. Seven out of 10 deaths among Americans each year are from chronic diseases and one out of two Americans has at least one chronic illness (Centers for Disease Control and Prevention [CDC], 2010).

Societal influences and individual lifestyle choices have negatively influenced health. In two important research articles describing the actual causes of death (nongenetic), smoking has remained the leading cause of death in the United States since 1990 (McGinnis & Foege, 1993; Mokdad, Marks, Stroup, & Gerberding, 2004). Poor diet, physical inactivity, alcohol consumption, microbial agents, toxic agents, motor vehicle crashes, incidents involving firearms, sexual behaviors, and illicit use of drugs follow smoking as actual causes of death. Cigarette smoking remains the nation's leading cause of death with almost 450,000 deaths in the United States each year attributed to this cause (CDC, 2009). Smoking causes deaths from lung and other cancers, chronic lung disease, heart disease, and stroke. Exposure to secondhand smoke causes premature death and disease in others who do not smoke themselves. Other smokeless tobacco use also causes cancer and other conditions.

Following closely behind tobacco use as a major health risk is obesity. The prevalence of obesity among adults shows upward trends and there have been increases in overweight children (CDC, 2009). One of every three adults and almost one in five children are obese (CDC, 2010). As researchers study the condition, long-term obesity has been associated with avoidable hospitalizations and substantial risk for health complications (Schafer & Ferraro, 2007). Obesity is associated with increased risk of diabetes, stroke, heart disease, some cancers, hypertension, osteoarthritis, gallbladder disease, and disability (CDC, 2009).

The CDC (2010) has maintained that four modifiable health-risk behaviors—smoking, poor diet, physical inactivity, and excessive alcohol consumption—are the major underlying causes of much of the illness, suffering, and early death related to chronic illness. These factors and the other modifiable behavioral risk factors listed previously are believed to be the genesis of heart disease, malignant neoplasm, cerebrovascular disease, diabetes mellitus, and other chronic diseases. One half of all deaths in the United States could be attributed to a limited number of largely preventable health behaviors and exposures (Mokdad et al., 2004). The U.S. spends more on health care than any other nation, yet the average life expectancy is far below many other developed countries that spend less on health care each year (CDC, 2009). The escalating healthcare costs, disease, and deaths associated with these factors make health promotion essential for all.

Defining Health Promotion in Chronic Illness

Health promotion is a multidimensional concept and focuses on maintaining or improving the health of individuals, families, and communities. Minimizing preventable health risk factors such as tobacco use, inadequate diets, and physical inactivity would substantially decrease the development and severity of many chronic diseases and conditions (Cory et al., 2010).

Health promotion for individuals with chronic or disabling conditions is commonly defined as efforts to create healthy lifestyles and a healthy environment to prevent secondary conditions, such as teaching people how to address their healthcare needs and increasing opportunities to participate in usual life activities. These secondary conditions can be the medical, social, emotional, mental, family, or community problems that an individual with a chronic or disabling condition likely experiences. Environmental factors that encompass healthy living include the policies, systems, social contexts, and physical surroundings that facilitate a person's participation in activities, including work, school, leisure, and community events (*Healthy People 2020*).

Health-promoting activities can be implemented at the public level or the personal level, and involve passive or active strategies (Greiner & Edelman, 2010). Passive strategies, such as those used in food industry sanitation, decrease infectious agents in foods and improve public health. National, state, and local public and private agencies are given the responsibility to provide passive strategies to promote health for their constituents. Active strategies, such as engaging in better personal nutrition or activity regimens, are dependent on the individual and/or family becoming involved (Edelman & Mandle, 2006). Although both strategies are essential, this chapter focuses primarily on active strategies for individuals with chronic illness and their families.

Health promotion applies to all individuals regardless of age or disability. The goal of health promotion is to increase the involved person's control over their health and to improve it. Leddy (2006) adds that health promotion is mobilizing strengths to enhance health, wellness, and well-being.

Health promotion in chronic illness involves individual behavioral change for positive lifestyle activities, accepting one's condition and making the necessary adjustments, decreasing the risk of secondary disabilities and preventing further disease, and striving for optimal health. Behavioral change becomes possible when environmental and political policies support the resources (Aro & Absetz, 2009).

Health promotion in chronic illness is important in maintaining and enhancing the function of the individual. It is also critical to prevent recurrence of some conditions. Often families direct their energies toward the illness rather than health. The illness and its cascade of effects alter family dynamics, usual roles, and patterns of life (Heinzer, 1998). Managing medicines, conserving physical and mental energy, keeping appointments with healthcare professionals, adjusting finances, and learning new resources will likely require substantial effort. These new stressors often overtax the individual, and activities to maintain a healthy lifestyle are often ignored. Preventive health screening for other conditions may be forgotten by the client and healthcare professional. Yet, health-promoting behaviors are crucial in the management of chronic conditions and are often the essential aspect in successful management. Individuals with chronic illness may develop comorbidities that could be avoided or minimized with early detection. Disease-specific preventive care needs and related physical, social, emotional, and spiritual well-being encompass health promotion for those with and without chronic illness. McWilliam, Stewart, Brown, Desai, and Coderre (1996) found in their phenomenological study exploring health and health promotion of 13 sample participants with chronic illness, "a dynamically changing and evolving endeavor that encompassed four components: fighting and struggling, resigning oneself, creatively balancing resources, and accepting" (p. 5).

Undoubtedly, chronic illness presents numerous challenges to health promotion. The potential for these activities and overall health remains largely untapped in many individuals with chronic illness. Creating new ways of accomplishing health promotion often remains an unfilled goal for nurses and their clients with chronic illness. Efforts must go beyond the individual's chronic illness and limitations to include holistic health that focuses on personal goals, evidence-based care tailored to the person, and a willingness to adjust the plan as needed. Determining individuals' perceptions of their condition, their aspirations, and their available resources, and supporting their efforts to achieve health promotion is an ongoing process. Leddy (2006) emphasizes that health promotion develops the individual strengths and environmental resources to find solutions rather than focusing solely on illness repair. Chronicity presents challenges to all those involved and can take precedence over other health considerations.

Nurses are ideally suited to promote the health of all individuals and their families. The holistic, caring perspective held by nurses provides opportunities to promote strengths at a time when others may perceive only threats to health. The consequences of failure to promote health are devastating. Additional morbidity, deaths, and financial strain for individuals, families, and society weigh heavy on the healthcare system. The rising healthcare costs and an aging population compound the problem. Sustained increases in out-of-pocket healthcare spending for Medicare recipients could make health care less affordable for all but the highest income individuals (Neuman, Cubanski, Desmond, & Rice, 2007).

ISSUES AND IMPACT

National Documents

One of the issues surrounding health promotion and disease prevention is compliance with national documents. Initiated almost 30 years ago with the publication of *Healthy People: The Surgeon General's Report on Health Promotion and Disease Prevention (1979)*, and subsequent publications *Healthy People: Objectives for the Nation (1980)*, *Healthy People 2000: National Health Promotion and Disease Prevention Objectives*, *Healthy People 2010, and Healthy People 2020*, *Healthy People* national documents build on one another and address select areas of health promotion with a vision for achieving improved health for all Americans. Each document was developed through a broad consultative process, made use of the best scientific knowledge available, and was designed to measure progress over time.

Healthy People 2010 and 2020

The *Healthy People* documents identify a comprehensive set of 10-year health objectives focusing on disease prevention and health promotion to achieve as a nation. *Healthy People 2010* remains as *Healthy People 2020* emerges. Many of the 2010 objectives have been retained or modified for the 2020 publication. The vision for *Healthy People 2020* is a society in which all people live long, healthy lives. The mission is to: 1) identify nationwide health improvement priorities; 2) increase public awareness and understanding of the determinants of health, disease, and disability and the opportunities for progress; 3) provide measurable objectives and goals that are applicable at the national, state, and local levels; 4) engage multiple sectors to take actions to strengthen policies and improve practices that are driven by the best available evidence and knowledge; and 5) identify critical research, evaluation, and data collection needs.

The four overarching goals are to: attain high quality, longer lives free of preventable disease, disability, injury, and premature death; achieve health equity, eliminate disparities, and improve the health of all groups; create social and physical environments that promote good health for all; and promote quality of life, healthy development, and healthy behaviors across all stages (*Healthy People 2020*). Topic areas for *Healthy People 2020* objectives are identified in **Table 16-1**. Each area has specific goals and potential relevance for individuals with chronic illness and their families.

One example of relevance for these individuals and families is disability and health. The specific goal for this focus area from *Healthy People 2020* is to promote the health and well-being of people with disabilities. People with disabilities are more likely to experience delays and other difficulties in receiving health screening and other health care, more likely to experience chronic diseases, use tobacco, not engage in fitness and other healthy activities, experience symptoms of psychological distress, and receive less social-emotional support. The *Healthy People 2020* objectives reinforce that people can have a disabling impairment or chronic condition at any point in life but these conditions do not define individuals, their health, or their

Table 16-1 **Topic Areas for** *Healthy People 2020*	
1. Access to Health Services	22. HIV
2. Adolescent Health	23. Immunization and Infectious Diseases
3. Arthritis, Osteoporosis, and Chronic Back Conditions	24. Injury and Violence Prevention
4. Blood Disorders and Blood Safety	25. Lesbian, Gay, Bisexual, and Transgender Health
5. Cancer	26. Maternal, Infant, and Child Health
6. Chronic Kidney Disease	27. Medical Product Safety
7. Dementias, including Alzheimer's disease	28. Mental Health and Mental Disorders
8. Diabetes	29. Nutrition and Weight Status
9. Disability and Health	30. Occupational Safety and Health
10. Early and Middle Childhood	31. Older Adults
11. Educational and Community-based Programs	32. Oral Health
12. Environmental Health	33. Physical Activity
13. Family Planning	34. Preparedness
14. Food Safety	35. Public Health Infrastructure
15. Genomics	36. Respiratory Diseases
16. Global Health	37. Sexually Transmitted Infections
17. Healthcare-Associated Infections	38. Sleep Health
18. Health Communication and Health IT	39. Social Determinants of Health
19. Health-Related Quality of Life and Well-Being	40. Substance Abuse
20. Hearing and Other Sensory or Communication Disorders	41. Tobacco Use
21. Heart Disease and Stroke	42. Vision

talents and abilities. The objectives highlight that people with chronic conditions: 1) be included in public health activities; 2) receive well timed interventions and services; 3) interact with their environment without barriers; and 4) participate in everyday life activities. Without these opportunities, people with disabilities and chronic conditions will continue to experience health disparities compared to the general population. Health promotion activities are relevant for all individuals and may decrease or eliminate further decline in health.

Another relevant *Healthy People 2020* topic is nutrition and weight status. The goal of this topic is to promote health and reduce chronic disease risk through the consumption of healthful diets and achievement and maintenance of healthy body weights. Individual behaviors, policies, and environments such as schools, worksites, healthcare organizations, and communities must work together to accomplish this goal.

Health promotion activities are relevant to all individuals, groups, communities, and to our nation as a whole. *Healthy People* documents emphasize the many similarities among individuals with disabilities as opposed to the differences among clinical diagnoses.

Developers of the documents have also considered caregiver issues as well as environmental barriers. Environmental factors affect the health and well-being of individuals with disabilities in many ways. For example, weather can hamper wheelchair mobility, medical offices and equipment may not be accessible, and shelters or fitness centers may not be staffed or equipped for people with disabilities. Compliance with the Americans with Disabilities Act (ADA) helps overcome some of these barriers.

Throughout the *Healthy People* documents, the U.S. Department of Health and Human Services (USDHHS) identifies objectives, such as the previous example of areas to address improvements in health status, risk reduction, public and professional awareness of prevention, delivery of health services, protective measures, surveillance, and evaluation, expressed in terms of measurable targets to be achieved by the targeted year. Full achievement of the goals and objectives of the *Healthy People* documents depends on a healthcare system reaching all Americans and integrating personal health care and population-based public health. The vision of *Healthy People* in healthy communities involves broad-based prevention efforts and moves beyond what happens in physicians' offices, clinics, and hospitals to environments in which a large portion of prevention occurs: to the neighborhoods, schools, workplaces, and families in which people live their daily lives.

Four foundational health measures will be used to monitor progress toward promoting health, preventing disease and disability, eliminating disparities, and improving quality of life. These measures include: 1) general health status such as life expectancy, healthy life expectancy, years of potential life lost, physically and mentally unhealthy days, self-assessed health status, limitation of activity, and chronic disease prevalence; 2) health-related quality of life and well-being, including physical, mental, and social health-related quality of life, well-being/satisfaction, and participation in common activities; 3) determinants of health including personal,

economic, social, and environmental factors that influence health status; and 4) disparities including measures of disparities and inequity based on race/ethnicity, gender, physical and mental ability, and geography. These determinants include biology, genetics, individual behavior, access to health services, and the environment. The *Healthy People* documents can be accessed at http://healthypeople.gov/.

Where Does the United States Stand?

The CDC (2010) reinforces that chronic diseases are among the most common, costly, and preventable of all health problems in the nation. Diseases such as heart disease, cancer, stroke, diabetes, and arthritis are the leading causes of death and disability. Seven out of 10 deaths among Americans each year are from chronic diseases. Almost one out of every two American adults has at least one chronic illness. Health disparities in chronic disease incidence and mortality are widespread among members of racial and ethnic minority populations.

Four modifiable health-risk behaviors—lack of physical activity, poor nutrition, tobacco use, and excessive alcohol consumption—are responsible for much of the morbidity and mortality. More than one-third of all adults do not meet recommendations for aerobic physical activity based on the 2008 Physical Activity Guidelines for Americans, and 23% report no leisure-time physical activity at all in the preceding month (USDHHS, 2009). In 2007, less than 22% of high school students and only 24% of adults reported eating five or more servings of fruits and vegetables per day. More than 43 million American adults smoke and 20% of high school students were current smokers in 2007 (CDC, 2011a). The 2005–2010 National Health Inter-view Surveys estimated that 45.3 million of U.S. adults were current cigarette smokers and 78.2% of these adults smoked every day. Non-Hispanic American Indians/Alaska Natives continued to have higher prevalence of smoking compared with other racial/ethnic groups. Smoking also continues to be higher in those with lower educational and income levels (CDC, 2011). The U.S. Surgeon General has issued a report on how tobacco smoke causes disease and the specific pathways by which tobacco smoke damages the human body (USDHHS, Office of the Surgeon General, 2010). The CDC National Center for Chronic Diseases and Health Promotion (2011a) emphasizes that lung cancer is the leading cause of cancer death, and cigarette smoking is related in almost all cases. Smoking causes about 90% of lung cancer deaths in men and almost 80% in women. Smoking also causes cancer of the larynx, mouth and throat, esophagus, bladder, kidney, pancreas, and others. Nearly 45% of high school students report consuming alcohol in the past 30 days, and more than 60% of those who drink report binge drinking within the past 30 days.

The CDC National Centers for Chronic Disease Prevention and Health Promotion (NCCDPHP) vision is that all people live healthy lives free from the devastation of chronic diseases (2011). The center's mission is to lead efforts that promote health and well-being through prevention and control of chronic diseases. The NCCDPHP strategic priorities are to:

- *Focus on well-being*: Increase emphasis on promoting health and preventing risk factors, thereby reducing the onset of chronic health conditions.
- *Health equity*: Leverage program and policy activities, build partner capacities, and establish tailored interventions to help eliminate health disparities.
- *Research translation*: Accelerate the translation of scientific findings into community practice to protect the health of people where they live, work, learn, and play.
- *Policy promotion*: Promote social, environmental, policy, and systems approaches that support healthy living for individuals, families, and communities.
- *Workforce development*: Develop a skilled, diverse, and dynamic public health workforce and network of partners to promote health and prevent chronic disease at the national, state, and local levels.

The NCCDPHP (2009) provides important health promotion and chronic disease information including statistics, state profiles, tools and resources. Its publication, *The Power of Prevention: Chronic Disease . . . the Public Health Challenge of the 21st Century,* is helpful in recognizing that chronic disease prevention must occur in multiple sectors and across individuals' entire lifespan.

In 2009, no state in the nation met the *Healthy People 2010* obesity target of 15%, and the self-reported overall prevalence of obesity had increased 1.1% points from 2007 (Sherry, Blanck, Galuska, Pan, & Dietz, 2010). These data undoubtedly give support to the alarm echoed by health professionals. The health status of the nation is summarized by Surgeon General Regina Benjamin as she calls on all Americans to help reverse the trend of obese and overweight adults and children in our nation. The priority should be health and wellness of our families and communities through focusing on healthy nutrition and regular physical activity and making the healthiest choices accessible to all citizens. (Further remarks may be found at http://www.surgeongeneral.gov/library/obesityvision/obesityvision2010.pdf.)

Online Resources

The CDC's website (http://www.cdc.gov) shares the goal of helping people live longer and healthier lives; it features health and safety topics on its home page. The website provides information on numerous diseases and conditions, emergency preparedness, environmental health, traveler's health, workplace safety, and other topics. One area, healthy living, is especially beneficial to consumers and healthcare providers for health in all life stages (further information is available at http://www.cdc.gov/HealthyLiving/).

The CDC has additional focus areas such as emphasizing the importance of a healthy diet and eating in moderation for the general population (http://www.cdc.gov/nutrition/everyone/basics/foodgroups.html); it includes further information on nutrition, which is available for healthcare providers (http://www.cdc.gov/nutrition/professionals/index.html). The National Physical Activity Plan (http://www.cdc.gov/physicalactivity/index.html) is a comprehensive set of policies, programs, and initiatives that aim to increase physical activity in all segments of the American population. The CDC encourages all people to learn how to prevent disease and improve their quality of life, helping to do so through providing this information. It recommends that people know their family history and how genes and personal history could put their health at risk.

Another website (http://healthfinder.gov/) provides a quick guide to healthy living, personal health tools, health news, locating health providers, and other information promoting health.

A variety of screening recommendations are provided from reputable sources such as the American Heart Association, the CDC, National Cancer Institute, National Heart Lung and Blood Institute, and the Agency for Healthcare Research and Quality (AHRQ). People can review the recommendations and share their history information with their healthcare professionals to determine what tests and screenings are appropriate for them. Healthy Men (http://www.ahrq.gov/healthymen/) is an AHRQ resource that helps men learn what preventive medical tests they need and when to get them. The website also provides the latest recommendations on screening for colorectal cancer, abdominal aortic aneurysms, and other conditions. It also includes information on immunizations, daily healthy choices, tips on communication with health providers, understanding prescriptions, and other sources of information for men's health.

These websites remind people, when faced with choices that may impact their health and the lives of those they love, that it is important to remember that there are options and resources to help them make healthy decisions. Related websites such as that for the U.S. Food and Drug Administration (FDA) provide information for people to make better informed decisions, for example, in taking medications (www.fda.gov/usemedicinesafely), and the Surgeon General offers information for protecting yourself from secondhand tobacco smoke (www.surgeongeneral.gov/library/second-handsmoke/factsheets/factsheet3.html).

The CDC's Healthy Communities Program called "Steps Communities" has been taking local action to reverse trends in health risk factors for obesity and chronic disease since 2003 (CDC, 2011b). Each of the Steps Communities implements chronic disease prevention and health promotion activities appropriate for the needs and context of its own community. They are showing, through effective interventions, what communities can do to reduce the burden of obesity, diabetes, and asthma, and producing local success in reducing the prevalence of three related health risk factors: physical inactivity, poor nutrition, and tobacco use and exposure. (More information about how to include communities is available at http://healthfinder.gov/.)

Steps Communities have formed partnerships with traditional and nontraditional partners to extend the reach of their activities and to accelerate progress toward achieving better health outcomes. In addition, interventions are integrated across the public and private sectors—including community settings, schools, work sites, and healthcare settings. The communities funded through Steps are grouped into three categories: state-coordinated small cities or rural communities, large cities or urban communities, and tribes or tribal entities (more information is available at: http://cdc.gov/healthycommunitiesprogram/communities/steps.htm). In a recent report of Steps Communities that were funded nationwide to address six focus areas—obesity, diabetes, asthma, physical inactivity, poor nutrition, and tobacco use and exposure—a survey of outcomes from noninstitutionalized community members aged 18 years and older revealed that none of the communities achieved the *Healthy People 2010* objective of increasing to 91% the proportion of adults with diabetes who have at least an annual clinical foot examination. The majority of the communities did not meet the *Healthy People* objectives for annual dilated eye examinations or hemoglobin A1c. The majority of communities also did not meet the goal for asthma patients not to have had any symptoms during the preceding 30 days. However, the number of community residents who engaged in moderate or vigorous physical activity for 30 or more minutes at least five times a week or who reported vigorous physical activity for 20 or more minutes three times a week ranged from 40.6% to 69.8%, exceeding the *Healthy People 2010* objective of 50%. The prevalence of consumption of fruits and vegetables at least five times per day ranged from 14.6% to 37.6%. Only two of the communities reached the *Healthy People 2010* objective to reduce the proportion of adults who smoke and no communities reached the objective of increasing to 75% smoking cessation attempts by adult smokers. The findings of the report reflect considerable variation in health risk behaviors, chronic diseases, and use of preventive health screenings and other health promotion activities. The authors strongly encourage the need for preventive interventions at the community level and to design and implement policies that promote and encourage healthy behaviors (Cory et al., 2010). Decreasing smoking among adolescents and adults is a major health objective for our nation. The Institute of Medicine has issued a blueprint for further reducing tobacco use (several measures are available at http://www.nap.edu/catalog/11795.html). Recently, a large meta-analysis identified smoking as a risk factor for prostate cancer, with the heaviest smokers having a 24% to 30% greater risk of death than did non-smokers (Huncharek, Haddock, Reid, & Kupelnick, 2010).

The following guides are other national documents that serve as recommendations for screening and other preventive health care.

Guide to Clinical Preventive Services

The Guide to Clinical Preventive Services includes the U.S. Preventive Services Task Force (USPSTF) recommendations on screening, counseling, and preventive medication topics, as well as clinical considerations for each topic. Sponsored since 1998 by the AHRQ, the USPSTF is an independent panel of experts in primary care and prevention that systematically reviews the evidence of effectiveness and develops recommendations for clinical preventive services. The task force rigorously evaluates clinical research to assess the merits of preventive measures. The clinical categories are cancer; heart and vascular disease; injury and violence; infectious diseases; mental health conditions and substance abuse; metabolic, nutrition, and endocrine conditions; musculoskeletal conditions; obstetrics and gynecologic conditions; pediatric disorders; and vision and hearing disorders. (More information is available at http://www.ahrq.gov/clinic/uspstfix.htm.)

Guide to Community Preventive Services

The Guide to Community Preventive Services serves as a filter for scientific literature on specific health problems that have a large-scale impact on groups of people who share a common community setting. This guide summarizes what is known about the effectiveness, economic efficiency, and feasibility of interventions to promote community health and prevent disease. The Task Force on Community Preventive Services, an independent decision-making body convened by the USDHHS, makes recommendations for the use of various interventions based on the evidence gathered in rigorous and systematic scientific reviews of published studies conducted by review teams for the guide. The findings from the reviews are published in peer-reviewed journals and also are made available online. The task force has published more than 100 findings across 16 topic areas, including tobacco use, physical activity, cancer, oral health, diabetes, motor vehicle occupant injury, vaccine-preventable diseases, prevention of injuries due to violence, and social environment. (More information is available at www.thecommunityguide.org.)

Challenges

These documents and other resources illustrate that health promotion and disease prevention are essential for all Americans. The nation needs to continually work toward the goals; however, to do so will require changes in the healthcare system. Providing chronic health care once the disease has occurred is only a segment of the needed care. Many of the risks to health—obesity, diabetes, hypertension, heart disease, cancer, and other chronic conditions—often result from failure to engage in preventive care. More closely articulated preventive, public health, and policy programs are needed to promote a healthy life. Other factors, including genetics and environmental risks, contribute to chronic illness.

Health promotion can and should occur before the onset of chronic illness, and as early as possible. Health promotion ideally occurs throughout one's life and in concert with chronic conditions through the end of life. Health promotion is a lifetime activity and can include end-of-life planning for individuals and their significant others. Preparing for the physical and psychosocial changes that accompany death requires attention before crisis events. Preparation, dissemination, and discussion of advance directives with significant others can help set clear boundaries for honoring the wishes of clients (Rainer & McMurry, 2002).

Barriers

Reported barriers to health screening and other preventive care must be addressed. Unhealthy behaviors continue to increase in the United States, putting people more at risk for initial chronic illness and deterring health promotion practices among those with chronic illnesses.

The CDC (2010) reports that more than one-third of all U.S. adults do not meet recommendations for aerobic physical activity and 23% report no leisure-time physical activity at all during the preceding year. In 2007, only 24% of U.S. adults and 22% of high school students ate five or more fruits and vegetables each day. Cigarette smoking is responsible for about 440,000 deaths in the United States each year. More deaths are caused each year by tobacco use than by all deaths from HIV/AIDS, alcohol use, motor vehicle injuries, suicide, and murder combined. Exercising regularly, eating a healthy diet, and not using tobacco can help people prevent and manage chronic diseases. However, many people in the United States do not have easy access to healthy foods and safe, convenient places to exercise. These barriers have led to increasingly sedentary lifestyles for the majority of Americans.

CASE STUDY

S.B. is a 55-year-old man with hypertension, type 2 diabetes, and hyperlipidemia. Mr. B. completed the 11th grade and worked as a mechanic until he could join the military. He served his country for 2 years and returned home. He lives at home with his wife of 35 years. Both he and his wife smoke, are overweight, and have sedentary jobs outside the home. Having raised three children, they now enjoy staying home and watching television together in the evenings. Neither has a physical exercise regimen even though both were told to increase exercise at their last medical appointment. S.B.'s last hemoglobin A1c was 8.1. He was scheduled for a colonoscopy but did not go for the appointment, stating he could not understand the informational brochure he was given. He reports he did receive a flu immunization this fall.

Discussion Questions

1. What are two health literacy implications of the preceding case?
2. How would you tailor a health-promotion program for S.B.?
3. What theoretical framework would be useful for the health-promotion program?

Other barriers exist for health screening. Kelly and colleagues (2007) identified fear and embarrassment as commonly cited client barriers to screening for colorectal cancer. Less than 44% of their study population of Appalachians in the state of Kentucky underwent colorectal cancer screening consistent with guidelines. These researchers identified establishing trust and educating clients, use of resources like educational materials, and finding inexpensive and easy ways to screen as the most productive way to overcome the barriers.

Little is known about how health screening and other preventive care affect outcomes. Norman and colleagues (2007) emphasized that we do not know what survivors of diseases like breast cancer must do to prevent recurrence. Data are needed on lifestyle change from prediagnosis to postdiagnosis, changes over time after diagnosis, and identification of potential lifestyle risk factors.

Health promotion has not been addressed well in the care of clients with numerous chronic health conditions. Capella-McDonnall (2007) reported that despite the recent focus on health promotion for persons with disabilities, adults who are visually impaired have not received adequate attention. Two conditions, being overweight or obese and not being physically active, are problems for many persons with disabilities, including those who are visually impaired.

Problems with health literacy are commonplace in our society. Health literacy is the capacity to obtain, process, and understand basic health information and services needed to make appropriate health decisions (U.S. Department of Health and Human Services, Office of Disease Prevention and Health Promotion, 2007). Nine out of 10 adults may lack the skills needed to manage their health and disease prevention. Poor health outcomes and less frequent use of preventive services are linked with low literacy. Individuals with low literacy are more likely to skip important preventive screening such as colonoscopy, Pap smears, and mammograms, and are less likely to receive protective measures such as flu immunizations. Persons with low literacy are more likely to have chronic illness and are less able to manage it effectively. More preventable hospitalizations and use of emergency services are found among clients with chronic illness with limited literacy skills. People with limited literacy skills often lack knowledge about the nature and causes of disease and may not understand the relationship between lifestyle factors such as smoking, lack of exercise and inadequate nutrition, and poor health outcomes.

Other barriers to health screening and preventive care include associated costs; lack of knowledge/understanding; negative beliefs/attitudes; lack of access, especially for those with limited geographical and/or functional ability; and other factors addressed in the models/theories/frameworks discussed in the following section.

Models/Theories/Frameworks

An entire body of literature has evolved around the models/theories relating to health behavior change. Considerable research has demonstrated success in changing behavior with smoking cessation, alcohol abuse, and others using these theories. The most often used theories in 193 articles on health behavior literature published in 10 leading public health, medicine, and psychology journals from 2000 to 2005 were the Transtheoretical Model, Social Cognitive Theory, and Health Belief Model (Painter, Borba, Hynes, Mays, & Glanz, 2008). In these articles, most (68.1%) involved research that was informed by theory; others applied theory, tested theory, and sought to develop theory. The examples that follow are theories/models that may be useful in assessing change within chronic illness.

The Transtheoretical Model (TTM) by Prochaska, Redding, and Evers (2002) incorporates the processes and principles of change from several major theories in psychotherapy and human behavior. The stages of change within the model include: 1) precontemplation (no intention to change in the foreseeable future); 2) contemplation (intention to change in the next 6 months); 3) preparation (intention to take action within the next 30 days and some behavioral steps to change); 4) action (has changed behavior for less than 6 months); and 5) maintenance (has changed behavior for more than 6 months). These stages represent a temporal dimension to change and are helpful in identifying timing of change interventions. A last stage—6) termination (individual who possesses total self-efficacy is no longer susceptible to temptation of unhealthy behavior)—is rarely used, as few individuals reach this level. In the TTM Model, individuals weigh the pros and cons of changing (decisional balance) and determine their confidence (self-efficacy) that they can cope with high-risk situations without relapsing to unhealthy or high-risk behavior specific to the situation.

The 10 processes of change of the TTM Model are activities that people use to progress through the stages of change. They include 1) consciousness raising (increasing awareness of the behavior); 2) dramatic relief (experiencing increased emotions followed by reduced effect if appropriate action is taken); 3) self-reevaluation (assessing one's image with and without the unhealthy behavior); 4) environmental reevaluation (assessing how one's social environment is affected by the unhealthy behavior); 5) self-liberation (believing and committing to change); 6) helping relationships (building support for healthy behavior change); 7) counterconditioning (learning that healthy behaviors can replace unhealthy behaviors); 8) contingency management (increasing reinforcement and probability that healthy behaviors will be repeated); 9) stimulus control (removing unhealthy behavior cues and adding healthy behavior cues); and 10) social liberation (increasing social opportunities to foster behavior change) (Prochaska et al., 2002, pp. 103–104). The TTM Model has been used in numerous studies including those involving smoking cessation, mammography screening, alcohol avoidance, and exercise and stress management. The TTM Model has been beneficial in tailoring interventions for the most appropriate stage of change.

The Theory of Reasoned Action (TRA) and the Theory of Planned Behavior (TPB) offer another framework for examining factors that determine behavioral change. The framework focuses on motivational factors as determinants of the person's likelihood of performing a specific behavior. The TRA provides the rationale that the person's beliefs and values determine whether the person intends to change behavior. The TPB adds that perceived behavioral control of facilitating or constraining conditions will affect intention and behavior. Beliefs affecting behavior differ widely among persons, groups, and even specific behaviors of the same individual. Use of the models is helpful in understanding the likelihood of people performing a specific healthier behavior and can provide a framework for interventions. These theories can be applied along with others to design and deliver behavioral change to improve research and practice (Montano & Kasprzyk, 2002).

The Health Belief Model (HBM) has been one of the most widely used conceptual frameworks to explain change in health behavior and to provide a framework for interventions (Janz, Champion, & Strecher, 2002). The components of the HBM have been revised many times since its inception in the 1950s. Once a model to explain readiness to obtain chest x-ray screening for tuberculosis, the model has evolved beyond screening behaviors to include preventive actions, illness behaviors, and sick-role behavior. The HBM Model now purports that individuals will take action to prevent, to screen for, or control ill-health conditions if there is perceived susceptibility (persons regard themselves as susceptible to the condition), if there is perceived severity (persons believe it would have potentially serious consequences), if there are perceived benefits (persons believe that a course of action available to them would be beneficial in reducing either their susceptibility to or the severity of the condition), and if the perceived barriers can be overcome (persons believe that the anticipated barriers to [or costs of] taking the action are outweighed by its benefits (Janz et al., 2002). Determining strategies to activate persons' readiness to change (cues to action) can include providing information and awareness campaigns. Like TTM, self-efficacy is an integral concept of the HBM. Researchers have tested interventions to increase positive change for each concept.

The Health Promotion Model (HPM) integrates constructs from the Expectancy-Value Theory and Social Cognitive Theory and provides a nursing perspective to depict the multidimensional nature of persons pursuing health (Pender, Murdaugh, & Parsons, 2002). The HPM purports that behavior change will occur if there is positive personal value and a desired outcome. The HPM has been revised since its initial development in the early 1980s and is considered an approach-oriented or competence model. The authors report that the HPM is different from the HBM discussed earlier, as it eliminates the negative source of motivation, fear or threat, from major motivating sources for health behavior change. The authors emphasize that elimination of the personal threat motivational factor provides applicability of the model across the lifespan. Self-efficacy is a major construct of HPM, and assumptions of the model require an active role of the person "in shaping and maintaining health behaviors and in modifying the environmental context for health behaviors" (Pender et al., 2002, p. 63). The HPM has been a framework for studies predicting its general health-promoting abilities and for specific health behaviors including hearing protection, exercise, and nutrition (Pender et al., 2002).

Theory and models are important in the understanding of health promotion and why people behave the way they do. Theory is also important in identifying variables that change these behaviors and help retain the new behaviors. The importance of identifying mediating variables is often overlooked. Understanding relationships among variables could help refine health behavior theories and design intervention studies.

In a recent study, researchers examined the role of perceived susceptibility on colorectal cancer screening intention and behavior (McQueen et al., 2010). Perceived susceptibility is a psychosocial variable in several health promotion theories and is viewed as a motivating factor in behavioral change, but there is disagreement on how its mechanism affects behavior. Results of this study showed perceived susceptibility was not limited to direct effects, but was independent of perceived benefits, was mediated by the change in family influence, and moderated the change in perceived barriers and self-efficacy.

Ongoing work on theory and relationships between variables helps advance the understanding of health promotion and behavioral change. Some authors believe theory development has not kept pace with the evolution of health promotion practice (Crosby & Noar, 2010). Some of this disparity relates to problems such as 1) theory is not grounded in practice; 2) theory is at the individual level and simplistic without attention to the contextual nature of human behavior and environment; and 3) theory is inaccessible to practitioners who are facing increased demands to prevent disease and promote health (Crosby & Noar, 2010). Remedies that allow for the complexity of theory development for the future are daunting but something to aspire to. Health care frequently uses broad-stroke approaches to health promotion interventions in hopes that some health behaviors will change. Further development of theory will better frame questions surrounding health promotion. Caution should accompany new theory development as misleading data can exaggerate the theories' predictive accuracy (Weinstein, 2007). Often studies in health promotion are based on correlational data with variables such as beliefs, attitudes, self-efficacy, intentions, diet, nutrition, preventive measures, and other human behaviors. While these studies may provide descriptive information, correlations do not infer causation. Theory development needs to be carefully designed. Theory must be tested in practice-based contexts, allow cross-cultural transfer, be more inclusive of environmental changes, and effectively serve

health promotion practice (DiClementi, Crosby, & Kegler, 2009).

INTERVENTIONS

Chronic diseases account for 70% of the 1.7 million deaths that occur in the United States each year. These diseases also cause major limitations in daily living for almost 1 in 10 Americans, or about 25 million people (CDC, 2011a). Although chronic diseases are among the most common and costly health problems, they are also among the most preventable. Adopting healthy behaviors such as eating nutritious foods, being physically active, and avoiding tobacco use can prevent or control the devastating effects of these diseases (NCCDHP, 2011).

Nurses have been leaders in health promotion since the time of Florence Nightingale, whose pioneering work with the use of statistics demonstrated the positive effect of improved sanitation on the health of injured soldiers. Nurses have also led the healthcare profession in recognizing that health is a state of physical and mental wellness and that it is impossible to separate the former from the latter. (Calloway, 2007, p. 105).

Olshansky (2007), editor of the *Journal of Professional Nursing*, emphasizes that nurses are the most appropriate health professionals to address health promotion. Nursing has role models within our profession such as Nola Pender who developed the HPM described previously. Nursing literature abounds with textbooks, articles, and other publications that include nursing's role in health promotion to individuals, families, communities, and populations. Yet, nurses cannot assume sameness for chronically ill persons, and nurses cannot assume resources are equally available to all. People with chronic illness may view health differently and have different goals defined within their limits of their illness.

Selected Examples of Health Promotion Interventions

A review of the literature provides examples of health promotion interventions for clients with chronic illness. The following discussion illustrates that much is yet to be examined. In an international study, Huang, Chou, Lin, and Chao (2007) analyzed survey data including the Health-Promoting Lifestyle Profile and quality of life data of 129 outpatients from a medical center who had systemic lupus erythematosus. These researchers found that a health-promoting lifestyle could not enhance the physical component summary of quality of life directly without an improvement in the fatigue disability, but a health-promoting lifestyle had a significant effect on the mental component summary of quality of life. This illustrates that although the physical aspects of the chronic condition may not improve without other physical changes, there can be improvements in psychological health.

Siarkowski (1999) emphasized the importance of including health promotion and illness management when working with insulin-dependent diabetes mellitus in children and their families. Siarkowski reviewed existing research and revealed factors that put children and their families at risk for poor adaptation. Health promotion is critical to minimize these risks.

Hope has been recommended as a health-promoting force. Hollis, Massey, and Jevne (2007) identified hope-enhancing strategies and sources to improve one's health. Blue (2007) studied 106 adults at risk for diabetes and found the theory of planned behavior to be useful in explaining their healthy eating intentions and physical activity.

Health-promoting activities such as prevention of injuries may make the difference in whether one is able to live with chronic conditions. One example is preventing falls. Falls are one of the most common causes of injuries in older adults. These preventable accidents cause loss of independence, enormous financial costs, and possibly death. One evidence-based program to prevent falls is exemplified in Ory and colleagues' (2010) analysis of community-dwelling older adults who participated in a Matter of Balance/Volunteer Lay Leader model intended to reduce fear of falling and increase physical activity of participants.

Motivational Interviewing

Motivational interviewing incorporates behavior change principles to promote healthy activities. Four guiding principles underscore motivational interviewing: 1) resist the righting reflex that helping professionals often have to set things right and assume patients are wrong; 2) understand and explore the patient's own motivation; 3) listen with empathy; and 4) empower the patient, encouraging hope and optimism (Rollnick, Miller, & Butler, 2008, p. 7). Brodie and Inoue (2005) demonstrated the effectiveness of motivational interviewing over a traditional exercise program in increasing reported physical activity in older adults with chronic heart failure. Jackson, Asimakopoulou, and Scammell (2007) demonstrated in an experimental study of 34 clients with type II diabetes that motivational interviewing and behavior change training significantly increased the participants' physical activity and stage of change.

Motivating Factors

Providing performance incentives, both financial and nonfinancial, have been explored in an effort to change behaviors in individuals and in communities. The following principles are helpful in guiding the development of any incentive design: 1) identify the desired outcome, 2) identify the behavior change that leads to the desired outcome, 3) determine the potential effectiveness of the incentive in achieving the behavior change, 4) link an incentive directly to the behavior or outcome, 5) identify possible adverse effects of the incentive, and 6) evaluate changes in the behavior or outcome in response to the incentive (Haverman, 2010). Researchers using a randomized study of 51 adults, all age 50, demonstrated that modest financial incentives were an effective approach for increasing physical activity among sedentary older adults (Finkelstein, Brown, Brown, & Buchner, 2008).

In a review of 26 studies (8 randomized controlled trials and 18 observational), use of pedometers have significantly increased physical activity and significantly decreased body mass index and blood pressure (Bravata et al., 2007). The use of pedometers as a motivating factor with chronically ill persons capable of using a pedometer and the long-term effect of pedometers are yet to be investigated. Motivating factors have been identified in theories/models/frameworks, and positive motivators such as those in the HPM are congruent with nursing philosophical bases. Challenges for the future are to continue the testing and use of such frameworks in the health-promoting activities of persons and families with chronic illness.

Health Coaching

Health coaching is emerging as a new approach for preventing exacerbations of chronic illness and supporting lifestyle changes. This method partners health coaches with clients to enhance self-management strategies. It is being piloted by Medicare for clients with congestive heart failure and diabetes (Huffman, 2007). Holland, Greenberg, Tidwell, and Newcomer (2003) described the success of the California Public Employees Retirement System (CalPERS) Health Matters program using a community-based health coaching program operating in Sacramento. Criteria for eligibility included one or more qualifying chronic health condition, being 65 or older, and other program criteria. The program uses a menu of disability-prevention strategies, with health coaching, patient education on the self-management of chronic illness, and fitness. The program helps link participants to existing community, health plan, and self-directed programs. It encourages their participation in the programs developed for the project.

The Self-Management of Care model is used for lifestyle coaching programs based on collaborative goal setting and self-management health education (Rohrer, Naessens, Liesinger, & Litchy, 2010). A study examined the usefulness of self-rated health metrics in assessing telephonic coaching programs targeting weight, exercise, stress, and nutrition. While these coaching programs showed positive improvements in all of the lifestyle interventions, the self-rated health metrics were correlated with improvements only in weight loss and exercise programs. Therefore, the coaching programs were successful, but self-ratings may not demonstrate the improvements in all areas (Rohrer et al., 2010).

Mass Media Campaigns

Beaudoin, Fernandez, Wall, and Farley (2007) used a mass media campaign of high-frequency paid television and radio advertising, as well as bus and streetcar signage to promote walking and fruit/vegetable consumption in a low-income, predominantly African American urban population in New Orleans. These researchers found over 5 months of the campaign, a significant increase in message recall measures and positive attitudes toward walking and toward fruit/vegetable consumption. It is unknown how many persons with chronic illness were included. It is likely many persons were at risk for future chronic illness. These efforts demonstrate population efforts to improve health that may be researched with chronic illness populations.

Snyder (2007) reviewed existing meta-analyses for effectiveness of health communication campaigns, and found that the average health campaign affects the intervention community by about five percentage points. Snyder concluded that successful campaigns that are likely to change nutrition behaviors need to include specific behavioral goals for the intervention, identification of the target population, communication activities and channels that will be used, provision of message content and presentation, and provision of techniques for feedback and evaluation.

Web-Based Programs

Verheijden, Jans, Hildebrandt, and Hopman-Rock (2007) found that Web-based behavioral programs often reach those who need them the least. However, obese people were more likely to participate in follow-up than people of normal body weight. The researchers proposed that the Web-based programs are a nonstigmatizing way of addressing the problem and suggested that weight management is better suited for this delivery method than many other health-related areas. Although this study was based in the

Netherlands, it provides a source of potential research for other countries with similar health-promotion problems. Successful Web-based interventions improve health knowledge and are effective in changing behaviors. These Web-based interventions have been implemented primarily through interactive messaging and information dissemination but are wide open for expansion (Annang, Muilenburg, & Strasser, 2010).

Contracts

Burkhart, Rayens, Oakley, Abshire, and Zhang (2007) found in their randomized, controlled trial of 77 children with persistent asthma that the intervention group who received asthma education plus contingency management, including a contingency contract, tailoring, cueing, and reinforcement, significantly increased adherence to asthma self-management over the control group who received asthma education without the contingency management. However, in 30 trials involving 4691 participants, Cochrane authors concluded that there is limited evidence that contracts can improve patients' adherence to health-promotion programs. Large, well controlled studies are needed to recommend contracts in preventive health programs (Bosch-Capblanch, Abba, Prictor, & Garner, 2007).

Health Literacy

Improving the use of health information is paramount in health-promotion programs. The USDHHS, Office of Disease Prevention and Health Promotion (2007) provides a summary of the best practices for healthcare professionals to improve health literacy through providing effective communications and health services that are usable. **Table 16-2** outlines these practices.

Table 16-2 Improving Health Literacy Interventions	
When providing health information, is the information appropriate for the user?	Identify intended users of the information and services.
	Evaluate the users' knowledge prior to, during, and after the introduction of information and services.
	Acknowledge cultural differences and practice respect.
When providing health information, is the information easy to use?	Limit the number of messages. Keep it simple, and, in general, limit the information to no more than four main messages.
	Use plain language. Use familiar language and an active voice. Avoid jargon. See www.plainlanguage.gov for more information.
	Focus on the behavior that you want the person to change.
	Supplement instructions with visuals to help convey your message.
	Make written communication easy to read by using large font and use of headings and bullets to break up text; limit line length to between 40 and 50 characters.
	Improve Internet information by using uniform navigation, organizing information to minimize searching and scrolling, including interactive features. Apply user-centered design principles and conduct usability testing.
When providing health information, are you speaking clearly and listening carefully?	Ask open-ended questions.
	Use a medically trained interpreter for those who do not speak English or have limited ability to speak or understand English.
	Use words and examples that make the information relevant to the person's cultural norms and values.
	Check for understanding using a "teach-back" method to enhance communication.
Improve the use of health services.	Improve usability of health forms and instructions including plain language forms in multiple languages.
	Improve the accessibility of the physical environment including universal symbols, clear signage, and easy flow-through healthcare facilities.
	Establish a patient navigator program of individuals who can help patients access services and appropriate healthcare information.
Build knowledge to improve health decision making.	Improve access to accurate and appropriate health information.
	Increase self-efficacy and facilitate health decision making.
	Partner with educators to improve health curricula.
Advocate for health literacy in your organization.	Make the case for health literacy improvement.
	Identify how low health literacy affects programs.
	Incorporate health literacy into mission and planning.
	Establish accountability by including health literacy improvement in program evaluation.

Nath (2007) reviewed the literature between 1990 and mid-2006 for overcoming inadequate literacy in diabetes self-management and other chronic illnesses. The importance of culturally appropriate health literacy, improvement in self-efficacy, improved communication, and quality computer-assisted instruction were discussed as essential elements in tailoring health education. Nurses were recommended to address barriers related to inadequate literacy by: 1) increasing sensitivity to the problem; 2) developing literacy-assessment protocol; 3) creating and evaluating materials for target populations; 4) providing clear communication; 5) including health literacy in nursing curricula; 6) fostering decision making with patients, and 7) conducting research about literacy.

Additional Studies

Using telehealth to improve access, students in a community setting applied self-efficacy theory to help low-income older adults with chronic health problems to increase their practices of health promotion (Coyle, Duffy, & Martin, 2007). Although faculty and students favorably evaluated the activity, measurement of patient outcomes was not conducted. Like Web-based programs, the effects of telehealth require further research.

Program design of health-promotion programs can significantly influence the participation of all individuals. Warren-Findlow, Prohaska, and Freedman (2003) demonstrated factors that influenced participation and retention in an exercise intervention study targeted to African American and white older adults with multiple chronic illnesses. These researchers found that eligible participants who did not enroll were

more likely to be diabetic and younger than age 60. Seventy percent of the enrolled participants remained in the program after 1 year. The attrition was related to program site, functional status, and having a high school degree. Attrition was not associated with chronic illness. The researchers concluded that group-specific efforts tailored for the group can be successful in recruiting and retaining participants.

Feldman and Tegart (2003) explored older African American women with arthritis and their motivations and struggles with health promotion. These reflections provide helpful suggestions as nurses develop health promotion programs for clients with chronic illness.

Miller and Iris (2002) found that socialization and social support were central to the participation of older adults with chronic illness who participated in a wellness program. In this study, participants recognized that chronic disease did not prohibit living a healthy lifestyle. The White Crane Model of Healthy Lives for Older Adults used in this study contributed to understanding the way older adults view health for themselves. This model is also thought to be helpful in developing program evaluation measures.

A diet and exercise program to reduce cardiovascular disease risk was used with employees regardless of presence of chronic illness. There were significant differences between pre- and post-intervention for lipid profiles and weight. Self-reported levels of participation in the diet were significantly related to improvement in the low-density lipoprotein (LDL) levels (White & Jacques, 2007).

The addition of health promotion to the usual care of frail older home-care clients was studied in Canada by Markle-Reid, Weir,

Browne, Roberts, Gafni, and Henderson (2006). These researchers found that proactively providing health promotion to older adults with chronic health needs enhanced quality of life but did not increase the overall costs of health care. Better mental health functioning, reduction in depression, and enhanced perceptions of social support were reported in the experimental group. The researchers concluded that their finding underscored the need to provide health promotion for older clients receiving home care.

Age differences were found when researchers randomly assigned 111 young adults aged 18 to 36 and 104 older adults aged 62 to 86 to read health pamphlets with identical factual information for healthy eating but containing either emotional or nonemotional goals for the healthy behavior. Basing their study on socioemotional selectivity theory and health promotion, the theory contends that as individuals get older, they perceive time as being increasingly limited so emotionally meaningful goals with more immediate payoffs will be chosen over future-oriented goals. Older adults in this study evaluated health messages that contained emotional goals rather than the nonemotional, future-oriented or neutral goals, more positively and the messages were better remembered and led to greater behavioral changes than in the younger adults. While cautioning generalization, these findings may suggest that health professionals should emphasize emotionally meaningful benefits when disseminating health messages to older adults (Zhang, Fung, & Ching, 2009). Similar results may be found in future studies of individuals with chronic illness, especially those perceiving time as being increasingly limited.

The adverse effects of obesity on chronic disease were supported when strong positive associations of age, gender, race/ethnicity, body mass index, and comorbidities were found with type II diabetes, hypertension, and hyperlipidemia (Crawford et al., 2010). African Americans were found to have the highest prevalence of diagnosed type II diabetes and hypertension and Caucasians were found to have the highest prevalence of diagnosed hypertension. The direct associations between body mass index and disease prevalence was consistent for both genders and across all racial/ethnic groups.

A shift from preventive home-care nursing functions to acute inpatient care functions has resulted in fragmented, expensive care for older adults with chronic illness, rather than comprehensive and proactive care that is more likely to improve health outcomes. Providing the most appropriate services to older adults was the impetus for this study. A two-armed, single-blind, randomized controlled trial of 288 older frail adults with chronic health needs, aged 75 and older, were evaluated in a Canadian study (Markle-Reid et al., 2006). The model of vulnerability by Rogers (1997) provided the theoretical basis for the study. Participants were randomly assigned to the usual home care or a "proactive" nursing health-promotion intervention that included a health assessment combined with regular home visits or telephone contacts, health education about management of illness, coordination of community services, and use of empowerment strategies to enhance independence. Of the 288 patients randomly assigned at baseline, 242 completed the study (120 with the proactive nursing intervention, 122 in the control group). Results demonstrated that proactively providing the intervention group with nursing health promotion significantly resulted in better mental health functioning ($P = 0.009$), a reduction in depression ($P = 0.009$), and enhanced perceptions of social support ($P = 0.009$), while not increasing the overall costs of health care. Findings supported the need to provide nursing services for health promotion for older patients receiving home care. Implications from this study support that health-promotion efforts are productive in improving health outcomes and can be cost effective.

Many areas remain for further research to measure the effect of health-promoting frameworks and interventions with individuals/families with chronic illness. The earlier discussion provides a sampling of the current literature.

Guidelines

There are numerous easily accessible guidelines for health promotion, health screening, and preventive care at the National Guideline Clearinghouse website (www.guidelines.gov) and other sources. Examples of guidelines are discussed here.

Immunizations are one of the most important discoveries in human history. Vaccines have helped save millions of lives worldwide and millions of dollars each year in unnecessary healthcare expenditures (Infectious Diseases Society of America, 2011). However, there are unacceptably low rates of coverage among adults and children in the United States. The influenza vaccine alone can save thousands of lives by providing protection for persons with chronic illness. Immunized healthcare providers can decrease transmission of influenza to chronically ill persons. Recommended immunization schedules and information are easily obtained from the CDC.

Several organizations provide guidelines that include health promotion for chronic conditions. Self-management education programs such as diabetes self-management education (DSME) are outlined in the diabetes national standards (Kulkarni, 2006). Nurses are encouraged to use evidence-based guidelines as they practice.

OUTCOMES

The desired outcome for individuals with chronic illness and their families is to maintain and improve their overall health. Health-promotion activities should target the major causes of death—tobacco use, poor diet, physical inactivity, alcohol consumption, microbial agents, toxic agents, motor vehicle crashes, incidents involving firearms, sexual behaviors, and illicit use of drugs. These causes are responsible for the majority of deaths in the United States. Measures are needed to research outcomes of health-promoting interventions across populations and disabilities. Further efforts to make activities accessible and studies to evaluate their effectiveness are encouraged. The challenge of the coming years will be to link existing and future research studies to practice.

Evidence-Based Practice Box

Researchers in a recent study (Mayer et al., 2010) examined the healthcare costs and participation in a community-based health program for older adults. The program, called Enhance-Wellness, was designed to prevent disabilities and improve health and functioning. Earlier studies (Leveille et al., 1998; Phelan et al., 2002) demonstrated increased physical activity, improvements in health status, no decrease in functional status, and other positive health outcomes of the Enhance-Wellness program. Leveille and colleagues reported a multi-component disability prevention and disease self-management program led by a geriatric nurse practitioner improved function and reduced inpatient utilization in chronically ill older adults. Phelan and colleagues demonstrated the health enhancement program reduced disability risk factors, improved health status, maintained functional status, and did not increase self-reported healthcare use. However, costs were not examined until a retrospective study (Mayer et al., 2010) in which program participants (N = 218) were matched for age and gender to nonprogram individuals (N = 654) and evaluated for 1 year after they began the program. Healthcare costs were $582 lower among the program participants than nonparticipants, but the differences were not significant. The preventive services score was significantly higher for participants, suggesting a stronger tendency of program participants to receive preventive services. Results of this study indicate that those participating in the health-promoting program did not cost more than nonparticipants. Future studies may show a significant decrease compared to nonparticipants and studies that reveal combined positive health outcomes with reduced costs will undoubtedly add support to companies and communities to develop and maintain health promotion programs.

Numerous free resources are available through the federal government and other organizations. Many have been described throughout this chapter. Nurses are instrumental in promoting health. Stemming from our earliest work, nurses recognize the importance of health promotion. Like many other countries, health promotion and disease prevention is paramount in our costly, fragmented healthcare systems. There are substantial but missed opportunities for promoting health and extending the lifespan that present an international challenge. Countries in Europe are struggling with strategies to improve the health of their aging populations as well as control costs. Italy has one of the oldest populations in the world with more than 20% of its population older than age 65 (Besdine & Wetle, 2010). Italy, like the United States, must be proactive in finding ways to minimize chronic illnesses and keep people healthy. Nurses and other health professionals must meet the challenge in designing and evaluating effective interventions that promote health and are accessible for all people.

STUDY QUESTIONS

Describe the importance of health promotion in chronic illness for all people.
Name the three major actual causes of death in the United States.
What is the goal of health promotion?
Identify a theory/model/framework useful in working with chronically ill individuals who need to change an unhealthy behavior.

(continues)

Study Questions (Cont.) www

Discuss national documents that address health promotion and disease prevention.

What interventions can nurses use to promote health in persons with chronic illness?

For a full suite of assignments and additional learning activities, www use the access code located in the front of your book and visit this exclusive website: **http://go.jblearning.com/larsen**. If you do not have an access code, you can obtain one at the site.

REFERENCES

Annang, L., Muilenburg, J. L., & Strasser, S. M. (2010). Virtual worlds: Taking health promotion to new levels. *American Journal of Health Promotion, 24*(5), 344–346.

Aro, A. R., & Absetz, P. (2009). Guidance for professionals in health promotion: Keeping it simple—but not too simple. *Psychology and Health, 24*(2), 125–129.

Beaudoin, C. E., Fernandez, C., Wall, J. L., & Farley, T. A. (2007). Promoting healthy eating and physical activity short-term effects of a mass media campaign. *American Journal of Preventive Medicine, 32*(3), 217–223.

Besdine, R. W., & Wetle, T. F. (2010). Improving health for elderly people: An international health promotion and disease prevention agenda. *Aging Clinical and Experimental Research, 22,* 219–230.

Blue, C. L. (2007). Does the theory of planned behavior identify diabetes-related cognitions for intention to be physically active and eat a healthy diet? *Public Health Nursing, 24*(2), 141–150.

Bosch-Capblanch, X., Abba, K., Prictor, M., & Garner, P. (2007). Contracts between patients and healthcare practitioners for improving patients' adherence to treatment, prevention and health promotion activities. *Cochrane Database of Systematic Reviews 2007, 2,* 1–61.

Brodie, D. A., & Inoue, A. (2005). Motivational interviewing to promote physical activity for people with chronic heart failure. *Journal of Advanced Nursing, 50*(5), 518–527.

Bravata, D. M., Smith-Spangler, C., Sundaram, V., Glenger, A. L., Lin, N., Lewis, R., et al. (2007). Using pedometers to increase physical activity and improve health. *Journal of the American Medical Association, 298,* 2296–2304.

Burkhart, P. V., Rayens, M. K., Oakley, M. G., Abshire, D. A., & Zhang, M. (2007). Testing an intervention to promote children's adherence to asthma self-management. *Journal of Nursing Scholarship, 39,* 133–140.

Calloway, S. (2007). Mental health promotion: Is nursing dropping the ball? *Journal of Professional Nursing, 23*(2), 105–109.

Capella-McDonnall, M. (2007). The need for health promotion for adults who are visually impaired. *Journal of Visual Impairment & Blindness, 101*(3), 133–145.

Centers for Disease Control and Prevention. (2009, November 13). Cigarette smoking among adults and trends in smoking cessation—United States, 2008. *MMWR Weekly, 58*(44), 1227–1232. Retrieved September 23, 2010, from: http://www.cdc.gov/mmwr/preview/mmwrhtml/mm5844a2.htm

Centers for Disease Control and Prevention. (2011). Vital signs: Current cigarette smoking among adults aged >18 years- United States, 2005–2010. *Morbidity and Mortality Weekly Report, 60*(35), 1207–1212. Retrieved September 9, 2011 from http://www.cdc.gov/mmwr/preview/mmwrhtml/mm6035a5.htm?s_cid=mm6035a5_w

Centers for Disease Control and Prevention. (2010). *Chronic diseases and health promotion.* Retrieved November 8, 2010, from: http://www.cdc.gov/chronicdisease/overview/index.htm

Centers for Disease Control and Prevention, Healthy Communities program (2011b). *Steps Communities.* Retrieved September 9, 2011, from http:/www.cdc.gov/healthycommunitiesprogram/communities/steps/

Centers for Disease Control, National Center for Chronic Disease Prevention and Health Promotion. (2011a). *Four common causes of chronic disease.* Retrieved

September 9, 2011 from http://www.cdc.gov/chronic-disease/overview/index.htm

Centers for Disease Control, National Center for Chronic Disease Prevention and Health Promotion. (2011b). Retrieved September 9, 2011 from http://www.cdc.gov/chronicdisease/about/index.htm

Centers for Disease Control and Prevention, National Center for Chronic Disease Prevention and Health Promotion. (2009). *The power of prevention: Chronic disease. . . the public health challenge of the 21st century.* Retrieved November 8, 2010, from: http://www.cdc.gov/chronicdisease/overview/pop.htm

Cory, S., Ussery-Hall, A., Griffin-Blake, S., Easton, A., Vigeant, J., Balluz, et al. (2010, September 24). Prevalence of selected risk behaviors and chronic diseases and conditions—Steps communities, United States, 2006–2007. *Morbidity and Mortality Weekly Report, 50*(SS-8), 1–9.

Coyle, M. K., Duffy, J. R., & Martin, E. M. (2007). Teaching/learning health promoting behaviors through telehealth. *Nursing Education Perspective, 28*(1), 18–23.

Crawford, A. G., Cote, C., Couto, J., Daskiran, M., Gunnarson, C., Haas, et al. (2010). Prevalence of obesity, type II diabetes mellitus, hyperlipidemia, and hypertension in the United States: Findings from the GE Centricity electronic medical record database, *Population Health Management, 13*(3), 151–161.

Crosby, R., & Noar, S. M. (2010). Theory development in health promotion: Are we there yet? *Journal of Behavioral Medicine, 33*(4), 259–263.

DiClemente, R. J., Crosby, R. A., & Kegler, M. C. (2009). Issues and challenges in applying theory in health promotion practice and research: Adaptation, translation, and global application. In R. J. DiClemente, R. A. Crosby, & M. C. Kegler (Eds.), *Emerging theories in health promotion practice and research* (2nd ed., pp. 551–568). San Francisco: Jossey-Bass.

Edelman, C. L., & Mandle, C. L. (2006). *Health promotion throughout the lifespan* (6th ed.). St. Louis: Mosby.

Feldman, S. I., & Tegart, G. (2003). Keep moving: Conceptions of illness and disability of middle-aged African-American women with arthritis. *Women & Therapy*, 127–144.

Finkelstein, E. A., Brown, D. S., Brown, D. R., & Buchner, D. M. (2008). A randomized study of financial incentives to increase physical activity among sedentary older adults. *Preventive Medicine, 47*(2), 182–187.

Greiner, P. A., & Edelman, C. L. (2010). In C. L. Edelman & C. L. Mandle (Eds.), *Health promotion throughout the lifespan* (7th ed., pp. 3–25). St. Louis: Mosby.

Haverman, R. H. (2010). Principles to guide the development of population health incentives. *Preventing Chronic Disease Public Health Research, Practice, and Policy, 7*(5), 1–5. Retrieved September 8, 2010, from: http://www.cdc.gov/pcd/issues/2010/sep/10_0044.htm

Healthy People 2020. (2011). *Improving the healthy Americans.* Retrieved September 11, 2011, from http:www.healthpeople.gov/2020/default.aspx

Healthy People 2010. (n.d.) Retrieved September 11, 2011, from http://www.healthypeople.gov/2010

Heinzer, M. M. (1998). Health promotion during childhood chronic illness: A paradox facing society. *Holistic Nursing Practice, 12*(2), 8–17.

Holland, S. K., Greenberg, J., Tidwell, L., & Newcomer, R. (2003). Preventing disability through community-based health coaching. *American Journal of the Geriatrics Society, 51,* 265–269.

Hollis, V., Massey, K., & Jevne, R. (2007). An introduction to the intentional use of hope. *Journal of Allied Health, 36*(1), 52–56.

Huang, H. C., Chou, C. T., Lin, K. C., & Chao, Y. F. (2007). The relationships between disability level, health-promoting lifestyle, and quality of life in outpatients with systemic lupus erythematosus. *Journal of Nursing Research, 15*(1), 21–32.

Huffman, M. (2007). Health coaching: A new and exciting technique to enhance patient self-management and improve outcomes. *Home Healthcare Nurse, 25*(4), 271–274.

Huncharek, M., Haddock, S., Reid, R., & Kupelnick, B. (2010). Smoking as a risk factor for prostate cancer: A meta-analysis of 24 prospective cohort studies. *American Journal of Public Health, 100*(4), 693–701.

Infectious Diseases Society of America. (2011). *Immunization/vaccination.* Retrieved August 25, 2011, from: http://www.idsociety.org/Content.aspx?id=6346

Jackson, R., Asimakopoulou, K., & Scammell, A. (2007). Assessment of the transtheoretical model as used by dietitians in promoting physical activity in people with type 2 diabetes. *Journal of Human Nutrition and Diet, 20,* 27–36.

Janz, N. K., Champion, V. L., & Strecher, V. J. (2002). The health belief model. In K. Glanz, B. K. Rimer, & F. M. Lewis (Eds.), *Health behavior and health education theory, research, and practice* (3rd ed., pp. 45–66). San Francisco: Jossey-Bass.

Kelly, K. M., Phillips, C. M., Jenkins, C., Norling, G., White, C., Jenkins, T., et al. (2007). Physician and staff perceptions of barriers to colorectal cancer screening in Appalachian Kentucky. *Cancer Control: Journal of the Moffitt Cancer Center, 14*(2), 167–175.

Kulkarni, K. D. (2006). Value of diabetes self-management education. *Clinical Diabetes, 24*(2), 54.

Leddy, S. K. (2006). *Health promotion: Mobilizing strengths to enhance health, wellness, and well-being.* Philadelphia: F.A. Davis.

Leveille, S. G., Wagner, E. H., Davis, C., Grothaus, L., Wallace, J., LoGerfo, M. et al. (1998). Preventing disability and managing chronic illness in frail older adults: A randomized trial of a community-based partnership with primary *care. Journal of the American Geriatrics Society, 46*(10), 1191–1198.

Markle-Reid, M., Weir, R., Browne, G., Roberts, J., Gafni, A., & Henderson, S. (2006). Health promotion for frail older home care clients. *Journal of Advanced Nursing, 54*(3), 381–395.

Mayer, C., Williams, B., Wagner, E. H., LoGerfo, J. P., Cheadle, A., & Phelan, E. A. (2010). Health care costs and participation in a community-based health promotion program for older adults. *Preventing Chronic Disease Public Health Research, Practice, and Policy, 7*(2), 1–7.

McGinnis, J. M., & Foege, W. H. (1993). Actual causes of death in the United States. *Journal of the American Medical Association, 270*, 2207–2212.

McQueen, A., Vernon, S. W., Rothman, A. J., Norman, G. J., Myers, R. E., & Tilley, B. C. (2010). Examining the role of perceived susceptibility on colorectal cancer screening intention and behavior. *Annals of Behavioral Medicine, 40*, 205–217.

McWilliam, C. L., Stewart, M., Brown, J. B., Desai, K., & Coderre, P. (1996). Creating health with chronic illness. *Advances in Nursing Science, 18*(3), 1–15.

Miller, A., & Iris, M. (2002). Health promotion attitudes and strategies in older adults. *Health Education & Behavior, 29*(2), 249–267.

Mokdad, A. H., Marks, J. S., Stroup, D. F., & Gerberding, J. L. (2004). Actual causes of death in the United States, 2000. *Journal of the American Medical Association, 291*, 1238–1245.

Montano, D. E., & Kasprzyk, D. (2002). The Theory of Reasoned Action and the Theory of Planned Behavior. In K. Glanz, B. K. Rimer, & F. M. Lewis (Eds.), *Health behavior and health education theory, research, and practice* (3rd ed., pp. 67–98). San Francisco: Jossey-Bass.

Nath, C. (2007). Literacy and diabetes self-management. *American Journal of Nursing, 107*(6 Supplement), 43–54.

Neuman, P., Cubanski, J., Desmond, K. A., & Rice, T. H. (2007). How much 'skin in the game' do Medicare beneficiaries have? The increasing financial burden of health care spending, 1997–2003. *Health Affairs, 26*(6), 1692–1701.

Norman, S. A., Potashnik, S. L., Galantino, M. L., DeMichele, A. M., House, L., & Localio, A. R. (2007). Modifiable risk factors for breast cancer recurrence: What can we tell survivors? *Journal of Women's Health, 16*(2), 177–190.

Olshansky, E. (2007). Nurses and health promotion. *Journal of Professional Nursing, 23*(1), 1–2.

Ory, M. G., Smith, M. L., Wade, A., Mounce, C., Wilson, A., & Parrish, R. (2010). Implementing and disseminating an evidence-based program to prevent falls in older adults, Texas, 2007–2009. *Preventing Chronic Disease Public Health Research, Practice, and Policy, 7*(6), 1–6. Retrieved November 2, 2010, from: www.cdc.gov/pcd/issues/2010/nov/09_0224.htm

Painter, J. E., Borba, C. P., Hynes, M., Mays, D., & Glanz, K. (2008). The use of theory in health behavior research from 2000 to 2005: A systematic review. *Annals of Behavioral Medicine, 35*, 358–362.

Pender, N. J., Murdaugh, C. L., & Parsons, M. A. (2002). *Health promotion in nursing practice* (4th ed.). Upper Saddle River, NJ: Prentice Hall.

Phelan, E. A., Williams, B., Leveille, S., Snyder, S., Wagner, E. H., & LoGerfo, J. P. (2002). Outcomes of a community-based dissemination of the health enhancement program. *Journal of the American Geriatrics Society, 50*(9), 1519–1524.

Prochaska, J. O., Redding, C. A., & Evers, K. E. (2002). The transtheoretical model and stages of change. In K. Glanz, B. K. Rimer, & F. M. Lewis (Eds.) *Health behavior and health education theory, research, and practice* (3rd ed., pp. 99–120). San Francisco: Jossey-Bass.

Rainer, J. P., & McMurry, P. E. (2002). Caregiving at the end of life. *Journal of Clinical Psychology, 58*, 1421–1431.

Rogers, A. C. (1997). Vulnerability, health and health costs. *Journal of Advanced Nursing, 26*, 65–72.

Rohrer, J. E., Naessens, J. M., Liesinger, J., & Litchy, W. (2010). Comparing diverse health promotion programs using overall self-rated health as a common metric. *Population Health Management, 13*(2), 91–95.

Rollnick, S., Miller, W. R., & Butler, C. C. (2008). *Motivational Interviewing in health care: Helping patients change behavior.* New York: Guilford Press.

Schafer, M. H., & Ferraro, K. F. (2007). Long-term obesity and avoidable hospitalization among younger, middle-aged, and older adults. *Archives of Internal Medicine, 167*, 2220–2225.

Sherry, B., Blanck, H. M., Galuska, D. A., Pan, L., & Dietz, W. H. (2010, August 6). Vital signs: State-specific obesity prevalence among adults-United States, 2009. *Morbidity and Mortality Week Report, 59*(30), 951–955.

Siarkowski, K. (1999). Children's adaptation to insulin dependent diabetes mellitus: A critical review of the literature. *Pediatric Nursing, 25*(6), 6–27.

Snyder, L. B. (2007). Health communication campaigns and their impact on behavior. *Journal of Nutrition Education and Behavior, 39*(2) Suppl: S32–S40.

U.S. Department of Health and Human Services (2009). *2008 physical activity guidelines for Americans.* Retrieved September 11, 2011, from http://www.health.gov/paguidelines

U.S. Department of Health and Human Services, Office of Disease Prevention and Health Promotion (2007). *Quick guide to health literacy.* Retrieved August 25, 2011, from: http://www.health.gov/communication/literacy/quickguide/

U.S. Department of Health & Human Services, Office of the Surgeon General. (2010). *A report of the Surgeon General: How tobacco smoke causes disease—The biology and behavioral basis for smoking—Attributable disease fact sheet.* Retrieved February 7, 2011, from: http://www.surgeongeneral.gov/library/tobaccosmoke/factsheet.html.

Verheijden, M. W., Jans, M. P., Hidebrandt, V. H., & Hopman-Rock, M. (2007). Rates and determinants of repeated participation in a Web-based behavior change program for healthy body weight and healthy lifestyle. *Journal of Medical Internet Research, 9*(1), e1.

Warren-Findlow, J., Prohaska, T. R., & Freedman, D. (2003, March). Challenges and opportunities in recruiting and retaining underrepresented populations into health promotion research. *The Gerontologist,* 37–47.

Weinstein, N. D. (2007). Misleading tests of health behavior theories. *Annals of Behavioral Medicine, 33*(1), 1–10.

White, K., & Jacques, P. H. (2007). Combined diet and exercise intervention in the workplace: Effect on cardiovascular disease risk factors. *Journal of the American Association of Occupational Health Nurses, 55*(3), 109–114.

Zhang, X., Fung, H., & Ho-hong Ching, B. (2009). Age differences in goals: Implications for health promotion. *Aging & Mental Health, 13*(3), 336–348.

CHAPTER 17

APRNs in Chronic Illness Care

Ann Marie Hart

INTRODUCTION

Advanced practice registered nurses (APRNs) play an integral role in the care and well-being of individuals and families experiencing chronic illnesses. The complex nature of chronic illness, with care focused primarily on maximizing function and well-being as opposed to cure and recovery, is particularly suited to nursing's holistic focus (Lupari, Coates, Adamson, & Crealey, 2011; Saxe et al., 2007). APRNs are involved in every facet of chronic illness care from making an initial diagnosis, providing early anticipatory guidance, and coordinating care to monitoring for disease progression, managing medications, and problem-solving complications (e.g., adverse treatment effects, caregiver fatigue, reimbursement issues). Truly, there is no aspect of chronic illness for which APRNs are not well suited to assist in and enhance the lives of those experiencing it.

APRN Defined

For almost 5 decades, APRNs have been involved in the health and care of patients, families, and communities. In 2008, more than 250,000 APRNs were licensed to practice in the United States—just over 8% of the entire population of licensed registered nurses (U.S. Department of Health and Human Services Health Resources and Service Administration, 2010). As the numbers of APRNs have increased, so too have their capabilities and specialties, making the need for a unified regulatory model paramount. In 2008, after 4 years of dialogue and collaboration among leaders from the APRN Consensus Work Group and the National Council of State Boards of Nursing (Stanley, Werner, & Apple, 2009), an important and visionary document was published: *Consensus Model for APRN Regulation: Licensure, Accreditation, Certification, and Education*. In addition to establishing regulatory guidance for APRNs, the model also provides a legal definition of APRN that underscores the commonalities inherent in all APRN practice. Thus far, the model has been well received and has provided much needed clarification and direction for current and future APRN education and practice.

According to the Consensus Model (APRN Consensus Work Group & the National Council of State Boards of Nursing [APRN CWG & NCSBN], 2008, pp. 7–8), an APRN is defined as a registered nurse (RN) who:

1. has completed an accredited graduate-level education program preparing him/her for one of the four recognized APRN roles: certified registered nurse anesthetist (CRNA), certified nurse-midwife (CNM), clinical nurse

specialist (CNS), or certified nurse practitioner (CNP);

2. has passed a national certification examination that measures APRN, role, and population-focused competencies and who maintains continued competence as evidenced by recertification in the role and population through the national certification program;

3. has acquired advanced clinical knowledge and skills preparing him/her to provide direct care to patients, as well as a component of indirect care; however, the defining factor for all APRNs is that a significant component of the education and practice focuses on direct care of individuals;

4. (whose) practice builds on the competencies of RNs by demonstrating a greater depth and breadth of knowledge, a greater synthesis of data, increased complexity of skills and interventions, and greater role autonomy;

5. is educationally prepared to assume responsibility and accountability for health promotion and/or maintenance as well as the assessment, diagnosis, and management of patient problems, which includes the use and prescription of pharmacologic and non-pharmacologic interventions;

6. has clinical experience of sufficient depth and breadth to reflect the intended license; and

7. has obtained a license to practice as an APRN in one of the four APRN roles.

The Consensus Model provides detailed descriptions for each of the four APRN roles, and the reader is encouraged to review the model for specific role-related information. Although one might envision chronic illness care falling only under the purview of the CNS and CNP, chronic illness has no boundaries and frequently enters the realm of care provided by CNMs and CRNAs. For example, CNMs encounter chronic illness when they are providing prenatal care to women with comorbidities such as diabetes, mental illness, and inflammatory bowel disease, as well as when they are providing care to non-pregnant women with illnesses such as endometriosis, polycystic ovarian disease, and breast cancer. Similarly, CRNAs routinely provide anesthesia services to individuals experiencing chronic illness, as well as analgesia to individuals experiencing chronic pain conditions (see **Figure 17-1** for the APRN Regulatory Model).

APRN Education

Similar to regulation, APRN education has also experienced a watershed event. In October 2004 after recognizing the additional knowledge and skill set required for advanced practice nursing, the American Association of Colleges of Nursing (AACN) published a landmark document, *AACN Position Statement on the Practice Doctorate Nursing* that called for the Doctor of Nursing Practice (DNP) to be the entry-level degree for all advanced practice nursing roles. Unlike the PhD degree, the DNP does not prepare graduates to conduct original research. Rather the DNP is a practice-focused doctorate that prepares nurse clinicians for the highest level of nursing practice. Since the AACN's call for doctoral education for APRNs, more than 100 nursing programs in 37 states have developed DNP programs (AACN, 2011a) and many more DNP programs are under development. While most practicing APRNs were initially educated at the

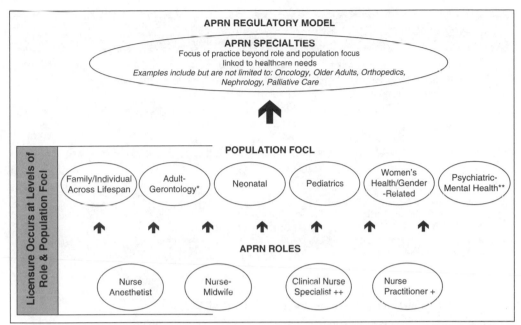

*The population focus, adult-gerontology, encompasses the young adult to the older adult, including the frail elderly. APRNs educated and certified in the adult-gerontology population are educated and certified across both areas of practice and will be titled Adult-Gerontology CNP or CNS. In addition, all APRNs in any of the four roles providing care to the adult population, e.g. family or gender specific, must be prepared to meet the growing needs of the older adult population. Therefore, the education program should include didactic and clinical education experiences necessary to prepare APRNS with these enhanced skills and knowledge.

**The population focus, psychiatric/mental health, encompasses education and practice across the lifespan.

+The certified nurse practitioner (CNP) is prepared with the acute care CNP competencies and/or the primary care CNP competencies. At this point in time the acute care and primary care CNP delineation applies only to the pediatric and adult-gerontology CNP population foci. Scope of practice of the primary care or acute care CNP is not setting specific but is based on patient care needs. Programs may prepare individuals across both sets of roles; the graduate must be prepared with the consensus-based competencies for both roles and must successfully obtain certification in both the acute and the primary care CNP roles. CNP certification in the acute care or primary care roles must match the educational preparation for CNPs in these roles.

++The Clinical Nurse Specialist (CNS) is educated and assessed through national certification processes across the continuum from wellness through acute care.

FIGURE 17-1   APRN Regulatory Model.

master's level, since 2004 many have either obtained or are now pursuing DNP education. The hope is that future generations of APRNs will all be doctorally prepared and competent in the eight essentials of DNP education (AACN, 2006). (See **Table 17-1.**)

Core Competencies of Advanced Practice Nursing

Although the consensus regulatory model (APRN CWG & NCSBN, 2008) and the AACN's (2004) position statement were both watershed

Table 17-1   Essentials of Doctor of Nursing (Practice) Education for Advanced Practice Nursing

I. Scientific Underpinnings for Practice[1]
II. Organizational and Systems Leadership for Quality Improvement and Systems Thinking
III. Clinical Scholarship and Analytical Methods for Evidence-Based Practice
IV. Information Systems/Technology and Patient Care Technology for the Improvement and Transformation of Health Care
V. Healthcare Policy for Advocacy in Health Care
VI. Interprofessional Collaboration for Improving Patient and Population Health Outcomes
VII. Clinical Prevention and Population Health for Improving the Nation's Health
VIII. Advanced Nursing Practice[2]

1. Includes natural and social sciences that make up the theoretical and scientific foundation for nursing practice
2. Education specific to the general and specific clinical role of the APRN (e.g., CNP role and family nurse practitioner [FNP] specialty)

Source: American Association of Colleges of Nursing (2006). *The essentials of doctoral education for advanced nursing practice.* Washington, DC: Author.

events for APRNs, no similar consensus has been reached regarding the conceptual underpinnings of advanced practice nursing. However, lack of conceptual consensus should not be construed as a dearth of work or quality scholarship in this area. Indeed, numerous nursing scholars have provided us with a rich body of literature as they have struggled to identify and articulate the essence of advanced practice nursing—that is how advanced practice nursing builds upon, yet is uniquely different from, basic nursing practice. Although it is beyond the scope of this chapter to summarize and critique the entire conceptual body of literature related to advanced practice nursing, six core competencies have been identified that are particularly useful for discussing the practice role of the APRN, particularly when caring for patients and families experiencing chronic illness (Hamric, 2009):

1. Expert coaching and guidance
2. Consultation
3. Research
4. Clinical, professional, and systems leadership
5. Collaboration
6. Ethical decision making

These six competencies have been espoused by and/or reflected in the work of multiple scholars and organizations including but not limited to the AACN (2006), Hamric (2009), Mantzoukas & Watkinson (2006); the National Association of Clinical Nurse Specialists [NACNS] (2004, 2009); and the National Organization of Nurse Practitioner Faculties [NONPF] (2006) and are described as "core competencies" by Hamric (2009) in her conceptual definition of advanced practice nursing (see **Figure 17-2**).

APRN CORE COMPETENCIES IN CHRONIC ILLNESS CARE

Although the six aforementioned core competencies underlie all APRN practice, they are by no means unique to APRNs. Basic-prepared nurses may also demonstrate them. What distinguishes these competencies from basic-prepared nursing is that they are essential to (i.e., required for) APRN practice. In other words, if an APRN

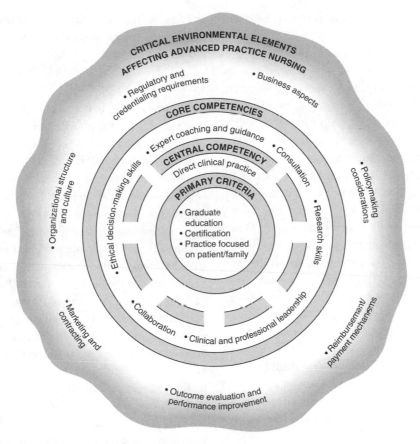

FIGURE 17-2 Hamric's Model of Advanced Practice Nursing.

is not proficient in or does not consistently strive to demonstrate all of these competencies in his or her practice, he or she is technically *not* providing advanced practice nursing care. The expectation is that these six competencies are consistently demonstrated in the APRN's routine practice. As such, these competencies serve as an excellent framework for discussing the role of the APRN in chronic illness care.

Expert Coaching and Guidance

Coaching and guidance are essential to the provision of chronic illness care. On the surface, this competency seems straightforward and the experienced nurse may assume he or she does this well and with "expertise." It is easy to assume proficiency with this competency; most nurses interact with and teach patients frequently during their daily patient care activities. Upon closer examination, there is more to coaching and guidance than meets the eye. Spross (2009) reminds us that the verb "coach" stems from the word's origins as a carriage used to facilitate the safe transmission of individual(s) from one point to another. Transferring this to nursing practice, coaching is "interpersonal work that helps people who are facing personal transitions or journeys" (p. 161), such as those associated with chronic illnesses.

The phenomenon of expert coaching is complex. In addition to establishing rapport, actively listening, and expressing empathy, expert APRN coaching requires clinical competence, and creative problem solving, as well as knowledge and skill regarding how best to assist individuals who are experiencing crisis, desiring change, or even expressing apathy toward an illness or situation. For example, to assist a middle-aged adult female with obesity and poorly controlled type II diabetes who desires to lose weight and bring her glycosolated hemoglobin level (HgbA1c) to goal range, the APRN must demonstrate expertise regarding the pathophysiology of diabetes and the complications associated with poor control. He or she must also be thoroughly familiar with current evidence regarding diabetes care parameters and treatments. In addition, the APRN should possess knowledge of and experience with efficacious diabetes education strategies, as well as the transtheoretical stages of change model (DiClemente & Prochaska, 1982; Norcross, Krebs, & Prochaska, 2011; Prochaska, 1979), motivational interviewing (Miller & Rollnick, 1992; Rollnick, Miller, & Butler, 2007), and other evidence-based behavioral change techniques.

Clinical Competence

To provide expert coaching and guidance in chronic illness care, APRNs must be knowledgeable regarding the illness(es) of interest and experienced enough to anticipate the informational and emotional needs of the patient and his or her family members. Going beyond asking the patient and family what they "want to know" and anticipating what they "need to know" is a critical aspect of the APRN's coaching skills

and requires that the APRN be intimately familiar with the illness of interest, its progression, and its management.

Creative Problem Solving

Just as no one asks to have a chronic illness, no one asks to have the myriad problems that are often associated with chronic illness. Expert coaching in chronic illness care often involves assisting patients and families who may be angry, despondent, anxious, confused, or desperate. Thus, it is critical that the APRN be willing to set aside his or her routine "script" or "protocol" and be able to create a revised plan that takes into consideration the unique needs, styles, and interests of the patient or family. Examples of creative educational and coaching strategies for chronic illness management that are gaining support in the research literature are group appointments for diabetes mellitus (Edelman et al., 2010); the use of lay-leaders for diabetes mellitus, hypertension, arthritis, and chronic pain (Foster, Taylor, Eldridge, Ramsay, & Griffiths, 2009); and the use of mobile phone technology for conditions such as diabetes and hypertension (Yoo et al., 2009).

Consultation

Although the APRN will often consult with other APRNs and members of the healthcare team, an essential feature of the role is that APRNs also serve as consultants to other professionals (e.g., nurses, physicians, mental health providers). There are a number of ways in which consultation may be categorized; however, in chronic illness care APRNs primarily provide consultations related to direct patient care. They either see a patient or make specific recommendations to the consultee (i.e., basic-prepared nurse, team of nurses, or nonnursing provider) on how best to proceed with the patient's care, or they assist the consultee with formulating an effective plan of care. Regardless of whether the APRN sees the actual patient or not, the aim of APRN-directed consultation is to assist the consultee in providing patient care.

Acting as a consultant requires that the APRN have expertise in a particular area and be respected for this expertise. Barron and White (2009, p. 196) pose seven principles of professional APRN consultation that espouse the collaborative, professional, and transparent nature of APRN consultation:

1) The consultation is usually initiated by the consultee.
2) The relationship between the consultant and consultee is nonhierarchical and collaborative.
3) The consultant always considers contextual factors when responding to the request for consultation.
4) The consultant has no direct authority for managing patient care.
5) The consultant does not prescribe but rather makes recommendations.
6) The consultee is free to accept or reject the recommendations of the consultant.
7) The consultation should be documented.

Research

Gone are the days when APRNs can avoid "research" by choosing to work in clinical practice settings. For more than half a century, nurses have worked to base their care in research-based evidence. Now with the accessibility of current and comprehensive electronic research databases (e.g., Cummulative Index to Nursing and Allied Health Literature [CINAHL] and the National Library of Medicine [through PubMed]), the

ability to truly bridge the research–practice gap is no longer an impossible dream.

In most healthcare settings since 2000, the term *research* has been replaced by the term *evidence*, and evidence-based practice (EBP) has become a priority goal of all allied health professionals, including APRNs. EBP is most commonly defined as the integration of three components: 1) best research evidence, 2) clinician expertise, and 3) patient preferences and values (Strauss, Richardson, Glasziou, & Haynes, 2005; Melnyk & Fineout-Overholt, 2010). To date, the EBP literature has primarily focused on how to develop compelling clinical questions, as well as how to search for and critique original research studies and systematic reviews. Very little has been published regarding how to best evaluate clinician expertise and patient values or how to "integrate" clinician expertise and values with research findings. Fortunately, APRNs have a long history of providing patient-centered care. Similarly, the development and recognition of nurse expertise has been well established and documented (e.g., Benner, 1984; De Jong et al., 2010; Foley, Kee, Minick, Harvey, & Jennings, 2002; Gorman & Morris, 1991).

By definition, EBP does not elevate or promote the status of research evidence above clinician expertise or patient values. However, EBP does require a moderate degree of competency in basic statistics, research terminology, and research design, which unlike clinician expertise and patient values, are areas that are not as easily gained or mastered from experiential practice. Thus it is critical that APRNs value research, master basic research skills, and utilize these skills on a routine basis.

Depalma (2009) describes three sub-components to the research competency for APRNs. These skills are also echoed in the AACN's

Essentials of Doctoral Education for Advanced Nursing Practice (2006) and *Essentials of Master's Education in Nursing* (2011):

1) Interpretation and use of research findings and other evidence in clinical decision making
2) Evaluation of practice
3) Participation in collaborative research

Interpretation and Use of Research Findings and Other Evidence in Clinical Decision Making

We live in exciting times, where a wealth of high-quality research exists to help inform and guide ARPN practice. Although not every clinical scenario has been fully researched and a fresh set of unanswered questions arises from each new study, much of the work facing APRNs is supported by research. Indeed it is rare for the APRN, particularly the APRN working with individuals experiencing chronic illnesses, not to have relevant research to draw upon. Thus it is critical for APRNs to be able to competently search for and critically evaluate the research literature, especially as it applies to their own area of clinical expertise.

Having a mechanism to remain aware of current research findings is an all important first step toward competency in research. At present, a growing number of services exist to facilitate this. Some examples include daily electronic "Smart Briefs" from the American Nurses Association, the American Academy of Nurse Practitioners (AANP), and Physician's First Watch. In addition, many other professional nursing organizations offer weekly or monthly electronic research updates to members.

Participation in professional journal clubs is another avenue for APRNs to remain current

regarding the research literature and has the added benefit of being able to dialogue with others about research and how it applies to clinical practice. Professional journal clubs may be sponsored by a workplace organization or organized "off site" by a group of like-minded colleagues. They may occur in a variety of formats including face-to-face monthly meetings, email discussions, wikis, or blogs. Several professional organizations and journals are now hosting electronic journal clubs to subscribers, for example the *AANP Virtual Journal Club* and the *Cochrane Journal Club*. There are a number of excellent publications regarding the value of and how to initiate a professional journal club, and the interested reader is encouraged to review these (e.g., Deenadayalan, Grimmer-Somers, Prior, & Kumar, 2008; Dobrzanska & Cromack, 2005; Honey & Baker, 2011; Hughes, 2010; Lizarondo, Kumar, & Grimmer-Somers, 2010; Luby, Riley, & Towne, 2006).

In addition to having access to research findings related to chronic illness, APRNs must also be able to critically evaluate these findings and determine whether and/or how the findings apply to practice. Simply put, critically appraising the research literature requires the ability to evaluate the validity of a single study's methodology and the meaningfulness of its findings, while simultaneously synthesizing findings from multiple studies across the literature. Obviously, there is nothing "simple" about this process, and similar to many clinical skills, research appraisal is an acquired process that requires adequate education and experience. A variety of excellent courses, workshops, and websites exist to assist APRNs with developing the skills to be able to critically evaluate research evidence (see **Table 17-2**). Having an EBP mentor or EBP team to consult

Table 17-2 Examples of Useful Resources for Evidence-Based Skill Development
• Academic Center for Evidence-Based Practice   http://www.acestar.uthscsa.edu/
• Agency for Healthcare Research and Quality (AHRQ)   http://www.ahrq.gov/
• Center for the Advancement of Evidence-Based Practice   http://nursingandhealth.asu.edu/evidence-based-practice/index.htm
• Cochrane Collaboration   http://www.cochrane.org/
• Duke University Evidence-Based Practice – Center for Clinical Health Policy Research   http://clinpol.duhs.duke.edu/modules/chpr_rsch_prac/index.php?id=1
• Institute for Johns Hopkins Nursing   http://www.ijhn.jhmi.edu/
• McMaster's University Evidence-based Practice Center   http://hiru.mcmaster.ca/epc/
• Oregon Evidence-Based Practice Center   http://www.ohsu.edu/xd/research/centers-institutes/evidence-based-practice-center/
• Vanderbilt Evidence-Based Practice Center   http://medicineandpublichealth.vanderbilt.edu/center.php?userid=1043409&home=1

with and a supportive work environment are also invaluable to the successful acquisition of EBP skills (Aitken et al., 2011; Fineout-Overholt & Melnyk, 2010).

Similarly, APRNs' practices should reflect an awareness of current research findings, which requires that they have and maintain mechanisms to remain current on the latest research literature. At present a variety of mechanisms exist to facilitate this, including daily or electronic research alerts from organizations such as the American Academy of Nurse Practitioners and Journal Watch (see **Table 17-3**). Fortunately, a variety of possibilities are available including APRNs being able to dialogue with other professionals, as well as patients, regarding research evidence.

Evaluation of Practice

In addition to basing care on research-based evidence, APRNs who work with individuals

Table 17-3 Evidence-Based Resources for APRNs
• AHRQ email updates   http://www.ahrq.gov/clinic/epcix.htm
• American Academy of Nurse Practitioners' Smart Brief   http://www.smartbrief.com/aanp/
• American Nurses Association's Smart Brief   http://www.smartbrief.com/ana/
• Cochrane Collaboration   http://www.cochrane.org/
• Journal Watch   http://www.jwatch.org/
• National Guidelines Clearinghouse   http://www.guideline.gov/
• Prescriber's Letter   http://www.prescribersletter.com
• UpToDate   http://www.uptodate.com

experiencing chronic illnesses should be routinely evaluating their clinical practice and practice-related outcomes. These types of evaluations not only ensure quality but also provide data that can be used by researchers and stakeholders (i.e., consumers, insurers, healthcare agencies) who are studying or evaluating care provided by APRNs. Evaluation of APRN practice may revolve around any number of professional aspects including but not limited to scope and standards of practice, role and job descriptions, and evidence-based guidelines and national quality indicators (Depalma, 2009). For example, APRNs who work with adults and children experiencing diabetes could evaluate their own practices to ensure that they are supported by (i.e., contained within) national and state scopes and standards for practice. Similarly, these APRNs could also evaluate specific aspects of diabetes management for adherence rates (e.g., influenza vaccination, microalbuminuria, and retinopathy screening) and attainment of goal disease indicators (e.g., HgbA1c, blood pressure, and lipids).

Practice evaluations may occur using a variety of mechanisms. For example, checklists can be developed to compare national and state standards to a particular agency's APRN job descriptions and evaluation criteria. Another example is conducting chart or electronic reviews of specific care practices (e.g., foot or retina evaluations in patients with diabetes) or patient outcomes (e.g., HgbA1c or lipid levels), which would need to be conducted in accordance with the Health Insurance Portability and Accountability Act (HIPAA, 1996).

Regardless of how or what practice parameters are evaluated, it is essential that APRNs utilize evaluative data to improve their practices. Thus it is critical that the evaluative process be understood and supported by all participating providers (e.g., APRNs, basic-prepared nurses,

technicians, and care providers). Similarly, it is important that data are reported in a clear, standardized fashion and that an established process for quality improvement/harm reduction be followed (e.g., using the principles of Continuous Quality Improvement [McLaughlin & Kaluzny, 2005] or Total Quality Management [Kelly, 2006]; see also Carman et al., 2010).

Participation in Collaborative Research

In addition to being able to interpret and apply research findings and evaluate and improve care based on research-based evidence, APRNs should also be able to participate and collaborate in research activities related to their area of clinical expertise. Although APRNs do not need to design and oversee research studies, they should possess general knowledge about research paradigms and phases of the research process (Burns & Grove, 2010; Polit & Beck, 2006). Perhaps most importantly, APRNs need to be interested in research and earnestly desire to contribute to research knowledge by developing collaborative relationships with nurse scientists and others who are studying aspects of interest to APRN practice.

Evidence-Based Practice Box

How Low Should We Go? HgbA1c Goals in Adults with Type 2 Diabetes Mellitus Early results from the U.K. Prospective Diabetes Study (UKPDS, 1998) demonstrated a significant association between lower HgbA1c values and reduction in the development of microvascular disease (i.e., nephropathy, neuropathy, retinopathy) but *not* macrovascular disease (i.e., coronary artery disease and cerebrovascular disease) in adults with type 2 diabetes. Because myocardial infarction (MI) is a leading cause of death amongst individuals with type 2 diabetes, there has been much controversy and continued research regarding intensive glucose control and coronary artery disease. A 10-year follow-up study of the original UKPDS subjects found that individuals who had originally been assigned to tight glycemic control group (HgbA1c 7.0 vs. 7.9) had significantly reduced rates of both MI (15–33% depending on treatment, $p < 0.01$) and all cause mortality (13–27% depending on treatment, $p \leq 0.007$) (Holman, Paul, Bethel, Matthews, & Neil, 2008). In addition, the PROactive trial found a 28% reduced rate of fatal and nonfatal MI ($p = 0.045$) in the group randomized to intensive treatment (HgbA1c 7.0 vs. 7.6) (Erdmann et al., 2007). However, the ACCORD (2008, HgbA1c 6.4 vs. 7.5), ADVANCE (2008, HgbA1c 6.3 vs. 7.0), and VADT (2009, HgbA1c 6.9 vs. 8.4) trials found no relationship between intensive HgbA1c lowering and reduction in coronary artery disease. Furthermore, the ACCORD trial, which studied patients with type II diabetes, who had either pre-existing coronary artery disease or other cardiovascular risk factors, found an increased risk for all cause mortality in patients who were in the intensive treatment arm (HR 1.22, 95% CI, 1.01–1.46, $p = 0.04$) with more cases of fatal MI and congestive heart failure.

Despite these conflicting findings, results of two meta-analyses suggest that intensive HgbA1c lowering is associated with a modest reduction in nonfatal MI (Turnbull et al., 2009; Tkac, 2009).

Additionally, researchers are exploring other potential causes between intensive glycemic lowering and increased coronary artery disease, including the relationship between severe hypoglycemia and vascular events (Riddle et al., 2010; Zoungas et al., 2010).

Debate and research regarding target HgbA1c levels in patients with type 2 diabetes are ongoing. For now, the American Diabetes Association (2011) recommends a general glycemic goal of HgbA1 $\leq$ 7% in nonpregnant adults with type 2 diabetes but urges providers to consider less stringent HgbA1c goals in patients with a history of severe hypoglycemia, history of coronary artery disease, progressive macrovascular or microvascular complications, limited life expectancy, or other complications. Thus APRNs who care for adult patients with type 2 diabetes should develop individual patient HgbA1c goals only after obtaining a thorough assessment. The APRN should also reassess the patient on a regular basis for tolerance issues and historical changes related to the set HgbA1c goal. In addition, the APRN should periodically scan the research literature for updates related to glycemic goals in patients with type 2 diabetes.

Clinical, Professional, and Systems Leadership

Although the APRN Consensus document (APRN Consensus Work Group and the National Council of State Boards of Nursing, 2008) does not specifically refer to the APRN as a leader, leadership qualities are evident in the common APRN definition. The Consensus document clearly distinguishes APRNs from basic-prepared nurses not only by their advanced education, but also by their high degree of autonomy, accountability for diagnosis and management of patient problems, and ability to synthesize complex data. Additionally, the AACN's "Essentials" documents master's (2011) and doctoral (2006) nursing education include leadership. As Spross and Hanson (2009) aptly note, "Not all APRNs are comfortable with the idea of being leaders, but leadership is not an optional activity" (p. 250).

APRNs have the opportunity to demonstrate leadership in four key domains: 1) clinical practice environments, 2) professional organizations, 3) healthcare systems, and 4) healthcare policy (Spross & Hanson, 2009), all of which are applicable to nurses who work in chronic illness care. The four domains are described individually; however, chronic illness care is complex and there is frequent overlap among the domains.

Clinical Leadership

Clinical leadership is the hallmark of APRN practice, and most APRNs demonstrate clinical leadership on a daily basis. Clinical leadership involves ensuring that all of the APRN's clients (i.e., patients, families, and communities) receive high-quality care. These patients may be the APRN's own clients or may represent clientele associated with the APRN's place of work (e.g., clinic, department, unit). APRNs provide clinical leadership as role models and leaders on patient care teams. They also lead on an individual basis, when patients, families, and communities meet with them for private consultation. In chronic illness management, clinical leadership means striving for the best care possible, even when

resources and time are scarce. Clinical leadership requires a high degree of intellect, creativity, and autonomy. It also requires experience, knowledge of the best available research evidence and healthcare systems, and a strong set of interpersonal and collaborative skills.

Professional Leadership

Professional leadership differs from clinical leadership in that it does not directly relate to the care of a particular individual or family (or in the case of a public/community health CNS, a particular community). However, its indirect effects significantly impact patient care, thus its importance cannot be understated. Professional leadership involves mentorship of junior nurses and APRNs, collaboration with colleagues (both like-minded colleagues and others!), and *active* participation in professional organizations. The goal of professional leadership is to ensure that all patients receive excellence in clinical care, and, thus similar to clinical leadership, all APRNs should be engaging in some degree of professional leadership.

Systems Leadership

Systems leadership involves leading at an organizational or delivery system level. Opportunities for quality systems leadership are available regardless of whether the APRN is responsible for an entire organization, a department, or a seemingly small component of an organization (e.g., patient care team, journal club, quality improvement initiative). However, true systems leadership does not occur in a vacuum and requires that the APRN have a mature understanding and appreciation of the complexity of a particular system and a desire to improve it. For example, an APRN leading a patient care team would be demonstrating systems leadership when he or she recognizes that the seemingly unique care aspects required by a particular patient might also be needed by other patients and works with the system to ensure accessibility and equity of information, resources, and services. Entrepreneurial leadership also falls under the domain of systems leadership and occurs when the APRN leader critically evaluates his or her opportunities and takes the initiative to practice outside of the traditional employment setting (i.e., hospital, physician-run clinic).

Health Policy Leadership

Health policy leadership refers to policies and laws related to patient care, public health, and nursing practice (i.e., both basic and advanced practice nursing). To be a leader in health policy, the APRN must analyze health systems data, possess advanced negotiation and communication skills, and maintain knowledge of the associated politics and stakeholders. Although not all APRNs are expected to engage in health policy leadership, all APRNs should maintain a keen interest in policies that affect patient care and APRN practice. In addition, all APRNs should develop mechanisms for staying abreast of current health policy and practice issues (e.g., via electronic mailing lists) and work to support those APRNs who are leaders in the health policy domain (e.g., write legislators, vote).

Despite differences in clinical, professional, systems, and health policy leadership domains, all four domains build upon the common concepts of mentorship and empowerment, innovation and change agency, and activism (Spross & Hanson, 2009). Thus even though an APRN may initially pursue an advanced practice role to become a clinical leader, with experience, continued education, and mentoring, the APRN may find that he or she is interested and well suited for leadership roles in nonclinical domains, using the same concepts that defined his or her clinical leadership. By engaging in professional, systems, and health policy leadership, the mature APRN is essentially recognizing that he or she is not the "end-all" of good patient care and has a responsibility to the future of good nursing care.

Collaboration

Frequently confused with consultation or referral, collaboration goes way beyond the notion of giving and receiving advice and is a fairly complex and sophisticated competency to master. Hanson and Spross (1996) define collaboration as:

> A dynamic, interpersonal process in which two or more individuals made a commitment to each other to interact authentically and constructively to solve problems and learn from each other to accomplish identified goals, purposes, or outcomes. The individuals recognize and articulate the shared values that make this commitment possible. (p. 232)

Due to its interpersonal nature, true collaboration cannot occur in the absence of willing partners, thus one could argue that collaboration should not be evaluated at the individual APRN level. However, components of effective collaboration—including clinical competence, interpersonal skills, respect for others, and recognition of and respect for differing values— are amenable to the individual APRN's prerogative and may be improved upon and evaluated (Hanson & Spross, 2009).

In chronic illness care facilitated by an APRN, collaboration primarily refers to the interpersonal processes that occur between the APRN and the patient and/or family, as well as among the APRN and other members of the patient's healthcare team (e.g., home health nurse, physical therapist, social worker, specialty physician). Unlike care provided for by "multidisciplinary" or "interdisciplinary" teams, which represent disciplines working side by side but in different ways, truly collaborative team members are committed to one another, the patient, and his or her family.

Ethical Decision Making

The complex nature of working with patients and families experiencing chronic illness often gives rise to ethical dilemmas (i.e., situations where two or more moral principles are in conflict and the best course of action is not immediately apparent). Examples of ethical dilemmas related to chronic illness care include issues related to inadequate pain management, abuse and neglect in the elderly or those with severe disabilities, decision making in patients experiencing early dementia, end-of-life decisions in patients who do not have adequate advance directives, and working with colleagues who are not competent. Although basic-prepared nurses frequently encounter and need to be prepared to handle ethical dilemmas, APRNs are often looked upon as leaders and consultants to help resolve particularly complicated or disturbing issues.

In order for the APRN to develop competency in dealing with complicated ethical dilemmas, he or she must possess maturity, excellent communication and collaboration skills, and have experience working through ethical dilemmas. The APRN should also be knowledgeable of the traditional moral principles underlying nursing and bioethics (Beauchamp & Childress, 2008; see **Table 17-4**). However, in recent decades, ethicists have become increasingly cognizant of the limitations of principlism (i.e., principle-based ethics) and have recognized the contributions offered by

Table 17-4   Traditional Moral Principles Underlying Ethics in Health Care

Moral principle	Description
Respect for autonomy	Duty to respect individual values and choices
Beneficence	Duty to do good
Nonmaleficence	Duty to prevent or remove harm
Justice	Duty to treat others equally

Source: Beauchamp, T. L., & Childress, J. F. (2008). *Principles of biomedical ethics*. (6th ed.) New York: Oxford University Press.

alternative ethical approaches such as casuistry and narrative ethics, which focus on critically examining existing dilemmas by comparing them to similar previous situations (Jecker, 2012). Other alternative ethical approaches that may assist APRNs who are providing chronic illness care include virtue and care-based ethics, which place emphasis on the virtue (i.e., care) employed by the moral agent (i.e., APRN) as well as the relationships that may be impacted by the dilemma (i.e., family members, caregivers, employers, etc.) (Armstrong, 2006; Arries, 2006; Cooper, 1991).

APRNs working with patients and families experiencing chronic illness are encouraged to familiarize themselves with the ethical references cited. It may also help to be aware of the four phases that Hamric and Delgado (2009) have identified for mastery of the ethical decision-making competency: 1) knowledge development, 2) knowledge application, 3) creating an ethical environment, and 4) promoting social justice within the healthcare system (see **Table 17-5**). Finally, the wise APRN will also recognize that important ethical dilemmas should not be solved in isolation and will develop and utilize a formal

Table 17-5 Phases of Development of Core Competency for Ethical Decision Making

Phase	Knowledge	Skill/Behavior
Phase 1: Knowledge development— Moral sensitivity	• Ethical theories • Ethical issues in specialty • Professional code • Professional standards • Legal precedent • Moral distress	• Sensitivity to ethical dimensions of clinical practice • Values clarification • Sensitivity to fidelity conflicts • Gather relevant literature related to problems identified • Evaluate practice setting for congruence with literature • Identify ethical issues in the practice setting and bring to the attention of other team members
Phase 2: Knowledge application— Moral action	• Ethical decision-making frameworks • Mediation/facilitation strategies	• Apply ethical decision-making models to clinical problems • Use skilled communication regarding ethical issues • Facilitate decision making by using select strategies • Recognize and manage moral distress in self and others
Phase 3: Creating an ethical environment	• Preventive ethics • Awareness of environmental barriers to ethical practice	• Role model collaborative problem solving • Mentor others to develop ethical practice • Address barriers to ethical practice through system changes • Use preventive ethics to decrease unit-level moral distress
Phase 4: Promoting social justice within the healthcare system	• Concepts of justice • Health policies affecting specialty population	• Ability to analyze the policy process • Advocacy, communication, and leadership skills • Involvement in health policy initiatives supporting social justice

Source: Hamric, A. B., & Delgado, S. A. (2009), Ethical decision making. In A. B. Hamric, J. A. Spross, & C. M. Hanson (Eds.), *Advanced practice nursing: An Integration Approach* (4th ed., pp. viii–xi). St. Louis, MO: Saunders Elsevier.

and/or informal network of mentors with which to explore thoughts and options.

Summary

The aforementioned six competencies (i.e., expert coaching and guidance, consultation, research, leadership, collaboration, and ethical decision making) are critical to the quality of chronic illness care regardless of whether the care is delivered directly by the APRN or delivered by RNs and other caregivers who work with APRNs. It is also important to note that meeting a competency or group of competencies is *not* a one-time goal. APRNs must continually strive to demonstrate these competencies, particularly when a change is made that significantly impacts patient care delivery, the nursing profession, and the healthcare system.

CONTRIBUTIONS OF APRNs IN CHRONIC ILLNESS CARE

Within the nursing profession, it is common knowledge that APRNs have made significant contributions to individuals and families experiencing chronic illness. Over the last few decades, the general public has also become aware of the APRN role, and there is an overall sense that patients and families experiencing chronic illness value the care they receive from APRNs. Despite these positive perceptions, little research has been conducted to quantify or validate the contributions made by APRNs in chronic illness care, and most of the existing data reflect care provided by CNPs who work in primary care settings (Grumbach, Hart, Mertz, Coffman, & Palazzo, 2003; Larsen, Palazzo, Berkowitz, Pirani, & Hart, 2003; Swartz et al., 2003). While data exist to support that CNPs are in fact practicing in long-term care settings (Rosenfeld, Kobayashi, Barber, & Mezey, 2004), there are no data regarding their outcomes or contributions to patients in long-term care.

Little data also exist regarding chronic illness care provided by CNSs, CNMs, and CRNAs. Upon a closer examination of CNS-delivered care, the literature is difficult to assess due to confusion in nursing role terminology. For example, a sizable amount of the literature reflects that "specialty" or specially trained nurses are effective in the management of heart failure (e.g., Case, Haynes, Holaday, & Parker, 2010; Duffy, Hoskins, & Dudley-Brown, 2005; Jolly et al., 2007; Phillips, Singa, Rubin, &

Jaarsma, 2005; Shearer, Cisar, & Greenberg, 2007; Turner et al., 2008); however, it is unclear from reading these studies whether the nurses were CNSs, other types of APRNs, or basic-prepared nurses who received additional training. Unfortunately, the confusion in nursing terminology also exists in the literature related to asthma (Griffiths et al., 2004; Xu et al., 2010), oncology (Cruickshank, Kennedy, Lockhart, Dosser, & Dallas, 2008; Eicher, 2005; Ritz et al., 2000), and stroke (Burton & Gibbon, 2005; Ellis, Rodger, McAlpine, & Langhorne, 2005).

Clinical Outcomes and Patient Satisfaction

The most common chronic illnesses for which APRN care (primarily provided by CNPs) has been studied include diabetes, hypertension, and dyslipidemia. With rare exception, these data have shown that patients who receive primary care from CNP-prepared APRNs have clinical outcomes (e.g., laboratory and blood pressure values) similar to patients who receive primary care services from physicians. Satisfaction with care has generally been found to be higher among patients seen by CNPs; however, not all studies reflect this finding and some indicate that satisfaction is higher with physician-delivered care (see **Table 17-6)**

IMPROVING APRN-DELIVERED CHRONIC ILLNESS CARE

Despite the growth in the number of APRNs, the APRN Consensus Model, the DNP degree, and a small but impressive body of literature indicating that APRNs deliver high quality primary care, there is still much work to do, mainly around the aforementioned research and collaboration competencies. Additionally, strong leadership at the

Table 17-6	Seminal APRN Outcome			
Study	**Design**	**Subjects**	**Length of follow up**	**Primary results**
Houweling et al. (2011)	RCT: Adults with type 2 diabetes randomized to NP or GP	N = 206	14 months	• No differences with regard to hemoglobin A1c, blood pressure, and lipid values • Subjects in NP group experienced some deterioration in QOL scores. No QOL decrease seen in GP subjects • Subjects in NP group more satisfied with care than those in GP group
Dierick-van Daele et al. (2009)	RCT: Adults randomized to NP or GP	N = 1501	6 months	• No differences in health status, medical resources utilized, or use of practice guidelines • Subjects in NP group had more follow-up consultations • NP consultations longer than GP consultations • No differences in patient satisfaction
Laurant et al. (2004)	Systematic review	NA—reviewed 16 studies	Average follow up ≤ 12 months	• No appreciable differences between patients cared for by physicians or nurses with regard to health outcomes, process of care, resource utilization, or cost • Patient satisfaction higher with NP care • NP consultations longer than physician consultations • Patient satisfaction higher with NP-led care
Lenz et al. (2004)	RCT: 2-year follow-up patients originally enrolled in two groups, Physician or Nurse Practitioner	N = 406	2 years	• No differences were found between the groups in health status, disease-specific physiologic measures, use of specialist, emergency room visits, or inpatient services • No differences in patient satisfaction
Mundinger et al. (2000)	RCT with subjects randomized to NP or physician	N = 1316	6 months; 1 year	• No differences between patients cared for by NPs and MDs with regard to: 1) patients' health status, 2) physiologic test results for patients with chronic conditions such as diabetes or asthma, 3) health services utilization, 4) satisfaction after initial appointment • For patients with hypertension, the diastolic value was lower for NP patients (82 vs 85 mm Hg; $p = 0.04$). • Satisfaction ratings at 6 months differed for 1 of 4 dimensions measured (provider attributes), with physicians rated higher (4.2 vs. 4.1 on a scale where 5 = excellent; $p = 0.05$); no differences in patient satisfaction at 1 year

GP—general practitioner; NA—not applicable; NP—nurse practitioner; QOL—quality of life; RCT—randomized controlled trial professional and the systems level is warranted in order to ensure that these competencies are continuing to be met.

Improving Research

Evidence-Based Practice

Broad electronic access to original research is a fairly recent development, thus many APRNs may find that they lack the necessary skills for searching and critiquing the research evidence. In a large national study of practicing RNs' preparedness for EBP (n = 1097), Pravikoff, Tanner, and Pierce (2005) found that more than 58% had never searched CINAHL or MEDLINE (a component of PubMed). In addition, 59% indicated that they had not identified a researchable problem within the last year and 72% had not read a research report within the last year. RNs in this study identified that their most frequent sources of information were colleagues and peers (51.3%), journals or books (42.4%), the Internet (33.3%), and conferences or workshops (31.9%). Although 9% of the RNs in this study indicated having a master's degree, it is unknown how many of the respondents were APRNs. As well, the data were not analyzed by educational level. Similarly, Koehn, and Lehman (2008) conducted a national study of registered nurses in the United Kingdom and found widespread misunderstandings of EBP and that 52% of the nurses did not subscribe to or read nursing journals. Although these studies are somewhat dated, their results are still noteworthy. Many of today's RNs and APRNs are not adequately prepared and/or do not value research-based evidence.

The first decade of the 21st century has witnessed an explosion of EBP resources, including books, journal articles, workshops, and websites, many of which are high quality (see Table 17-3). However in order to learn about and ultimately practice EBP, the APRN must first possess an appreciation for and a desire to seek out research-based evidence. Because many nurses were educated prior to the EBP era, this appreciation will likely need to be role-modeled by early adopters of and leaders in EBP, a process Melnyk and Fineout-Overholt (2010) refer to as "Step 0: Cultivate a spirit of inquiry" in their seven-step EBP process. However, if the APRN is practicing in an environment or setting that is void of EBP role models, then he or she will need to initiate the leadership to become knowledgeable in this realm through courses, immersion workshops, formal mentoring programs, and more (see **Table 17-7**).

Research Agenda

In addition to possessing solid EBP skills, APRNs need to lead the initiative to influence APRN-related research agendas, with the first

Table 17-7   Steps of the EBP process
0. Cultivate a spirit of inquiry.
1. Ask a burning clinical question in PICOT format (PICOT—Patient population, Intervention or Issue of interest, Comparison intervention or group, Outcome, and Timeframe).
2. Search for and collect the most relevant best evidence.
3. Critically appraise the evidence.
4. Integrate the best evidence with one's clinical expertise and patient preferences and values in making a practice decision or change.
5. Evaluate outcomes of the practice decision or change based on evidence.
6. Disseminate the outcomes of the BP decision or change.

Source: Melnyk, B. M., & Fineout-Overholt, E. (2010). Making the case for evidence-based practice and cultivating a spirit of inquiry. In B. M. Melnyk & E. Fineout-Overholt (Eds.), *Evidence-based practice in nursing & healthcare: A guide to best practice* (2nd ed., pp. 3–24). Philadelphia: Lippincott.

step being to put APRNs on the research "radar." The body of research literature regarding the contributions of APRNs to patient care, let alone chronic illness care, is currently small, confusing, and in some cases, nonexistent, causing APRNs to be referred to as "invisible champions" (Kleinpell, 2007) and "missing in action" (Morgan, Strand, Ostbye, & Albanese, 2007). Currently, APRN data are not included in the National Ambulatory Medical Care Survey (Hsiao, Cherry, Beatty, & Rechtsteiner, 2007), and although CNPs were included in the most recent National Hospital Ambulatory Medical Care Survey (Hing, Hall, Ashman, & Xu, 2010; Niska, Bhuiya, & Xu, 2010), their care-related data were not separated from physician data.

In this era of performance-based care, APRNs must document that their care leads to better patient outcomes. To accomplish this, practicing APRNs need to partner with nurse researchers, universities, and grant-funding agencies to ensure that the importance of this type of research is realized and that it is designed and carried out in a manner that best reflects the uniqueness of APRN-delivered care.

Similarly, APRNs need to influence research agendas related to patient care. By definition, experienced APRNs are practice experts, who should possess researchable ideas related to the nature and delivery of chronic illness care. It is also critical for APRNs to share their clinical observations with researchers and work collaboratively with them on study designs so that these observations can be objectively evaluated and disseminated to improve chronic illness care.

APRN-Sensitive Outcomes

Establishing research outcomes that are reflective and sensitive to the unique care provided by APRNs should also be a priority for APRNs. With rare exceptions, most of the current research

studies related to APRN care have measured traditional medical outcomes (i.e., lab values, vital signs, and other measures of disease). While medical outcomes are important, they do not reflect the unique care contributions offered by APRNs, including indicators such as symptom resolution and reduction, adherence to treatment plan, knowledge of patients and families, trust of care provider, collaboration among care providers, frequency and type of procedures ordered, and quality of life (Ingersoll, McIntosh, & Williams, 2000). Similarly, research related to APRN-directed chronic illness care should reflect theories and models that guide chronic illness care such as the Chronic Care Model (Dancer & Courtney, 2010; Wagner et al., 2001).

Improving Collaboration

Clinical Competence

Clinical competence is the foundation of respectful working relationships in health care and is arguably the most critical component of effective collaboration. Although the existing data suggest that APRNs are clinically competent, there are essentially no data regarding their knowledge of or adherence to evidence-based clinical recommendations for chronic illnesses. However, considering what we know about physicians' knowledge regarding and adherence to evidence-based recommendations for illnesses such as chronic obstructive pulmonary disease (Yawn & Wollan, 2008), cardiovascular disease (Doroodchi et al., 2008), and diabetes (Hayes, Fitzgerald, & Jacober, 2008), there is likely room for clinical competency improvement in APRNs as well.

In terms of education, a national study of CNPs' perceptions of their initial preparedness for practice indicated that only 10% felt they were well prepared for practice after completing their basic CNP education and that 51% felt they were somewhat or minimally prepared (Hart & Macnee,

2007). Although similar research regarding educational preparation is not available for CNSs, CNMs, and CRNAs, it is likely that these APRN graduates also feel inadequately prepared for practice, most likely due to the lack of opportunities for formal post-graduate residencies. In fact, 87% of the respondents in Hart and Macnee's study indicated that they would have taken advantage of a 1-year post-graduate residency, even if this meant being paid less and having to relocate. Fortunately, the need for post-graduate nurse residency programs (including APRNs) is starting receiving attention in the literature (e.g., Burman et al., 2009; Flinter, 2005) and was one of eight recommendations made by the Institute of Medicine (2010) in their report, *The Future of Nursing: Leading Change, Advancing Health*. In addition to formal residency programs, it is hoped that APRN programs will utilize the move to the DNP to reconceptualize and improve clinical education (Burman et al., 2009).

Transdisciplinary Collaboration

To improve competency in collaborative skills, APRNs are also encouraged to review recent advances in the concepts of collaboration and the benefit of integrated care. Over the last 2 decades, the concept has grown from *multidisciplinary* collaboration, which recognizes the contributions of other disciplines; to *interdisciplinary* collaboration, in which members from different disciplines share care responsibilities for a patient; and more recently to *transdisciplinary* collaboration, where members from different disciplines are committed to engaging with and learning from each other, as well as working together across boundaries to plan and provide integrated patient services (Glittenberg, 2004; Maitland, 2010; Verdejo, 2001). When APRNs and members from other disciplines view and approach patient care from a transdisciplinary perspective, the outcomes are typically positive for patients and family members and the experience is often transformative for the involved clinicians as well (Hanson & Spross, 2009).

Integrated Care Models

Integrated care models utilize the principle of transdisciplinary collaboration to provide patient care services. These models are still in their infancy and have primarily been designed for patients who are experiencing both a chronic physical and mental illness, combining primary care and behavioral health services. Preliminary studies of integrated models for patients with chronic illnesses such as diabetes, HIV, depression, and substance abuse have shown that integrated care models are both efficacious and cost effective (Bogner & de Vries, 2010; Katon et al., 2010; Schouten, Niessen, van de Pas, Grol, & Hulscher, 2010), and APRNs are encouraged to pursue integrated care opportunities.

CASE STUDY

You are an APRN working with a new patient, Kate Jackson, a 62-year-old Caucasian woman, who presents to you because she hears that you are "good with train wrecks like me." Kate brings in a copy of her medical records, which show that she has a history of multiple comorbid chronic illnesses, including obesity, type 2 diabetes mellitus, essential hypertension, Parkinson's disease, stage 2 chronic kidney disease, obstructive sleep apnea, major depressive disorder, and

CASE STUDY   (Continued)

chronic pain in her lower back and knees stemming from degenerative disc disease and osteoar-thritis. She has been treated for most of these illnesses for the past decade; with the exception of the Parkinson's disease, which was diagnosed 1 year ago and has caused her to have a resting tremor and shuffling gait. In addition, 2 years ago, she was diagnosed with stage 1 chronic kid-ney disease, which has since progressed to stage 2, despite her having fairly well controlled diabetes (HgbA1cs between 6.5 and 7) and hypertension (average readings 120/75). Current medications include metformin 1000 mg twice daily, insulin glargine 23 units subcutaneously at bedtime, Lisinopril 10 mg every day, Hydrochlorothiazide 12.5 mg every day, pravastatin 40 mg at bedtime, Sinemet (combination carbidopa and levodopa) 25/100 four times per day, fluoxetine 20 mg twice daily, MS Contin 30 mg twice daily, hydrocodone/acetaminophen 10/325 mg i–ii by mouth every 6 hours as needed, and Senokot-S (standardized Senna concen-trate with docusate sodium 50 mg) 2 tablets twice daily. She also receives CPAP therapy at night. She has been on all of these medications for the last 2 years, with the exception of the Sinemet, which was started after being diagnosed with Parkinson's disease.

Kate says that she has been seeing a family practice physician in town for the last 5 years and was fairly satisfied with his care until she was diagnosed with Parkinson's disease. Since that time, her back and knee pain have worsened, but apparently her physician told her, "there is nothing more I can do to help you with your pain," and, "with all of your mobility issues, we need to start transitioning you to the nursing home." Kate gets teary when she shares this with you and says, "I know I'm a mess, but I really love living at home and don't want to go to the nursing home."

Past Medical History (PMH)

Kate has no known history of cardiac or vascular disease. Her only surgery was a cholecystec-tomy 10 years ago. She had a screening colonoscopy at age 50 that was normal; however, she has not had one since then due to mobility issues. No history of abnormal Pap smears or mam-mograms; however, her last Pap and mammogram were more than 3 years ago.

Family History

Parents were both obese but had no health problems when they died. Maternal grandparents lived to be in their 90s and died of "old age." Paternal grandfather died of metastatic prostate cancer at age 75. Maternal grandmother died of a "massive stroke" at age 81.

Social History

Kate earned a bachelor's degree in journalism when she was 22 and worked for 30 years as a grant writer and business consultant. She reports that she has "always" been overweight but

(continues)

CASE STUDY   (Continued)

was able to wear normal size clothes and get around without difficulty until about 15 years ago, when she started traveling 5 days a week for her work and eating out most of the time. Over the course of 5 years, she gained 150 pounds and started having significant pain and mobility problems, which eventually led to her disability status. She has tried multiple weight-loss regimens throughout her life but has not been successful with any of them. She no longer eats out and primarily eats the food she receives from Meals on Wheels as well as some other grocery items that friends bring to her. However, she has significant mobility issues related to her pain and Parkinson's disease and continues to have a BMI of 56. She receives Medicare and Social Security Supplemental income. She lives alone in a low-income housing apartment and receives Home Health Services several times a week to help her with bathing and house-work. She uses a walker with ambulation. She wears a "lifeline" at all times and says that she had to use it 6 months ago when she fell in the shower and couldn't get up. Since then, she has not attempted to bathe alone and waits for the home health aide to assist her with this.

Kate was an only child and both of her parents died in an auto accident when she was 45. She has a few distant cousins that she exchanges Christmas cards with and talks to on the phone several times a year; however, they all live several hundred miles away and the last time that she saw any of them was at a family reunion 5 years ago. She identifies with being heterosexual, but never married and does not have an intimate partner. She has no children. She indicates that she is a Christian and used to attend services at a local Methodist church until a couple of years ago when it became too difficult for her to drive, and she sold her car. She continues to have some friends from church who visit her and offer to take her to church. However, she goes to church and leaves her home very infrequently due to her extreme mobility problems and con-cern regarding falling. Kate denies current or past use of alcohol, tobacco, or other illicit drugs.

Objective

As you talk with Kate, she answers all questions appropriately. She is neatly groomed, orga-nized, and seems to easily recall relevant facts related to her health care. Her affect is generally happy; however, she is clearly concerned about her future living arrangements and gets teary when she talks about living away from home.

Discussion

1) How would you go about assessing and prioritizing Kate's care needs (both today and in the future)? How does current research-based evidence fit into this?

2) Consider each of the 6 APRN competencies discussed in this chapter and presented in Figure 17-2. Which of these competencies are most challenged by this case, and how would you go about trying to meet them as you work with Kate?

3) How would a transdisciplinary team look at Kate? Think about the available resources and providers in your own community or those that you could consult with by telehealth.

CASE STUDY (Continued)

How could you provide transdisciplinary care with these individuals versus multi- or interdisciplinary care?

4) What outcomes are most important as you assess Kate's care? Identify both traditional medical outcomes and APRN-sensitive outcomes. What outcomes are your highest priority and why?

5) The family physician that Kate has been seeing prior to her consultation with you today apparently told her that nothing more could be done regarding her pain management. What are your thoughts regarding her pain management? What does the research-based evidence say about using opioids to manage non-malignant chronic pain, especially in individuals with multiple comorbidities?

SUMMARY AND CONCLUSIONS

APRNs have a long history of providing quality care to individuals and families experiencing chronic illness. Each of the four APRN roles (CNM, CNP, CNS, and CRNA) is involved in chronic illness care to some extent. Although there is no agreed-upon conceptual consensus for APRN-delivered care, APRN practice requires competence in the six areas of 1) expert coaching and guidance; 2) consultation; 3) research; 4) clinical, professional, and systems leadership; 5) collaboration; and 6) ethical decision making (Hamric, 2009).

Since 2000, significant strides have been made to APRN regulation and education. Together these changes help unify and strengthen APRN practice. Despite these strides, there is still much work for APRNs to do, particularly with regard to the research and collaboration competencies.

Regarding research, APRNs need to work to ensure that the chronic illness care provided by APRNs is studied and documented. This care should be studied using traditional medical outcomes and outcomes that are sensitive to advanced nursing care. Additionally, all APRNs need to be proficient in research as it relates to

interpreting and applying EBP, the new gold standard in health care.

With regard to collaboration, recent research evidence indicates that transdisciplinary collaboration and integrated care services for patients experiencing chronic illness may be more efficacious and cost effective than traditional care led by a single provider. Thus it is critical that APRNs commit themselves to working with and learning from members of other disciplines as they develop and provide patient care services.

In closing, the reader is reminded that APRN certification and licensure do not ensure that the APRN is engaging in advanced practice nursing. What distinguishes advanced practice nursing from basic nursing is that the six aforementioned competencies are *always* reflected in the APRN's practice. In this spirit, this chapter is closed with the challenge offered to APRNs and APRN educators:

There is still much work to be done: not all APN students are educated to practice with the competencies described here; too many nurses are in APN roles without the necessary credentials or competencies, and thus true advanced practice nursing is not demonstrated. (Hamric, Spross, & Hanson, 2009, p. x)

For a full suite of assignments and additional learning activities, use the access code located in the front of your book and visit this exclusive website: **http://go.jblearning.com/larsen**. If you do not have an access code, you can obtain one at the site.

REFERENCES

Aitken, L. M., Hackwood, B., Crouch, S., Clayton, S., West, N., Carney, D., et al. (2011). Creating an environment to implement and sustain evidence-based practice: A developmental process. *Australian Critical Care,* (epub ahead of print). doi:10:1016/j.aucc.2011.01.004.

American Association of Colleges of Nursing. (2004). *AACN position statement on the practice doctorate in nursing.* Washington, DC: Author.

American Association of Colleges of Nursing. (2006). *The essentials of doctoral education for advanced nursing practice.* Washington, DC: Author.

American Association of Colleges of Nursing (2011a). *Doctor of Nursing Practice (DNP) Programs.* Retrieved February 8, 2011 from http://www.aacn. nche.edu/dnp/dnpprogramlist.htm#AL

American Association of Colleges of Nursing. (2011b). *The essentials of master's education in nursing.* Washington, DC: Author.

American Diabetes Association. (2011). Standard of medical care in diabetes—2011. *Diabetes Care, 34,* S11–S61.

APRN Consensus Work Group & the National Council of State Boards of Nursing APRN Advisory Committee. (2008). *Consensus model for APRN regulation: Licensure, accreditation, certification & education.* Retrieved August 29, 2011, from: http://www.aacn.nche.edu/education/pdf/APRNReport.pdf

Armstrong, A. E. (2006). Towards a strong virtue ethics for nursing practice. *Nursing Philosophy, 7,* 110–124.

Arries, E. (2006). Virtue ethics: An approach to moral dilemmas in nursing. *Curationis, 28,* 64–72.

Barron, A. M., & White, P. A. (2009). Consultation. In A. B. Hamric, J. A. Spross, & C. M. Hanson (Eds.). *Advanced practice nursing: An integrative approach* (4th ed., pp. 191–216). St. Louis, MO: Saunders Elsevier.

Beauchamp, T. L., & Childress, J. F. (2008). *Principles of biomedical ethics* (6th ed.). New York: Oxford University Press.

Benner, P. (1984). *From novice to expert: Excellence and power in clinical nursing practice.* Menlo Park, CA: Addison-Wesley.

Bogner, H. R., & de Vries, H. F. (2010). Integrating type 2 diabetes mellitus and depression treatment among African Americans: A randomized controlled pilot trial. *Diabetes Educator, 36,* 284–292.

Burman, M. D., Hart, A. M., Conley, V., Brown, J., Sherard, P., & Clarke, P. N. (2009). Doctor of nursing practice: Reconceptualizing advanced nursing practice. *Journal of the American Academy of Nurse Practitioners, 2,* 11–17.

Burns, N., & Groves, S. K. (2010). *Understanding nursing research: Building an evidence-based practice* (5th ed.). Philadelphia: W.B. Saunders.

Burton, C., & Gibbon, B. (2005). Expanding the role of the stroke nurse. *Journal of Advanced Nursing, 52,* 640–650.

Carman, J. M., Shortell, S. M., Foster, R. W., Hughes, E. F., Boerstler, H., O' Brien, J. L., et al. (2010). Keys for successful implementation of total quality management in hospitals. *Health Care Management Review, 35,* 283–293.

Case, R., Haynes, D., Holaday, B., & Parker, V. G. (2010). Evidence-based nursing: The role of the advanced practice registered nurse in the management of heart failure patients in the outpatient setting. *Dimensions in Critical Care Nursing, 29,* 57–62.

Cooper, M. D. (1991). Principle based ethics and the ethics of care: A creative tension. *Advances in Nursing Science, 14,* 22–31.

Cruickshank, S., Kennedy, C., Lockhart, K., Dosser, I., & Dallas, L. (2008). Specialist breast care nurses for supportive care of women with breast cancer. *Cochrane Database of Systematic Reviews.* Issue 1. Art.No.:CD005634.

Dancer, S., & Courtney, M. (2010). Improving diabetes patient outcomes: framing research into the chronic care model. *Journal of the American Academy of Nurse Practitioners, 22,* 580–585.

Deenadayalan, Y., Grimmer-Somers, K., Prior, M., & Kumar, S. (2008). How to run an effective journal club: A systematic review. *Journal of Evaluation in Clinical Practice, 14,* 898–911.

De Jong, M. J., Benner, R., Benner, P., Richard, M. L., Kenny D. J., Kelley, P., et al. (2010). Mass casualty care in an expeditionary environment: Developing local knowledge and expertise in context. *Journal of Trauma Nursing, 17,* 45–58.

DePalma, J. A. (2009). Research. In A. B. Hamric, J. A. Spross, & C. M. Hanson (Eds.). *Advanced practice nursing: An integrative approach* (4th ed., pp. 217–248). St. Louis, MO: Saunders Elsevier.

DiClemente, C. C., & Prochaska, J. O. (1982). Self-change and therapy change of smoking behavior: A comparison of processes of change in cessation and maintenance. *Addictive Behavior, 7,* 133–142.

Dierick-van Daele, A. T. M., Metsemakers, J. F. M., Derckx, W. C. C., Spreeuwenberg, C., & Vrijhoef, J. J. M. (2009). Nurse practitioners substituting for general practitioners: Randomized controlled trial. *Journal of Advanced Nursing, 65,* 391–401.

Dobrzanska, L., & Cromack, D. (2005). Developing a journal club in the community setting. *British Journal of Community Nursing, 10,* 376–377.

Doroodchi, H., Abdolrasulnia, M., Foster, J. A., Foster, E., Turakhia, M. P., Skelding, K. A., et al. (2008). Knowledge and attitudes of primary care physicians in the management of patients at risk for cardiovascular events. *BMC Family Practice, 9,* 42–50.

Duffy, J. R., Hoskins, L. M., & Dudley-Brown, S. (2005). Development and testing of a caring-based intervention for older adults with heart failure. *Journal of Cardiovascular Nursing, 20,* 325–333.

Edelman, D., Fredrickson, S. K., Melnyk, S. D., Coffman, C. J., Jeffreys, A. S., Datta, S., et al. (2010). Medical clinics versus usual care for patients with both diabetes and hypertension: A randomized trial. *Annals of Internal Medicine, 152,* 689–696.

Eicher, M. R. (2005). Nursing expertise in breast cancer care: A systematic review on the effectiveness of specialised nurse interventions. *Pfledge, 18,* 353–363.

Ellis G., Rodger, J., McAlpine, C., & Langhorne, P. (2005). The impact of stroke nurse specialist input on risk factor modification. *Age and Aging, 34,* 389–392.

Erdmann , E., Dormandy, J. A., Charbonnel, B., Massi-Benedetti, M., Moules, I. K., Skene, A. M., et al. (2007). The effect of pioglitazone on recurrent myocardial infarction in 2,445 patients with type 2 diabetes and previous myocardial infarction: Results from the PROactive Study. *Journal of the American College of Cardiology, 49,* 1772–1780.

Fineout-Overholt, E., & Melnyk, B. M. (2010). ARCC Evidence-based practice mentors: The key to sustaining evidence-based practice. In B. M. Melnyk & E. Fineout-Overholt (Eds.), *Evidence-based practice in nursing & healthcare: A guide to best practice* (2nd ed., pp. 344–351). Philadelphia: Lippincott Williams & Wilkins.

Flinter, M. (2005). Residency programs for primary care nurse practitioners in federally qualified health centers: A service perspective. *Online Journal of Issues in Nursing, 10,* 6.

Foley, B. J., Kee, C. C., Minick, P., Harvey, S. S., & Jennings B. M. (2002). Characteristics of nurses and hospital work environments that foster satisfaction and clinical expertise. *Journal of Nursing Administration, 32,* 273–282.

Foster, G., Taylor, S. J. C., Eldridge, S., Ramsay, J., & Griffiths, C. J. (2009). Self-management education programmes by lay leaders for people with chronic conditions. *Cochrane Database of Systematic Reviews.* Issue 4. Art. No.: CD005108. DOI: 10.1002/14651858.CD005108.pub2.

Glittenberg, J. (2004). A transdisciplinary, transcultural model for health care. *Journal of Transcultural Nursing, 15,* 6–10.

Gorman, M., & Morris, A. (1991). Developing clinical expertise in the care of addicted patients in acute care settings. *Journal of Professional Nursing, 7,* 246–253.

Griffiths, C., Foster, G., Barnes, N., Eldridge S., Tate H., Begum S., et al. (2004). Specialist nurse intervention to reduce unscheduled asthma care in a deprived multiethnic area: The east London randomised controlled trial for high risk asthma (ELECTRA). *British Medical Journal, 328,* 144–147.

Grumbach, K., Hart, L. G., Mertz, E., Coffman, J., & Palazzo, L. (2003). Who is caring for the underserved? A comparison of primary care physicians and nonphysician clinicians in California and Washington. *Annals of Family Medicine, 1,* 97–104.

Hamric, A. B. (2009). A definition of advanced practice nursing. In A. B. Hamric, J. A. Spross, & C. M. Hanson (Eds.), *Advanced practice nursing: An integrative approach* (4th ed., pp. 75–94). St. Louis, MO: Saunders Elsevier.

Hamric, A. B., & Delgado, S. A. (2009). Ethical decision making. In A. B. Hamric, J. A. Spross, & C.M. Hanson (Eds.), *Advanced practice nursing: An integrative approach* (4th ed., pp. 315–346). St. Louis, MO: Saunders Elsevier.

Hamric, A. B., Spross, J. A., & Hanson, C. M. (2009). Preface. In A. B. Hamric, J. A. Spross, & C. M. Hanson (Eds.), *Advanced practice nursing: An integrative approach* (4th ed., pp. viii–xi). St. Louis, MO: Saunders Elsevier.

Hanson, C. M., & Spross, J. A. (1996). Collaboration. In A. B. Hamric, J. A. Spross, & C. M. Hanson (Eds), *Advanced practice nursing: An integrative approach* (pp. 229–248). Philadelphia: Saunders.

Hanson, C. M. & Spross, J. A. (2009). Collaboration. In A. B. Hamric, J. A. Spross, & C. M. Hanson (Eds.), *Advanced practice nursing: An integrative approach* (4th ed., pp. 283–314). St. Louis, MO: Saunders Elsevier.

Hart, A. M., & Macnee, C. L. (2007). How well are NPs prepared for practice?: Results of a 2004 questionnaire study. *Journal of the American Academy of Nurse Practitioner, 19,* 35–42.

Hayes, R. P., Fitzgerald, J. T., & Jacober, S. J. (2008). Primary care physician beliefs about insulin initiation in patients with type 2 diabetes. *International Journal of Clinical Practice, 62,* 860–868.

Health Insurance Portability and Accountability Act (HIPAA). (1996). Public Law 104–191. Retrieved March 25, 2011, from: http://aspe.hhs.gov/admnsimp/pl104191.htm

Hing, E. Hall, M. J., Ashman, J. J., & Xu, J. (2010). National hospital ambulatory medical care survey: 2007 outpatient department summary. *National Health Statistics Report, 28.*

Holman, R. R., Paul, S. K., Bethel, M. A., Matthews, D. R., & Neil, H. A. W. (2008). 10-year follow-up of intensive glucose control in type 2 diabetes. *New England Journal of Medicine, 359,* 1577–1589.

Honey, C. P., & Baker, J. A. (2011). Exploring the impact of journal clubs: A systematic review. *Nurse education today* (epub ahead of print). doi:10.1016/j.nedt.2010.12.020

Houweling. S. T., Kleefstra, N., van Hateren, K. J. J., Groenier, K. H., Meyboom-deJong, B., & Bilo, H. J. G. (2011). Can diabetes management be safely transferred to practice nurses in a primary care setting? A randomised controlled trial. *Journal of Clinical Nursing, 20,* 1264, 1272.

Hsiao, C., Cherry, D. K., Beatty, P. C., & Rechtsteiner, E. A. (2007). National ambulatory medical care survey: 2007 summary. *National Health Statistics Reports, 27.*

Hughes, J. (2010). Developing a journal club that impacts practice. *Gastroenterology Nursing, 33,* 66–68.

Ingersoll, G. L., McIntosh, E., & Williams, M. (2000). Nurse-sensitive outcomes of advanced practice, *Journal of Advanced Nursing. 32,* 1272–1281.

Institute of Medicine. (2010). *The future of nursing: Leading change, advancing health.* Washington, DC: The National Academies Press.

Jecker, N. S. (2012). Applying ethical reasoning: philosophical, clinical, and cultural challenges. In N. S. Jecker, A. R. Jonsen, & R. A. Pearlman (Eds.), *Bioethics: An introduction to the history, methods, and practice* (3rd ed., pp. 127–139). Sudbury, MA: Jones & Bartlett.

Jolly, K., Tayor, R. S., Lip, G. Y. H., Greenfield, S. M., Davies, M. K., Davis, R. C., et al. (2007). Home-based exercise rehabilitation in addition to specialist heart failure nurse care: Design, rationale and recruitment to the Birmingham Rehabilitation Uptake Maximisation study for patients with congestive heart failure (BRUM-CHF): A randomised controlled trial. *BMC Cardiovascular Disorders, 7,* 9–17.

Katon, W. J., Lin, E. H., Von Korff, M., Ciechanowski, P., Ludman, E. J., Young, B., et al. (2010). Collaborative care for patients with depression and chronic illnesses. *New England Journal of Medicine, 363,* 2611–2620.

Kelly, D. L. (2006). *Applying quality management in health care: A systems approach* (2nd ed.). Chicago: Health Administration Press.

Kleinpell, R. (2007). APNs: Invisible champions. *Nursing Management, 38,* 18–22.

Koehn, M. L., & Lehman, K. (2008) Nurses' perceptions of evidence-based nursing practice. *Journal of Advanced Nursing, 62,* 209–215.

Larsen, E. H., Palazzo, L., Berkowitz, B., Pirani, M. J., & Hart, L. G. (2003). The contribution of nurse practitioners and physician assistants to generalist care in Washington State. *Health Services Research, 38,* 1033–1050.

Laurant, M., Reeves, D., Hermens, R., Branspenning, J., Grol, R., & Sibbald, B. (2004). Substitution of doctors by nurses in primary care. *Cochrane Database of Systematic Reviews,* 18:CD001271. Doi: 10.1002/14651858.CD001271.pub2.

Lenz, E. R., Mundinger, M. O., Kane, R. L., Hopkins, S. C., & Lin, S. X. (2004). Primary care outcomes in patients treated by nurse practitioners or physicians: Two-year follow-up. *Medical Care Research and Review, 61*, 332–351.

Lizarondo, L., Kumar, S., & Grimmer-Somers, K. (2010). Online journal clubs: An innovative approach to achieving evidence-based practice. *Journal of Allied Health, 39*, e17–e22.

Luby, M., Riley, J. K., & Towne, G. (2006). Nursing research journal clubs: Bridging the gap between practice and research. *Medsurg Nursing, 15*, 100–102.

Lupari, M., Coates, V., Adamson, G., & Crealey, G. E. (2011). 'We're just not getting it right': How should we provide care to the older person with multi-morbid chronic conditions. *Journal of Clinical Nursing, 20*, 1225–1235.

Maitland, M. E. (2010). A transdisciplinary definition of diagnosis. *Journal of Allied Health, 39*, 306–313.

Mantzoukas, S., & Watkinson, S. (2006). Review of advanced nursing practice: The international literature and developing generic features. *Journal of Clinical Nursing, 16*, 28–37.

McLaughlin, C. P. & Kaluzny, A. D. (2005). *Continuous quality improvement in health care.* Sudbury, MA: Jones & Bartlett.

Melnyk, B. M., & Fineout-Overholt, E. (2010). Making the case for evidence-based practice and cultivating a spirit of inquiry. In B. M. Melnyk & E. Fineout-Overholt (Eds.), *Evidence-based practice in nursing & healthcare: A guide to best practice* (2nd ed., pp. 3–24). Philadelphia: Lippincott.

Miller, W. R., & Rollnick, S. P. (1992). *Motivational interviewing: Preparing people to change addictive behavior.* New York, NY: Guildford Press.

Morgan, P. A., Strand, J., Ostbye, T., & Albanese, M. A. (2007). Missing in action: Care by physician assistants and nurse practitioners in national health surveys. *Health Services Research, 42*, 2022–2037.

Mundinger, M. O., Kane, R. L., Lenz, E. R., Totten, A., Tsai, W., Cleary, P., et al. (2000). Primary care outcomes in patients treated by nurse practitioners or physicians: A randomized trial. *Journal of the American Medical Association, 283*, 59–68.

National Association of Clinical Nurse Specialists (NACNS). (2004). *Statement on clinical nurse specialist practice and education* (2nd ed.). Philadelphia, PA: Author.

National Association of Clinical Nurse Specialists (NACNS). (2009). *Core practice doctorate clinical nurse specialist competencies.* Philadelphia, PA: Author.

National Organization of Nurse Practitioner Faculties (NONPF). (2006). *Domains and core competencies of nurse practitioner practice.* Washington, DC: Author.

Niska, R., Bhuiya, F., & Xu, J. (2010). National hospital ambulatory medical care survey: 2007 emergency department summary. *National Health Care Statistics Report, 26.*

Norcross, J. C., Krebs, P. M., & Prochaska, J. O. (2011). Stages of change. *Journal of Clinical Psychology, 67*, 143–154.

Phillips, C. O., Singa, R. M., Rubin, H. R., & Jaarsma, T. (2005). Complexity of program and clinical outcomes of heart failure disease management incorporating specialist nurse-led heart failure clinics. a meta-regression analysis. *European Journal of Heart Failure, 16*, 333–341.

Polit, D. F., & Beck, C. T. (2006). *Essentials of nursing research: Methods, appraisal and utilization* (6th ed). Philadelphia: Lippincott, Williams, & Wilkins.

Pravikoff, D. S., Tanner, A. B., & Pierce, S. T. (2005). Readiness of nurses for evidence-based practice. *American Journal of Nursing, 105*, 40–51.

Prochaska, J. O. (1979). *Systems of psychotherapy: A transtheoretical analysis.* Homewood, IL: Dorsey.

Riddle, M. C., Ambrosius, W. T., Brillon, D. J., Buse, J. B., Byington, R. P., Cohen, R. M., et al. (2010). Epidemiologic relationships between A1c and all-cause mortality during a median 3.4-year follow-up of glycemic treatment in the ACCORD trial. *Diabetes Care, 33*, 983–990.

Ritz, L. J., Nissen, M. J., Swenson, K. K., Farrell, J. B., Sperduto, P. W., Sladek, M. L., et al. (2000). Effects of advanced nursing care on quality of life and cost outcomes of women diagnosed with breast cancer. *Oncology Nursing Forum, 27*, 923–932.

Rollnick, S. P., Miller, W. R., & Butler, C. C. (2007). *Motivational interviewing in health care: Helping patients change behavior.* New York, NY: Guilford Press.

Rosenfeld, P., Kobayashi, M., Barber, P., & Mezey, M. (2004). Utilization of nurse practitioners in long-term care: Findings and implications of a national survey. *Journal of the American Directors Association, 5*, 9–15.

Saxe, J. M., Janson, S. L., Dennehy, P. M., Stringari-Murray S., Hirsch, J. E., & Waters, C. M. (2007).

Meeting a primary care challenge in the United States: Chronic illness care. *Contemporary Nurse, 26,* 94–103.

Schouten, L. M., Niessen, L. W., van de Pas, J. W., Grol, R. P., & Hulscher, M. E. (2010). Cost-effectiveness of a quality improvement collaborative focusing on patients with diabetes. *Medical Care, 48,* 884–891.

Shearer, N. B. C., Cisar, N., & Greenberg, E. A. (2007). A telephone-delivered empowerment intervention with patients diagnosed with heart failure. *Heart & Lung, 36,* 159–169.

Spross, J. A. (2009). Expert coaching and guidance. In A. B. Hamric, J. A. Spross, & C. M. Hanson (Eds.), *Advanced practice nursing: An integrative approach* (4th ed., pp. 159–190). St. Louis, MO: Saunders Elsevier.

Spross, J. A., & Hanson, C. M. (2009). Clinical, professional, and systems leadership. In A. B. Hamric, J. A. Spross, & C. M. Hanson (Eds.), *Advanced practice nursing: An integrative approach* (4th ed., pp. 249–282). St. Louis, MO: Saunders Elsevier.

Stanley, J. M., Werner, K. E., & Apple, K. (2009). Positioning advanced practice nurses for health care reform: Consensus on APRN regulation. *Journal of Professional Nursing, 25,* 340–348.

Strauss, S. E., Richardson, W. S., Glasziou, P., & Haynes, R. B. (2005). *Evidence-based medicine: How to practice and teach EBM* (3rd ed.). Edinburgh: Churchill Livingstone.

Swartz, M. K., Grey, M., Allan, J. D., Ridenour, N., Kovner, C., Hinton Walker, P., & Marion, L. (2003). A day in the lives of APNs in the U.S. *Nurse Practitioner, 28,* 32–39.

Tkac, I. (2009). Effect of intensive glycemic control on cardiovascular outcomes and all-cause mortality in type 2 diabetes: Overview and metaanalysis of five trials. *Diabetes Research and Clinical Practice, 86S,* S57–S62.

Turnbull, F. M., Abraira, C., Anderson, R. J. Byington, R. P., Chalmers, J. P., Duckworth, W.C., et al. (2009). Intensive glucose control and macrovascular outcomes in type 2 diabetes, *Diabetologia, 52,* 2288–2298.

Turner, D. A., Paul, S., Stone, M. A., Juarez-Garcia, A., Squire, I., & Khunti, K. (2008). Cost-effectiveness of a disease management program for secondary prevention of coronary artery disease and heart failure in primary care. *Heart, 94,* 1601–1606.

U.K. Prospective Diabetes Study Group. (1998). Intensive blood-glucose control with sulphonylureas or insulin compared with conventional treatment and risk of complications in patients with type 2 diabetes, *Lancet, 352,* 837–853.

U.S. Department of Health and Human Services Health Resources and Service Administration. (2010). *The registered nurse population: Findings from the 2008 national sample survey of registered nurses.* Retrieved August 29, 2011, from: bhpr.hrsa.gov/healthworkforce/rnsurveys/rnsurveyfinal.pdf

Verdejo, T. (2001). Leading into the 21st century: Changing the vision and leading toward success. *Seminars for Nurse Managers, 9,* 115–118.

Wagner, E. H., Austin, B. T., Davis. C., Hindmarsh, M., Schaefer. J., & Bonomi, A. (2001). Improving chronic illness care: translating evidence into action. *Health Affairs, 20,* 64–78.

Xu, C., Jackson, M., Scuffham, P. A., Wootton, R., Simpson, P., Whitty, J., et al. (2010). A randomized controlled trial of an interactive voice response telephone system and specialist nurse support for childhood asthma management. *Journal of Asthma, 47,* 768–773.

Yawn, B. P., & Wollan, P. C. (2008). Knowledge and attitudes of family physicians coming to COPD continuing medical education. *International Journal of Chronic Obstructive Pulmonary Disease, 3,* 311–317.

Yoo, H. J., Park, M. S., Kim, T. N, Yang, S. J., Cho, G. J,, Hwang T. G., et al. (2009). A ubiquitous chronic disease care system using cellular phones and the internet. *Diabetic Medicine, 26,* 628–635.

Zoungas, S., Patel, A., Chalmers, J., DeGalan, B. E., Li, Q., Billot, L., et al. (2010). Severe hypoglycemia and risks of vascular events and death. *New England Journal of Medicine, 363,* 1410–1418.

CHAPTER 18

Complementary and Alternative Therapies

Pamala D. Larsen

INTRODUCTION

The use of complementary and alternative treatments has continued to increase in the United States (National Center for Complementary and Alternative Medicine [NCCAM], 2008a). What motivates an individual with chronic illness to try nontraditional therapies? If the traditional allopathic approach is not able to provide a treatment that relieves human suffering and improves quality of life, should healthcare providers help individuals with chronic illnesses find nonallopathic treatments that may help? What is the role of government in balancing the safety of healthcare treatments with an individual's right to access alternative or complementary treatments? Addressing these questions in a scholarly, evidence-based manner assists the healthcare professional in providing improved health care for clients with chronic illnesses.

Definitions

Complementary and alternative medicine (CAM) are labels used to describe diverse medical and healthcare systems, practices, and products that are not generally considered part of conventional (Western or allopathic) medicine (NCCAM, 2008a). The boundaries of CAM and conventional medicine are dynamic, and over time, some CAM practices may be labeled as conventional medicine. Alternative medicine refers to therapies used in place of conventional medicine. Complementary medicine, sometimes called integrative medicine, refers to using alternative medicine with conventional treatment (NCCAM, 2008a). Self-healing is the primary concept in CAM practices. External sources merely mobilize the body's inner resources for healing (Micozzi, 2011).

Users

The National Health Interview Survey (NHIS) provides rich data on the use of CAM. The 2007 survey of 23,393 adults was conducted to determine usage. Nearly 4 of 10 adults (38.3%) and 11.8% of children under age 18 had used CAM therapies in the last 12 months (Barnes, Bloom, & Nahin, 2008). The 2007 survey expanded the 2002 survey by increasing the number of CAM therapies in the survey from 27 to 36 as well as the number of diseases treated with CAM from 73 to 81. The structure of this survey was quite different from the 2002 survey. The 36 CAM therapies were grouped into five broad categories: alternative medical systems, biologically based therapies, manipulative and body-based therapies, mind–body therapies, and energy healing therapies. This survey followed the taxonomy of unconventional health care proposed by Kaptchuk and Eisenberg (2001), meaning that folk medicine practices, stress management courses, support groups, and religious (faith) healing—for example, praying for one's own health or having others pray for one's health—were not included in the definition of CAM in this report (Barnes et al., 2008; Nahin, Barnes, Stussman, & Bloom, 2009). This differs significantly from the 2002 NHIS survey where prayer for self and prayer for others were included. The most frequently cited therapies in the 2007 survey included: nonvitamin, nonmineral natural products (17.7%); deep-breathing exercises (12.7%); meditation (9.4%); chiropractic or osteopathic manipulation (8.6%); massage (8.3%); and yoga (6.1%) (Barnes et al., 2008, p. 2). From 2002 to 2007, there was increased use of mind–body therapies, acupuncture, massage therapy, and naturopathy. There was a significant decrease in the use of the Atkins diet.

Reasons for Use

Individuals with chronic illnesses often feel frustrated with disease-focused, fragmented, time-limited traditional allopathic care. As a result, they may turn to alternative or complementary practitioners, who may take more time to listen and evaluate not only their health problems but their entire lives. Specifically, these nontraditional healthcare services are noted for extensive clinical evaluations that focus on understanding individuals and their experiences in dealing with a chronic illness; continuity with care providers over time; active participation in care by clinicians, patients, and their family members; choice of individualized services; provision of hope; open communication and information sharing; and an emphasis on the meaning and spiritual components of dealing with chronic illnesses

(Bezold, 2005; Oguamanam, 2006; Saydah & Eberhardt, 2006).

The most commonly reported health problems treated by CAM in the 2007 NHIS survey included: musculoskeletal problems, including back pain or problems (17.1%); neck pain or problems (5.9%); joint pain or stiffness or other joint condition (5.2%); arthritis (3.5%); and other musculoskeletal conditions (1.8%) (Barnes et al., 2008, p. 4). These data are relatively unchanged from 2002. The use of CAM to treat head or chest colds showed a marked decrease from 2002 to 2007 (9.5% to 2.0%). A small increase in CAM use was seen in treating cholesterol problems. Lastly, data from the 2007 survey were consistent with the 2002 data demonstrating that CAM use was more prevalent among women, adults aged 30 to 69; higher levels of education; individuals who were not poor; adults living in the West; former smokers; and adults who were hospitalized within the last year (Barnes et al., 2008, p. 4).

More than two-thirds of CAM users do not tell their physicians or healthcare providers about using these therapies (Briggs, 2007). Perhaps this is because when clients do tell their clinicians about their choices, they might scold them, become angry and defensive, or dismiss clients' reasons for seeking additional care instead of exhibiting understanding behaviors. This lack of empathy may result in future reluctance to tell conventional practitioners about nonstandard treatments as well as loss of trust in allopathic providers (Oguamanam, 2006; Sleath, Callahan, DeVellis, & Sloane, 2005).

Costs

In 2007 adults in the United States spent $33.9 billion dollars out of pocket on visits to CAM practitioners and purchases of CAM products, classes, and materials. Practitioner costs totaled $11.9 billion dollars (35.2%). The remaining $22.0 billion dollars (64.8%) included costs associated with relaxation techniques; homeopathic medicine; yoga, tai chi, and qigong classes; and self-care costs to include nonvitamin, nonmineral natural products (Nahin et al., 2009, p. 3). Approximately 75% of visits to CAM practitioners and total costs related to visits to CAM providers were associated with manipulative and body-based therapies (chiropractic or osteopathic manipulation, massage, and movement therapies) (p. 6).

Overview of NCCAM

A national initiative established in 1991 to evaluate alternative treatments led to the establishment of the Office of Alternative Medicine (OAM) at the National Institutes of Health (NIH). In 1998 the OAM became the National Center for Complementary and Alternative Medicine (NCCAM).

The role of the NCCAM is to explore CAM practices using rigorous scientific methods and build an evidence base regarding the safety and effectiveness of such practices. This mission is achieved through basic, translational, and clinical research; research capacity building and training; and education and outreach programs. There are four foci of the NCCAM: 1) advancing scientific research, 2) training CAM researchers, 3) sharing new information, 4) supporting integration of proven CAM therapies (NCCAM, 2010a). The NCCAM has authored a number of pamphlets/publications, which can also be found online, for the public to further describe CAM, including *Evaluating Web-based Health Resources* (2011a); *Selecting a CAM Practitioner* (2011b); and *Using Dietary Supple-ments Wisely* (2011c). Many other patient and family materials are available.

The NCCAM receives its budget through the National Institutes of Health (NIH). The budget rose steadily from 1999 (when it became an institute) to 2005; the financial year (FY) budget in 2005 was $123.1 million dollars and for FY2010 it was $128.8 million dollars. The NCCAM (2011d) recently released its third strategic plan, *Exploring the Science of Complementary and Alternative Medicine: Third Strategic Plan 2011–2015.* The five strategic objectives include:

- Advance research on mind and body interventions, practices, and disciplines
- Advance research on CAM natural products
- Increase understanding of "real world" patterns and outcomes of CAM use and its integration into health care and health promotion
- Improve the capacity of the field to carry out rigorous research
- Develop and disseminate objective, evidence-based information on CAM interventions (NCCAM, 2011d)

As one can see, many of the strategic objectives are focused on research. In exploring the literature for this chapter, the lack of rigorous research was evident. Textbooks on CAM seem somewhat incomplete, with old references or a lack of references. Because of these concerns, the research cited in this chapter has been carefully screened.

Common Treatment Modalities

The NCCAM groups CAM practices into broad categories. These include: 1) natural products, 2) mind–body medicine, 3) manipulative and body-based practices, and 4) other CAM practices (NCCAM, 2008a). Each of these categories encompasses a wide range of subcategories. Many CAM practices may fit into more than one category.

Natural Products

Natural products include a variety of herbal medicines (also known as botanicals), vitamins, minerals, and other "natural products." Many of these products are sold as dietary supplements. Natural products also include probiotics—live microorganisms (usually bacteria) that are similar to microorganisms normally found in the human digestive tract. Probiotics are available in foods such as yogurts or in dietary supplements. In the 2007 NHIS survey, this category of CAM was the most frequently used with 17.7% of those surveyed using natural products (Barnes et al., 2008).

The federal government regulates dietary supplements primarily through the U.S. Food and Drug Administration (FDA). The regulations for dietary supplements are not the same as those for prescription or over-the-counter drugs. In general, the guidelines are less strict. For example, a manufacturer does not have to prove the safety and effectiveness of a dietary supplement before it is marketed. Once a dietary supplement is on the market, the FDA monitors safety and product information, and the Federal Trade Commission (FTC) monitors advertising (NCCAM, 2008a).

The NCCAM website provides a series of fact sheets on herbs and botanicals and includes common names, uses, potential side effects, and other resources for more information. The fact sheets are included in a free booklet published by NIH and NCCAM (2011e).

The National Standard (http://www.natural-standard.com) was founded by healthcare providers and researchers to provide quality evidence-based information about CAM. Each Natural Standard monograph on CAM is prepared using a variety of electronic databases including the Cochrane Library and MEDLINE.

Their findings on herbs and supplements is compiled in a book, *Davis's Pocket Guide to Herbs and Supplements* (Ulbricht, 2011). This source includes information on more than 600 products. It is organized like a traditional pharmacology pocket guide.

Another source of information about natural products is the Natural Medicines Comprehensive Database (http://naturaldatabase.therapeuticresearch.com/). This website states it is unbiased, scientific clinical information on complementary, alternative, and integrative therapies.

Dietary supplements are defined under the Dietary Supplement Health and Education Act of 1994 (Zarowitz, 2010a). Manufacturers need to register themselves pursuant to the Bioterrorism Act with the FDA before producing or selling supplements. The United States Pharmacopeia (USP) is also involved in CAM because it has established criteria for levels of evidence that can be used to evaluate the literature on efficacy and safety of dietary supplements. Only products with moderate to high quality evidence are approved by the USP (p. 125).

Older adults are the largest per capita consumers of prescription medications and over-the-counter (OTC) complementary and alternative medicines in the United States (Qato et al., 2008). Part of this could be due to the increase in chronic disease as we age, as well as efforts to counter undesirable effects of the aging process. The combination of an OTC dietary supplement and a prescribed medication could have serious side effects, particularly in the older adult. In a Mayo Clinic study of 1795 adults averaging 55 years of age, there were 107 dietary supplement–drug interactions of significance (cited in Zarowitz, 2010b), The five supplements accounting for 68% of the interactions were kava, garlic, ginkgo biloba, St. John's wort, and valerian. The prescription medications most frequently implicated included: warfarin, sedatives/hypnotics, antidepressants, insulin, oral antidiabetic agents, hepatotoxic medications, oral contraceptives, and tramadol. Additionally, more than 78 dietary supplements have some effect on the CYP enzymes most commonly involved with drug metabolism (Zarowitz, 2010b).

Mind–Body Medicine

For practitioner-based therapies, there is no standardized, national system for credentialing CAM practitioners. The extent and type of credentialing vary greatly from state to state. Some CAM practitioners (e.g., chiropractic) are licensed in all or most states. Other CAM practitioners are licensed in few states or not at all (NCCAM, 2008a).

Mind–body practices focus on interactions among the brain, mind, body, and behavior. The intent is to use the mind to affect physical functioning and thus promote health. There are a wide variety of practices within this category. The main practices include: meditation, yoga, acupuncture, deep-breathing exercises, guided imagery, hypnotherapy, progressive relaxation, Qigong, and tai chi (see Table 18.1). Acupuncture is also a component of energy medicine, manipulative and body-based practices, and traditional Chinese medicine (NCCAM, 2008a). Use of three of these practices—deep-breathing exercises, meditation, and yoga—increased significantly in the 2007 NHIS survey compared with the 2002 NHIS survey.

Acupuncture has been practiced in China and other Asian countries for thousands of years. It has been practiced in the United States for 200 years. The FDA approved the acupuncture needle as a medical device in 1996 (National Cancer Institute, 2011). Acupuncture has been used in a

Table 18-1 Mind–Body Medicine

Approach	Therapeutic Method	Rationale
Meditation	Refers to a group of techniques such as mantra meditation, relaxation response, mindfulness meditation, and Zen Buddhist meditation; elements include a quiet location, specific comfortable position, focus of attention, and an open attitude	Practice is believed to result in a state of greater calmness and physical relaxation and psychological balance due to person learning to focus attention
Yoga	Combines physical postures, breathing exercises, meditation, and the spirit	Enhances stress-coping mechanism and mind–body awareness
Acupuncture	Thin needles are inserted superficially on the skin in various patterns and left in place for 8 to 20 minutes	Points along channels of energy are manipulated to restore balance; acupuncture is part of Traditional Chinese Medicine

Sources: National Center for Complementary and Alternative Medicine. (2007a). *Acupuncture: An introduction.* Retrieved August 30, 2011, from: http://nccam.nih.gov/health/acupuncture/introduction.htm; National Center for Complementary and Alternative Medicine. (2008c). *Yoga for health: An introduction.* Retrieved August 30, 2011, from: http://nccam.nih.gov/health/yoga/introduction.htm#keypoints; National Center for Complementary and Alternative Medicine. (2006a). *Meditation: An introduction.* Retrieved August 30, 2011, from: http://nccam.nih.gov/health/meditation/overview.htm#keypoints.

wide variety of chronic conditions. A review of the Cochrane Database reveals three systematic reviews on acupuncture. Reviews include depression, chronic asthma, and stroke rehabilitation. The 2010 update of the original 2005 systematic review of acupuncture for depression now includes data from 30 studies. These 30 studies included 2812 participants in the meta-analysis. Two clinical trials found acupuncture may have an additive benefit when combined with medication compared to medication alone. However, the authors' conclusion was that there was insufficient evidence to recommend the use of acupuncture for people with depression. Further, the results are limited by the high risk of bias in the majority of trials meeting inclusion criteria (Smith, Hay, & Macpherson, 2010).

An updated review of a 2003 review of randomized clinical trials of acupuncture for chronic asthma included 12 studies with 350 participants meeting the inclusion criteria. Trial reporting was poor and trial quality inadequate. The conclusion of the authors was there was no change in the 2003 conclusion of insufficient evidence to make any recommendations of acupuncture in asthma treatment. (McCarney, Brinkhaus, Lasserson, & Linde, 2009)

Five clinical trials of 368 participants met the inclusion criteria in a systematic review of acupuncture and stroke rehabilitation. These trials included both ischemic and hemorrhagic stroke in the subacute or chronic stage. There was no evidence of any effects of acupuncture on subacute or chronic stroke. This was an update to a 2006 Cochrane review (Wu et al., 2009).

Manipulative and Body-Based Practices

These practices focus on the structures and systems of the body and include the bones and joints, soft tissues, and circulatory and lymphatic systems. Spinal manipulation (chiropractic) and massage therapy are the primary practices within this area. (NCCAM, 2008b). See Table 8-2.

Massage therapy is based on the principle that body tissues will function at optimal levels when arterial supply and venous and lymphatic drainage are unimpeded. Massage is designed to reestablish proper fluid dynamics through the skin, muscles, and fascia, although nerve pathways may sometimes be included (Coughlin & Delany, 2011). Massage is generally applied in the direction of the heart to stimulate increased venous and lymphatic drainage from the involved tissues with muscles being addressed in groups. Different combinations of techniques are used depending on the objectives of the treatment; however, all five basic techniques are of the passive variety, meaning that the practitioner does all of the work (Coughlin & Delany, 2011).

A 2011 review of Cochrane Systematic Reviews revealed several reviews of massage therapy, all associated with a specific disorder. One condition that is typically associated with the use of massage therapy is low back pain. Massage in the Cochrane review was defined as soft tissue manipulation using hands or a mechanical device on any body part. Thirteen randomized trials with 1596 participants were included in the review (Furlan, Imamura, Dryden, & Irvin, 2008). The authors concluded that massage might be beneficial for patients with subacute and chronic nonspecific low back pain, especially when combined with exercises and education.

The main emphasis of chiropractic care is on the spine and its effects to the central nervous system, the autonomic nervous system, and the peripheral nervous system. Chiropractors

Table 18-2	**Manipulative and Body-Based Practices**	
Approach	**Therapeutic Method**	**Rationale**
Massage	Encompasses many techniques. Therapists press, rub, and manipulate the muscles and other soft tissues of the body.	Numerous theories about how massage therapy may affect the body. One is the gate control theory that suggests that massage helps to block pain signals to the brain. Other theories suggest that massage stimulates the release of certain chemicals in the body
Reflexology	A practice in which pressure is applied to points on the foot and sometimes the hand with the intent to promote relaxation or healing in other parts of the body	There are "reflex" areas on the feet and hands that correspond to specific organs (e.g., tips of the toes and the head)
Chiropractic medicine	Adjustments, high-velocity, and low-amplitude thrusts are made on the spinal column. Focuses on the relationship between body's structure, mainly the spine, and its functioning	Rearranging displaced structures promotes healing, improves functioning, and decreases pain.

Source: National Center for Complementary and Alternative Medicine. (2006c). *Massage therapy: An introduction.* Retrieved August 30, 2011, from: http://nccam.nih.gov/health/massage/massageintroduction.htm; National Center for Complementary and Alternative Medicine. (2010b). *Irritable bowel syndrome and CAM: At a glance.* Retrieved August 30, 2011, from: http://nccam.nih.gov/health/digestive/IrritableBowelSyndrome.htm; National Center for Complementary and Alternative Medicine. (2007b). *Chiropractic.* Retrieved August 30, 2011, from: http://nccam.nih.gov/health/chiropractic/; National Center for Complementary and Alternative Medicine. (2006b). *What is reflexology?* Retrieved August 30, 2011, from: http://altmedicine.about.com/od/therapiesfromrtoz/a/Reflexology.htm

emphasize that adjusting the spinal joints and resolving subluxations restore normal nerve function and optimal health (Freeman, 2009). A Cochrane systematic review examined 12 studies involving 2887 participants with low back pain who were using combined chiropractic interventions. The authors concluded that combined chiropractic interventions slightly improved pain and disability in the short-term and pain in the medium-term for acute and subacute lower back pain. However, there is no current evidence that supports or refutes that these interventions provide a clinically meaningful difference for pain or disability when compared with other interventions (Walker, French, Grant, & Green, 2010).

Other CAM Practices

This broad category includes:

- Western and Eastern movement therapies such as Pilates, Rolfing, and the Feldenkrais method
- Traditional healers

- Manipulation of energy fields, such as magnet therapy, qigong, Reiki, and healing touch
- Whole medical systems such as Ayurvedic medicine, traditional Chinese medicine, homeopathy, and naturopathy (see Table 18-3)

Chronic Disease and CAM

Increasing numbers of individuals with chronic disease are using complementary and/or alternative medicine. When traditional (i.e, Western) approaches to treating and managing chronic

Table 18-3   Other CAM Practices

Approach	Therapeutic Method	Rationale
Qigong	Self-initiated moving meditation consisting of movement, self-massage, meditation, and breathing. It is a combination of Qi (life-force, energy, creativity, consciousness, breath, function) and gong (cultivation or practice over time).	Qigong puts the body into the relaxation/ regeneration state where the autonomic nervous system is predominately in the parasympathetic mode.
Traditional Chinese medicine	All aspects of the person are interconnected and interact with the environment. Acupuncture, herbs, and nutrition are used to promote health and internal and external balance.	Health and healing result from determining and resolving imbalances of energy flow in the body. Central to TCM is yin-yang theory; qi which circulates in the body through a system of pathways called meridians; the use of 8 principles to analyze symptoms and categorize conditions and 5 elements to explain how the body works (these elements correspond to organs and tissues in the body)
Homeopathic Medicine	A whole medical system based on the principle of similars (or "like cures like"). Remedies are made from naturally occurring substances from plants, minerals, or animals. Common remedies include red onion, arnica, and stinging nettle plant.	This whole medical system seeks to stimulate the body's ability to heal itself by giving very small doses of highly diluted substances based on the principle of similars.
Reiki	Japanese technique for stress reduction and relaxation that promotes spiritual healing and self-improvement; administered through laying on of hands	An unseen "life force energy" flows through us and is what causes us to be alive. If that energy is low, the likelihood of getting sick or feeling stress is high. Reiki is not taught in the traditional sense of the word, but is transferred to a student during an "attunement" in a Reiki class given by a Reiki master.

Sources: Qigong Institute. (2004–2011). *What is Qigong?* Retrieved August 30, 2011, from: http://www.qigonginstitute.org/ html/qigonghealth.php#AboutQigong; International Center for Reiki Training. (1990–2011). *What is Reiki?* http://www.reiki. org/FAQ/WhatIsReiki.html; NCCAM. (2009b). *Traditional Chinese medicine: An introduction.* Retrieved September 11, 2011, from http://nccam.nih.gov/health/whatiscam/chinesemed.htm; NCCAM. (2009a). *Homeopathy: An introduction.* Retrieved September 11, 2011, from http://nccam.nih.gov/health/homeopathy/; NCCAM. (2006d). *Reiki: An introduction.* Retrieved September 11, 2011, from http://nccam.nih.gov/health/reiki/introduction.htm

disease, whether benign or terminal, are ineffective, individuals and their families begin looking for alternatives. This section of the chapter focuses on two conditions of morbidity and mortality in the United States: hypertension and cancer.

Hypertension

Researchers examined the adverse effects of complementary and alternative medicine use on antihypertensive medication adherence in 2180 adults age 65 and older. CAM use was described as health food, herbal supplements, and relaxation therapy. In this cohort of managed care patients, CAM use was associated with low adherence to antihypertensive medication among blacks, but not whites (Krousel-Wood et al., 2010).

Jain and Mills (2010) conducted a systematic review of biofield therapies (Reiki, therapeutic touch, and healing touch) on hypertension. There was little evidence that biofield therapies reduced systolic blood pressure, and conflicting evidence that biofield therapies reduced diastolic blood pressure when compared with no treatment (p. 12).

In a study to assess the efficacy of acupuncture for treatment of essential hypertension, Kim and Zhu (2010) found no evidence to support the role of acupuncture in individuals with hypertension. Further, they noted that there was a lack of rigorous trials and needed better designed and powered studies to reach any conclusions.

Acupuncture, as a part of Traditional Chinese Medicine, has been used to treat hypertension in China for a long time. However, how this mechanism works is unclear. A group of Chinese researchers have created an intervention protocol through the Cochrane Hypertension Group. This review, created by Yang and colleagues (2010), will quantify blood pressure–lowering effects of acupuncture in adults with primary hypertension. Unique to this review is that studies that are included must have a control group of either placebo or sham acupuncture or no treatment.

CANCER

Jain and Mills (2010) conducted a systematic review of 66 clinical studies examining the use and effectiveness of biofield therapies (Reiki, therapeutic touch, and healing touch) in a variety of individuals with different chronic conditions. In their review they noted that there was moderate evidence (Level 2) for positive effects on acute cancer pain. There was conflicting evidence for longer term pain, cancer-related fatigue, quality of life, and physiologic indicators of the relaxation response (p. 10).

Complementary and alternative therapies are often used in symptom management in individuals with cancer. Boon, Olatunde, and Zick (2007) reported that 80% of their sample of 1434 women with breast cancer used CAM for symptom management (p. 58). To better understand this statistic, Wyatt, Sikorskii, Wills, and An (2010) used secondary data analysis in a sample of 222 Stage I and Stage II stage breast cancer patients to explore the association of CAM use, spending on CAM therapies, demographic variables, surgical treatment, and quality of life. Overall 58.2% of the women used CAM—specifically the biologically based therapies—77 women used vitamins, 25 used audiotapes, 18 used massage, and 17 used spiritual healing. Alternative medical systems were used in 13 women. Counts from individual therapies do not add up to the total category type because some women used more than one CAM therapy. Individuals reporting lower quality of life are highly likely to use CAM therapies (Wyatt et al., 2010).

Telephone interviews were conducted to ascertain CAM use among breast cancer (BRCA) mutation carriers enrolled in a high-risk breast and ovarian cancer screening study. Of the 164 BRCA 1 or BRCA 2 women in the analysis, 78% reported CAM use of prayer and lifestyle diet as the most commonly reported modalities. Using three or more CAM therapies was reported in 34% of the women. CAM use was associated with older age, higher education level, and higher levels of ovarian cancer worry (Mueller et al., 2008).

In a study funded by the National Cancer Institute, NCCAM, and the National Institute on Aging, researchers examined the interface between allopathic medical providers and CAM providers in a sample of older women with breast cancer. The qualitative study interviewed 44 women who were approximately 5 years post-diagnosis. For all but four women, a diagnosis of breast cancer was not the catalyst for CAM use. The women highly valued their simultaneous relationships with both their CAM provider and their biomedical provider. Although the study focused on the interface of different practitioners, core results of the study reflected on broader beliefs of health, illness, and aging (Adler, Wrubel, Hughes, & Beinfield, 2009).

There are frequently studies in the literature on the use of CAM to prevent cancer, treat cancer, and control symptoms. In the October 2010 *NCCAM Clinical Digest,* the focus of the issue was "Cancer and CAM: What the Science Says." The following is a summary of the findings:

- A 2007 review of clinical trials looking at the effectiveness of multivitamin/mineral supplements for cancer prevention found that few such trials have been conducted and that the results of most large-scale trials have been mixed. According to the National Cancer Institute, the following

have been studied but have not been shown to lower the risk of cancer: vitamins B_6, B_{12}, E, and C; beta-carotene; folic acid; and selenium.

- A 2008 review of 20 clinical trials found no convincing evidence that antioxidant supplements prevent gastrointestinal cancer, but did find indications that some might actually increase overall mortality. The review looked at beta-carotene, selenium, and vitamins A, C, and E. Selenium alone demonstrated some preventive benefits.

- Research from the National Cancer Institute notes that higher intake of calcium may be associated with reduced risk of colorectal cancer, but concludes that the available evidence does not support taking calcium supplements to prevent colorectal cancer.

- A 2008 review of the research concluded that some botanicals used in Ayurvedic medicine and Traditional Chinese Medicine may have a role in cancer treatment. However, scientific evidence is limited as much of the research on botanicals and cancer treatment is in the early stages.

- It is unclear whether the use of vitamin and mineral supplements by patients with cancer is beneficial or harmful. There is a concern that some supplements might interfere with the cancer treatment.

- A 2008 evidence-based review of clinical options for managing nausea and vomiting in cancer patients noted that electroacupuncture was an option to be considered. A study of 380 patients with advanced cancer concluded that massage therapy may offer some limited relief for these patients. A 2008 review of botanical research concluded that some botanicals have shown promise in managing the side effects of cancer treatment. However, the reviewers did not find sufficient evidence to recommend any specific treatment (NCCAM, 2010a).

ISSUES

Issues concerning alternative and complementary therapies include research, dissemination of information, legislative matters, and quackery.

Research

The mission of the NCCAM is to define, through rigorous scientific investigation, the usefulness and safety of complementary and alternative medicine interventions and their roles in improving health and health care (2011b). The NCCAM funds scientific research on CAM and the training of CAM researchers. In fiscal year 2010, the budget of the NCCAM was $128.8 million. Despite what may seem like a large budget, NCCAM was able to fund only 12% of the proposals that it received (2008 data).

There are challenges in designing rigorous research studies to evaluate alternative and complementary therapies. Determining the correct therapy, amount to be administered, and population to receive the treatment is essential in order to test effectiveness, but is particularly challenging when these parameters are not standardized in the practice arena. Criticisms of research on alternative and complementary treatments include the following: Studies often do not use hypothesis testing, large numbers of subjects, or randomly assign subjects to treatment and control groups; and they often rely on subjective responses from clients rather than objective measures.

Bausell (2009) reviewed 45 CAM efficacy randomized controlled trials (RCTs) from four high-impact journals: *New England Journal of Medicine*, *Journal of the American Medicine Association*, *Annals of Internal Medicine,* and *Archives of Internal Medicine*. Bausell's review was based on three validity criteria: the existence of a placebo control, moderate attrition rates, and 50 or more participants in each group of the sample. Of the 26 trials meeting all three criteria, only two were judged to be supportive of the CAM therapy, while more than half (55.5%) of the 19 trials failed to meet one or more of the criteria reported positive results (p < 0.001). Of the two positive high validity trials, one was funded and authored by the herbal company marketing the product tested, and one used a placebo control group of questionable credibility (p. 349).

In several systematic reviews generated by the Cochrane Collaboration, it was noted that bias was present. Although there may have been many studies examined in a systematic review, Cochrane authors often note that there are few randomized clinical trials that meet study criteria. Walker and colleagues (2010), in their review of chiropractic and low back pain, note that of the studies they reviewed, there were none that looked at chiropractic interventions versus no treatment. Kim and Zhu (2010), in their review of acupuncture and hypertension, note that there was a lack of rigorous trials. Further, Jain and Mills (2010), in their systematic review, stated that the studies were of average quality and met minimum standards required for validity. Only 6 out of 67 studies reviewed reported an effect size. It is noted that their review reports a lower overall study quality than previous authors have.

Examples of NCCAM–funded research include: randomized study of tai chi in the management of chronic heart failure; randomized study of the effects of massage on the immune system of preterm infants; analysis of U.S. health surveys to examine CAM use among racial and ethnic minorities; research center grants to establish research centers to support basic and clinical research on botanicals and acupuncture (NCCAM, 2011c).

CASE STUDY

Mrs. Martin, a 70-year-old woman, developed rheumatoid arthritis when she was 18 years old. Her first symptoms were swelling in her left knee and ankle. She had just relocated from a rural community to a college town, where she worked as a secretary full-time and attended college part-time. She was in a great deal of pain when she went to see a physician. The physician drained her knee, performed various diagnostic tests, and informed her that she had rheumatoid arthritis. She was told to take 12 aspirin throughout the course of each day. No education regarding her illness, prognosis, or the potential side effects of her medication were provided. She was shy, deferred to authority figures, and was unprepared to advocate for herself.

She took a leave of absence from her job for a month, returned to the rural community in which she was raised, and rested. Her father had died when she was 4 years old. Her mother had an 8th-grade education. Her two older brothers and sisters lived nearby but were not actively involved in her life. After she had rested and began to feel a little better, she returned to her secretarial job and continued taking classes. Her left knee and both of her ankles remained swollen and painful, and the same symptoms developed in her fingers, wrists, and elbows. She had her knee drained and injected with steroid medication every other month; however, in a short time it would swell again. She felt fatigued and in pain.

Several years after her diagnosis, she married and had two children. During the course of her pregnancies, her arthritis symptoms totally resolved. After each of her children was born, her symptoms immediately came back. As the years went by, she was followed closely by her primary care physician and saw a number of internists and rheumatologists. She took a variety of nonsteroidal anti-inflammatory agents.

Her joints were periodically drained and injected with a steroid. She tried gold shots without any relief. She went to physical therapists and was careful to eat a healthy and well balanced diet. Over time, her wrists, elbows, fingers, and feet developed joint deformities and contractures. Despite the deformities and pain, she maintained an active lifestyle and balanced her household and maternal duties.

When she was 35, Mrs. Martin's symptoms became so severe that she was unable to do any work and was bedridden for 6 months. Because of her severe pain, she cried most of the time that she was awake. Her primary care doctor was empathetic but unable to help her. He referred her to a rheumatologist who failed to help relieve her suffering, but told her, "You're doing fine for having a case of rheumatoid arthritis that is so aggressive."

Mr. Martin began to actively read about arthritis and search for ways to help relieve some of his wife's suffering. The couple tried a number of dietary programs without success. One day a friend mentioned to Mr. Martin that he knew of a woman with rheumatoid arthritis who had been in a wheelchair and was now walking. Mr. Martin tracked the woman down, and she told him about an alternative treatment for arthritis that seemed miraculous and had changed her life.

CASE STUDY   (Continued)

Because this was an alternative treatment, governmental regulations prohibited it from being provided in the United States. Against the advice of her rheumatologist, Mrs. Martin went to Canada with her husband for therapy. Within 3 days, Mrs. Martin's pain and swelling were reduced. She was walking, had resumed her household duties, and felt more energetic and in less pain than she had felt in her adult life. The contractures that had developed did not go away, so she began to use an alternative treatment weekly—massages to help with mobility, muscle relaxation, and pain minimization.

Over the years, primary care physicians had not been willing to prescribe Mrs. Martin's alternative treatment, requiring her to travel yearly to get her medication. However, they have been amazed at the change in her health status. Currently, although several newer allopathic treatments for rheumatoid arthritis are available, she does not see a rheumatologist. In order to determine if any of these allopathic treatments were appropriate for her, Mrs. Martin consulted with seven different rheumatologists. Each chastised her for her long-term use of an alternative, unproven therapy and was unwilling to discuss transitioning her to one of the newer allopathic treatments unless she completely stopped her existing medication (in order for them to do several months of work-up). Consequently, since she is functioning well, considering the severity and length of time that she has had her disease, Mrs. Martin has opted to continue alternative treatment. She also has an array of vitamins, healthy nutrition, exercise, and rest. Mrs. Martin has been on this alternative regimen for 35 years. She adjusts her dosage daily in response to the presence of symptoms and continues to walk a half a mile each day, drive a car, do much of her own housework, and participate in social activities such as going to the opera.

Discussion Questions

1. What motivated Mrs. Martin to begin using alternative treatment for her rheumatoid arthritis?
2. What worked well for Mrs. Martin in the allopathic healthcare system, and what did not work well?
3. Healthcare professionals were absent from Mrs. Martin's care; what are some of the ways that they could have—or should have—been involved in her care?
4. How will you help individuals who have chronic illnesses and choose to use alternative treatments to meet their healthcare needs?
5. What would you do if you or one of your family members developed a chronic illness that was continuing to cause worsening disability and suffering and allopathic healthcare providers were unable to offer effective treatment options?
6. What is the healthcare professional's role in advocating for expanded practice, changes in the healthcare system, and an open-minded approach with regard to alternative treatments for individuals with chronic illnesses?

This case study was developed by Dr. Lisa Onega.

Barriers to research of nontraditional treatments include limited funding; lack of needed research skills among practitioners; lack of access to computers, academic libraries, and statistical support; problems obtaining suitable numbers of subjects; difficulty in comparing and interpreting research; and methodological issues such as individualized treatment and lack of control subjects for comparison. Ultimately, allopathic medicine demands scientific validation of the efficacy of a treatment on composite groups of patients using experimental and control groups, whereas nonallopathic therapies emphasize holistic, individualized treatment that is qualitative in nature. Therefore, the two therapeutic paradigms may lend themselves to different types of evaluative research (Boozang, 2003; Oguamanam, 2006).

Individuals with chronic illnesses who have had positive outcomes using nontraditional therapies believe their experiences to be valid and significant. They reject the dismissal of their results as anecdotal and inconsequential and support increased case study methodology to validate and explain their experiences (Boozang, 2003; Isaacs, 2007).

Dissemination of Information

Journals developed for healthcare practitioners to address alternative, complementary, and integrative treatments include: *Alternative Therapies in Health and Medicine, Complementary Therapies in Medicine, Evidence Based Complementary and Alternative Medicine, Journal of Alternative and Complementary Medicine, BMC Complementary and Alternative Medicine, Journal of Holistic Nursing,* and *Research in Complementary Medicine.*

Coelho, Pittler, and Ernst (2007) in an effort to categorize knowledge dissemination and compare it with previously published categorizations from 1995 and 2000, examined the 2005 contents of six major journals that publish research on alternative, complementary, and integrative treatments. Fewer articles than in previous years were about clinical trials (1995 had 28%, 2000 had 23%, and 2005 had 22%). Several additional journals were also reviewed, which had not previously been included in the 2000 and 1995 investigations. With these articles included (n = 363), only 19% of the manuscripts were classified as clinical trials. None of the journals published meta-analyses, and only 4% of the articles included a systematic review of the state of the science. The most common articles were about general alternative, complementary, and integrative topics (20%), phytomedicine (standardized herbal treatments) (14%), and homeopathy (11%). This survey of the literature indicates that although the number of individuals with chronic illnesses is increasing, the evidence-based literature testing nonallopathic therapies to treat these individuals is decreasing. Clinicians who want to provide safe and effective options for their clients and families are in a quandary because they know that hope and options are essential both for treatment of disease and for healing the human spirit; however, they also know that scientific evaluation of treatment modalities is necessary.

Legislative Matters

Legal matters related to alternative and complementary therapies are discussed in the next two sections—paradigm issues and those specific to advanced practice nurses.

Paradigm Issues

Some critics of allopathic health care have argued that physicians, out of self-interest, have convinced legislators to restrict the scope of practice of alternative and complementary healthcare providers and limit choices for individuals with chronic illnesses. They believe that because physicians work closely with hospitals, pharmaceutical companies, and reimbursers, they have persuaded these organizations to avoid partnering with nontraditional healthcare providers. Therefore, according to these critics, physicians, hospitals, pharmaceutical companies, and reimbursers have influenced policy and legislation to limit these practices and, when possible, to prosecute nonphysician practitioners who offer competitive healthcare services (Boozang, 1998; Cuellar, Cahill, Ford, & Aycock, 2003).

Ultimately, a clash exists between proponents of the allopathic healthcare paradigm and proponents of the alternative and complementary healthcare paradigm. Advocates of the allopathic healthcare paradigm believe that governmental regulation is based on scientific evidence, promotes safety, and ensures that the treatment provided to persons with chronic illness is effective. Advocates of the nonallopathic healthcare paradigm believe that individuals should have access to information and treatment, the freedom to evaluate benefits and risks, and ultimately decide for themselves their form of health care (Cuellar et al., 2003; Oguamanam, 2006).

Advanced Practice Nursing Issues

Advanced practice nurses (APN) providing care to individuals with chronic illnesses are often concerned about whether activities related to alternative and complementary treatment fall within acceptable legal parameters. In addition, they are worried about liability protection as it relates to nontraditional therapies (College of Registered Nurses of British Columbia, 2006; Cuellar et al., 2003). For example, individuals with chronic illness who feel that they have exhausted allopathic options may ask an APN to prescribe or administer nonallopathic treatments. Clinicians may feel persuaded by anecdotal evidence, compassion for clients and their families, and the belief that the treatment is in their scope of practice; however, they may be concerned about how their state board of nursing or their malpractice insurers would view their prescribing or administering of the requested treatment. Contacting the board of nursing and their malpractice insurer to obtain other perspectives may provide useful feedback about the desired treatment and assist the APN in making wise decisions (Cuellar et al., 2003).

APNs should be aware that states differ regarding licensure of nonallopathic practitioners. For example, acupuncturists can refer to a website that describes the laws/regulation of acupuncture in each state (Acupuncture.com, 2011). There is no current uniform licensing or professional standards for the practice of homeopathy in the United State. The licensing of homeopaths varies from state to state. Licensure as a homeopathic physician is available only to medical doctors and doctors of osteopathy in Arizona, Connecticut, and Nevada. Some states explicitly include homeopathy within the scope of practice of chiropractic, naturopathy, physical therapy, dentistry, nursing, and veterinary medicine (NCCAM, 2009a).

Quackery

Although research verifying the effectiveness of most alternative, complementary, and integrative treatments is inadequate, practitioners have the responsibility to provide information regarding the known benefits and risks of the treatment (Chez & Jonas, 2005; Cuellar et al., 2003). When healthcare providers misrepresent treatments to consumers, they are committing fraud (Cuellar et al., 2003).

Boozang (1998) defines quackery as treatment that is implausible, unscientific, unproven, or disproved. She notes, however, that some non-allopathic treatments, although not yet adequately evaluated (unproven), may be helpful to clients. She emphasizes the importance of heightened informed consent for any treatments outside of the accepted standard of care. Cuellar and colleagues (2003) state that clinicians have a duty to present both traditional and nontraditional perspectives and assert that informed consent means providing information about allopathic and non-allopathic treatment options along with benefits, risks, and uncertainties associated with each choice.

Professional Education

Medical schools are realizing the importance of including alternative, complementary, and integrative therapies in curricula. In 1998, 63% of medical schools offered at least one course dedicated to this content and 37% offered two or more (Helms, 2006).

Nursing schools have been slower to include classes in alternative and complementary treatments. This material is often integrated throughout graduate and undergraduate curricula; however, few schools provide dedicated courses. Several schools have made a noteworthy commitment to nonallopathic theories. The University of Minnesota has incorporated alternative, complementary, and integrative content and research into its undergraduate, masters', and doctoral programs in nursing. The University of California at San Francisco was the first nurse practitioner program in the country to include this material in its curriculum. In order to prepare advanced practice nurses to properly care for individuals with chronic illnesses, nursing education needs to instruct students about these therapies (Helms, 2006).

For health professionals and consumers, the NCCAM has a page on its website listing alerts and advisories, many of which involve natural products. For example, 2011 advisories include:

- FDA warns consumers to stop using Soladek vitamin solution
- Recall of U-Prosta dietary supplement
- "Black Ant" contains undeclared drug ingredient
- Beware of fraudulent weight-loss "dietary supplements"
- Biotab Nutraceuticals, Inc., issues a voluntary recall of specific lots of the nutritional supplement EXTENZE (Men's Regular) (NCCAM, 2011f)

Ethical Decision Making

Healthcare professionals working with individuals who have chronic illnesses may experience ethical decision-making challenges related to the use of nonallopathic treatment. The following is one example. Thinking about one's values, beliefs, and rationale for decision-making will help prepare the advanced practice nurse for those unexpected and difficult challenges.

CASE STUDY

Dr. Smithton—A 58-Year-Old Man with Amyotrophic Lateral Sclerosis

Dr. Thomas Smithton, a 58-year-old man, is a professor and owns a successful mathematical consulting business. Thomas has been happily married for 32 years to his wife, Patricia, who is a geologist. They have three children—Samuel, who is 30, married, has two children, and lives across the country; Jenna, who is 27, married, and lives in another state; and Ben, who is 25 and in graduate school in another state. Although their children are grown and do not live nearby, Thomas and Patricia maintain a close relationship with them.

Throughout his adult life, Thomas has tried to maintain a healthy balance between work and family. He visits relatives once a year, has several good friends, and has many acquaintances. He eats healthy foods and exercises at a gym twice a week. He has never smoked cigarettes, used illegal drugs, or used alcohol excessively. He describes himself as a "high-energy person" and functions well on about 6 hours of sleep a night.

Thomas has been seeing Ms. Mason, a family nurse practitioner, for physical examinations and episodic visits for 15 years. He has excellent preventive health care and health habits. Thomas is known to Ms. Mason to always be on time for appointments, prepared, cooperative, and highly motivated. Ms. Mason considers him to be "the model patient, just an all around great guy." She provides care for the entire family and says that, "the whole family is special." She feels that long-term relationships like these are what make being an advanced practice nurse meaningful and rewarding.

About 2 years ago, Thomas set up an appointment with Ms. Mason because he was feeling weak, had tripped over the carpet several times, and was dropping things. Ms. Mason did a neurologic and muscle evaluation, laboratory work (including blood and urine studies with high-resolution serum protein electrophoresis, thyroid and parathyroid hormone levels, and 24-hour urine collection for heavy metals), and X-rays. She also referred him to a neurologist for further evaluation. The neurologist diagnosed him with amyotrophic lateral sclerosis (ALS), also known as Lou Gehrig's disease.

Thomas has been a model patient in living with his ALS; however, his illness has progressed. About a year and a half ago he took disability from his job at the university, and several months later closed his consulting business. Patricia took family medical leave for 6 months to modify their house for a person with a disability, made sure that business and legal matters such as power of attorney and advance directives were updated, and hired around-the-clock, live-in care. She has gone back to work out of financial necessity. Thomas's treatment team includes physical, occupational, and speech therapists; rehabilitation specialists; and two neurologists. He now uses a motorized wheelchair and is unable to feed himself or do any activities of daily living on his own.

(continues)

CASE STUDY   (Continued)

Thomas's mind remains alert, and he and his wife have used the Internet to look for treatment options. They recognize that gold treatment is a long shot but have spoken to three individuals with ALS in different states who have experienced remission using gold treatment. These individuals have sent information regarding their dosage and where they obtained their medication. In addition, Thomas and Patricia have read information from homeopathic, alternative, and anecdotal sources that explain the rationale, procedures, dosing, and prescribing information for gold in ALS treatment. They have provided this information to their two neurologists, who have dismissed their requests to have this information reviewed.

Thomas and Patricia have a long-standing relationship with Ms. Mason; they trust her and know that she cares about them as individuals, so they share the information that they have gathered with her and ask her if she would be willing to order gold treatment for Thomas. They say that they understand that she may feel uncomfortable with this request, but they ask her to put herself in their position, think about the evidence that they have provided, and make a fair-minded decision. They also state that they will be happy to sign any type of form stating that they understand that this is not the usual treatment but that under the circumstances, they want to take the risk because they feel that the risk of trying this treatment outweighs the benefit of not trying the treatment.

Nurse practitioners in the state in which Ms. Mason works are independent. They are governed exclusively by the Board of Nursing. They do not practice under the supervision of physicians or as physician extenders. They are expected to abide by the regulations of the Board of Nursing and provide care within their scope of practice. Ms. Mason contacts the Board of Nursing to obtain further clarification. The board representative says that if she is knowledgeable about a treatment and deems it to be appropriate, she should document her rationale and provide the treatment. Ms. Mason contacts her malpractice insurance company, but is unable to speak with a lawyer. The service representative tells her that careful documentation of care is necessary. She consults a trusted colleague and asks him about the case. He says that there is "no way" that he would ever prescribe a medication that was not approved by the FDA.

Ms. Mason cares about Thomas. She has worked with him for 15 years and knows that he is a thorough, reliable, and careful person. She understands that he is suffering from an incurable disease and that allopathic treatments offer no hope. She believes that trust and offering hope are the most valuable interventions that an advanced practice nurse can provide to a person with a chronic illness. She has talked to both Thomas and Patricia and knows that they are not looking for a cure or a miracle; they are looking for some relief of suffering, improved quality of life, and a little extra time together. She worries that other practitioners may question her judgment and even file a complaint against her to the Board of Nursing. Because she has not spoken to

CASE STUDY (Continued)

Thomas and Patricia's children about this treatment, she is concerned that one of them may be angry about their father's illness and may file a lawsuit against her at some point in the future.

Discussion Questions

1. What should Ms. Mason do? What would you do?
2. How do ethical principles affect your decision?
3. How can you, as a practitioner, emotionally support the family even though you do not believe they should participate in the gold treatment?
4. How do your own values and beliefs influence your decisions in this situation?

This case study was developed by Dr. Lisa Onega.

INTERVENTIONS

Healthcare professionals considering the role of alternative and complementary treatment in the care of individuals with chronic illnesses need to be aware of their life experiences and feelings, promote wise decision making, deliver safe and effective care, and be informed about legal issues.

Self-Reflection

Healthcare professionals need to be aware of their own feelings about alternative and complementary treatments as they relate to chronic illness. Typically, most healthcare professionals are comfortable with complementary treatment; however, personal experience influences how they view alternative therapies that replace allopathic methods. Understanding one's own experiences and beliefs is essential in order to be present with individuals with chronic illnesses and understand their fears, concerns, motivations, and needs, without burdening them with personal biases that may inhibit them from making the wisest choices for their circumstances (Burman, 2003).

Decision Making

Healthcare professionals espouse individualized, holistic, and healing care; this requires considering the unique aspects, goals, and needs of each individual with a chronic illness. It is essential to partner with patients and view them as human beings, not cases with diseases (Burman, 2003; Chez & Jonas, 2005; Helms, 2006; Sleath et al., 2005; Wagner et al., 2005). Care should be accessible, affordable, compassionate, effective, efficient, evidence based, patient focused, safe, and timely (Bezold, 2005; Chez & Jonas, 2005). To facilitate wise decision making on the part of the patient, the healthcare professional should address the following information with their patients:

- Find out all information about safety of the product.
- Look for warning signs; if it sounds too good to be true, it probably is.

- Be alert for new information; do your research on the CAM modality.
- Never try to diagnose or treat your own condition.
- Talk to your healthcare provider.
- Ask your healthcare provider for advice.
- Make a plan with your healthcare provider; how will the therapy fit into your medical treatment plan?
- Be open and honest.
- Ask your healthcare provider if he or she can refer you to someone knowledgeable about CAM.
- Share information you have about your therapy with your healthcare provider.
- Tell your healthcare provider about any CAM you are using and its benefits.
- Obtain licensing requirements for CAM practitioners in the state.
- Visit the CAM practitioner before your treatment and observe how the patients are treated.
- Consider the cost of the therapy, and talk with your insurance company to find out whether services are covered.
- Ask the CAM provider important questions such as: Have you ever treated conditions like mine? Is the treatment effective? How long will it take for me to see results? Are you willing to work with my healthcare provider? (Cuella, Rogers, & Hisghman, 2007).

Although these teaching instructions were originally created for older adults, they apply to everyone.

Legal Implications

Healthcare professionals wishing to incorporate alternative or complementary treatments into their activities should be certain that therapies comply with federal, state, and local licensure and regulatory requirements. Close adherence to governmental requirements is challenging but necessary, as many of the individuals monitoring adherence to these requirements may have little understanding of nontraditional therapies (Burman, 2003; Cuellar et al., 2003; Helms, 2006).

Although individuals with chronic illnesses often use alternative or complementary treatments, healthcare professionals are challenged to maintain a balance between providing these therapies and protecting the public from potentially harmful interventions. Education about nonallopathic treatments can enable healthcare professionals to intelligently differentiate between clinical innovations that do not harm individuals and offer them hope and fraudulent or harmful treatments that rob individuals of dignity and economic resources (Burman, 2003; Cuellar et al., 2003; Cuellar et al., 2007; Sleath et al., 2005).

Healthcare professionals should share conceptual and evidence-based information about alternative and complementary treatments with colleagues, legislators, and reimbursers. Regulatory reform to facilitate a flexible scope of practice with rigorous competency requirements will not only ensure public safety but will also enable clinicians to practice to the full extent of their preparation, improve access to nontraditional therapies, and promote cost-effective treatment options. Although existing state practice acts vary, they do not prohibit healthcare professionals from providing nonallopathic treatments. As knowledge increases, state practice acts need to be revised to incorporate healthcare professionals' rights to provide these services (Burman, 2003; Cuellar et al., 2003).

Evidence-Based Practice Box

Researchers in the United Kingdom explored how 35 patients integrated CAM and orthodox medicine (OM) or traditional medicine in self-managing their chronic illness (Brien et al., 2011). Semistructured interviews were conducted with individuals who had a chronic benign condition for 12 months or longer and who were using CAM practices along with traditional medicine. Seven categories were developed from the interview data and included: 1) using CAM to maintain OM use, 2) using OM to support long-term CAM use, 3) using CAM to reduce OM, 4) using CAM to avoid OM, 5) using CAM to replace OM, 6) maximizing relief using both CAM and OM, and 7) returning to OM. These seven categories were neither mutually exclusive nor static. Changes in clients' behavior occurred over time and were related to their treatment experiences which either reinforced existing beliefs or inspired new beliefs (p. e94). Clients used OM and CAM practices and integrated both approaches in managing their chronic illness. Given the nature of clients' decisions and beliefs changing over time, an ongoing discussion between CAM and OM practitioners is necessary..

Source: Brien, S. B., Bishop, F. L., Riggs, K., Stevenson, D., Freire, V., & Lewith, G. (2011, February). Integrated medicine in the management of chronic illness: A qualitative study. *British Journal of General Practice*. doi: 10.3399/bjgp11X556254

OUTCOMES

Healthcare professionals caring for individuals with chronic illnesses need to balance an open-minded view of alternative and complementary treatments with a scientific, evidence-based perspective. Healthcare professionals are in a unique position to bridge the gap between allopathic and nonallopathic health care by melding compassion, flexibility, and commitment to scientific and clinical excellence with common sense.

Individuals with chronic diseases are not having their needs met by the existing healthcare system, which is hampered by the dichotomous relationship between traditional and nontraditional schools of thought. The disciplinary perspective of healthcare professionals enables them to offer these individuals alternative and complementary options that address their specific circumstances.

ACKNOWLEDGMENT

Many thanks to Lisa Onega for her contribution to this chapter in the previous edition.

STUDY QUESTIONS

Why do individuals with chronic illnesses use nontraditional treatments?

What are the four categories of alternative and complementary treatments outlined by the NCCAM?

How common is using nonallopathic therapy in the United States?

Why is researching alternative and complementary treatments challenging?

(continues)

Study Questions (Cont.)   WWW

What are some of the legislative issues associated with nontraditional treatments?

How do nursing and medical school curricula differ regarding alternative and complementary treatments?

How does self-awareness regarding nonallopathic therapies relate to providing unbiased care for individuals with chronic illnesses?

How can healthcare professionals help individuals with chronic illnesses make decisions regarding alternative and complementary treatments?

What factors need to be considered when providing safe and effective nonallopathic interventions to individuals with chronic illnesses?

What legal issues do healthcare professionals need to consider when providing nontraditional treatments?

For a full suite of assignments and additional learning activities,   WWW
use the access code located in the front of your book and visit this exclusive website: **http://go.jblearning.com/larsen**. If you do not have an access code, you can obtain one at the site.

REFERENCES _____

Acupuncture.com. (2011). *State laws*. Retrieved August 30, 2011, from: http://www.acupuncture.com/statelaws/statelaw.htm#2

Adler, S. R., Wrubel, J., Hughes, E., & Beinfield, H. (2009). Patients' interactions with physicians and complementary and alternative medicine practitioners: Older women with breast cancer and self-managed health care. *Integrative Cancer Therapy, 8*(1), 63–70.

Barnes, P. M., Bloom, B., & Nahin, R. L. (2008). *Complementary and alternative medicine use among adults and children: United States, 2007* (National Health Statistics Reports, No. 12). Hyattsville, MD: National Center for Health Statistics.

Bausell, R. B. (2009). Are positive alternative medical therapy trials credible? Evidence from four high-impact medical journals. *Evaluation and the Health Professions, 32*(4), 349–369.

Bezold, C. (2005). The future of patient-centered care: Scenarios, visions, and audacious goals. *The Journal of Alternative and Complementary Medicine, 11*(Suppl. 1), 77–84.

Boon, H. S., Olatunde, F., & Zick, S. M. (2007). Trends in complementary/alternative use by breast cancer survivors: Comparing survey data from 1998 and 2005. *BMC Women's Health, 30*(7), 4.

Boozang, K. M. (1998). Western medicine opens the door to alternative medicine. *American Journal of Law and Medicine, 24*(2–3), 185–212.

Boozang, K. M. (2003). National policy on CAM: The White House Commission report. *The Journal of Law, Medicine and Ethics, 31*(2), 251–261.

Brien, S. B., Bishop, F. L., Riggs, K., Stevenson, D., Freire, V., & Lewith, G. (2011, February). Integrated medicine in the management of chronic illness: A qualitative study. *British Journal of General Prac*tice. doi: 10.3399/bjgp11X556254

Briggs, J. (2007). Audio file about the 2007 National Health Interview survey CAM use data. Retrieved August 30, 2011, from: http://nccam.nih.gov/news/multimedia/audio/nhisaudio.htm

Burman, M. E. (2003). Complementary and alternative medicine: Core competencies for family nurse practitioners. *Journal of Nursing Education, 42*(1), 28–34.

Chez, R. A., & Jonas, W. B. (2005). Challenges and opportunities in achieving healing. *The Journal of Alternative and Complementary Medicine, 11*(Suppl. 1), 3–6.

Coelho, H. F., Pittler, M. H., & Ernst, E. (2007). An investigation of the contents of complementary and alternative medicine journals. *Alternative Therapies in Health and Medicine, 13*(4), 40–44.

College of Registered Nurses of British Columbia. (2006). Complementary and alternative health care: The role of the nurse. *Nursing-bc, 38*(3), 20–22.

Coughlin, P., & Delany, J. (2011). Massage and touch therapies. In M. Micozzi (Ed.), *Fundamentals of complementary and alternative medicine* (4th ed., pp. 211–231). St. Louis: Saunders Elsevier.

Cuellar, N. G., Cahill, B., Ford, J., & Aycock, T. (2003). The development of an educational workshop on complementary and alternative medicine: What every nurse should know. *The Journal of Continuing Education in Nursing, 34*(3), 128–135.

Cuellar, N. G., Rogers, A. E., & Hisghman, V. (2007). Evidenced based research of complementary and alternative medicine (CAM) for sleep in the community dwelling older adult. *Geriatric Nursing, 28*(1), 46–52.

Freeman, L. (2009). Chiropractic. In L. Freeman (Ed.), *Mosby's complementary and alternative medicine: A research based approach* (3rd ed., pp. 283–309). St. Louis: Mosby Elsevier.

Furlan, A. D., Imamura, M., Dryden, T., & Irvin, E. (2008). Massage for low back pain. *Cochrane Database of Systematic Reviews*, Issue 4. Art..No:. CD001929. doi: 10.1002/14651858. CD001929.pub2

Helms, J. E. (2006). Complementary and alternative therapies: A new frontier for nursing education? *Journal of Nursing Education, 45*(3), 117–123.

Isaacs, L. L. (2007). Evaluating anecdotes and case reports. *Alternative Therapies in Health and Medicine, 13*(2), 36–38.

Jain, S., & Mills, P. J. (2010). Biofield therapies: Helpful or full of hype? A best evidence synthesis. *International Journal of Behavioral Medicine, 17*, 1–16.

Kaptchuk, T. J., & Eisenberg, D. M. (2001). Varieties of healing, 2: A taxonomy of unconventional healing practice. *Annals of Internal Medicine, 135*(3), 196–204.

Kim, L. W., & Zhu, J. (2010). Acupuncture for essential hypertension. *Alternative Therapies in Health and Medicine, 16*(2), 18–29.

Krousel-Wood, M. A., Muntner, P., Joyce, C.J., Islam, T., Stanley, E., Holt, E. W., et al. (2010), Adverse effects of complementary and alternative medicine use on antihypertensive medication adherence: Findings from CoSMP. *Journal of the American Geriatric Society, 58*(1), 54–61.

McCarney, R. W., Brinkhaus, B., Lasserson, T. J., & Linde, K. (2009). Acupuncture for chronic asthma. *Cochrane Database of Systematic Reviews*, 2003, Issue 3, Art. No.: CD000008. doi: 10.1002/14651858. CD000008. pub2

Micozzi, M. (2011). Characteristis of complementary and alternative medicine. In M. Micozzi (Ed.), *Fundamentals of complementary and alternative medicine* (4th ed., pp. 1–8). St. Louis: Saunders Elsevier.

Mueller, C. M., Mai, P. L., Bucher, J., Peters, J. A., Loud, J. T., & Greene, M. H. (2008). Complementary and alternative medicine use among women at increased genetic risk of breast and ovarian cancer. *BMC Complementary and Alternative Medicine, 8*. doi:10.1186/1472-6882-8-17.

Nahin, R. L., Barnes, P. M., Stussman, B. J., & Bloom, B. (2009). *Costs of complementary and alternative medicine (CAM) and frequency of visits to CAM practitioners: United States, 2007* (National Health Statistics Reports, no. 18). Hyattsville, MD: National Center for Health Statistics.

National Cancer Institute. (2011). Acupuncture (health professional version). Retrieved August 30, 2011, from: http://www.cancer.gov/cancertopics/pdq/cam/acupuncture/healthprofessional/page1

National Center for Complementary and Alternative Medicine. (2006a). *Meditation: An introduction*. Retrieved August 30, 2011, from: http://nccam.nih.gov/health/meditation/overview.htm#keypoints

National Center for Complementary and Alternative Medicine. (2006b). *What is reflexology?* Retrieved August 30, 2011, from: http://altmedicine.about.com/od/therapiesfromrtoz/a/Refl exology.htm

National Center for Complementary and Alternative Medicine. (2006c). *Massage therapy: An introduction*. Retrieved August 30, 2011, from: http://nccam.nih.gov/health/massage/massageintroduction.htm

National Center for Complementary and Alternative Medicine. (2006d). *Reiki: An introduction*. Retrieved September 11, 2011, from http://nccam.nih.gov/health/reiki/introduction.htm

National Center for Complementary and Alternative Medicine. (2007a). *Acupuncture: An introduction*. Retrieved August 30, 2011, from: http://nccam.nih.gov/health/acupuncture/introduction.htm

National Center for Complementary and Alternative Medicine. (2007b). *Chiropractic*. Retrieved August 30, 2011, from: http://nccam.nih.gov/health/chiropractic/

National Center for Complementary and Alternative Medicine. (2008a). *CAM basics: What is complementary and alternative medicine?* Retrieved August 30, 2011, from: http://nccam.nih.gov/health/whatiscam/#types

National Center for Complementary and Complementary Medicine. (2008b). *Manipulative and body-based practices.* Retrieved August 30, 2011, from: http://nccam.nih.gov/health/whatiscam/#manipulative

National Center for Complementary and Alternative Medicine. (2008c). *Yoga for health: An introduction.* Retrieved August 30, 2011, from: http://nccam.nih.gov/health/yoga/introduction.htm#keypoints

National Center for Complementary and Alternative Medicine. (2009a). *Homeopathy: An introduction.* Retrieved September 11, 2011, from http://nccam.nih.gov/health/homeopathy/

National Center for Complementary and Alternative Medicine. (2009b). *Traditional Chinese medicine: An introduction.* Retrieved September 11, 2011, from http://nccam.nih.gov/health/whatiscam/chinesemed.htm

National Center for Complementary and Alternate Medicine. (2010a). *Cancer and CAM: What the science says.* Retrieved September 11, 2011, from http://www.nccam.nih.gov/health/providers/digest/cancer_science.htm

National Center for Complementary and Alternative Medicine. (2010b). *Irritable bowel syndrome and CAM: At a glance.* Retrieved August 30, 2011, from: http://nccam.nih.gov/health/digestive/IrritableBowelSyndrome.htm

National Center for Complementary and Alternative Medicine. (2011a). *Alerts and advisories.* Retrieved August 30, 2011, from: http://nccam.nih.gov/news/alerts

National Center for Complementary and Alternative Medicine (2011b). *NCCAM exploring the science of complementary and alternative medicine: Third strategic plan: 2011–2015.* Retrieved August 30, 2011, from:http://nccam.nih.gov/about/plans/2011/

National Center for Complementary and Alternative Medicine. (2011c). *Grants and funding.* Retrieved August 30, 2011, from:http://nccam.nih.gov/grants/getfacts/

National Center for Complementary and Alternative Medicine. (2011d). *Evaluating web-based healthresources* (NCCAM Pub No. D437). Retrieved August 30, 2011, from: http://nccam.nih.gov/health/webresources/

National Center for Complementary and Alternative Medicine. (2011e). *Herbs at a glance.* Retrieved August 30, 2011, from: http://nccam.nih.gov/health/herbsataglance.htm

National Center for Complementary and Alternative Medicine. (2011f). *Selecting a CAM practitioner* (NCCAM Publication No. D346). Retrieved August 30, 2011, from: http://nccam.nih.gov/health/decisions/practitioner.htm

National Center for Complementary and Alternative Medicine. (2011g). *Using dietary supplementswisely* (NCCAM Publication No. D426). Retrieved August 30, 2011, from: http://nccam.nih.gov/health/supplements/wiseuse.htm

Oguamanam, C. (2006). Biomedical orthodoxy and complementary and alternative medicine: Ethical challenges of integrating medical cultures. *The Journal of Alternative and Complementary Medicine, 12*(5), 577–581.

Qato, D. M., Alexander, G. C., Conti, R. M., et al. (2008). Use of prescription and over-the-counter medications and dietary supplements among older adults in the United States. *Journal of the American Medical Association, 300*, 286–778.

Qigong Institute. (2004–2011). *What is Qigong?* Retrieved August 30, 2011, from: http://www.qigonginstitute.org/html/qigonghealth.php#AboutQigong

Qigong Saydah, S. H., & Eberhardt, M. S. (2006). Use of complementary and alternative medicine among adults with chronic diseases: United States 2002. *The Journal of Alternative and Complementary Medicine, 12*(8), 805–812.

Sleath, B., Callahan, L., DeVellis, R. F., & Sloane, P. D. (2005). Patients' perceptions of primary care physicians' participatory decision-making style and communication about complementary and alternative medicine for arthritis. *The Journal of Alternative and Complementary Medicine, 11*(3), 449–453.

Smith, C. A., Hay, P. P., & Macpherson, H. (2010). Acupuncture for depression. *Cochrane Database of Systematic Reviews* 2010, Art No. CD004046.

Ulbricht, C. (2011). *Davis's pocket guide to herbs and supplements.* Philadelphia: Davis.

Wu, H. M., Tang, J., Lih, X. P., Lau, J., Leung, P. C., Woo, J., & Li, Y. (2009). Acupuncture for stroke rehabilitation. *Cochrane Database of Systematic Reviews*, Issue 3, Art. No.:CD004131. doi: 10.1002/14651858. CD004131. pub2.

Wagner, E. H., Bennett, S. M., Austin, B. T., Greene, S. M., Schaefer, J. K., & Vonkorff, M. (2005). Finding common ground: Patient-centeredness and evidence-based chronic illness care. *The Journal of Alternative and Complementary Medicine, 11*(Suppl. 1) 7–15.

Walker, B. F., French, S. D., Grant, W., & Green S. (2010). Combined chiropractic interventions for low back pain. *Cochrane Database of Systematic Reviews 2010*, Issue 4. Art No.:CD005427. doi: 10.1002/14651858. CD005427.pub2.

Wyatt, G., Sikorskii, A., Wills, C. E., & An, H. S. (2010). Complementary and alternative medicine use, spending, and quality of life in early stage breast cancer. *Nursing Research, 59*(1), 58–65.

Yang, J., Feng, Y., Ying, L., Liu, G .J., Chen J., Ren, Y. L., & Liang, F. R. (2010). Acupuncture for hypertension (protocol). *Cochrane Database of Systematic Reviews 2010*, Issue 11. Art.No.:CD008821. doi: 10.1002/14651858. CD00821

Zarowitz, B. (2010a). Complementary and alternative medicine. *Geriatric Nursing, 31*(2), 123–125.

Zarowitz, B. (2010b). Complementary and alternative medicine: Dietary supplement interactions with medication. *Geriatric Nursing, 31*(3), 206–211.

PART IV

Impact of the System

CHAPTER 19

Models of Care

Pamala D. Larsen

INTRODUCTION

As the population age 65 and older increases and the healthcare system sees more individuals with chronic illness, healthcare providers and third-party payers are examining how to care for individuals with chronic disease long term. Increasingly we hear about disease management models that have demonstrated better patient outcomes than "usual care." Less well publicized, however, is nursing's role in caring for individuals with chronic disease. For some of us, it has always made sense that chronic care should be nursing's domain, particularly as the profession looks at care as opposed to cure.

The United States continues to outspend similar nations in health care. As noted in Chapter 1, however, more money does not translate into better patient outcomes or better value for the consumer. Phrases heard today are "value-based" and "value-added"—whether in manufacturing, architecture, engineering, or now health care. What is the value of the health care that the patient is receiving? Robinson (2008) defines value in health care as measured in terms of contributions of health care minus the attendant costs, with costs and contributions conceptualized broadly (p. 11).

As of March 2010, the United States has a new healthcare reform bill in place. Will it be successful? Will it make a difference? Does it address the "real" issues of our healthcare system? There are already calls to repeal the bill after only a year in existence. Clearly, health care is at a crossroads with or without the Affordable Care Act (ACA) and at the core of that crossroads is chronic care. How do we effectively provide quality care to those with chronic conditions?

This chapter provides an overview of models and frameworks that provide care for individuals with chronic illness and their families.

Historical Perspectives

In 1983, diagnosis-related groups (DRGs) for reimbursement were initiated for all Medicare patients. This was the direct result of trying to find a better way to pay care providers than the retrospective payment system that was in place from 1965 to 1983. Furthermore, healthcare costs were escalating and it seemed that paying care providers prospectively, per diagnosis group, would decrease costs. DRGs were implemented using the International Classification of Diseases, Ninth Revision, Clinical Modifications (ICD-9-CM). ICD-9-CM coding classified diseases, symptoms, and procedures with individual codes. Although DRGs were used initially only for Medicare patients, third-party payers use the coding (now in its 10th revision with plans for an 11th in 2015) as well.

With the advent of DRGs, acute care facilities soon developed clinical pathways or care algorithms for patients with a diagnosis that matched a specific DRG. Patients with heart failure, myocardial infarction, appendectomy, cholecystectomy, stroke, diabetes, and so forth were placed within standard care plans, care maps, clinical pathways, or algorithms (the name varied in each institution) as a way to monitor these patients and make sure they were "on track" for discharge. Because the hospital was to be paid a certain amount of money for each individual with a specific condition, it was critical that patients were treated swiftly and effectively and discharged in a timely manner. Although one would not consider DRGs a disease or illness management model, this change to Medicare in the 1980s has influenced how we manage care today.

IMPACT

The direct and indirect costs associated with providing appropriate care for someone with multiple chronic conditions cannot be overstated (see Chronicity, Chapter 1). Fully 23% of Medicare beneficiaries with five or more chronic conditions account for 68% of the program's funding (Anderson, 2005). From a cost perspective alone, the need to provide high quality care efficiently hailed the advent of both formal and informal disease management programs. Disease management programs may originate from federal and state agencies as well as from for-profit and not-for-profit companies.

Disease Management Versus Illness Management

The majority of models available today for patient care are disease management models.

These models monitor the physiologic markers of disease, the measurement of one's glycosylated hemoglobin (HbA1c), the forced expiratory volume (FEV) of a patient with chronic obstructive pulmonary disease (COPD), the number of medications prescribed to a patient, the number of visits to the healthcare provider, and so forth. However, looking at the disease, the pathophysiology, and the required medications is only one part of caring for the patient, and, quite frankly, that is the easier part—the measurable part. The illness experience of an individual patient, the uniqueness of the patient, and the patient's living situation, social support, and coping mechanisms—whether effective or ineffective—are the other components of the patient's life that disease management programs do not address.

INTERVENTIONS

During the mid to late 1990s, many disease management companies were formed, with most having the goal of providing cost-effective care to those with chronic conditions. By 1999 there were 200 companies nationwide offering disease management services for such conditions as diabetes, asthma, and heart failure (Bodenheimer, 2003). Most of these programs did not originate within healthcare institutions but were outsourced to outside firms. Today, few of those companies exist or are profitable, primarily because their focus was on one specific disease, when typically the older adult population has multiple chronic conditions. As an example, fewer than one half of the rehospitalizations among patients initially hospitalized with heart failure are actually attributed to heart failure. The other hospitalizations are related to conditions that predispose to heart failure such as coronary artery disease, hypertension, COPD, and so forth (DeBusk, West, Miller, & Taylor, 1999). Disease management companies offered programs that were just that, programs, with neither a systems approach nor an integration of these programs into a healthcare system or institution. In addition, a number of those disease management programs were based on physician specialty practice and not primary care. As we look at older adults, they may have several chronic conditions necessitating going to several different specialty physicians. Therefore, programs based on specialty practice typically did not work.

Most of the literature today looks at disease management models versus illness management models. However, in most studies, the definition of disease management and the components of each program vary, making it hard to compare programs and health outcomes of participants. When performing a meta-analysis or systematic review, it becomes difficult to figure out inclusion criteria for studies, because each program is different. Furthermore, when looking at outcomes, what specific component of the program "makes a difference" in the health outcome or is it the combination of components acting interdependently?

Mattke, Seid, and Ma (2007), in their analysis of disease management programs, suggest in broad terms that disease management refers to a system of coordinated healthcare interventions and communications to help patients address chronic disease and other health conditions. Disease management programs are "big business," with 96% of the top 150 U.S. payers offering some form of disease management service and 83% of more than 500 major U.S. employers using programs to help individuals manage their health (as cited in Mattke et al., 2007, p. 670). Revenues associated with these programs have grown significantly from $78 million in 1997 to nearly $1.2 billion in 2005 and projected to top $1.8 billion by the end of 2008 (Mattke et al., 2007). What are the health outcomes of spending $1 to 2 billion a year? Are these programs making a difference in health outcomes, and, if so, are they reducing costs in other areas?

In their review of three evaluations of large-scale, population-based programs, 10 meta-analyses, and 16 systematic reviews covering 317 studies, Mattke and colleagues (2007) found consistent evidence of improved processes of care and disease control, but no conclusive support of improved health outcomes. In addition, when the costs of the programs and/or interventions were accounted for and then cost savings subtracted, there was no evidence of a net reduction in medical costs (pp 675–676).

TRICARE Management Activity, who administers healthcare benefits for U.S. military service personnel, retirees, and their dependents, developed a disease management program for beneficiaries with diabetes. A quasi-experimental approach assessed the program's impact for 37,370 beneficiaries ages 18 to 64 living in the United States. Beneficiaries were categorized as "uncontrolled" or "controlled" based on past medical claims. The study compared observed outcomes to predicted outcomes in the absence of diabetes management. Results indicated that total annual medical savings per participant averaged $783. More active participation in the program was associated with lower medical costs (Dall et al., 2010).

Buntin Jain, Mattke, and Lurie (2009) suggest that results from disease management programs may be skewed because of selection bias. Selection bias includes patients being recruited into programs because they are likely to attain quality and cost benefits (typically the more engaged patient interested in self-management). The conundrum is whether the disease management program itself causes the results or whether it is the selection of the appropriate patients that make the difference (Buntin et al., 2009).

Chronic Care Model

The best known model for providing care to those with chronic disease is the chronic care model (CCM). Work on this model began in the early 1990s with Dr. Edward Wagner, an internist and director of the Seattle-based MacColl Institute for Healthcare Innovation at the Center for Health Studies, Group Health Cooperative. Wagner identified three issues in providing care to those with chronic illness through primary care (Wielawski, 2006):

1. Primary care offices are set up to respond to acute illnesses rather than anticipate and respond proactively to patients' needs (which is what individuals with chronic illness need).
2. Patients with chronic illness are not adequately informed about their conditions and they are not supported in the self-care of their conditions beyond the physician's office.
3. Physicians are too busy to educate and support patients with chronic illness to the degree needed for them to stay healthy. (p. 5)

Wagner's (1998) solution was to replace the physician-centered office with a structure that supported a team of professionals that collaborated with the patient in his or her care. Early implementation of his model took place with 15,000 patients with diabetes at the Group Health Cooperative, a 590,000-member health maintenance organization in Seattle. During 5 years, the percentage of patients with up-to-date screening improved; blood sugar levels and the regularity of monitoring improved; patients reported higher satisfaction with their care; and admission to acute care facilities decreased.

During this period of time in the mid to late 1990s, Wagner and associates partnered with The Robert Wood Johnson Foundation (RWJ) to further develop the model. The model was refined and published in its current form in 1998. Improving Chronic Illness Care (2006–2011), a national program through RWJ, was launched in 1998 with the CCM as its core (**Figure 19-1**). The CCM is not a model for individual care, but for large populations of individuals. It does not redesign patient care, but redesigns clinical practices that are delivering care by implementing system and process change.

A 2009 Intervention Review of an earlier Cochrane Review supported the use of the CCM with clients with both type I and type II diabetes. Forty-one studies with a total of 48,000 clients were involved in the review. Renders and colleagues (2000) concluded that multifaceted professional interventions can enhance the performance of healthcare professionals in managing clients with diabetes. Although using the model enhanced process outcomes, the effect on client health outcomes was less clear.

Studies from 2000 through 2009 were reviewed to determine the impact of the CCM in redesigning care. For this review, a CCM–based intervention was defined as an intervention that integrated changes that involved most or all of the six areas of the model: self-management support, decision support, delivery system design, clinical information systems, healthcare organization, and community resources (Coleman, Austin, Brach, & Wagner, 2009). Eighty-two

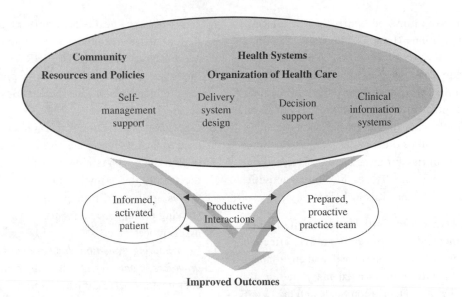

FIGURE 19-1 The Chronic Care Model.
Source: Wagner, E.H. (1998). Chronic disease management: What will it take to improve care for chronic illness? *Effective Clinical Practice*, 1, 2–4.

studies were retained for the final study. Published evidence suggests that practices redesigned in accord with the CCM generally improve the quality of care and the outcomes for patients with various chronic illnesses (Coleman et al., 2009, p. 81).

Although the CCM is a model for primary medical care, Jacelon, Furman, Rea, Macdonald, & Donaghue (2011) have adapted the model for long-term care. The six constructs of the CCM were implemented to create a model for high-quality chronic disease care.

Guided Care

Using the CCM as a basis, researchers at Johns Hopkins University developed a care model, Guided Care, to improve the quality of life and efficiency of resource utilization for older adults with multiple chronic conditions. Guided Care

enhances the use of primary care (versus specialty care) and utilizes the following seven principles of chronic care: disease management; self-management; case management; lifestyle modification; transitional care; caregiver education and support; and geriatric evaluation and management (Boyd et al., 2007, p. 697). What is unique about the Guided Care model is the use of registered nurses specially trained in Guided Care concepts, who, in turn, use a computerized electronic health record (EHR) in working with two to five primary care physicians to meet the needs of 50–60 older adults with multiple comorbidities. The Guided Care Nurse (GCN) is based in the primary care physician's office, and performs eight clinical activities, guided by scientific evidence and the patients' priorities (p. 698). Pilot versions of Guided Care included several of the eight core activities. The first major application of guided care occurred in a cluster-randomized controlled trial (RCT) through Johns Hopkins University. The study utilized 8 sites (49 physicians) in the Baltimore–Washington, DC area, with 904 patients in either the experimental group of Guided Care or the control group (usual care) (Boult et al., 2008). Patients eligible for the study were those 65 years old or older and ranking in the upper quartile of risk for using health services during the coming year. The eight clinical activities performed by the GCN included:

1. *Assessment.* Initial assessments include medical, functional, cognitive, affective, psychosocial, nutritional, and environmental. Other tools used may include the Geriatric Depression Scale and the CAGE alcoholism scale. The client is also asked what his or her priorities are for improved quality of life.
2. *Planning.* The EHR merges the assessment data with evidence-based practice guidelines to create a preliminary care guide that manages and monitors the patients' health conditions. The GCN and the primary care physician then personalize the care guide with input from the patient and family. The end result is a patient-friendly version of the plan called "My Action Plan," written in lay language and given to the patient.
3. *Chronic disease self-management (CDSM).* The GCN encourages the patient's self-efficacy in the management of his or her chronic conditions. The patient is referred to a free, local 15-hour CDSM course led by trained lay people and supported by the GCN. In this program—developed by Kate Lorig and associates at Stanford University—the patient learns how to operationalize the action plan.
4. *Monitoring.* The GCN monitors each patient at least monthly by telephone to address issues promptly. The EHR plays an important role in the monitoring by providing reminders about each patient (Boyd et al., 2007).
5. *Coaching.* Motivational interviewing is used to facilitate the patient's participation in care along with reinforcing adherence to the action plan (Boyd et al., 2007). The GCNs are trained in motivational interviewing principles and strategies to assist in this process.
6. *Coordinating transitions between sites and providers of care.* The GCN is the primary coordinator of care for patients in this program, and is thus responsible for the care transitions that occur between home, the emergency room, hospitals, long-term care facilities, and other care settings.
7. *Educating and supporting caregivers.* The GCN works with family or other unpaid caregivers of the patients to educate and support them. This may include individual or group assistance, support group meetings, or ad hoc telephone consultation (Boyd et al., 2007).
8. *Accessing community resources.* Determining appropriate community resources for the patient, such as Meals on Wheels, transportation needs, and so forth are key functions of the GCN. The idea is not to duplicate services, but to utilize the services available in the community.

In April 2008, 6 months into the RCT, data suggested that the Guided Care model provided improved quality of care, reduced medical care costs, and there was high satisfaction in both the primary care physicians and the GCNs (Boult et al., 2008). Based on these early results, two of the managed care partners in the trial, Kaiser Permanente and Johns Hopkins HealthCare, agreed to continue to pay the costs of the GCNs for an additional year. However, 18-month outcomes demonstrated few results. The study looked at the use of health services and included 850 older patients at high risk for using healthcare in the future. The only statistically significant overall effect of guided care was a reduction in episodes of home health care (Boult et al., 2011).

Program of All-Inclusive Care for the Elderly (PACE)

Although the Program of All-Inclusive Care for the Elderly (PACE) was not specifically developed for individuals with chronic illness, it is obvious that the majority of older adults accessing this program could have at least one chronic condition. PACE is a capitated benefit authorized by the Balanced Budget Act (BBA) of 1997 that offers comprehensive health care to older adults. PACE is modeled after the successful On Lok Senior Health Services program in San Francisco. The On Lok model showed successful outcomes in a number of demonstration projects funded through the Centers for Medicare & Medicaid Services (CMS), then known as the Health Care Financing Administration (HCFA), in the 1980s and 1990s. PACE is a permanent entity within the Medicare program that enables states to provide PACE services to Medicaid beneficiaries as a state option.

Participants in PACE must be 55 years of age, live in a PACE service area, and be certified as eligible for nursing home care. The program allows most of its participants to receive services while they continue to live at home. Capitated financing allows care providers to deliver all services that the participants need, rather than those that are limited under Medicare

and Medicaid fee-for-service systems (www.cms.hhs.gov/pace/). PACE becomes the sole source of services for the Medicare and Medicaid eligible enrollees. As of 2011 there were 58 PACE providers located in 26 states.

Mukamel and colleagues (2007) attempted to determine what program characteristics of PACE were associated with the risk-adjusted health outcomes of mortality, functional status, and self-assessed health. The research examined 3,042 newly enrolled persons in 23 PACE programs over a 4-year period (1997 to 2001). There were a number of program characteristics that were significantly associated with better functional outcomes. These included: a medical director who was a trained geriatrician; medical directors who spent time providing direct patient care; programs with effective interdisciplinary teams; teams composed of more aides than professionals; the same ethnicity of participant and team member; and larger and older PACE programs (Mukamel et al., 2007).

Fewer program characteristics were associated with participant self-assessed health outcomes. Higher staffing levels, having more diverse services, and having a match between the ethnicity of the participant and the staff member were associated with higher self-assessed health outcomes (Mukamel et al., 2007, p. 524).

Centers for Medicare & Medicaid

Since 1999 seven disease management demonstration and pilot programs have been conducted by the CMS for the traditional fee-for-service Medicare program. These programs have included 300,000 beneficiaries in 35 programs (Bott, Kapp, Johnson, & Magno, 2009). Programs ranged in size from 257 in a case management demonstration to 200,000 in the

Medicare Health Support Organizations. Some programs targeted beneficiaries with specific chronic illnesses, while others focused on high-cost or high-risk beneficiaries regardless of diagnosis, while others were a combination. These disease management programs have been defined as a system of coordinated healthcare interventions and communications for populations with conditions in which patient self-care efforts are significant. The goal was to improve the health status of the population, improve satisfaction with the care, and reduce total healthcare costs—net of fees and the programs' implementation costs. A disease management intervention that was effective but increased spending would not be an option to add to traditional Medicare. Evaluations are now complete on 20 programs, and evaluations are pending on the other 15.

Results from the CMS demonstration projects have not shown widespread evidence of improvement in compliance with evidence-based care, satisfaction for providers or beneficiaries, or broad behavior change (Bott et al., 2009, p. 92). Only a few programs produced financial savings net of fees. Foote (2009) suggests that the CMS needs to develop a new strategy with its demonstration projects. In 2007 CMS healthcare expenditures totaled $418 billion. The need for CMS to "get it right" cannot be overstated.

The CMS is currently testing the patient-centered medical home (PCMH) model in the multipayer Advanced Primary Care Practice Demonstration and the Federally Qualified Health Centers Advanced Primary Care Practice Demonstration. The CMS also plans to test the PCMH model under the Innovation Center created by Section 3021 of the Patient Protection and Affordable Care Act (CMS, 2011).

The ACA established a voluntary program for accountable care organizations (ACO) under the CMS (to be available by January 2012). ACOs are provider groups that accept responsibility for the cost and quality of care delivered to a specific population of patients cared for by the groups' clinicians (Shortell, Casalino, & Fisher, 2010, p. 1293). ACOs are seen as a way to reduce the rate of increases in healthcare costs over time while improving the coordination and quality of patient care. ACOs will be largely based on physician practices that may be organized as PCMHs (Shortell et al., p. 1294). Other ACOs could include hospitals, home health agencies, and nursing homes.

The ACA also established a Center for Medicare and Medicaid Innovation. The center's mission is to help transform the Medicare, Medicaid, and Children's Health Insurance Programs (CHIP) to deliver better health care, better health, and reduced costs through improvement for CMS beneficiaries, and in so doing, help to transform the healthcare system for all Americans (Center for Medicare & Medicaid Innovation, n.d., para 1), The Innovation center was given flexibility and resources to rapidly test innovative care and payment models and scale up successful models.

Health Promotion

It would seem that prevention of chronic diseases would surely save dollars versus dealing with the diseases themselves. Unfortunately data do not support this idea. Russell (2009) summarizes the cost-effectiveness analysis of many preventive treatments. For example, the accumulated costs of treating hypertension are nonetheless greater than the savings of preventing heart disease and stroke, because many individuals, not all of whom would suffer heart disease or a stroke, must take medication for many years (Russell, 2009, p. 43). Another more recent analysis shows that cost-effectiveness varies by type of medication, although no drug reduces medical spending (Russell, 2009).

The Diabetes Prevention Study showed that lifestyle changes can prevent diabetes. The program provided diet and exercise plans that were backed by nutritionist visits and physical training sessions. Over 4 years, only 11% of those in the intervention group developed diabetes as compared with 23% in the control group. Even so, "the program adds to medical costs: $143,000 per healthy year in 2000" (Russell, 2009, p. 44).

Patient-Centered Medical Homes

The American Academy of Pediatrics (AAP) first used the term *medical home* to refer to an environment for children with special needs. More recently the AAP along with the American Academy of Family Physicians, the American College of Physicians, and the American Osteopathic Association have refined the concept and expanded it to the care of all patients. There is widespread agreement that primary care is in crisis. Patients are not satisfied with their care, and purchasers and insurers are disappointed with its cost and quality. There are many highly effective primary care practices, but many that are poorly organized and not able to provide timely, quality care (PCMH, 2010). Fifty percent of all patients do not understand what their primary care physician is telling them because visits are too short to address their concerns. Coordination between primary care physicians, specialists, and hospitals is often lacking, and each is unaware of the others' treatment plans (PCMH, 2010). Many believe that the PCMH can address these issues. Although initially focused on the physician–patient relationship, the concept has evolved to emphasize team-based care.

As defined by the four medical societies, PCMHs support the following principles:

- Each patient receives care from a personal physician.
- Care has a whole-person orientation.
- Safe, high-quality care is provided.
- There is enhanced access to care.
- The payment recognizes the added value provided to patients who have a PCMH. (Abrams, Davis, & Haran, 2009)

No one set of criteria exists to identify medical homes. However, many states have developed their criteria based on the joint principles agreed to by the four medical societies. The National Committee for Quality Assurance (NCQA; see www.ncqa.org) developed the Physician Practice Connections Patient-Centered Medical Home standards in parallel with the four medical societies' efforts. The NCQA (2011) sees the medical home concept as strengthening the physician–patient relationship and replacing episodic care with coordinated care. The NCQA released its latest standards for the PCMH program on January 31, 2011. They include:

- Access and communication
- Patient tracking and registry functions
- Care management
- Self-management support
- Electronic prescribing
- Test tracking
- Referral tracking
- Performance reporting and improvement
- Advanced electronic communications (NCQA, 2011)

A health policy brief issued by *Health Affairs* in September 2010 identified that there are more than 100 demonstration projects testing the effectiveness of PCMHs (PCMH, 2010). Additionally, 31 states are planning or implementing medical home pilots within Medicaid or CHIP, and at least 12 states have developed medical home initiatives that involve multiple payers. One fifth of medical homes recognized by the NCQA are sole practices, although it is much more common for large practices to be medical homes (Abrams, Schor, & Schoenbaum, 2010).

TransforMed, funded by the American Academy of Family Physicians, launched a 24-month project in June of 2006 through May 2008, with 36 family medicine practices across the country. The practices were small, independent practices that wished to become PCMHs. Practices were randomized into "facilitated intervention" and "self-directed" (Nutting et al., 2011). Findings from the project revealed that practices made:

> heroic efforts and attempted to implement as many model components as possible over the two-year life of the project. . . . Many of the chronic care and health IT components may be implemented by highly motivated practices. Nevertheless, even with extensive assistance from their facilitator, the availability of expert consultation, and the incentive of being in a national spotlight, two years was not long enough to implement the entire model and to transform work processes. (Nutting et al., 2011, p. 440)

Interestingly, the article seems to be more focused on the processes involved rather than the patients. Isn't the end result of medical homes better patient outcomes?

Self-Management Programs

The term *self-management* initially appeared in a book by Thomas Creer on the rehabilitation of children with chronic illness (Lorig & Holman,

2003). Creer and colleagues used the concept to indicate that the patient was an active participant in their care. Creer and Holroyd (2006) state that self-management differs from adherence in that "self-management places greater emphasis on the patient's active role in decision-making, both inside and outside the consultation room" (p. 8). Self-management is also seen as different from disease management. Creer and Holroyd view disease management as being more focused on healthcare professionals' algorithms and interventions to standardize care as opposed to self-management, which emphasizes the patients' involvement in defining the problems.

Lorig and colleagues' (1999) work at Stanford University has conceptualized best what we know about self-management programs. Her work is based on Corbin and Strauss's (1992) framework of medical management, role management, and emotional management. These concepts, along with how the chronic condition is perceived by the patient and family, are hallmarks of Lorig's work. Lorig's framework for self-management programs includes five core self-management skills: problem solving, decision making, resource utilization, forming of a patient–healthcare provider partnership, and taking action (Lorig & Holman, 2003).

Empirical results of self-management programs have been mixed. What follows are examples of the literature in this area.

- Lorig and colleagues (1999) studied 952 patients, 40 years of age and older with a diagnosis of heart disease, lung disease, stroke, or arthritis in a 6-month-long RCT. The Chronic Disease Self-Management Program (CDSMP) consisted of seven, weekly 2.5-hour sessions on making management choices and achieving success in reaching self-selected goals as opposed to prescribing specific behavior changes (Lorig et al., 1999, p. 7). Outcome measures included health behaviors, health status, and health service utilization. At 6 months, the experimental group demonstrated improvements in weekly minutes of exercise, frequency of cognitive symptom management, communication with physicians, and self-reported health. Participants also had decreased fatigue and disability and less social/role-activity limitations with less health distress, fatigue, and disability. There were no differences between the groups in pain/physical discomfort, shortness of breath, or psychological well-being (Lorig et al., 1999, p. 5).

- In a more recent study of the CDSMP, researchers, using data from previous CDSMPs in English and Spanish, examined whether there were statistically significant interactions between baseline status and randomization in estimating 6-month changes in health status (Ritter, Lee, & Lorig, 2011). The researchers were looking for moderators that might affect outcome variables. Results demonstrated no moderating factors that consistently predicted improved health outcomes.

- Warsi, Wang, LaValley, Avorn, and Solomon (2004) conducted a systematic review of the literature from 1964 to 1999 and reviewed 71 clinical trials. Diabetic patients had reductions in HbA1c levels and improvements in systolic blood pressure, and asthmatic patients experienced fewer attacks. Arthritis self-management education programs were not associated with statistically significant effects. Warsi and colleagues found a large number of limitations with the studies they reviewed. The methods of conducting (i.e., study design) and reporting

these trials were suboptimal. There was also evidence of publication bias (Warsi et al., 2004, p. 1648).

- Chodosh and colleagues (2005) assessed the effectiveness of self-management programs with a meta-analysis design. Of the 780 studies screened, 53 met the researchers' criteria for inclusion. Self-management interventions led to statistically and clinically significant results of decreased HbA1c (amounting to a decrease of .81%), a decrease of 5 mm Hg in systolic blood pressure, and a decrease of 4.3 mm Hg in diastolic blood pressure. There were no significant results for participants with osteoarthritis in either pain or function. Their conclusion was that the studies had variable quality, making it difficult to analyze, and there was possible publication bias present (pp. 435–436). In addition, it was not clear what constituted a self-management program.

A Cochrane Review on self-management programs, led by lay leaders, was completed in 2007. The review included 17 studies with 7,442 individuals with chronic conditions such as arthritis, diabetes, hypertension, and chronic pain. Many of the programs were similar, but differed in the condition they were for and the outcomes that each researcher reported. Overall, the programs led to modest, short-term improvements in patients' confidence to manage their condition and perceptions of their own health. There were increases in the amount of aerobic exercise by participants. While there were some improvements in pain, disability, fatigue, and depression, the changes were not clinically significant. The programs did not improve quality of life for the individuals, alter the number of doctor visits for these individuals, or reduce hospitalizations (Foster, Taylor, Eldridge, Ramsay, & Griffiths, 2007).

Transitional Care

Naylor, Aiken, Kurtzman, Olds, & Hirschman (2011) conducted a systematic review of literature and summarized 21 randomized clinical trials of transitional care interventions targeting adults with chronic illness. Transitional care is defined as a broad range of time-limited services designed to ensure healthcare continuity, avoid preventable poor outcomes among at-risk populations, and promote the safe and timely transfer of patients from one level of care to another or from one type of setting to another (Coleman & Boult, 2003). Transitions have been associated with increased rates of potentially avoidable hospitalizations. A 2009 study reported that approximately 20% of Medicare beneficiaries discharged from hospitals were rehospitalized within 30 days and that 34% were readmitted within 90 days (as cited in Naylor et al., 2011).

The review (Naylor et al., 2011) of transitional care provided 21 studies focusing on adults with chronic illness transitioning from an acute care hospital to another setting. There was a mean sample size of 377 subjects among the studies. A variety of primary and secondary outcomes in five categories were reported: health outcomes, quality of life, patient satisfaction or perception of care, resource use, and costs. Among the 21 studies, all but one reported positive findings in at least one category (p. 749).

The 21 interventions discussed in the articles (Naylor et al., 2011) varied in terms of their nature, point of initiation, intensity, and duration. The largest group of studies could be characterized as comprehensive discharge planning and follow up with (4 studies) or without (3 studies) home visits. The remainder dealt with disease or case management (4 studies), education or psychoeducation (2 studies), peer support (2 studies), telehealth facilitation (1 study), post-discharge geriatric assessment (1 study), and intensive primary care (1 study)

(p. 749). Eighteen of the studies designated a nurse, most frequently an advanced practice nurse (10 studies), as the intervention's clinical manager or leader. A variety of primary and secondary outcomes in five categories were reported. Overall, the authors concluded that there is a robust body of evidence supporting the benefits of transitional care. Studies of nine interventions demonstrated a positive effect on at least one measure of readmissions; eight of the nine reduced all-cause readmission through at least 30 days after discharge (p. 751). Three studies effectively reduced readmissions for at least 6 or 12 months after discharge. Each of these three studies included a focus on patient self-management (Naylor et al., 2011).

Section 3026 of the ACA establishes the Community-Based Care Trans-itions Program (Naylor et al., 2011). The program will provide $500 million from 2011 to 2015 to health systems and community organizations that provide at least one transitional care intervention to high-risk Medicare beneficiaries.

Other

In a systematic review and meta-analysis of COPD management programs, Peytremann-Bridevaux, Staeger, Bridevaus, Ghali, and Burnand (2008) reviewed nine RCTs, one controlled trial, and three uncontrolled before–after trials (that met their definition of a disease management program). These programs demonstrated modest improvement in exercise capacity, health-related quality of life, and decreased hospital admissions. However, the researchers caution that it is unclear which specific component(s) of the program had the most benefit for the clients. Again, the study struggled with defining and identifying the components of the disease management programs, because each program in the review was slightly different.

CASE STUDY

Mary Brown is an 80-year-old widow living alone on her farm 5 miles from town in a western rural state. Mrs. Brown's town, with a population of 10,000, has a critical access hospital. She lives in the farmhouse that she moved to when she married 60 years ago. She would like to stay there as long as possible, but after her hip replacement surgery last fall, her mobility is not as good as it used to be. She is mildly hypertensive and is on medication. Her type II diabetes is under control with diet and medication. She has lots of friends in the community, but her grown children live several states away.

Because of her isolation and age, she might be considered "at risk."

Discussion Questions

1. What are Mrs. Brown's "at-risk" variables?
2. What self-management tasks should be initiated with her?
3. What does Mrs. Brown need? What are her potential needs? This is a small community with few resources available. Be creative and develop a model of care for her.

Collaborative Care

A single-blind RCT involving 214 participants in 14 primary care clinics was conducted in Washington state. Patients were randomly assigned to the usual-care group or to the intervention group, in which a medically supervised nurse, working with each patient's primary care physician, provided guideline-based collaborative care management with the goal of controlling risk factors for chronic disease (Katon et al., 2010). The primary outcomes were lowering HbA1c, low-density lipoprotein (LDL), and systolic blood pressure levels, and measuring scores from the Symptom Checklist-20, a depression tool. Compared with the control group, patients in the intervention group had greater overall 12-month improvement across HbA1c, LDL, systolic BP, and the Symptom Checklist-20.

VNS CHOICE Program

In the early 1990s, the state of New York explored several options to increase the range of community services available to the older adult population. Managed long-term care (MLTC) is the result of that initiative (Dehm & McCabe, 2007). Visiting Nurse Service (VNS) CHOICE operates under a contract with the New York State Department of Health and is licensed by the state as a managed care organization. The program receives a fixed per-member, per-month premium from the state at a rate that is negotiated with the MLTC plan annually. All covered services, care management, and administrative costs are paid for and managed through this monthly payment. The average VNS CHOICE member is 81 years old, female, and lives with either a family member or alone. Most members speak English, Spanish, or Chinese. The average member has 3.6 chronic illnesses, the most common being hypertension, diabetes, osteoarthritis and related disorders, and heart disease. The cornerstone of the VNS CHOICE program is a care management model that links home- and community-based services, acute care, and long-term care with the assistance of an interdisciplinary team. Currently the plan covers 9,700 individuals with plans to expand the MLTC area (Dehm & McCabe, 2007).

Telephone Disease Management

This diabetes disease management program used the telephone as the source of education in a sample of 1,220 Medicare+Choice recipients older than age 65 in Ohio, Kentucky, and Indiana (Berg & Wadhwa, 2007). There were 610 intervention group members matched to a control group of the same number of members. The disease management program used a structured, evidence-based telephonic nursing intervention to provide patient education, counseling, and monitoring services. The self-management intervention plan included risk stratification, formal scheduled nurse education sessions, 24-hour access to a nurse counseling and symptom advice telephone line, printed action plans, workbooks, medication compliance and vaccination reminders, physician alerts, and signs and symptoms of complications. The participants in the study were high users of services, with rates of hospitalization of 605 of 1,000 in the intervention group and 612 of 1,000 in the control group. Emergency room visits were also high with 700 of 1,000 in both groups during the baseline period (Berg & Wadhwa, 2007, p. 230). The groups were well matched and could be assumed to be moderately ill to severely ill older adults with diabetes.

The intervention group had significantly lower rates of acute service utilization compared with the control group: 23.8% increase in angiotensin-converting enzyme (ACE) inhibitor use, 13.3% increase in blood glucose regulator use, 11.8% increase in HbA1c testing, 10.3% increase in lipid panel testing, 26% increase in eye exams, and 35.5% increase in microalbumin tests (Berg & Wadhwa, 2007, p. 226).

Another study used the telephone for disease management in patients with heart failure (Smith, Hughes-Cromwick, Forkner, & Galbreath, 2008). This study examined the cost-effectiveness of the approach versus the patient outcomes. Adult subjects with documented systolic heart failure or diastolic heart failure ($n = 1,069$) were randomized into one of three study groups: usual care, disease management, or augmented disease management. Subjects in the intervention arms were assigned a disease manager who was an RN and performed patient education and medication management with the patient's primary care provider for the full 18 months of the study. Subjects in the augmented disease management group also received in-home devices for enhanced self-monitoring. These data were electronically transmitted to the disease manager. Although the program produced statistically significant survival advantages among all patients, analyses of direct and intervention costs showed no cost savings associated with the intervention. It also did not reduce healthcare utilization of the subjects (Smith et al., 2008).

Evidence-Based Practice Box

Guided care, a model of care developed from the Chronic Care Model (CCM), was evaluated in a randomized controlled trial in the Washington, DC/Baltimore, Maryland area. Eligible patients from 3 healthcare systems were cluster-randomized to receive guided care or usual care for 20 months between November 1, 2006 and June 30, 2008. Eight services were provided by guided care nurses working in partnership with patients' primary care physicians: comprehensive assessment, evidence-based care planning, monthly monitoring of symptoms and adherence, transitional care, coordination of healthcare professionals, support for self-management, support for family caregivers, and enhanced access to community services. The study included 850 older patients at high risk for using health care in the future. The only statistically significant overall effect of guided care was a reduction in episodes of home health care. In a preplanned analysis, guided care also reduced skilled nursing facility admissions among Kaiser-Permanente patients.

Source: Boult, C., Reider, L., Leff, B., Frick, K. D., Boyd, C. M., Wolff, J. L., et al. (2011). The effect of guided care teams on the use of health services. *Archives of Internal Medicine, 171*(5), 460–466.

Online Disease Management

A retrospective, quasi-experimental cohort design evaluated program participants in an online disease management program (through Blue Cross Blue Shield) and a matched cohort of nonparticipants. The study was conducted with 413 online participants and 360 nonparticipants. The online program was a commercially available, tailored program for chronic disease self-management. Healthcare costs per person per year were $757 less than predicted for participants relative to matched nonparticipants, yielding a return on investment of $9.89 for every dollar spent on the program (Schwartz et al., 2010).

Patient Advocacy Case Management

Service use and costs were examined in eight studies using the patient advocacy case management model of care with frail older adults or those with chronic illness. Results from the systematic review identified that this model of care did not increase service use and costs and was effective in decreasing service use and costs in two studies (Oeseburg, Wynia, Middel, & Reijneveld, 2009).

Shared Care

Smith, Allwright, and O'Dowd (2007) completed a systematic review for the Cochrane Database on "shared care." These authors considered "shared care" as the combined management or joint participation of primary care physicians and specialty care physicians in planning the delivery of care for a client. Twenty studies were identified for chronic disease management, with 19 of them being RCTs. The results were mixed. The authors concluded that there was insufficient evidence to demonstrate significant benefits from shared care, apart from improving prescribing medications.

OUTCOMES

With any model of care for individuals and families with chronic conditions, an expected outcome is that both the disease and illness experience are managed appropriately and some cost savings are realized. This chapter has demonstrated mixed results for the models currently in practice. It is still unclear how the U.S. Health System should be organized to provide care for those with chronic illness. Because a high percentage of chronic illness affects older adults, the CMS has been at the forefront in developing programs or models of care through their demonstration projects. So far there have been few, if any, positive results. Are PCMHs the answer? Only time will tell if these entities make a difference.

What is not "measured" in these models is how these programs or models of care affect the illness experience of the individual and family. Can we say that because an individual with a chronic illness has a lower HbA1c, or has not been hospitalized within the last 6 months, or checks his blood glucose level regularly, has a better quality of life or experiences more life satisfaction, or in the terms of Strauss and colleagues (1984), is successful at normalizing his or her life?

STUDY QUESTIONS

What are the benefits of disease management models of care?

Identify the issues involved with a disease management model of care for an older adult.

How do we as nurses care for individuals and families and their *illness experience* within a disease management model?

After reading about different models of care in this chapter, what do you think should be included in a model of care for an older adult with multiple comorbidities?

Study Questions (Cont.)

How do self-management components of care fit within a disease management program?

What role does (or should) the advanced practice nurse have in disease management?

INTERNET RESOURCES

Chronic Disease Self-Management Program, Stanford University: patienteducation.stanford. edu/programs/cdsmp.html

Commonwealth Fund: www.commonwealthfund. org

Guided Care: www.guidedcare.org

Improving Chronic Illness Care: www.improving-chroniccare.org

PACE: http://www.medicare.gov/Nursing/ Alternatives/Pace.asp

For a full suite of assignments  and additional learning activities, use the access code located in the front of your book and visit this exclusive website: **http://go.jblearning.com/larsen**. If you do not have an access code, you can obtain one at the site.

REFERENCES

Abrams, M., Davis, K., & Haran, C. (2009). Can patient-centered medical homes transform health care delivery? Retrieved September 8, 2011, from: http://www.commonwealthfund.org/Content/From-the-President/2009/Can-Patient-Centered-Medical-Homes-Transform-Health-Care-Delivery.aspx

Abrams, M., Schor, E. L., & Schoenbaum, S. (2010). How physician practices could share personnel and resources to support medical homes. *Health Affairs, 29*(6), 1194–1199.

Anderson, G. F. (2005). Medicare and chronic conditions [Electronic version]. *New England Journal of Medicine, 353*(3), 305 309.

Berg, G. D., & Wadhwa, S. (2007). Health services outcomes for a diabetes disease management program for the elderly [Electronic version]. *Disease Management, 10*(4), 226–234.

Bodenheimer, T. (2003). Interventions to improve chronic care: Evaluating their effectiveness. *Disease Management, 6*(2), 63–71.

Boult, C., Reider, L., Frey, K., Leff, B., Boyd, C.M., Wolff, J. L., et al. (2008). Early effects of "guided care" on the quality of health care for multimorbid older persons: A cluster-randomized controlled trial. *Journal of Gerontology: Medical Sciences, 73A*(3), 321–327.

Bott, D. M., Kapp, M. C., Johnson, L. B., & Magno, L. M. (2009). Disease management for chronically ill beneficiaries in traditional Medicare. *Health Affairs, 28*(1), 86–98.

Boult, C., Reider, L., Leff, B., F rick, K. D., Boyd, C. M., Wolff, J. L., et al. (2011). The effect of guided care teams on the use of health services: Results from a cluster-randomized controlled trial. *Archives of Internal Medicine, 171*(5), 460–466.

Boyd, C. M., Boult, C., Shadmi, E., Leff, B., Brager, R. Dunbar, L., et al. (2007). Guided care for multimorbid older adults. *The Gerontologist, 47*(5), 697–704.

Buntin, M. B., Jain, A. K., Mattke, S., & Lurie, N. (2009) Who gets disease management? *Journal of General Internal Medicine, 24*(5), 649–655.

Center for Medicare & Medicaid Innovation. (n.d.). About the Innovation Center. Retrieved September 8, 2011, from: http://innovations.cms.gov

Centers for Medicare & Medicaid Services. (2011). Medicare demonstrations. Retrieved September 8, 2011, from: http://www.cms.gov/DemoProjectsEvalRpts/MD/itemdetail.asp?filterType=none&filterByDID=-99&sortByDID=3&sortOrder=descending&itemID=CMS1199 247&intNumPerPage=10

Chodosh, J., Morton, S. C., Mojica, W., Maglione, M., Suttorp, M. J., Hilton, L., et al. (2005). Meta-analysis: Chronic disease self-management programs for older adults [Electronic version]. *Annals of Internal Medicine, 143*, 427–438.

Coleman, E. A., & Boult, C. (2003). Improving the quality of transitional care for persons with complex care needs. *Journal of the American Geriatrics Society, 51*(4), 556–557.

Coleman, K., Austin, B. T., Brach, C., & Wagner, E. H. (2009). Evidence on the chronic care model in the new millennium. *Health Affairs, 28(*1), 75–85.

Corbin, J., & Strauss, A. (1992). A nursing model for chronic illness management based upon the trajectory framework. In P. Woog (Ed.), *The chronic illness trajectory framework: The Corbin and Strauss nursing model* (pp. 9–28). New York: Springer.

Creer, T., & Holroyd, K. A. (2006). Self-management of chronic conditions: The legacy of Sir William Osler. *Chronic Illness, 2*, 7–14.

Dall, T. M., Roary, M., Yanag, W., Zhanag, S., Zhang, S., Chen, Y. J., et al. (2010). Health care use and costs for participants in a diabetes disease management program, United States, 2007–2008. *Preventing Chronic Disease, 8*(3). Retrieved September 8, 2011, from: http://www.cdc.gov/pcd/issues/2011/may/10_0163.htm

DeBusk, R., West, J., Miller, N., & Taylor, C. (1999). Chronic disease management: Treating the patient with disease(s) vs. treating the disease(s) in the patient. *Archives of Internal Medicine, 159*, 2739–2742.

Dehm, K., & McCabe, S. (2007). Managing care for adults with chronic conditions: The VNS CHOICE Model. *Policy & Practice*, 14–17.

Foote, S. M. (2009). Next steps: How can Medicare accelerate the pace of improving chronic care? *Health Affairs, 28*(1), 99–102.

Foster, G., Taylor, S. J. C., Eldridge, S., Ramsay, J., & Griffiths, C. J. (2007). Self-management education programmes led by lay leaders for people with chronic health conditions. *Cochrane Database of Systematic Reviews, 17*(4), CD005108. doi: 10.1002/14651858.CD005108.pub2

Improving Chronic Illness Care. (2006–2011). Chronic care model. Retrieved from http://www.improvingchroniccare.org/index.php?p=The_Chronic_Care_Model&s=2

Jacelon, C., Furman, E., Rea, A., Macdonald, B., & Donaghue, L. C. (2011). Creating a professional practice model for postacute care. *Journal of Gerontological Nursing, 37*(3), 53–60.

Katon, W. J., Lin, E., Von Korff, M., Ciechanowski, P., et al. (2010). Collaborative care for patients with depression and chronic illness. *New England Journal of Medicine, 363*(26), 2611.

Lorig, K., & Holman, H. R. (2003). Self-management education: History, definition, outcomes and mechanisms. *Annals of Behavioral Medicine, 26*(1), 1–7.

Lorig, K. R., Sobel, D. S., Steward, A. L., Brown, B. W., Bandura, A., Ritter, P., et al. (1999). Evidence suggesting that a chronic disease self-management program can improve health status while reducing hospitalization: A randomized trial. *Medical Care, 37*(1), 5–14.

Mattke, S., Seid, M., & Ma, S. (2007). Evidence for the effect of disease management: Is $1 billion a year a good investment? *American Journal of Managed Care, 13*, 670–676.

Mukamel, D. B., Peterson, D. R., Temkin-Greener, H., Delavan, R., Gross, D., Kunitz, S. J., et al. (2007). Program characteristics and enrollees' outcomes in the Program of All-Inclusive Care for the Elderly (PACE). *The Milbank Quarterly, 85*(3), 499–531.

National Committee for Quality Assurance. (2011). Patient-centered medical home 2011. Retrieved September 11, 2011, from: http://www.ncqa.org/tabid/1302/Default.aspx

Naylor, M. D., Aiken, L. H., Kurtzman, E. T., Olds, D. M., & Hirschman, K. B. (2011). The importance of transitional care in achieving health reform. *Health Affairs, 30*(4), 746–754.

Nutting, P. A., Crabtree, B. F., Miller, W. L., Stange, K. C., Stewart, E., & Jaen, C. (2011). Transforming physician practices to patient-centered medical homes: Lessons learned from the national demonstration project. *Health Affairs, 39*(3), 439–445.

Oeseburg, B., Wynia, K., Middel, B., & Reijneveld, S. A. (2009). Effects of case management for frail older people or those with chronic illness: A systematic review. *Nursing Research, 58*(3), 201–210.

Patient-centered Medical Homes. (2010). *Health Affairs*. Retrieved September 11, 2011, from: http://www.healthaffairs.org/healthpolicybriefs/brief.php?brief_id=25

Peytremann-Bridevaux, I., Staeger, P., Bridevaus, P. O., Ghali, W. A., & Burnand, B. (2008). Effectiveness of chronic obstructive pulmonary disease management programs: Systematic review and meta-analysis. *The American Journal of Medicine, 121*, 433–443.

Renders, C. M., Valk, G. D., Griffin, S. J., Wagner, E., vanEijk, J. T., & Assendelft, W. J. J. (2000). Interventions to improve the management of diabetes mellitus in primary care, outpatient and community settings. *Cochrane Database of Systematic Reviews.* (4), CD001481. doi: 10.1002/14651858.CD001481.

Ritter, P. L., Lee, J., & Lorig, K. (2011). Moderators of chronic disease self-management programs: Who benefits? *Chronic Illness, 7*(2), 162–172.

Robinson, J. C. (2008). Slouching toward value-based health care [Electronic version]. *Health Affairs, 27*(1), 11–12.

Russell, L. B. (2009). Preventing chronic disease: An important investment, but don't count on cost savings. *Health Affairs, 28*(1), 42–45.

Schwartz, S. M., Day, B., Wildenhaus, K., Silberman, A., Wang, C., & Silberman, J. (2010). The impact of an online disease management program on medical costs among health plan members. *American Journal of Health Promotion, 25*(2), 126–133.

Shortell, S. M., Casalino, L. P., & Fisher, E. S. (2010). How the center for Medicare and Medicaid innovation should test accountable care organizations. *Health Affairs, 29*(7), 1293–1298.

Smith, B., Hughes-Cromwick, P. F., Forkner, E., & Galbreath, A. D. (2008). Cost-effectiveness of telephonic disease management in heart failure [Electronic version]. *The American Journal of Managed Care, 14*(2), 106–115.

Smith, S. M., Allwright, S., & O'Dowd, T. (2007). Effectiveness of shared care across the interface between primary and specialty care in chronic disease management. *Cochrane Database of Systematic Reviews*, (3), CD004910. doi: 10.1002/14651858.CD004910.pub2.

Strauss, A., Corbin, J., Fagerhaugh, S., Glaser, B., Maines, D., Suczek, B., & Wiener, C. (1984). *Chronic illness and the quality of life* (2nd ed.). St. Louis: Mosby.

Wagner, E. H. (1998). Chronic disease management: What will it take to improve care for chronic illness? *Effective Clinical Practice, 1*, 2–4.

Warsi, A., Wang, P. S., LaValley, M., Avorn, J., & Solomon, D. H. (2004). Self-management education programs in chronic disease. A systematic review and methodological critique of the literature]. *Archives of Internal Medicine, 164*(15), 1641–1649.

Wielawski, I. M. (2006). Improving chronic illness care. In S. L. Isaacs & J. R. Knickman (Eds.), *To Improve Health and Health Care, 10, The Robert Wood Johnson Foundation Anthology* (pp. 1–17). Princeton, NJ: Robert Wood Johnson Foundation.

CHAPTER 20

Home Health Care

Cynthia S. Jacelon

INTRODUCTION

The home healthcare industry delivers a variety of services to individuals with chronic health problems living in homes within communities. Services can be divided into two types: 1) skilled healthcare providers, under the direction of a physician's order and supported by third-party reimbursement, and 2) "supportive community services" (SCS), including support for instrumental activities of daily living and personal care (Capitman, 2003). Individuals and agencies provide SCS on a fee-for-service basis. It is common that healthcare providers and SCS workers simultaneously provide services to clients, often through the same agency. The focus of this chapter is on the roles of nurses and other skilled healthcare providers in the home.

Home health nurses provide nursing care to clients with acute and/or chronic illnesses, as well as meet the terminal care needs of clients in their place of residence. The overall goal of care is to enhance quality of life or support clients at the end of life (American Nurses Association [ANA], 2008). Home health nurses use holistic strategies to work with clients, families, and informal caregivers to manage disease or disability. They practice highly independently, often being the only professional care provider in the home. The specialty of home health nursing differs from other nursing specialties in that care is

provided in the client's home; the duration and frequency of care is dependent upon the care delivery model and the holistic needs of the client, family, and caregivers; and the nurse must have advanced knowledge of healthcare payment systems and cost containment (ANA, 2008).

History of Home Care

William Rathbone, a wealthy British businessman and philanthropist, founded the first district nursing association. The district nursing services combined therapeutic nursing care and education for healthful living practices. Working with Florence Nightingale, he advocated for district nursing throughout England in the mid 1880s (Stanhope & Lancaster, 2010) and founded a visiting nurses training school to ensure that nurses had the necessary knowledge and skills to work successfully in a community setting (Hitchcock, Schubert, & Thomas, 2003).

The visiting nurse model established in England was adapted by the United States as a means of addressing some of the serious public health problems of the late 19th century. Large American cities faced many challenges associated with increasing numbers of immigrants entering the country. Poverty-stricken communities with congested living conditions quickly gave rise to epidemics of infectious diseases such as tuberculosis, smallpox, scarlet fever, typhoid, and typhus (Schoen & Koenig, 1997).

The first visiting nurse associations (VNAs) to provide care in the needy person's home were established in the United States in Buffalo (1885), Philadelphia (1886), and Boston (1886). Charitable activities, supported by wealthy people, funded settlement houses and early VNAs. One of the early settlement houses in the United States began through the efforts of Lillian Wald and Mary Brewster (Stanhope & Lancaster, 2010).

Funded by the Metropolitan Life Insurance Company (Murkofsky & Alston, 2009), Lillian Wald and Mary Brewster revolutionized the concept of public health nursing (Hitchcock et al., 2003). Lillian Wald is credited with developing the title *public health nurse*, and with that title the focus of nursing care was broadened to encompass not just the health of individuals but also the health, social, and economic needs of the community as a whole. In 1893 Wald and Brewster co-founded the first organized public health nursing agency, New York City's Henry Street Settlement. The settlement house provided a unique combination of social work, nursing, and social activism (Schoen & Koenig, 1997). The focus was public education to improve maternal and child health, communicable disease control, nutrition, and mental health. By 1911 Metropolitan Life Insurance Company had established the first national system of insurance for home care (Murkofsky & Alston, 2009).

The roles of the visiting nurse and public health nurse became more distinct by the late 1920s. Visiting nurses, employed by the private sector and financed by charity and public contributions, clearly were the "hands-on" providers of bedside nursing care in the home setting. Public health nurses, employed primarily by government health departments, focused their attention on promoting health and preventing disease in the broader community. Although their areas of concentration differed, both groups of nurses functioned independently in the delivery of nursing care outside of an institutional setting and shared the common goal of promoting, maintaining, and restoring health in the community (Hitchcock et al., 2003; see **Table 20-1**).

Successes achieved by the collective efforts of visiting nurses, public health nurses, and public health services created a shift in the focus of health care in the first half of the 20th century. Successes in teaching hygiene and decreases in immigration reduced the threat of communicable disease. Success in the community combined with advances in technology and hospital care led to changes in the populations served by home health nurses. During the 1930s and 1940s, fewer clients received care from visiting nurses (Reichley, 1999). However, hospitals quickly realized that although they were the providers of acute care, they were also becoming the providers of care for individuals with long-term chronic disorders. As a result, hospitals began searching for ways to control the increasing costs incurred by chronic illness care.

Establishment of New York City's Montefiore Hospital Home Care Program in 1947 provided one alternative to care of clients needing healthcare interventions outside of an acute care setting. The Montefiore Program, a "Hospital Without Walls," created a model of hospital-linked, home-delivered care utilizing the professional services of physicians, nurses, and social workers (Gundersen, 1999). This hospital-based homecare model demonstrated significant cost savings over in-hospital care and served as the catalyst for the resurgence of home health care as we know it today (Reichley, 1999). The focus for home care from Montefiore was not only the clients' illness, with its subsequent chronic state, but also their

Table 20-1 Similarities and Differences Between Public Health Nursing and Home Health Nursing		
Similarities		
Setting	Nursing care is provided to clients in their residences or in a community environment.	
Independent nature of practice	Nurses practice independently outside of institutions.	
Control and environment	Client is an active participant in care decisions. Control is shifted to the client. Environment empowers the client.	
Family-centered care	The family is considered as a unit of care. Family members contribute significantly to client care.	
Broad goals	Public health and home health services strive to promote, maintain, and restore health in the community.	
Differences	**Public Health Nursing**	**Home Health Nursing**
Focus of intervention	Population	Individual/family
Caseload acquisition	Case finding in community at large	Referral by physician
Interventions	Continuous	Episodic
Orientation	Wellness Primary prevention	Illness Secondary prevention Rehabilitation Tertiary prevention
Entry into services	Risk potential Social diagnosis	Medical diagnosis

Source: Hitchcock, J., Schubert, P., & Thomas, S. (Eds.). (2003). *Community health nursing: Caring in action* (2nd ed., p. 480). Albany, NY: Delmar. Reprinted with permission of Cengage Learning/Nelson Education.

holistic needs. Social workers addressed the clients' social needs and overall well-being and were interested in clients' families, including their role in providing for the clients' health care (Lundy & Janes, 2001).

For more than half a century, philanthropists, public charities, and contributions raised by the VNAs funded homecare services. In 1966 the federal government began providing for homecare services as a benefit of the new legislation known as Medicare. Medicare allowed for the expansion of homecare services to many people, particularly the elderly who did not have access to such care. In 1973 the Medicare homecare benefit was expanded to include disabled Americans regardless of age. However, homecare advocates became increasingly concerned that the narrowness of homecare legislation limited services as a means of avoiding the excessive costs of providing the full range of services that many clients needed (Reichley, 1999).

Between 1980 and 1996 the home healthcare industry experienced a 400% increase in Medicare-sponsored home care. During that time period, the number of agencies certified to bill Medicare rose by 200% (Montauk, 1998). This was a direct result of many reimbursement changes affecting hospitals. In an effort to control the cost of care in acute care hospitals, Congress passed the Social Security Amendments of 1983 to initiate the prospective payment system (PPS) for inpatient services (Stanhope & Lancaster, 2010). Therefore, federal government shifted reimbursement to a PPS based on diagnosis-related groups (DRGs). With reimbursement for hospital care now predetermined by client diagnosis, hospitals responded to the significant revenue reductions by decreasing the average length of stay for clients. The direct consequence was shorter hospital stays and increased referrals to home care (Stanhope & Lancaster, 2010).

However, in 1997 Congress targeted home health care as a place to reduce healthcare expenditures. The passage of the Balanced Budget Act of 1997 (BBA) imposed stricter limits on Medicare reimbursement for homecare services and required the Medicare administration to develop a PPS (Murkofsky & Alston, 2009). The BBA narrowed the definition of those individuals eligible to receive homecare services to those individuals who were deemed "homebound." Under these guidelines, Medicare recipients were no longer eligible for home care if they were able to leave home for any reason other than medical services (Maurer & Smith, 2005). The number of persons eligible for Medicare homecare funding declined by 50% between 1997 and 2000 (Maurer & Smith, 2005). Today, the industry continues to provide holistic care in a fiscally restrained environment. Under the PPS implemented in 2000, agencies were paid a set amount for each 60-day episode of care regardless of the number of visits provided. These payments are case-mix adjusted so the agency received more money for clients requiring more care (Murkofsky & Alston, 2009).

THEORETICAL FRAMEWORKS FOR MANAGEMENT OF CHRONIC ILLNESS IN HOME CARE

Homecare nurses provide intermittent care and rely heavily on clients' ability to self-manage their health problems. As such, the nurse is in a unique position to apply frameworks for practice that help the nurse work with clients to promote independence. Mid-range theories, applied in homecare settings to help promote client's self-management of chronic health problems, conceptualize nursing care as based in relationships and coaching, and provide guidelines for collaborative decision making, are presented here. Also included are models for community-based care of clients with chronic illness and hospice care.

Self-Management and Family Management of Chronic Conditions

The framework for self- and family management of chronic conditions is designed to provide a structure for understanding factors influencing the ability of individuals and their families to manage chronic illness (Grey, Knafl, & McCorkle, 2006; Tanner, 2004; see **Figure 20-1**). The components of the framework are: self-management; risk and protective factors including condition factors, individual factors, psychosocial characteristics, family factors, and the environment.

Self- and family management of chronic illness is defined as the decisions and activities that individuals make on a daily basis to manage

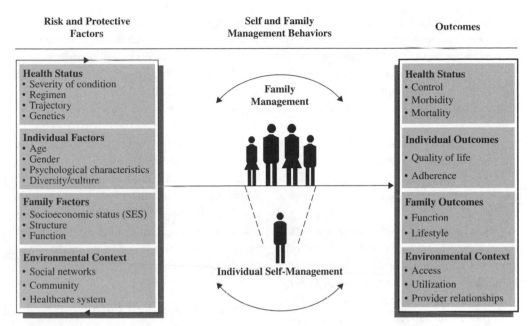

Risk and Protective Factors

Self and Family Management Behaviors

Outcomes

FIGURE 20-1   Self-management and Family Management Framework.
Source: Grey, M., Knafl, K., & McCorkle, R. (2006). A framework for the study of self- and family management of chronic conditions. *Nursing Outlook*, 54, 278–286. Reprinted with permission by: Elsevier Inc.

their chronic health problems (Improving Chronic Illness Care, 2007; Grey et al., 2006; Ryan & Sawin, 2009). For some individuals, particularly those who are older or have cognitive deficits, engaging in self-management will be an ongoing challenge (Tanner, 2004). The nurse is challenged to help the client manage at the level of his or her ability (Jacelon, Furman, Rea, Macdonald, & Donoghue, 2011). The concept of self-management extends the responsibility of individuals with chronic illness beyond compliance and adherence to managing an ongoing condition within the context of their daily lives. In home care it is imperative that the nurse consider both the client's ability to self-manage and the family's ability to support the individual's self-management (Grey et al., 2006).

The ability of individuals and families to manage chronic illness depends on the severity of the condition, the treatment regimen, the course of the disease, individual and family characteristics, and the environment in which individuals will manage their disease (Grey et al., 2006). The severity of the illness from the perspective of the individual with the chronic illness may not be the same as the nurse's perception. The meaning of the condition and the implications for management may be affected by the meaning of the illness to the individual and family. The etiology of the condition (e.g., a lifestyle disease such as emphysema as a result of smoking or a genetically determined disease) will affect the ability for self-management. The implications for the family in these situations may cause guilt or concern for the susceptibility of other family members. The treatment regimen for a chronic illness may be complex, requiring significant lifestyle adjustment. Individual factors such as the person's age, psychosocial situation, functional ability, self-perceived ability to manage the illness, education, and socioeconomic status all contribute to the individual's ability for self-management. Careful assessment by the nurse is imperative in providing care. Once an assessment is complete, the homecare nurse is in a position to coach the individual or family in management of the illness.

In the model of self-management and family management, outcomes can include improved condition symptoms, and improved individual and family outcomes such as better disease management, improved quality of life, or improved self-efficacy (Grey et al., 2006). The main goal of the model is to help the individual improve his or her health, using the broadest definition of health possible. The homecare nurse will want to support the self- and family's self-management, teach them the skills needed to improve health, and coach the individual and family on incorporating those activities into their daily lives.

Coaching as a Technique to Enhance Self-management and Family Management

The homecare nurse is in an excellent position to coach the client and family in the management of the chronic illness. Coaching, or motivational interviewing, is a strategy in which the nurse uses a combination of providing education, collaborative decision making, and empowerment to help clients manage their health needs (Butterworth, Linden, & McClay, 2007; Huffman, 2007, 2009). Health coaching has its roots in substance abuse counseling and has been found to be a relatively

short-term, successful strategy. Health coaching is a client-centered approach to care with the focus on the issues and barriers to self-management.

To employ health coaching, the home health nurse begins by asking the client what he or she is most concerned about. In this way, the nurse can capitalize on the client's interest in resolving or managing a particular problem. The next step is to validate the client's feelings about his or her capacity to manage the problem. Following this, the nurse might help the client develop solutions to the problem by asking about what strategies the client has tried in the past, and what strategies he or she might like to try (Huffman, 2007).

Relationship-Based Care

In this model, relationship is the basis of nursing practice (Doane, 2002). Individuals are "viewed as contextual beings who exist in relation with other people and with social, cultural, political, and historical processes" (Doane & Varcoe, 2007, p. 198). Every day nurses engage in relationships with clients, other nurses, and healthcare professionals. This network of relationships forms a web of mutual dependencies (Doane & Varcoe, p. 193). Relationship-based care is a model of human relating that reflects this web of interactions within the context of humanistic values (Hartrick, 1997). In the past, models of nursing care have been based on behavioral models in which the nurse learns a set of communication skills and applies those skills when interacting with clients. This model is unique in that it is based on the recognition of the relational nature and complexity of human experience (Hartrick, 1997, p. 524). Rather than enhancing communication between nurse and client, applying communication techniques may impede communication because the nurse may be focused on performing these techniques, and unable to be "in-caring-human-relation" (Hartrick, 1997, p. 525). According to this model, "health and healing are promoted through the development of an increasing openness to learning and growth, an increasing capacity to tolerate ambiguity and uncertainty, and an increasing experience of empowerment and choice" (Hartrick, 1997, p. 525). For clients with chronic illness, this model of human relation may provide a means for the client, family, and nurse to grow in relationships with each other as well as in the relationship with the chronic illness.

Relationship-based care is not founded on problem identification and resolution, but on responding to the client in a manner that acknowledges and supports the significance of the chronic illness as the client experiences it. Nursing action is based on five capacities: 1) initiative, authenticity, and responsiveness; 2) mutuality and synchrony; 3) honoring complexity and ambiguity; 4) intentionality in relating; and 5) re-imaging (Hartrick, 1997, p. 526).

Initiative, authenticity, and responsiveness address the nurse's active concern for others (Hartrick, 1997, p. 526). Within this model, these concepts are intertwined. The nurse takes the initiative to engage in relationship with the client. She or he is authentic, responding to the client and the situation in a way that is consistent with his or her personality, and showing emotions as they arise. Finally the nurse is responsive to the feelings, needs, and goals of the client. The nurse is mindful of her presence with the client and is attentive to the client with conscious listening.

The concepts of mutuality and synchrony explain the nature of relationships. Mutuality refers to the commonalities experienced by people in relationships. A mutual relationship is a negotiated, collaborative process where client and nurse both participate, make choices, and act (Doane & Varcoe, 2007, p. 193). These commonalities include shared visions and goals, while acknowledging differences in perspectives. Synchrony describes the rhythms naturally occurring in the relationship, including synchrony between internal and external patterns, and periods of silence (Hartrick, 1997, p. 526).

The nurse honors complexity and ambiguity by acknowledging the complexity of human experience. The nurse, in relation with the client, seeks to uncover the numerous and possibly conflicting elements of the experience. Through this process of discovery, the nurse and client begin to mutually make connections between seemingly disparate actions, feelings, and events. Through this process, the client and nurse are able to appreciate the relevance of the experience and make choices regarding the management of the disease process (Hartrick, 1997, p. 526).

Intentionality involves the nurse exploring his or her values and then maintaining consistency between personal values and values in use during professional practice. Each nursing moment is shaped by the actions and intentions of the nurse, the actions and responses of others, and by the contexts within which those interactions occur (Doane & Varcoe, 2007, p. 202). The intent of relational practice is to help clients understand the meaning of their health and healing experiences, and to discover choice and power within the experiences (Hartrick, 1997, p. 527). Re-imaging is the process of questioning the usual ways of being in the world. Through this process, the nurse can help clients transform their health and healing experiences and enhance their relational capacity (Hartrick, 1997, p. 527).

The nurse who engages in relational nursing practice makes a conscious commitment to act using the values and goals of the nursing profession to attend to each client's unique context and situation, helping that person grow in health. Difficulty and suffering can provide a vehicle for meaningful relationships, which is the basis for ethical decision making. In these situations, responsive nursing care creates the space for mutual experience, and for nurse and client to develop clarity and courage to act in health-promoting ways (Doane & Varcoe, 2007, p. 202).

In more recent work, Weydt (2010) identifies other characteristics necessary for effective relationship-based care. These include clinical proficiency, interdisciplinary communication and teamwork, and continuity of nurse/patient/family relationships. In home care where a primary nursing care model is common, building relationships with clients to improve their self-management of chronic disease can help clients maximize their quality of life.

Chronic Care Model of Disease Management

Individuals with chronic disease require a new strategy for health management. The Chronic Care Model (CCM) (**Figure 20-2**) was developed through a grant from the Robert Wood Johnson Foundation to change the way health care was delivered to individuals with chronic illness (Improving Chronic Illness Care, 2007). The model is designed to support the person with the chronic illness to self-manage his or her health using appropriate community and healthcare system resources. The home health nurse is in an excellent position to assist the client in managing his or her own health and chronic illness within this model (see Chapter 19).

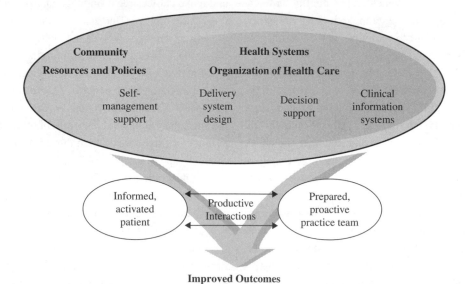

FIGURE 20-2 The Chronic Care Model.
Source: Wagner, E.H. (1998). Chronic disease management: What will it take to improve care for chronic illness? *Effective Clinical Practice*, 1, 2–4.

Traditionally, the healthcare system in the United States has been focused on providing acute care for acute illness in an episodic manner. Individuals with chronic illness require a proactive approach, combining self-management with effective use of community resources and the healthcare system (Improving Chronic Illness Care, 2007). Care is based on evidence-based protocols that are then tailored to the needs of the individual client. Common areas of difficulty for self-management include managing multiple medications, recognizing early warning signs of condition changes, coordinating and appearing for multiple physicians' appointments, understanding the plan of treatment, and coordinating support services (Meckes, 2005).

According to the CCM, healthcare systems need to retool to provide planned visits focused on maintaining wellness. In this model, clients are recognized as having the central role in managing their health. It is the role of healthcare providers to support clients' ability to self-manage their health (Improving Chronic Illness Care, 2007). The nurse can also affect the client's understanding of the disease process and choices for management. By being in the client's home, the homecare nurse has a unique perspective on the client's culture, and the meaning of the illness in his or her life.

Recently the CCM has been adapted to reflect care delivered by nurses in post-acute care settings such as home care (Jacelon et al., 2011). In this version of the model, the nurse and client are at the center of the model. The nurse and client form a team where the nurse coaches and advises the client in effective self-management techniques. The home healthcare nurse may act as a case manager, helping the client navigate complicated interactions with several medical care professionals, and guiding the client to seek medical care for condition changes in a timely manner. In addition, the nurse can encourage clients to engage with community organizations to help support their self-management strategies; these community agencies might include food programs and disease-focused organizations (e.g., the Alzheimer's Association).

Philosophy of Palliative and Hospice Care

Palliative care is a philosophy of care in which the focus is on promoting quality of life in the time an individual has left. According to the National Quality Forum (2006), palliative care refers to patient- and family-centered care that optimizes quality of life by anticipating, preventing, and treating suffering. The philosophy is applied across a wide variety of settings and professional fields. Palliative care, throughout the continuum of illness, involves addressing physical, intellectual, emotional, social, and spiritual needs and facilitating patient autonomy, access to information, and choice in the face of life-threatening illness. It incorporates symptom control, including pain management, supportive care, respite care, rehabilitation, and terminal care. The philosophy of palliative care can be applied whenever the client has a life-limiting chronic illness (World Health Organization [WHO], 2009).

While palliative care is a philosophy, hospice care is a particular type of care provided at the end of life. The focus of hospice is the belief that each person has the right to die pain-free and with dignity, and that family members and informal caregivers will receive the necessary support to allow people to do so (National Hospice and Palliative Care Organization, 2007). Hospice care is a constellation of services provided with the goal of providing comfort and symptom management at the end of life (Stuart, 2003). Hospice care is often provided in a specialized facility or in the individual's home. Recently hospice services have begun to be offered in nursing homes and some acute care facilities (Candy, Holman, Leurent, Davis, & Jones, 2011). Many home healthcare agencies offer hospice services in addition to their regular homecare services. As a clearly circumscribed level of care, Medicare pays for service to hospice clients on a per diem basis. Nonetheless, the hospice benefit is underutilized; only 20% of those people eligible use their hospice benefit (Stuart, 2003). In order to be eligible for the hospice benefit, physicians must determine that the client has fewer than 6 months to live, and the patient must forgo treatment that may extend life (see Chapter 22).

INTERVENTIONS

It is anticipated that the need for homecare services will increase as the population ages. Because of the unique characteristics required to be a successful homecare nurse, the shortage of qualified nurses in home care may be more severe than in other areas of the healthcare system (Ellenbecker, 2004). Homecare nurses must possess unique skills including "flexibility, creativity, and innovative approaches to situations and problems in the context of individual and environmental differences and widely varying resource availability" (ANA, 2008, p. 7). According to *Home Health Nursing Scope: and Standards of Practice* (ANA, 2008), the nurse best suited to homecare practice is the baccalaureate-prepared nurse. This is because of his or her broad-based education. Nurses prepared at the associate degree or diploma level are

typically members of the homecare team. All nurses engaged in home care are expected to advance their ability to meet client needs in the homecare setting. This goal is accomplished by supporting colleagues, structured preceptor programs, clinical experience, and lifelong learning (ANA, 2008). See **Table 20-2** for the ANA minimum qualifications for a homecare nurse.

Using grounded theory techniques, Neal (1998) developed a model of Home Health Nursing Practice. The model outlines three stages of proficiency in homecare nursing. At the first level, termed *dependency*, the nurse is typically new to the setting, overwhelmed by the complexity of the setting, and is dependent on support and assistance from others. As the nurse moves to the second phase, *moderate dependency*, he or she becomes less dependent on others, before finally moving to the phase of *autonomy*, where the nurse achieves confidence, self-assurance, and

Table 20-2   Minimum Qualifications of Homecare Nurses
A baccalaureate degree in nursing
Ability to incorporate communication and motivation skills and principles in the home health setting
Ability to apply critical thinking to physical, psychosocial, environmental, cultural, family, and safety issues
Ability to utilize clinical decision making in applying the nursing process to clients in their places of residence
Ability to practice as an effective member of an interdisciplinary team
Competency in applying care-management skills

Source: American Nurses Association. (2008). *Home health nursing: Scope and standards of practice.* Silver Springs, MD: Author.

autonomy in the role of a home health nurse (p. 23). Later, Neal used a triangulated design combining focus groups with one sample of homecare nurses and a survey with a second group to test and enhance the model (Neal, 2000).

Cultural Competence

As the older population grows, and diversity of individuals with chronic illness increases, there are persistent trends in usage of homecare services. Caucasians are more likely to use formal services than Hispanics, African Americans, and Asian Americans. However, it is difficult to tell if this pattern is a choice of the care recipient or if this trend represents a cultural bias of the care providers who refer individuals to home care (Young, 2003). It is critical for the homecare nurse to remember that when he or she is providing care in the client's home, he or she is a guest in the client's culture. In order to increase the likelihood of the client adopting the self-management strategies the nurse is offering, the nurse must find a way to connect the health care that he or she is offering with meaningful experiences that connect the client's experience.

Reimbursement in Home Care/Documentation

Skilled services that are reimbursable by third-party payers drive the homecare industry. The majority of skilled homecare services are paid for by health insurance, particularly Medicare and Medicaid. In 2000 Medicare and Medicaid paid for 72% of homecare services and 87% of hospice clients (Clark, 2008). In 2006 the percentage had increased to 77% with private insurance accounting for only 12% of costs. The remaining 10% were paid out of pocket by clients (Murkofsky & Alston, 2009). Usually, private insurance companies follow the guidelines set by Medicare. Therefore, changes in Medicare regulations and reimbursement have a major effect on the home healthcare industry.

Medicare establishes regulations that determine who is eligible to receive reimbursable homecare services. Accompanying the Medicare funding stream are strict regulations for client eligibility, homecare practice, and reimbursement mechanisms. Although the Medicare homecare benefit was designed to extend care to more people, access was difficult because only certain agencies could provide care, and restrictions limited who was eligible for care, which services clients could receive, and length of service. An additional burden on homecare agencies was a complex billing system that often resulted in extensive payment delays.

Agencies adhering to the Medicare guidelines to receive Medicare and Medicaid payment are classified as "certified." "Noncertified" home health agencies render home healthcare privately without consideration of the Medicare guidelines, and thus receive no payment from Medicare. A home health agency may choose to participate in the Medicare program and can receive payment from Medicare for those clients who meet the eligibility criteria. Agencies choosing not to participate in the Medicare program follow their respective state-established regulations that govern the provision of homecare services. However, as a quality measure, private payment agencies often follow the standards of adequate care as established by Medicare.

When a client's care can no longer be billed to Medicare, the agency is responsible for providing advanced notice to the physician and client, and assisting with finding other sources of care. The client can independently pay the agency. This arrangement provides an alternative to third-party reimbursed care. Since the inception of PPS, many long-term care clients have paid their own bills for care. As Medicare defines its payment criteria, it was never intended to pay for care other than short term, acute, intermittent, and skilled, so clients needing longer term services require other payment sources.

If a home health agency determines that a client can no longer be served because of costs, discontinuation of care may make the agency at risk for charges of client abandonment. The definition of abandonment is cessation of services by an agency to a client who continues to require care and for whom no provision has been made; nor has the client received proper and timely notice of impending discharge from service.

In the PPS, a specific dollar amount per client is given to a healthcare professional for delivery of services. The healthcare provider, in turn, becomes the coordinator of the individual's care and assumes responsibility for managing cost, risk, resources, and outcomes of care (Remington, 2000). Reimbursement amounts are determined by clinical assessment of the client's needs using the mandated assessment tool, Outcome Assessment System and Information Set (OASIS).

OASIS is an assessment tool designed to establish the national standard for collecting client outcome data that can be used to evaluate homecare services on an industry-wide basis. The tool is used to collect a combination of demographic, clinical, and functional client care data used in calculating Medicare payments to home health agencies.

The actual charges submitted by an agency are determined by the OASIS clinical scoring system, which assigns points to select items in the OASIS data set plus assigns additional points if therapy services are needed. The OASIS scoring system is intended to calculate Medicare

payments based on the severity and acuity of the client's condition, and, in this way, higher payments are provided for sicker clients. There are no limitations on the episodes of care that a client can receive. The OASIS has been used to measure outcomes from nursing interventions. However, in their evaluation of OASIS, Schneider, Barkauskas, and Keenan (2008) did not find it to be sensitive to the effects of home healthcare nursing, as measured by intervention intensity.

The influence of the implementation of the PPS in home health has been more stringent regulations about which services will be reimbursed, and for how long, in some instances. This may well limit access to care for certain vulnerable groups, such as the frail elderly and chronically ill individuals whose care is largely home based, and people who are human immunodeficiency virus (HIV) positive. Nurses and other healthcare providers must work even more closely with families to determine the kinds of services needed to foster self-care and the optimal timing of these services (Stanhope & Lancaster, 2010).

The individuals who use homecare services often have very complex health needs. In a study designed to determine which hospitalized clients were most likely to be referred for homecare services, Narsavage and Naylor (2000) found that those individuals most likely to be referred had more than one chronic illness (chronic obstructive pulmonary disease and congestive heart failure [CHF]), were unmarried, needed help with activities of daily living, and had a longer than average hospital stay.

The Future of Reimbursement

Since 2000, there has been increasing pressure by the government to slow the growth and costs of home care. Pay for performance demonstrations were instituted in seven states, and Congress has instituted several caps and restrictions on reimbursement (Murkofsky & Alston, 2009). At the same time the reimbursement for skilled services through Medicare is contracting, there is an initiative to move individuals out of long-term care institutions and provide supportive services in their homes. This initiative is funded by state Medicaid budgets and is an effort to reduce long-term care costs.

Although the Patient Protection and Affordable Care Act signed into law in March 2010 does not specifically mention homecare services, the act will affect services. The mandate that all individuals have health insurance may not have a major effect on home care, because private insurance accounts for only 12% of homecare revenue. However, the move to expand Medicaid to include all individuals with incomes up to 133% of the poverty level could mean an increase in Medicaid-covered services.

Two provisions in the new law will have a direct effect on home health care. First, beginning in January 2013, there is a provision to establish a national Medicare pilot program to develop and evaluate paying a bundled payment for acute, inpatient hospital services, physician services, outpatient hospital services, and post-acute care services for an episode of care that begins 3 days prior to a hospitalization and spans 30 days following discharge. If the pilot program achieves stated goals of improving (or not reducing) quality and reducing spending, CMS will develop a plan for expanding the pilot program beginning in 2016. The second provision, beginning in 2012, will create the Independence at Home demonstration program to provide high-need Medicare beneficiaries with primary care services in their home and allow participating teams of health professionals to share in any savings if they reduce preventable hospitalizations, prevent hospital readmissions, improve health outcomes, improve the efficiency of care, reduce the cost of healthcare services, and achieve patient satisfaction. (Kaiser Foundation, 2010).

Home Healthcare Agencies

Home care is a unique healthcare service, in that homecare practice is by definition in the home of the recipient of care. The living arrangements of the individual receiving care are an important consideration in determining the "goodness of fit" between the client's needs and the services provided (Hayes, 2002). The home health nurse uses primary, secondary, and tertiary prevention strategies in assisting clients and families with self-management and coordination of community resources. This is accomplished within the community in the home of the client (ANA, 2008).

Home healthcare practitioners and standards of practice are governed by state and federal legislation. Individual state regulations must be met for basic licensing of all home health agencies. If participation in the Medicare reimbursement program is desired, there are also federal regulations that govern Medicare certification and coverage of services (Conditions of Participation and HHA-11, respectively) that must be met. These federal mandates, along with individual state licensing or certification requirements, help ensure that home healthcare practitioners are qualified to provide their specialized services.

Language of Home Health Care

Several definitions are important in determining eligibility of patients and subsequent reimbursement by the home healthcare agency. Terms are defined by federal Medicare regulations and include the following: *homebound, primary services, continuing services*, and *dependent services*.

Federal Medicare regulations include the qualifications of clients for coverage of home health services. The client must be confined to the home or to an institution that is not a hospital or skilled nursing facility (SNF). Confined to the home does not mean the client must be bedridden. *Homebound*, or home confined, is defined as an inability to leave the home normally and that leaving would be taxing and require considerable effort and assistance. When the client does leave the home, the absences are infrequent and of relatively short duration, or to receive medical care. The client must be under the care of a physician and in need of skilled services on an intermittent-visit, not continuous, basis. The services must be provided in the client's home. Hospitals or nursing homes are not considered the client's home, but individuals living in assisted living facilities or other group living situations are eligible for home care (Murkofsky & Alston, 2009). Reimbursement is made to the homecare agency under the PPS. Medicare pays the homecare agency a set amount of money for each client whose diagnosis is one of 80 home health resource groups (Stanhope & Lancaster, 2010). In addition to primary skilled services, home health aides and social work services are covered as dependent services under Medicare regulations. The client must require a skilled service to receive a home health aide or social work services, and once the skilled service is no longer required, the home health aide and social work services are not covered. These dependent services can also be continued if occupational therapy (a continuing service) is to be provided to the client.

Home Healthcare Team

The home healthcare team consists of the client, physicians, nurses, physical therapists, occupational therapists, speech therapists, medical social workers, home health aides, and informal caregivers. Each member of the team possesses a special set of skills that collectively supports a comprehensive approach to assist the client in meeting his or her care needs.

Effective home care depends on groups of independent practitioners forming teams to provide services for clients. These practitioners have different skill sets and are not always all from the same agency. The multiple practitioners on the home healthcare team have the knowledge and skills to identify clients' needs and address those needs through management of complex plans of care (Marelli, 1998). Each practitioner must have a strong grasp of the rules and regulations that govern home health care, the ability to pay attention to detail, well-developed interpersonal skills, strong clinical skills, a working knowledge of the changing economics of health care, and the ability to effectively prioritize and time-manage challenging tasks and responsibilities.

Four models of team functioning have been identified: medical, multidisciplinary, interdisciplinary, and transdisciplinary (Mauk, 2007, p. 3). In a medical model team, the physician leader directs all functions of the team. Team members do not meet together but communicate through the physician. This team configuration is most common in acute care settings where the physician is in daily contact with the client. This model is not desirable in a homecare situation because the client may not be in contact with the physician; the care providers are in the client's home, and independent decision making is a hallmark of this type of care.

The second type of team is the multidisciplinary team. In this model, professionals work in parallel. Each provider develops goals for his or her interaction with the client, and coordination occurs at the supervisory level. The individuals who are providing care rarely communicate directly with each other. This model of care is common in long-term care settings in which a rigid bureaucratic structure exists. Multidisciplinary models also occur in homecare settings. However, the nature of home care is that practitioners work independently and may interact with other professionals on the team only sporadically (Gantert & McWilliams, 2004).

Transdisciplinary teams are found in rehabilitation settings where team members and the client are in proximity daily. In this model, the client and primary care provider work as a team with the counsel of all other team members (Mauk, 2007). Individual team members perform the interventions required for the client while the provider is with the client. Although this model is effective in rehabilitation settings, the nature of home care does not lend itself to this type of team function. The billing constraints in home care require that professionals perform the interventions within their scope of practice, and do not reimburse for care outside of that scope. This model works best in a capitated payment system, where the agency receives a predetermined amount of money for care regardless of who is providing the care.

The team configuration that is most effective in the home setting is the interdisciplinary team model. In an interdisciplinary team, professionals working with a client communicate directly with the client and each other. In this model, the client is an integral part of the team, and professionals collaborate with the client to establish goals for care (Mauk, 2007). Effective interdisciplinary team collaboration has been associated with benefits for both practitioner and client. These include increased provider autonomy and job satisfaction, and improved client outcomes and cost containment (Gantert & McWilliams, 2004).

Gantert and McWilliams (2004) identified three dimensions of interaction among interdisciplinary team members: networking, navigating, and aligning. Each dimension occurs along a continuum. The less interactive end of the continuum is representative of a multidisciplinary team, whereas the more interactive end is representative of a more interdisciplinary model. For networking, the continuum ran from isolation to connectedness. As communication among team members increased, so did feelings of connectedness among team members. Navigating had to do with how the team members trusted each other. The more contact team members had with each other, the more trust they exhibited with each other. Finally, the dimension of aligning described the strategies used to determine roles within the team. Team function ranges from the traditional organization hierarchy to a more fluid organization, where team members function autonomously and collaboratively (Gantert & McWilliams, 2004).

Coordination of Care

Care coordination is defined as services provided to individuals with chronic illness who are at risk for adverse outcomes and expensive care that remedy shortcomings in current health care by:

- Identifying medical, functional, social, and emotional needs that increase risk of adverse outcomes and expensive care.
- Addressing those needs through self-care education and optimization of medical treatment.
- Monitoring progress and identifying problems early (Mathematica Policy Research, 2000).

Homecare nurses and agencies are in an excellent position to incorporate the role of care coordinator into the role of the nurse because these high-risk individuals are often being treated by homecare nurses. Nurses have a well established relationship with physicians and the local healthcare system and are in an excellent position to incorporate technology into the plan of care through the use of telehealth strategies to augment care (Meckes, 2005).

Three major care coordination issues have been identified (Feldman, 2004). The first is coordination between the hospital and the homecare agency at discharge from the hospital or at admission to the hospital from the homecare agency. Transitions from one service to another are fraught with opportunities for miscommunication. The second issue for care coordination is strengthening the effectiveness and communication among the members of the interdisciplinary team (Feldman, 2004). The third issue is to improve the effectiveness of interaction between the formal and informal caregivers and to foster self-management (Feldman, 2004). This issue is described in more detail in the following.

The Program of All-Inclusive Care for the Elderly (PACE) provides for older adults with chronic illness, who are eligible for both Medicare and Medicaid, and who are living at home even though they qualify for nursing home care (Young, 2003). Through PACE, interdisciplinary teams assess individuals and provide comprehensive services across settings. By removing the financial barriers to coordination of care, the PACE concept unites the healthcare team around providing long-term care management in the least restrictive setting (Young, 2003).

Formal and Informal Caregivers

Unpaid assistance is provided to older individuals and those with chronic illness in at least 22.9 million households (21%) across the United States. By contrast, less than half (41%) of the individuals receiving informal care reported paying for services from professional care providers (National Alliance for Caregiving [NAC] & AARP, 2004). The NAC and AARP counted individuals as caregivers if they were older than 18 years of age and performed one of 13 activities for another adult—**Table 20-3** lists the 13 caregiving behaviors. Young (2003) reports that 73% of caregivers are women, with an average age of 46, and 64% work outside of the home.

In a study conducted at the Visiting Nurse Service of New York, researchers explored the effects of formal and informal caregiving on the recovery of the client, and the interaction between

Table 20-3   Informal Caregiver Behaviors

Instrumental Activities of Daily Living

Transportation (82%)

Grocery shopping (75%)

Housework (69%)

Managing finances (64%)

Preparing meals (59%)

Helping with medication (41%)

Managing services (30%)

Activities of Daily Living

Get in and out of a chair or bed (36%)

Dressing (29%)

Bathing or showering (26%)

Toileting (23%)

Eating (18%)

Incontinence (16%)

Source: National Alliance for Caregiving and American Association of Retired Persons. *Caregiving in the US; Executive summary*. Washington, DC: Author. Used with permission.

formal and informal caregivers. The findings identified gaps in the information and training received by informal caregivers (Feldman, 2004, p. 34) (see Chapter 10).

Assessing the ability of unpaid caregivers to support the individual with chronic illness is critical to developing an effective plan of care. Tanner (2004) developed a scale to be used with individuals with chronic health problems to determine the availability of family support. The Tanner Family Support Scale (TFSS) is a 13-item scale in which the individual agrees or disagrees with such statements as, "My family members do as much as they can to help me with my health problems when I need help" (Tanner, 2004, p. 314).

Often the home healthcare nurse and the recipient of care rely heavily on the informal caregiver. Collaboration and decision making often involve a triad rather than the usual nurse–client dyad (Dalton, 2003). However, the nurse must carefully negotiate the relationship to make sure that the recipient of care is not silenced (Dalton, 2003). Dalton (2005) identified three types of decisions commonly made about nursing care: program decisions (goals and content of care), operational control decisions (how the plan is implemented), and agenda decisions (timing and frequency of nursing visits and care delivery). Coalitions formed between two of the three parts of the triad can affect all care decisions. Homecare nurses should collaborate with both the client receiving care and informal caregivers to optimize the benefit of the available professional care. Leff (2004) found that clients demonstrated higher satisfaction with care when they were included in decision making regarding goals, the plan, who (which disciplines and personnel) will provide care, how often and what time of day visits would occur, the activities

occurring during the visit, how care is provided, and who will communicate with the physician (p. 298).

Information Technology and Telehealth

One of the fastest growing areas of home health care is telehealth. Assistive devices in the home have the potential to improve home safety, enhance independence, and reduce the risk for injury of individuals with chronic illness (Young, 2003). However, Medicare does not presently reimburse for telehealth home care. In addition, some individuals, both clients and care providers, are ambivalent about the use of monitoring technology in the home because of the potential invasion of privacy (Percival & Hanson, 2006). At the same time that home technology is exploding, home care is an industry that has embraced the use of technology such as cellular phones, laptop computers, the Internet, and telehealth (ANA, 2008). Appropriate use of information technology and telehealth can lead to enhanced quality of care, improved client and clinician safety, and increased productivity (American Telemedicine Association [ATA], 2011). Meanwhile, the ethical issues of privacy and data protection are significant (Percival & Hanson, 2006).

The ATA has defined telemedicine as "the use of medical information exchanged from one site to another via electronic communications to improve clients' health status" (ATA, 2011). Telemedicine may include distance monitoring of an individual's health status, routine consultations with healthcare providers, referrals to specialists for complex problems, and consumer health information sites on the Internet. However, at present, a telehealth visit may not be substituted for an in-person visit, and if telemedicine is to be used for a homecare client, the plan of care and the physician's order must specify the expected level of live visits and the expected level of telehome care (Pushkin, 2001).

Guidelines for telehealth programs have been developed, including generic guidelines for all home telehealth applications, interactive home telehealth guidelines, and telemonitoring (Britton, 2003). The generic guidelines should be included in all telehealth programs and include determining client-inclusion criteria, explaining the program and obtaining client consent, protection of individual's health information, home assessment for appropriateness of the plan, client/caregiver education, and a plan for performance improvement that includes the client (Britton, 2003). In addition, programs using interactive home telehealth should establish procedures to protect the client's privacy when he or she does not wish to be observed, and the plan of care must be guided by physician order and clearly outline the plan for live and virtual visits. Finally, for programs that use telemonitoring, formal care providers must be adequately trained, and the protocol for monitoring and for action when the client symptoms deviate from the normal parameters for that patient must be clearly established (Britton, 2003).

As the available technology expands, the efficacy of telemedicine and telehealth is being tested. In a study evaluating the effectiveness of a telemedicine intervention for clients with CHF who had recently been discharged from the hospital as opposed to a group of similar clients receiving the usual homecare services, researchers found that while the telemedicine intervention reduced the number of nursing visits, home health costs, and improved the client's self-perceived quality of life, it did not affect the number of re-admissions or visits to the emergency department (Myers, Grant, Lugn, Holbert, &

Kvedar, 2006). Unexpected findings included a need for ongoing education and support for the clients using the telehealth equipment throughout the treatment period. In addition, several potential research participants declined or withdrew from the study because they were anxious about using the equipment (Myers et al., 2006).

Telehealth is here to stay. In a Cochrane review of controlled clinical trials evaluating the efficacy of telehealth, Murray, Burns, See Tai, Lai, and Nazareth (2005) found that interactive health communication applications (IHCAs) had a positive effect on several aspects of functioning. The review included 3,739 clients involved in 24 randomized controlled clinical trials. Across studies, people with chronic illnesses using IHCAs had a better understanding of their health problems, and IHCAs had a positive effect on social support and behavioral and clinical outcomes. In addition, IHCAs were positively related to improved self-efficacy (Murray et al., p. 1).

Clinical Care Classification (CCC) System

The CCC was developed in 1991 by Saba and colleagues as a way of predicting resource needs and measuring the outcomes of home care (Saba, 1998). Since then, the system has gained credibility through independent research and use in clinical and educational settings (**Table 20-4**). The most recent update was in 2004 (Saba, 2004).

The classification system consists of two standardized, interrelated terminologies: one for nursing diagnosis and another for nursing interventions. The two terminologies are classified by 21 care components and organized into four health patterns: behavioral, functional, physiologic, and psychological, representing a comprehensive

Table 20-4   CCC System: 21 Care Components by Four Clinical Pattern
Health Behavioral Components
Medication
Safety
Health behavior
Functional Components
Activity
Fluid volume
Nutritional
Self-care
Sensory
Physiologic Components
Cardiac
Respiratory
Metabolic
Physical regulation
Skin integrity
Tissue perfusion
Bowel elimination
Urinary elimination
Life cycle
Psychological Components
Cognitive
Coping
Role relationship
Self-concept
Source: Saba, V. K. Clinical Care Classification (CCC) System. Retrieved from www.sabacare.com/. Used with permission.

approach to client care (Saba, 1998). The system was designed, in part, to facilitate computerized client recordkeeping and relating nursing diagnosis and interventions to client outcomes. It can be incorporated into an existing home healthcare record, and linked to reimbursement software (Saba, 1998, p. 12; more information on the CCC can be obtained at www.sabacare.com).

The home health industry is challenged to skillfully manage the risk, cost, resources, and outcomes of client care. All agency staff require a thorough education to be familiar with the rules and regulations for agency operations and how each staff member's skills and talents will be used to achieve agency goals. Clinicians need continuing education focused on maximizing the value of provided care. Accurate, thorough client assessments and rapid submission of these data are critical for the agency to obtain timely reimbursement.

OUTCOMES

The desired outcomes for home health care in the management of the client with chronic illness seem initially to be quite apparent. The positive effects of the health care delivered in the home to the client, as well as the positive effects of the caregiver support mechanisms that keep the client at home and do not necessitate institutionalization, are clearly important outcomes. However, the urgency of establishing outcome criteria that are stable and dependable in order to measure outcome attainment is essential to knowing if positive effects are occurring to the advantage of the client and caregiver or simply because there is no alternative to providing care.

Maurer and Smith (2005) have established nine possible outcome measures for evaluating the outcome attainment judged by changes in the population, the healthcare system within the community, or the environment. The identified outcome measures include 1) knowledge; 2) behaviors, skills; 3) attitudes; 4) emotional well-being; 5) health status (epidemiology); 6) presence of healthcare system services and components; 7) satisfaction or acceptance regarding the program interventions; 8) presence of policy allowing, mandating, and funding; and 9) altered relationship with the physical environment (p. 403).

Evaluating the outcomes of care rendered by any of the disciplines participating in home health care for the first five measures is inclusive in the care itself. The professionals and paraprofessionals who work within the home-care team function within and by delivering care using these first five principles, thereby making their use as measurement variables relatively easy and functional. The last four outcome measures, however, have been a continuous struggle for home health care throughout the 20th and now the 21st

centuries. These four measures are unpredictably influenced by the ups and downs of financial support, government regulations, management control in home health itself, and in the institutional care that passes clients on to in-home care.

Home health nurses can promote clients' self-management of their chronic diseases. The nurse can be effective in helping clients and their informal caregivers to maximize the support available to them. Using strategies such as coaching and telemedicine can help clients improve their self-care abilities. Resources such as protocols, care maps, and clinical pathways will become more useful, along with the incentive to explore advanced technologies such as point-of-service computers and telemedicine devices.

CASE STUDY

Ms. Lavoie is a 77-year-old woman with a diagnosis of CHF. She lives alone on the first floor of a two-family home in an urban neighborhood. She has lived in the same house for 57 years. Over that time, the neighborhood has declined around her. Now there are many boarded-up houses on her street. Ms. Lavoie was admitted to the hospital after an exacerbation of her cardiac symptoms. While in the hospital, the physician evaluated and adjusted her cardiac medications. It was determined that one of the contributing factors to the exacerbation of symptoms was Ms. Lavoie's diet. When interviewed at admission, it was clear that Ms. Lavoie had a poor understanding of her diet prescription.

After 5 days in the hospital, Ms. Lavoie was discharged from the hospital with orders for home care. Nurse Jones visited Ms. Lavoie for her intake interview within the regulated 48 hours after discharge from the hospital. At the first visit, Nurse Jones completed the admission assessment including self-management; risk and protective factors including condition factors, individual factors, psychosocial characteristics, family factors, and information about the neighborhood (environment). She collected the OASIS data, and began teaching Ms. Lavoie about her new medications. Nurse Jones created a chart written in large print with the name of each medication, the purpose of each, and when Ms. Lavoie should take the medication. Nurse Jones developed a 60-day plan of care for Ms. Lavoie that included the number of visits, medications, diet education, treatments, and client-focused goals. The plan included skilled nursing services for teaching Ms. Lavoie about her medications, diet, and management of CHF and monitoring disease process; physical therapy to increase her daily activity, balance, and safety in the home; a nurse's aide three times weekly for help with activities of daily

CASE STUDY   (Continued)

living; and a homemaker for assistance with instrumental activities of daily living. The nurse included telehealth services for close daily monitoring of Ms. Lavoie's CHF. The plan of care was subsequently signed by the physician.

Over the course of the first week of services, the nurse visited twice more to coach Ms. Lavoie on using the telehealth equipment for daily weight and blood pressure monitoring, self-medication management, and diet. The nurse and physical therapist coordinated their visits so that they visited together on day 3 after discharge and thereafter visited on alternate days to maximize the presence of health professionals in the home. In collaboration with Ms. Lavoie, Nurse Jones organized the care schedule so that during the first 2 weeks after discharge from the hospital, someone on the healthcare team (registered nurse, physical therapist, certified nursing assistant, homemaker) visited Ms. Lavoie each day. By the end of the first 2 weeks, Ms. Lavoie was stronger, was using the telehealth equipment to send her blood pressure information and weight to the homecare office daily and was making better diet choices. Nurse Jones determined that she could decrease her visits to weekly as did the physical therapist. Nurse Jones continued to monitor Ms. Lavoie using the telehealth system.

At the beginning of week 4, using the telehealth data, Nurse Jones noted a sharp increase in Ms. Lavoie's weight and blood pressure. Nurse Jones telephoned Ms. Lavoie and made an appointment for a visit. During the visit, Ms. Lavoie and Nurse Jones reviewed Ms. Lavoie's activities for the last 3 days. Ms. Lavoie reported that she had been feeling so much better that she had cooked one of her favorite meals, which may have been too salty. Nurse Jones reviewed the recipe with Ms. Lavoie and coached her on how to adjust the recipe so that there was less sodium, and how to divide the recipe into single servings and freeze them so that Ms. Lavoie did not eat the entire casserole for 8 every day until it was gone. In addition, Nurse Jones had Ms. Lavoie create a log where she could write down her weight and blood pressure every day so she could use the information to self-manage her health.

Over the next week, Ms. Lavoie's blood pressure and weight decreased, returning to baseline. The physical therapist determined that Ms. Lavoie had met her mobility goals. The plan was modified to discharge physical therapy and add walking to the certified nurse assistant activities. At week 6, the nurse helped Ms. Lavoie to transition from monitoring her blood pressure and weight on the telehealth equipment to using her own equipment, continuing to write down the results daily and looking for trends. Also during her visit at week 6, Nurse Jones discussed community resources that Ms. Lavoie might use to reduce her isolation and increase her activity outside the home.

Ms. Lavoie was discharged from homecare services 7 weeks after discharge from the hospital. She was competently self-managing her CHF. Ms. Lavoie was consistently taking her medication according to the prescription, she could manage her diet to control her sodium and fluid intake, and she had increased her daily activity to include a trip (using public transportation for individuals with disabilities that would pick her up at her house) to the mall to take a

(continues)

CASE STUDY   (Continued)

short walk. Nurse Jones had developed a relationship with Ms. Lavoie in which they worked together to improve. Nurse Jones used coaching as a primary teaching strategy.

Discussion Questions

1. Describe the theoretical framework that Nurse Jones used to provide care to Ms. Lavoie.
2. What effect did telehealth have on Ms. Lavoie's outcomes?
3. Discuss the 'team' concept used in Ms. Lavoie's care.
4. Describe the different patient education teaching strategies used in providing care to Ms. Lavoie.

Evidence-Based Practice Box

Bowles and Baugh (2007) conducted a synthesis of research published between 1995 and 2005 focused on using telehealth technology in the home. They identified 40 studies that used peripheral medical devices to deliver home care for adult clients with chronic illness. The word "telehomecare" was used to identify a subset of telemedicine technology that used a telecommunication device with medical peripherals to provide home visits between a client and nurse (p. 5). Mechanisms may include voice, video, or clinical data conveyed over telephone lines. Many types of devices are included in these categories such as computers, cameras, and medical devices including blood pressure cuffs and blood glucose monitors. Research reported in this review used telehomecare to enhance homecare services for clients with many diagnoses including diabetes, heart failure, hypertension, spinal cord injury, and chronic wounds, among others. Four themes were identified in the 19 articles in the review: 1) effects on adult clients, 2) chronic illness outcomes, 3) providers, and 4) costs.

In seven studies in the sample, adult clients were receptive to using telehomecare devices, and diabetic clients found the devices to be empowering. Although the clients reported satisfaction with the devices and found them easy to use, they reported a better understanding of their disease process when they met with a nurse in person. Other positive benefits of using the telehomecare equipment included client's increased sense of security as well as improved confidence; they felt the equipment was helpful in managing their chronic disease.

Telehomecare devices have been used effectively with clients with chronic disease. Positive outcomes include better management of diabetes; decreased rehospitalization rates for individuals with heart failure, diabetes, and spinal cord injury; and the ability to assess wounds from a distance. The findings of several studies indicated client's improved self-management, overall improved health, and a higher likelihood of being discharged from the hospital to home when telehomecare technology was being used. While the studies reviewed by Bowles and Baugh varied widely, there is evidence that telehomecare technology is effective for improving outcomes in older clients with heart failure and diabetes.

Three studies in the sample evaluated nurses' attitudes toward telehomecare technology. The nurses reported that the technology added dimensions to their relationships with clients, was effective and efficient for monitoring vital signs, increased productivity, and improved care. The nurses also reported that the complexity of the technology was sometimes a barrier.

The effect of telehomecare on cost of services was evaluated as an outcome measure in four studies. All investigators found that telehomecare has the potential to be cost effective. Initially the cost of care increased related to the cost of the equipment, but the cost of care decreased related to decreased hospital charges and travel costs to the provider.

The findings of the research reported in this synthesis are promising with respect to the efficacy of telehomecare. It is to be noted that most of the research reviewed had design issues such as small, nonrandomized samples; also, variations in the equipment used make assumptions across studies difficult. Nonetheless, it appears that telehomecare can improve the effectiveness of homecare services for clients with chronic health problems.

Source: Bowles, K. K., & Baugh, A. C. (2007). Applying research evidence to optimize Telehomecare. *Journal of Cardiovascular Nursing, 22*(1), 5–15.

Home Care Satisfaction Measures

In health care, objective measures of client satisfaction with care are often used as an indicator of positive outcomes. However, in home care, it has been more difficult to measure client satisfaction with care (Geron et al., 2000). Although some scales of client satisfaction have been adapted from acute care, few measures have been developed specifically for home care. The Home Care Satisfaction Measure (HCSM) is a 60-item instrument measuring overall satisfaction with home care and satisfaction with five common services (Geron et al., 2000). The HCSM is designed to measure satisfaction with homemaker and home health aide services, case management, home-delivered meal service, and grocery service. The instrument is designed so that each service can be measured separately or the scores summed for an overall measure of satisfaction. The HCSM can be completed in person or by telephone. It is to be noted that the HCSM evaluates client satisfaction with aspects of home care that are not usually covered by Medicare and private insurance.

With the establishment of capitation payment and agencies learning how best to serve the client within this system, along with increased Medicare support to both the individual client and to the caregiver, the desired outcomes of home health care should become more realistic. These outcomes should be more attainable as well. Outcomes evaluation and analysis can demonstrate that the home healthcare process results in appropriate, adequate, and effective client care.

Positive client outcomes require that homecare agencies become aware of the roles that clients, family, and caregivers play before the client is admitted for service. Homecare providers, clients, families, and caregivers must enter into partnerships to provide the care needed for the client. Informal care providers need to know the significance of their roles in the plan of care, and nurses must enlist these informal caregivers to continue to provide care. In turn, the client's family must understand what can be expected from agency services.

Several forces are coming to bear on the need for homecare services. As the population ages and individuals survive longer, chronic illness is increasing, and there is a social movement to decrease institutionalization in nursing homes in favor of keeping clients in their own communities. The homecare industry is in an excellent position to create partnerships with clients and families to help clients stay in their own environments and manage their chronic illness.

STUDY QUESTIONS   www

What is the goal of home care according to the ANA?

Describe how homecare nurses differ in practice from public health nurses.

Discuss the definition of *homebound* and how being homebound might affect an individual's ability to go to church regularly and how it might affect the provision of health care.

Describe the Self- and Family Management of Chronic Illness model. How might you apply the model to an individual with type I diabetes?

Discuss how the homecare nurse might use the CCM to provide care to a client with chronic illness.

How does including telehealth in the list of interventions affect the delivery of home care?

Discuss strategies the homecare nurse might use to help a client and his or her family manage the disease process.

Study Questions (Cont.)   www

What skills does a nurse need to be an effective homecare nurse?

How can the interdisciplinary team maintain effective communication in the home?

Discuss how nurses might use homecare outcome measures to improve the healthcare delivery system.

INTERNET RESOURCES   www

Centers for Medicare and Medicaid Services: http://www.cms.gov/oasis/

Home Healthcare Nurses Association: www.hhna.org

National Association for Home Care and Hospice: www.nahc.org

For a full suite of assignments and additional learning activities, www use the access code located in the front of your book and visit this exclusive website: **http://go.jblearning.com/larsen**. If you do not have an access code, you can obtain one at the site.

REFERENCES

American Nurses Association. (2008). *Home health nursing: Scope and standards of practice*. Silver Springs, MD: Author.

American Telemedicine Association. (2011). American telemedicine association. Retrieved September 12, 2011, from: http://www.americantelemed.org.

Bowles, K. K., & Baugh, A. C. (2007). Applying research evidence to optimize Telehomecare. *Journal of Cardiovascular Nursing, 22*(1), 5–15.

Britton, B. (2003). First home telehealth clinical guidelines. *Home Healthcare Nurse, 21*(1), 703–706.

Butterworth, S. W., Linden, A., & McClay, W. (2007). Health coaching as an intervention in health management programs. *Disease Management of Health Outcomes, 15*(5), 299–307.

Candy, B., Holman, A., Leurent, B., Davis, S., & Jones, L. (2011). Hospice care delivered at home, in nursing homes and in dedicated hospice facilities: A systematic review of quantitative and qualitative evidence. *International Journal of Nursing Studies, 48*, 121–133.

Capitman, J. (2003). Effective coordination of medical and supportive services. *Journal of Aging and Health, 15*(1), 124–164.

Clark, M. J. (2008). *Community health nursing: Advocacy for population health* (5th ed.). Upper Saddle River, NJ: Pearson.

Dalton, J. (2003). Development and testing of the theory of collaborative decision-making in nursing practice for triads. *Journal of Advanced Nursing, 50*(1), 22–33.

Dalton, J. (2005). Client-caregiver-nurse coalition formation in decision-making situations during home visits. *Journal of Advanced Nursing, 52*(3), 291–299.

Doane, G. (2002). Beyond behavioral skills to human-involved processes: Relational nursing practice and interpretive pedagogy. *Journal of Nursing Education, 41*(9), 400–404.

Doane, G., & Varcoe, C. (2007). Relational practice and nursing obligations. *Advances in Nursing Science, 30*(3), 192–205.

Ellenbecker, C. (2004). A theoretical model of job retention for home health care nurses. *Journal of Advanced Nursing, 47*(3), 303–310.

Feldman, P. (2004). Penny Feldman on home healthcare quality and research. *Journal for Healthcare Quality, 26*(3), 31–37.

Gantert, T., & McWilliams, C. (2004). Interdisciplinary team processes within an in-home service delivery organization. *Home Health Services Quarterly, 23*(3), 1–17.

Geron, S., Smith, K., Tennstedt, S., Jette, A., Chassler, D., & Kastern, L. (2000). The home care satisfaction measure: A client-centered approach to assessing the satisfaction of frail older adults with home care services. *Journal of Gerontology: Social Sciences, 55B*, 5.

Grey, M., Knafl, K., & McCorkel, R. (2006). A framework for the study of self- and family management of chronic conditions. *Nursing Outlook, 54*, 278–286.

Gundersen, L. (1999). There's no place like home: The home health care alternative. *Annals of Internal Medicine, 131*, 639–640.

Hartrick, G. (1997). Relationship capacity: The foundation for interpersonal nursing practice. *Journal of Advanced Nursing, 26*, 523–528.

Hayes, J. (2002). Living arrangements and health status in later life: A review of recent literature. *Public Health Nursing, 19*(2), 136–151.

Hitchcock, J., Schubert, P., & Thomas, S. (Eds.). (2003). *Community health nursing: Caring in action* (2nd ed.). Albany, NY: Delmar.

Huffman, M. (2007). Health coaching: A new and exciting technique to enhance patient self-management and improve outcomes. *Home Healthcare Nurse, 25*(4), 271–274.

Huffman, M. (2009). Health coaching: A fresh, new approach to improve quality outcomes and compliance for patients with chronic conditions. *Home Healthcare Nurse, 27*(8), 491–496.

Improving Chronic Illness Care. (2007). The chronic care model. Retrieved September 12, 2011, from: http://www.improvingchroniccare.org/index.php?p=The_Chronic_Care_Model&s=2

Jacelon, C. S., Furman, E., Rea, A., Macdonald, B., & Donoghue, L. C. (2011). Creating a professional practice model for post acute care: Adapting the Chronic Care Model for long-term care. *Journal of Gerontological Nursing, 37*(3), 53–60.

Kaiser Foundation. (2010). Summary of new health reform law. Retrieved September 12, 2011, from: http://www.kff.org/healthreform/8061.cfm.2/12/11.

Leff, E. (2004). Involving patients in care decisions improves satisfaction: An outcomes based quality improvement project. *Home Healthcare Nurse, 22*(5), 297–301.

Lundy, K., & Janes, S. (2001). *Community health nursing: Caring for the public's health*. Sudbury, MA: Jones and Bartlett.

Marelli, T. (1998). *Handbook of home health standards and documentation guidelines for reimbursement*. St. Louis: Mosby.

Mathematica Policy Research. (2000). *Best practices in coordinated care: Prepared for health care financing administration.* Retrieved September 12, 2011, from: http://www.mathematica-mpr.com/pdfs/bestsum.pdf

Mauk, K. (2007). *The specialty practice of rehabilitation: A core curriculum.* Glenview, IL: Association of Rehabilitation Nurses.

Maurer, F., & Smith, C. (2005). *Community public health nursing practice.* St. Louis: Elsevier Saunders.

Meckes, C. (2005). Opportunities in care coordination. *Home Healthcare Nurse, 23*(10), 663–669.

Montauk, S. (1998). Home health care. *American Family Physician, 58,* 1609–1614.

Murkofsky, R. L., & Alston, K. (2009). The past, present, and future of skilled home health agency care. *Clinical Geriatric Medicine, 25*(1), 1–17.

Murray, E., Burns, J., See Tai, S., Lai, R., & Nazareth, I. (2005). Interactive health communication applications for people with chronic disease. *Cochrane Database of Systematic Reviews,* (4), CD004274. DO004271:004210.001002/14751858.CD14004274, pub14651854.

Myers, S., Grant, R., Lugn, N., Holbert, B., & Kvedar, J. (2006). Impact of home-based monitoring on the care of patients with congestive heart failure. *Home Health Care Management and Practice, 18*(6), 444–445.

Narsavage, G., & Naylor, M. (2000). Factors associated with referral of elderly individuals with cardiac and pulmonary disorders for home care services following hospital discharge. *Journal of Gerontological Nursing, 26*(5), 14–20.

National Alliance for Caregiving and the American Association of Retired Persons. (2004). *Caregiving in the U.S.: Executive Summary.* Washington, DC: Author.

National Hospice and Palliative Care Organization. (2007). Caring connections. Retrieved January 14, 2008, from http://www.caringinfo.org/LivingWithAnIllness/Hospice.htm

National Quality Forum. (2006). A National Framework and Preferred Practices for Palliative and Hospice Care Quality. Retrieved September 12, 2011, from: http://www.qualityforum.org/Projects/n-r/Palliative_and_Hospice_Care_Framework/Palliative__Hospice_Care__Framework_and_Practices.aspx

Neal, L. (1998). *Rehabilitation nursing in the home health setting.* Glenview, IL: Association of Rehabilitation Nurses.

Neal, L. (2000). Validating and refining the Neal theory of home health nursing practice. *Home Health Care Management and Practice, 12*(2), 16–25.

Percival, J., & Hanson, J. (2006). Big brother of brave new world? Telecare and its implications for older people's independence and social inclusions. *Critical Social Policy, 26*(4), 888–909.

Pushkin, D. (2001). Telemedicine: Follow the money. *The Online Journal of Issues in Nursing, 6*(3). Retrieved September 12, 2011, from: http://www.nursingworld.org/MainMenuCategories/ANAMarketplace/ANAPeriodicals/OJIN/TableofContents/Volume62001/No3Sept01/Telemedicine.aspx

Reichley, M., (1999). Advances in home care: Then, now and into the future. *Success in Home Care, 3*(6), 10–18.

Remington, L. (2000, July/August). PPS is making people run out of excuses for a change. *The Remington report: Business and clinical solutions for home care and post-acute markers.* p. 13–15.

Ryan, P., & Sawin, K. J. (2009). The Individual and Family Self-Management Theory: Background and perspectives on context, process, and outcomes. *Nursing Outlook, 57*(4), 217–225.

Saba, V. K. (1998). Home health care classification system: An overview. *The Online Journal of Issues in Nursing, 3*(2). Retrieved September 12, 2011, from: http://www.nursingworld.org/MainMenuCategories/ANAMarketplace ANAPeriodicals/OJIN/TableofContents/Volume72002/No3Sept2002/ArticlesPreviousTopic/HHCCAnOverview.aspx

Saba, V. K. (2004). CCC System Version 2.0. Retrieved September 19, 2011, from www.sabacare.com/Framework

Schneider, J. S., Barkauskas, V., & Keenan, G. (2008). Evaluation of home health care nursing outcomes with OASIS and NOC. *Journal of Nursing Scholarship, 40*(1), 76–82.

Schoen, M., & Koenig, R. (1997). Home health care nursing: Past and present. *MedSurg Nursing, 6*(4), 230–234.

Stanhope, M., & Lancaster, J. (2010*). Foundations of nursing in the community: Community-oriented practice* (3rd ed.). St. Louis: Mosby.

Stuart, B. (2003). Transition management: A new paradigm for home care of the chronically ill near the end of life. *Home Health Care Management & Practice, 15*(2), 126–135.

Tanner, E. (2004). Chronic illness demands for self-management in older adults. *Geriatric Nursing, 25*(5), 313–317.

Young, H. (2003). Challenges and solutions for care of frail older adults. *The Online Journal of Issues in Nursing, 8*(2). Retrieved September 12, 2011, from: http://www.nursingworld.org/MainMenuCategories/ANAMarketplace/ANAPeriodicals/OJIN/TableofContents/Volume82003/No2May2003/OlderAdultsCareSolutions.aspx

Weydt, A. (2010). Mary's story, relationship-based care delivery. *Nursing Administration Quarterly, 34*(2), 141–146.

World Health Organization. (2009). Definition of palliative care. Retrieved September 12, 2011, from: http://www.who.int/cancer/palliative/definition/en/

CHAPTER 21

Long-Term Care

Susan J. Barnes and Kristen L. Mauk

INTRODUCTION

Long-term care (LTC) is an umbrella term that refers to a range of services that address the health, personal care, psycho-emotional, and social needs of persons with some degree of difficulty in caring for themselves. Although family members may assist those persons with age-related functional decline or those with disabilities, LTC is often needed as time progresses to bridge the gap in care. The ideal LTC services promote independence of the person for as long as possible and allow him or her to remain at home as appropriate. LTC may be required because of disability associated with birth defects, injury, or the aging process. The concept of LTC may best be visualized on a continuum. Between the two ends of the spectrum—independence with minimal assistance at home versus skilled care in the nursing home—are many alternatives and options.

Care needs may be minimal or extensive (**Figure 21-1**). LTC services are offered in a variety of settings, as discussed in greater detail in this chapter. There is a growing trend in community-based services. Often, persons visualize a nursing home setting when they think of LTC, but this setting is used by only a small portion of the population at any given time.

Nurses are in an excellent position to design and implement innovative, cost-effective, and visionary care modalities to provide high-quality LTC services for patients while preserving their dignity and personhood. Because of the holistic perspective that nurses have of the patient, family, and community, they are in an excellent position to act as change agents in the process of healthcare reform.

In 2005, approximately 9 million people used LTC services in the United States (Chandra, Smith, & Paul, 2006), and 3.7 million Medicare enrollees used paid or unpaid personal caregivers in 1999 (most current data available; Administration on Aging, 2011). The cost of providing health care to persons older than age 65 is three to five times greater than for younger persons. The changing demographics of the baby boomer generation entering the older age group will have a significant impact on the whole of society (Lomastro, 2006). "One of the CDC's [Centers for Disease Control and Prevention] highest priorities as the nation's health protection agency is to increase the number of older adults who live longer, high-quality, productive, and independent lives" (CDC & the Merck Foundation, 2007, p. i). In 2009, there were 39.6 million people over age 65 in America. By 2030, there will be approximately

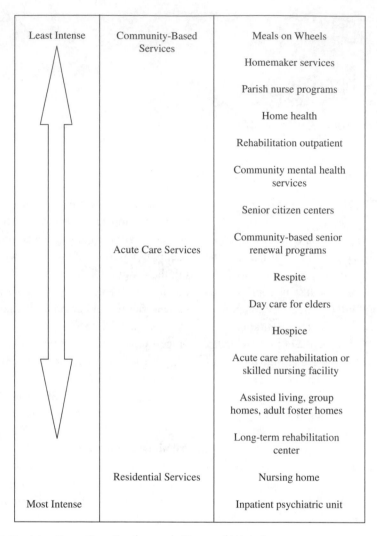

FIGURE 21-1   Long-Term Care Continuum in Terms of Intensity.

72.1 million older adults, more than twice the number in 2000 (Administration on Aging, 2011).

For many persons, increased age is accompanied by one or more chronic illnesses. Reported health conditions among those in the Health and Retirement Study (National Institute on Aging, 2007) included (in order of frequency): arthritis, hypertension, heart conditions, diabetes, psychological/emotional problems, cancer, chronic lung disease, and stroke. These chronic conditions represent many of the frequent complaints of older adults as they experience the aging process. The National

Interview Health Survey (National Center for Health Statistics, 2007) found that nearly one third of adults older than 75 had fair or poor health. As the incidence of chronic disease grows, deficits in a person's ability to perform self-care often follow, which can eventually lead to the need for LTC services. According to a document from the AARP (Houser, Fox-Grage, & Gibson, 2009), indicators of the need for LTC services include advanced age, living alone, poverty, less education, not owning a home, and not having a vehicle for transportation. The issue of LTC is sufficiently significant that the 2005 White House Conference on Aging focused on the "booming" dynamics of aging, tackling difficult issues relating to the baby boomer generation entering the older age group. The topics of the conference included promoting dignity, healthy independence, and financial security of older adults (Administration on Aging, 2008).

Historical Perspectives

Caring for a client with complex health needs over a long period continues to be a challenge for the healthcare system. Throughout history, consideration given to the quality of care for older adults or other vulnerable populations is seen as a reflection of societal values (Koop & Schaeffer, 1976). In societies with more fluid resources, vulnerable populations such as the frail elderly or individuals with chronic illness are better cared for because of the availability of assistance with health care (Kalisch & Kalisch, 2004). History has demonstrated that in societies under the strain caused by famine, war, or social upheaval, the vulnerable may not be able to survive because of malnutrition, lack of health care, and the lack of ability of the family unit to provide support.

A review of LTC in the United States reveals several significant events that have led to our current system of providing care. Prior to the 20th century, older adults in the United States were usually cared for within extended family units (DeSpelder & Strickland, 2011). Those without family to care for them might have gone to a facility supported by a religious organization or by charitable citizens, such as a poorhouse or almshouse. Changes in medical care altered hospital stays and allowed LTC to evolve, with group rest homes and private charitable homes providing care for chronically ill, dependent persons. Because life expectancies continued to increase, the demand for LTC increased. Political response came in the form of the Social Security Act in 1932, which provided services for the elderly and chronically ill. In 1951, the first White House Conference on Aging was held. The first conference (now held every 10 years, with the next slated for 2015) focused on issues that affected the quality of life of the aged person.

Title XVIII of the Social Security Act, which was passed in 1965 and was a part of the Great Society of President Lyndon B. Johnson, provided medical insurance for the elderly (Medicare) and further involved the federal government in health care (Centers for Medicare & Medicaid Services [CMS], 2011a). At the same time, in 1965, public policy was altered by the enactment of the Older Americans Act, which established aging networks throughout the states and funded community-based health services. Medicare opened the door for the government to dictate regulations and set the standard for care in formal caregiving settings. Evolution of the system included a restructuring of the Health Care Financing Authority into the CMS with the emphasis on improving the overall process of coordinating care of complex illness in the context of managed care (Administration on Aging, 2008).

Part of the Social Security Amendments of 1965 was Title XIX, Medicaid, to provide medical and health-related services for individuals and families with low incomes. Medicaid, a cooperative work between each state and the federal government, is the largest source of funds for services to the poor. Each state establishes its own eligibility standards, sets the rate of payment for services, and administers its own program (CMS, 2011a). Further changes in LTC were accomplished by Title XX of the Social Security Act Amendments, which made in-home services for medically indigent more widely available. In 1972 legislation was established that paid for intermediate care. The Omnibus Reconciliation Act, passed in 1987, included the Nursing Home Reform Act, which established high quality of care as a goal, along with the preservation of residents' rights in LTC facilities. Among the changes included was the requirement that comprehensive assessments of all nursing home residents were to be done to determine the functional, cognitive, and affective levels of the residents and to be used in planning care. In addition, more specific requirements for nursing, medical, and psychosocial services were designed to attain and maintain the highest possible mental and physical functional statuses by focusing on patient outcomes (Harrington, Carrillo, Blank, & O'Brian, 2010). Resident rights were also clearly defined. Organizations such as the National Association for Home Care and Hospice and others (Kempthorne, 2004) have seen the need for continued work on health policy in this area and have made LTC a high priority on the legislative agenda.

The Affordable Health Care Act passed in 2010 promotes a major overhaul of the existing healthcare funding system aimed at providing care to all Americans. This act is likely to undergo major revision before being funded and taking effect, but it will serve as a catalyst for change. (Updates may be found at the White House website: http://www.whitehouse.gov/healthreform.)

As Western culture has evolved, the family structure has been modified by the increasing number of women who work outside the home and are unavailable to care for aging parents (Gaugler & Teaster, 2006; Wagner, 2006). Current cultural values have made it less common for extended families to live together. However, Latino and Asian cultures often include extended families, with several generations living in the same household or nearby, which makes it possible for family members to look after the interests of vulnerable elder members and limits the need for formal LTC services (Leininger, 2002). In many cultures, the concept of the "double caregiver" adds enormous stress to women who work and provide care for a family and ailing parents (Remennick, 2001). However, current U.S. values emphasize single-family dwellings, dual-income families, and transient lifestyles, which have led to families no longer residing in the same area, often geographically separated by great distance. This culturally driven environment has created a high demand for services from an already inefficient LTC care system.

The Continuum of Care

Community-Based Long-Term Care

The premise of community-based LTC is to provide seamless, comprehensive programs to facilitate aging in place (Willging, 2006). However, much work needs to be done to operationalize the seamless aspect of transitions. There is a variety of services available within the LTC continuum. Current trends advocate using a case management approach to coordinate services and to ensure that individuals receive services in an efficient, timely fashion. Case management promotes aging in place with chronic illness, trying to keep a person in the home setting for a long as possible. The LTC system may be confusing to clients and families, but case managers can help to arrange and coordinate services such as Meals on Wheels, medical care, home health aides, and companion services. For older adults, the role of the geriatric care manager is an emerging one. Professional geriatric care managers (PGCMs) help families care for their older relatives while promoting independence. The National Association of Professional Geriatric Care Managers (2011) lists services that families might expect with a PGCM as follows:

- Conduct care-planning assessments to identify problems and to provide solutions.
- Screen, arrange, and monitor in-home help or other services, including assistance in hiring a qualified caregiver for home care.
- Provide short- or long-term assistance for caregivers living near or far away.
- Review financial, legal, or medical issues and offer referrals to geriatric specialists.
- Provide crisis intervention.
- Act as a liaison to families at a distance, overseeing care, and quickly alerting families to problems.
- Assist with moving an older person to or from a retirement complex, assisted care home, or nursing home.
- Provide consumer education and advocacy.
- Offer eldercare counseling and support.

Related services for the frail elder or individual with chronic illness could also include legal services, adult protective services, area councils on aging, ombudsman programs, senior centers, and elder-advocacy groups. Older adults with chronic illnesses that are rehabilitative may receive assistance with recovery through Medicare, which pays for inpatient and limited outpatient therapies ordered by a physician. Respite care for family members who care for loved ones with chronic illness and disability is also a community-based service.

The Program of All-Inclusive Care for the Elderly (PACE) is another community-based alternative that promotes aging in place (Boult & Wieland, 2010). This program is an evidence-based model of care whose services are often covered by Medicare and Medicaid. The National PACE Association (2011) states that the average user is 80 years old, and preliminary studies suggest that involvement in a PACE program may slow functional decline for older adults. The PACE model combines dollars from different funding streams to deliver a comprehensive set of services focused on the health and well-being of the individual (National PACE Association, 2011). The number of states with participating organizations has increased to 30 in the last few years (the list of states with programs is found on the PACE website at: http://www.npaonline.org). Continuing evaluation of this program in terms of cost benefit to the funding agencies may make it available on a wider scale.

Residential Long-Term Care Settings

Residential LTC facilities are formal, organized agencies that provide care for persons unable to live alone because of physical or other problems, but who do not require hospitalization. Persons living in residential care are not called patients, but residents, because the LTC setting is their home. The three most common types of residential LTC facilities are group homes, assisted-living centers, and nursing homes. Many retirement communities combine independent living facilities and assisted living facilities, although these represent two different levels of care. Those living independently in a retirement community may do so because of declining health caused by chronic illness, safety factors, frailty, and the need for socialization. The decision to move from one's own home to a community living situation is difficult and often involves the advice of family members who are concerned about the older adult's ability to live alone safely. LTC residents are a vulnerable population who tend to have more chronic illnesses and may require advocacy from health or social professionals.

Group homes. Group homes are also referred to as personal care homes, foster homes, domiciliary care homes, board and care homes, and congregate care homes. The philosophy embraces a home environment with a limited number of residents who share common characteristics in needing assistance with such things as activities of daily living, shopping, cleaning, and medication management. Much like a boarding house, the owner of the home provides services such as meals, laundry and cleaning, medication management, and a safe environment. These homes are licensed by the state. This type of care is most appropriate for those with uncomplicated medical problems. Payment for group homes can be private, although in some states, it may be covered by Welfare. The Robert Wood Johnson Foundation has sponsored research in creating innovative and livable homes under the Green House Project (more information may be found in the research literature and at: www.thegreenhouseproject.org).

Assisted-living centers. Persons in assisted living are those who require some type of help with activities of daily living. According to the National Center for Assisted Living (2011), there

are more than 900,000 individuals living in assisted living, and of those 64% require help with bathing, 39% need help with dressing, 26% need help with toileting, 19% need help with transferring, and 12% need help with eating. Of these residents, 81% need help with medication. Assisted living has taken over approximately 15% of what was previously the nursing home population (Kinosian, Stallard, & Wieland, 2007).

Because Medicare, Medicaid, and the U.S. Department of Veterans Affairs (VA) do not pay for assisted living, the cost for this living arrangement and services are paid for out of pocket. Assisted living centers may be found as free-standing facilities, as part of retirement communities, or attached to nursing homes to allow for smoother transition of care for those expected to need skilled nursing in the future.

The National Center for Assisted Living (2011) has summarized the characteristics of the 36,000 assisted living centers in the United States. The typical profile of a resident in assisted living is an 86-year-old woman who is ambulatory but needs help with at least two activities of daily living. Residents' average age in 2006 was 85 years, and the average length of stay was 28.3 months. One third of these residents will die, 59% will move into another nursing facility, and the remainder will return home or to other living situations. From these statistics, it is evident that although today's older adults value their independence, the frailties that accompany old age make it necessary for more than 900,000 people in the United States to have some assistance with everyday activities.

Although assisted living facilities are accountable to a board of directors and may employ a registered nurse (RN) consultant, the care is generally provided by aides, with licensed practical nurses (LPNs) used regularly to supervise daily services. Assisted living facilities provide autonomy for older adults, allowing them to live in a safe, home-like environment adapted for those with physical challenges. Assisted living provides personal space in the form of apartments or suites and also provides meals through community dining as well as transportation and social activities.

CASE STUDY

Mrs. Saltano is an 89-year-old widow who lived alone for 2 years after her husband of 51 years died of colorectal cancer. For most of their lives, Mr. and Mrs. Saltano lived in the same neighborhood and in the same house where they raised their five children. Mrs. Saltano planned to stay in the family home after her husband's death, but she experienced bouts of loneliness and social isolation, despite being an active member of her local church before and after his death. She began to experience the effects of chronic illnesses, including having a bilateral knee replacement because of pain and decreased mobility from arthritis, and taking more medications to control her high blood pressure and lower her cholesterol. With advancing age, Mrs. Saltano also developed diabetes and some mild memory loss that her children found concerning. After one visit with the family at Christmas, Mrs. Saltano's eldest daughter suggested that her mother explore the possibility of going to a retirement community designed for older adults.

Mrs. Saltano was absolutely opposed to leaving the home she had shared with her husband and where they had raised their family. She did not want to be in an "institution," as she called it, but she admitted to having begun to have difficulty driving as a result of failing vision, and said she did not feel safe living alone. Mrs. Saltano did consent to visit a nearby retirement community with two of her adult children and found that some old friends of hers who were also widowed were living there. Her friends seemed happy and active. The apartment she would have gave her privacy (and had its own kitchenette, refrigerator, and large bathroom) but also allowed the staff to check on her. Meals were served in a nice dining room with linen tablecloths and a formal menu, and a library, big screen TV, pool table, and exercise room were available. A beauty shop was on the premises, and transportation to doctors' offices and shopping was available for a nominal charge. Mrs. Saltano slowly warmed to the idea of moving to the continuous care retirement community, and so the arrangements were made. The quality of Mrs. Saltano's life improved significantly through socialization and activities in this new environment. Her adjustment to a change in living situation was facilitated by the attitudes of her children, the staff, and other residents.

Discussion Questions

1. What factors prompted Mrs. Saltano's children to encourage her to consider another living arrangement?
2. From the information in this chapter, was moving to a continuous care retirement community a prudent choice for Mrs. Saltano? Why or why not?
3. What problems and issues with adaptation to her new home is Mrs. Saltano likely to face?
4. What interventions might be helpful to assist with her adjustment?

Skilled nursing facilities or nursing homes. Nursing home is a term used to refer to a facility that has either skilled nursing services and/or intermediate care. Nursing homes are LTC facilities for individuals with chronic illness, who are medically frail, or who are disabled. The level of care may be described as residential, long-term, non-emergent, or custodial care. A number of facilities may include an intermediate care or rehabilitation unit for individuals who need assistance in re-establishing self-care abilities.

The majority of such agencies are "for profit." Exceptions are agencies generally associated with churches or other nonprofit organizations such as the VA. The Veterans Health Admini-stration (VHA) predicted that the number of veterans older than age 85 will double in the next decade and that the VHA–enrolled veterans in this oldest old age group will increase sevenfold, resulting in a 22–25% increase in both nursing home and community-based services. The VHA currently uses 90% of its LTC resources on nursing home care. For veterans, age and marital status were found to be significant predictors of the use of LTC services (Kinosian et al., 2007).

Agencies that receive income from the CMS are required to meet minimum state and federal standards. Standards address items such as: nutritional and fluid intake; provision of social interaction and activities; and support services such as physical therapy, rehabilitation therapy, housekeeping, and laundry services. There is a continued concern by those employed in LTC settings that facility structure and staffing are often based on minimal standards that contain costs instead of considering first what is desirable or needed for the client. However, as the baby boomer generation ages, it is expected that its interest in this issue will influence the creation of higher standards, and quality of care may improve in LTC facilities.

Approximately 5% of the elderly population reside in nursing homes in the United States, and 28% pay for their own care. Care in nursing homes may be funded by the individual (self-pay), insurance, Medicare (with limits), or Medicaid. To be eligible for Medicaid payment for residential care, the client must have limited assets with which to pay for the services required. Often an LTC resident will enter a nursing home, paying for services until his or her estate is spent down, and then Medicaid pays for care until the client's death (AARP, 2010).

Much of the care provided in the traditional nursing home setting is considered custodial care. Rehabilitative services are provided for those who have the capacity to regain function. Because the institutionalized individual may require a great deal of help with the physical aspects of care, such as bathing, dressing, eating, and space maintenance, the cognitive needs (emotional, psychological, and spiritual) may be considered less important. Activity programs are sometimes geared only toward one segment of the facility population. Care in LTC settings should include not only appropriate physical care, but also appropriate social and cognitive stimulation.

Long-Term Care Recipients—A Vulnerable Population

Vulnerable individuals are those who are at increased risk for loss of autonomy, loss of self-will, injustice, loss of privacy, and increased risk for abuse. A vulnerable adult is defined as an individual who is either being mistreated or is in danger of mistreatment and who because of age and/or disability is unable to protect him/herself (Teaster, 2002). A vulnerable individual can be described as one who has been judged by someone to be a nonperson. Examples of vulnerable persons in LTC may include those with physical or mental or emotional problems, the elderly, those with dementia, and those who have been in prison. In a culture that values youth, energy, strength, and the ability to work, many devalue elders or those with chronic illness. Laws and practices differ between states in the areas of abuse, neglect, and protective services. Ultimately, it is the care providers and administrators in LTC who are responsible for maintaining an environment that supports the unique personhood of the client and protects the vulnerable.

Many individuals requiring LTC have already lost some autonomy and self-will because of illnesses that affect the individual's ability to make decisions or carry out intentional behavior. Vulnerability is of special concern in these individuals. Decisions must be made for them regarding many aspects of life, such as eating, bathing, medication administration, socialization, and exercising religious practices. Some persons may benefit from the services of a guardian, discussed later in this chapter.

Abuse in the home or in a residential facility is an extreme threat to the autonomy of the client. If the nurse providing care is the first to observe signs and symptoms of mistreatment, reporting these observations to Adult Protective Services (APS) (or other public agency, as designated in the particular state) is required by law. In the home, the home healthcare nurse may be in a position to discover abuse and act as the primary advocate to prevent further abuse. The nurse may work with various agencies to ensure that appropriate intervention is made. Because elder mistreatment is often subtle, the nurse must be persistent in reporting signs until action is taken. If abuse or neglect of the community-based client is profound, a move to residential care may be indicated.

PROBLEMS AND ISSUES IN LONG-TERM CARE

There are a number of issues in LTC, ranging from overall system breakdown to individual treatment issues for clients in the system. The issues mentioned in this chapter are not an exhaustive list but can be considered an introduction to current problems.

Provision of Care

Along the continuum of LTC, problems in the provision of care include organization of services and access to care, gaps in public policy, funding, staffing, and standards of care. Specific issues vary within individual states or communities. It is imperative that the professional nurse involved in LTC is cognizant of the local and state issues that affect delivery and quality of LTC services. Being a political activist in order to further the issues of the recipients of LTC is also important.

Organization of Services

It was not surprising that the second most important resolution that came from the White House Conference on Aging in 2005 was the need for a more comprehensive and well-coordinated LTC strategy (Lomastro, 2006). In community-based LTC, the array of services in a given community may not be organized according to any hierarchy. Each specialized service, such as home care, elder daycare, hospice, or nutrition programs, was most likely begun in response to a specific need or business opportunity in the community. It is often necessary for a program of LTC to be pieced together from a number of different organizations to meet one client's needs. This is especially true for community-dwelling residents.

Partial help with this problem comes from the United Way, a nonprofit service-based agency. The United Way publishes a resource book in larger cities that describes community programs and services. (This publication can be obtained by calling the local United Way office or obtaining the list online at http://www.united-way.org.) This resource book assists clients, family, and care providers in identifying appropriate services, phone numbers, and eligibility requirements. Many times, individuals with chronic illness and their families are not aware that when they are involved with one system (such as a nursing home), they have access to other services (such as hospice). Individuals with chronic illnesses often view access to the LTC system as complicated and overwhelming. Those with chronic illnesses and their families may have a limited amount of energy to invest in problem solving and identifying the best options. Often, access to the LTC system is controlled by gatekeepers who have minimal training and experience with complex medical conditions. Rules may be seen as arbitrary, and appear to exclude the very individuals intended to benefit from programs.

With the utilization of more case management for individuals with chronic illness, whether through the local or federal VA, state health and human services divisions, or private companies, some progress is being made in assisting community-dwelling individuals to more effectively access LTC services. However,

for most clients and families, access to the LTC system remains confusing and complex.

Gaps in Public Policy

In the United States, the primary responsibility for paying for LTC services is with the individuals who need those services. Medicare pays for limited skilled nursing care, up to 100 days, associated with an acute illness requiring at least 3 days of hospitalization (Houser et al., 2009; Medpac, 2010). Partially because of the funding sources and partially because of the method of development of services, there are gaps that exist in LTC services. Much policy work needs to be done related to transitions that individuals experience moving from one type of service to another because no overall umbrella of comprehensive care exists. The current healthcare reform effort is at least partially aimed at making transitions more seamless. Pharmaceutical costs, extended home health care, and rehabilitative services are problematic for many in LTC. For those unable to self-pay, some go without services or medications.

Funding

Gaps in service and public policy are both related to funding issues. In 2009, $144 billion was paid by state and federal agencies to free-standing nursing home facilities (Harrington et al., 2010). Medicaid alone spent $94.5 billion on LTC services in 2005 (Houser et al., 2009). As previously mentioned, a significant number of residents in nursing homes and other residential care facilities pay privately for their care until their estate is spent down, at which time state and federal funding may take over (Houser et al., 2009). Many persons may be eligible for both Medicare and Medicaid. Although these persons do not generally report difficulty obtaining medical care, 58% of those who need LTC report their needs as being unmet. This problem has led to additional consequences such as falls (Komisar, Feder, & Kasper, 2005). Private insurance and nonprofit organizations also provide services for those in need of LTC. However, beyond the nursing home setting, piecing together a comprehensive LTC program for a frail elder with comorbidities who wishes to remain in the community is challenging. Certification for eligibility for certain benefits, such as extended home care, is strict and for a limited amount of time only.

Resources, whether private or public, are limited. Community-dwelling elders may be eligible for Medicare to pay for certain services, such as home health care, but only as long as some rehabilitation progress can be documented. Once progress stops, and the condition is considered chronic, the individual may have to pay privately for rehabilitative and home services. For individuals who have lived through the Great Depression, World War II, and other historical events that have required genuine frugality, spending nearly $100 to pay for less than an hour of a home visit from an agency RN is not a viable option. Many older adults from working class backgrounds do without needed care rather than pay privately. One study found that the greater the use of paid home care in a state, the less likely persons were to report unmet need (Komisar et al., 2005). This suggests that state policies can make a difference in the health care of their citizens.

It is important to consider the entitlement to care that older adults and those with chronic illness possess because of Social Security programs. These programs were designed to provide some comfort and security to the older individual. One view is that society has an obligation to provide for those in need, particularly the elderly, because of the labor and service that they have provided (Tobin & Salisbury, 1999). Another view is that society is obligated to provide care for frail and chronically ill elders because of the sanctity of all human life, and not simply because of work undertaken during the adult life. Philosophical origins play an important part not only in the establishment and continuation of programs, but also in setting standards for ongoing programs.

Alternative financing for LTC needs to be explored. Although both PACE (mentioned previously in this chapter) and social managed care plans offer alternatives to nursing homes and promote aging in place, it is evident that their scope and availability are significantly limited. In Arkansas, research revealed a need to expand health services because of unmet needs, suggesting policy recommendations to improve access to community-based care (Stewart, Felix, Dockter, Perry, & Morgan, 2006). In addition, a few strategies to fund LTC costs have arisen from the financial sector: reverse mortgages and life settlement. Both concepts focus on helping individuals liquidate assets (for example, a home or life insurance policy) to provide cash to privately pay to enter or remain in a facility (Feaster, 2006). It is only since 2000 that using one's life insurance as a financial tool to obtain relatively quick cash has been considered. However, individuals considering this option should consult with a financial adviser.

Staffing

Healthcare agencies that receive Medicare and Medicaid funding are licensed by each state or are accredited by a recognized accrediting agency. Each agency must meet requirements in staffing. Two main issues in staffing are the training of the staff member and the staff-to-client ratio (Harrington et al., 2010).

Standards for required staff training are often minimal. For example, medication aides working in an assisted-living center may be required to attend a 6-week training course, yet the medication regimens for the assisted-living center clientele may be extremely complex. For proper medication management, much more time is required to educate a person on the pharmacologic effects of medications, side effects, and complications. Although assisted-living centers are required to have an RN available, that one RN may act as a consultant for multiple centers under the same ownership umbrella. The actual individual who "supervises" the medication aides may be an LPN who works a 40-hour week.

Qualifications for the director or administrator of an assisted-living center are minimal and may be as little as possessing a GED and attending an industry-sponsored seminar lasting 2 weeks or less. The majority of staff working in such facilities may be minimally trained personnel, and client safety is a legitimate concern.

Staffing challenges in providing home health care are also significant. State requirements vary for home health aides, but no training program is more than 8–12 weeks in length. Often, aides are trained and then expected to work independently, with little supervision.

Staffing in nursing homes is a continuing issue. There is conclusive evidence that a positive relationship exists between nursing staffing and quality of nursing home care. Fewer RN and nursing assistant hours are associated with quality-of-care deficiencies (Arling, Kane, Mueller, Bershadsky, & Degenholtz, 2007; Harrington,

Zimmerman, Karon, Robinson, & Beutel, 2000). The turnover rate for nursing assistants can be as high as 40–100% in some facilities. High turnover rates have been associated with poor quality care (Castle, Engberg, & Men, 2007). Recruitment and retention of qualified nursing assistants is an ongoing problem. Creating an environment that promotes teamwork, addresses care-related stressors, promotes positive communication, reduces paperwork inefficiencies and staffing shortages, and has high organizational morale has been shown to increase job satisfaction and commitment to the organization, but there are many other factors to consider in the complex process of staff turnover in these settings (American Association of Colleges of Nursing [AACN], 2011; Arling et al., 2007; Cherry, Ashcraft, & Owen, 2007; Donoghue & Castle, 2006; Sikorska-Simmons, 2006). The decreasing level of RN staffing is also of growing concern, and yet reimbursements and prospective payments have been reduced in some cases, making it impossible to increase the number of RNs in residential facilities.

To complicate this situation, there is a projected shortage of healthcare professionals. Half of the RN workforce is at least 45 years old. It is estimated that by 2025 there will be a shortage of at least 260,000 RNs because of a number of significant factors, including the population growth, retirement of nurses in the current workforce, and the lack of faculty to educate willing students in nursing programs (Harrington, 2008).

Standards

Residential and community-based LTC facilities that accept government payments are regulated by federal and state mandates. Agencies and institutions involved in providing LTC that receive outside funding are required to meet certain standards and undergo regular inspection (Harrington et al., 2010).

Requirements change frequently. Part of the responsibility of both the facility administrator and the director of nursing in any LTC facility is to be aware of and implement changes that are made necessary as a result of changes in state and federal requirements. In home health agencies, the number and type of visits that can be reimbursed by insurance or Medicare are limited. If evidence in regard to why the visits were made and what health-related goal was achieved is unclear, the payer may bill the agency back for those services, which can be financially devastating to an organization.

Nursing homes undergo an initial survey to become certified and then undergo inspection no less than every 15 months with an average of every 12 months (Harrington et al., 2010). State surveyors evaluate both process and outcomes of nursing home care in several areas. Tags are assigned depending on the severity of the violation. If deficiencies are found, follow-up surveys may be conducted. If care is so poor that residents are deemed to be in danger, facilities can be fined large amounts of money, be prohibited from admitting any residents, and even be closed for severe violations. Agencies must demonstrate that the staff meet educational requirements, that residents are receiving adequate care, and that documentation is appropriate. Requirements vary for various types of agencies and are complicated. Most states post the results of surveys on a public website, where family members can access information and compare facilities when making decisions about placing loved ones into LTC. Current national survey results are available through the CMS website (http://www.cms.gov).

Standards address issues such as nursing care hours per client, nursing assessments, care plans, accidents, fall prevention, prevention of pressure sores, use of physical restraints, nutrition, use of certain medications, and housekeeping services. In addition, facilities are to provide care for residents in a manner that maintains dignity and respect by providing grooming, appropriate dress, and promotion of independence in dining; allowing private space and property; and interacting respectfully. For example, nursing staff must not perform any invasive assessment or task in a public area, but should take the resident to his or her room for procedures such as listening to lung sounds or checking a glucometer reading.

Harrington and colleagues (2010) point out that quality of care provided in nursing homes has long been a matter of great concern to consumers, professionals, and policymakers. If the regulation and inspection process is ignored, LTC residents may suffer. Examples of system failures can be found at both the local and state levels. Deficiency reports are readily available online through the CMS. The RN is at times required to act as an advocate for the residents and to ensure compliance with minimal standards.

Standards by which care is measured were outlined in 2002 by the CMS. The standards from 2002 have undergone major revision and the LTC (specifically nursing homes) system is currently undergoing change to incorporate the newest and most patient-oriented measurement standards (CMS, 2011b).

Ethical Issues in Long-Term Care

Individuals who are chronically ill or who are frail are a vulnerable population who are often at the mercy of the caregivers in the LTC system.

Healthcare professionals in LTC should have a solid understanding of the ethics involved in this type of care. Principles upon which decisions should be made include: autonomy, nonmaleficence, beneficence, and justice (Beauchamp & Childress, 2009; Jonsen, 2007). The manner in which these principles are executed in the professional nurse–client relationship can make a visible difference in the quality of life of the LTC resident. Some of the more common ethical issues are discussed herein.

Client Autonomy Versus Dependence

One principle of critical importance in LTC is autonomy. Healthcare professionals and caregivers should observe the particularly essential rule of bioethics: Respect the autonomy of persons (Jonsen, 2007). Autonomy is sometimes misapplied or ignored (Kane, Freeman, Caplan, Aroskar, & Urv-Wong, 1990). It is possible for an individual to gradually lose increments of his or her autonomy because of limitations imposed by sensory deprivation, immobility, weakness, and cognitive impairment (Mezey, Mitty, & Ramsey, 1997). Research suggests that even frail elderly individuals who are homebound have a greater sense of personal control than those in nursing homes (Crain, 2001), making those living in facilities at greater risk for loss of decision making and independence. Loss of autonomy and development of excess disability are a problem for many LTC clients.

Excess Disability

Disability that is in excess of what is attributable to a chronic condition is often an unwanted consequence of care (Slaughter, Eliasziw, Morgan, & Drummond, 2009). It suggests a dependence of a resident on a caregiver to perform a task the client has the ability to perform. This phenomenon

is a significant problem in the LTC setting. Depression, learned helplessness, and changes in sensorium contribute to increased dependence upon caregivers. Caregivers may be unintentional contributors to excess disability. Providing unnecessary assistance or an inappropriate type of assistance can contribute to residents' dependency. "Factors influencing excess disability include: a desire of the caregiver to be helpful; lack of knowledge and skill of the caregiver; and lack of time and staff" (Remsburg & Carson, 2006, p. 584). An example of excess disability is dressing assistance provided to nursing home residents. Aides often do the dressing activities for residents in order to save time, instead of allowing the residents to perform the activity at their own pace (Beck et al., 1997). This action moves the resident toward unnecessary and unwanted dependence.

Custodial Care

Using basic ethical principles, an issue arises whether providing minimal physical care for those with chronic illness is acceptable versus providing more comprehensive care extending beyond custodial physical care. This is particularly challenging in a residential LTC environment. As a result of regulation, funding, and staffing patterns for Medicare/Medicaid residential facilities, the goal inadvertently becomes custodial care.

Physical issues of the resident are important, but those issues should not be the only focus. Mental health needs should also be considered in the chronically ill and elderly populations. With limited attention to these needs, the client is at risk of suffering boredom, anxiety, and, consequently, depression. In 2004 persons age 65 and older accounted for 16% of suicide deaths, although they comprised only 12% of the entire population at that time (National Institute of Mental Health [NIMH], 2010). Suicide rates of non-Hispanic white men over age 85 are the highest in the nation (U.S. Department of Health and Human Services, 1999). Appropriate referral is a responsibility of the nurse who detects symptoms of emotional difficulties. Signs of depression include feeling nervous, empty, guilty, tired, restless, irritable, and unloved, and that life is not worth living. Physical symptoms associated with mental health problems include eating more or less than normal, sleep disturbances, headaches, stomachaches, and an increase in chronic pain (Varcarolis & Halter, 2010). The risk of depression in the elderly increases with the presence of chronic illness and a loss of physical function (NIMH, 2010). If symptoms of depression are present in an LTC client, services are available to provide assistance.

End-of-Life Decision Making

Difficult and complex decisions at end of life are an inherent component of LTC. Many older adults lack the resources, or lack knowledge of the available resources, that could help with decision making at end of life. Although most older adults are approached about completing written documents to outline treatment preferences, many choose not to do so. Making one's wishes known in the event of terminal illness or incapacity is one approach to preserving autonomy for the older adult. Family issues may impact the elder's willingness to do this.

In many states, an older person can make his wishes known by completing a document such as Five Wishes (Aging with Dignity, 2010). The Five Wishes program, sponsored by Aging with Dignity, is unique from other living will declarations, in that it addresses all aspects of the person's life: emotional, spiritual, personal, and medical (Aging with Dignity, 2010). This document is legally recognized in 42 states and allows the person to use his or her own lay language to express end-of-life desires. Five Wishes documents the following information for the older adult's family and doctors (Aging with Dignity, 2010):

- Which person should make healthcare decisions
- The kind of medical treatment the person wants and does not want
- How comfortable the person wishes to be made
- How the person wants others to treat him or her
- What the person wants loved ones to know

Cultural and religious beliefs play an important part in end-of-life decision making. There are some religions that dictate that everything should be done to preserve life and others that support allowing natural death. For example, African Americans are generally opposed to placing a loved one in a nursing home, preferring family members to die at home. Healthcare professionals should familiarize themselves with the major traditions and practices of their clients so that culturally appropriate care can be provided.

In a study of older community-dwelling adults (with a mean of 80.7 years of age), a durable power of attorney for health care had been completed by 60.8% of respondents before death. However, a startling finding of this research was that persons with lower levels of cognitive functioning were less likely to have completed an advance directive than those older adults with higher cognitive functioning (McGuire, Rao, Anderson, & Ford, 2007). This research underscores the need for healthcare professionals to address advance directives with persons while they are capable of expressing their end-of-life wishes.

Abuse and Neglect of Vulnerable Adults

The incidence of abuse and neglect of vulnerable adults is difficult to estimate. The National Association of Adult Protective Services Administrators (2005) estimated that anywhere between 500,000 and 5 million elders and other vulnerable adults in the United States were in some way victims of abuse. More current data indicate nearly 6 million cases of elder abuse every year (Elder Abuse Daily, 2010). It is believed that cases of abuse, neglect, or exploitation are grossly underreported because of fear, intimidation, lack of sound research, or other factors. Nursing home residents are particularly vulnerable to being victims of abuse (Lindbloom, Brandt, Hough, & Meadows, 2007).

Abuse can be categorized as domestic or institutional. Within these categories, physical, sexual, and emotional/psychological abuse may occur as well as neglect, self-neglect, abandonment, and financial exploitation (National Center for Elder Abuse, 2011). Because of longer life expectancies for those with chronic illness, it is very likely that the incidence of abuse will increase (Teaster, 2002). The individual with chronic illness, if cognitively competent, may be hesitant to discuss the mistreatment because he or she fears the loss of the relationship or other reprisal by the perpetrator. If the individual is not capable of expressing information regarding the abuse, identification may be by forensic evidence. Physical abuse is the actual assault of an individual, and evidence exists with the presence of unexplained bruises, fractures, cuts, or burns in various stages of healing. Sexual abuse also falls within this category. The victim of such treatment is in danger and

requires immediate advocacy. Physical abuse often escalates from neglect or other forms of abuse. Perpetrators often share similar characteristics such as lack of social support, history of being an abuse victim, and mental or emotional problems.

Neglect is defined as the lack of provision of basic necessities, such as food, water, and medical care. Neglect may be evidenced by poor hygiene, malnutrition or dehydration, pressure ulcers, and reports of being left in an unsafe condition or being left without resources to obtain necessary medications. Neglect can take place because of willful intention or because home management has become overwhelming to the client's aging spouse or family. This type of abuse may be seen more frequently in homes where the caregiver lacks the knowledge or resources to provide care. Neglect can include self-neglect, which is defined as an individual losing the will or the ability to properly care for himself. Abandonment is the extreme form of neglect.

The third type of elder abuse, exploitation, is defined as the use of an elder's resources without knowledge or consent for the gain of another. Signs of elder exploitation include the disappearance of monetary resources or the "taking over" of personal belongings without permission or consent (Fulmer, 1999). Financial abuse in the form of fraud or deception may also be considered exploitation and may come through family members who borrow money with no intention to repay it, or from mail fraud schemes that attempt to cheat persons out of money by promising prizes and rewards.

Each state has an APS to protect the rights and health of older people and people with disabilities who are in danger of being mistreated or neglected, unable to protect themselves, and have no one to assist them. APS is responsible for receiving the report of abuse, investigating the report, assessing the individual's risk, developing and implementing case plans, service monitoring, and evaluation. Some agencies may provide more in-depth services including housing, medical care, social support, and economic and legal services (National Association of Adult Protective Services Administrators, 2005). Healthcare professionals and paraprofessionals such as RNs, physicians, nurse aides, and homemaker aides are mandated by law to report suspected adult or elder abuse.

INTERVENTIONS

Theoretical Frameworks for Practice

Using a theoretical framework to plan and implement nursing care in an LTC setting helps the nurse to avoid doing things simply "because they have always been done that way." Nurses draw from the sciences and use physiologic theory, pharmacologic theory, and theories of communication, change, caring, grief and bereavement, and ethics. A theoretical framework explains or guides one's practice. Mid-range theories are those defined as specific to particular caregiving situations and that have measurable outcomes. Theoretical frameworks give direction in the choice of interventions so that nursing care is tailored to each client.

Several middle-range frameworks are appropriate for LTC. One example is "The Needs-Driven Dementia-Compromised Behavior Model." It can assist the care professional in understanding how to better interact with dementia clients (Algase et al., 1996). This model hypothesizes that problematic behaviors in dementia clients are a result of needs that, when

identified, can be addressed by the care provider, thereby avoiding a crisis. Such frameworks are helpful in assisting the care provider in solving problems encountered in the clinical area when dealing with LTC clients (Mitty & Flores, 2007a; Peterson & Bredow, 2004).

Any number of other mid-range theories may help enlighten the nurse's perspective on the LTC client and guide the planning of care. Examples include Kolcaba's (2003) Theory of Comfort which can help nurses understand the importance of comfort and the need for relief of problematic symptoms and achievement of ease in the patient's daily life; the Theory of Unpleasant Symptoms (Gift, 2004; originally developed by Lenz, Suppe, Gift, Pugh, & Milligan in 1995) also gives insight into a paradigm of understanding the challenges faced by those with chronic illness. Eakes (2004), building on previous researchers' work in the Theory of Chronic Sorrow, discusses clients facing the loss of interpersonal relationships as well as physical functioning. These theories and others are available to the healthcare provider working in LTC.

Admission and Assessment in the Long-Term Care Setting

Admission to a nursing home can be very distressing to anyone. From the individual's perspective, the move to a nursing home or even assisted living away from their personal home may symbolize the reality of the loss of health, autonomy, personal relationships, economic power, productivity, and independence. Adjustment to such facilities may evoke a mix of emotions. The stress of going into a facility in which one is surrounded by strangers can be difficult. In addition, the individual must adjust to schedules determined by others, instead of following routines established throughout a lifetime. In many nursing homes, eating and bathing schedules are relatively fixed. Although not ideal, the resident is often the one who must change expectations to make allowance for the workload of the nursing home staff.

The decision to move to a nursing home is usually made after much consideration by the client and family. The transition may be made more smoothly when the client retains as much participation in the process as possible. The client should be encouraged to have input into choosing the facility and in planning the move. Retention of personal items gives the individual a better sense of self in the new facility. Admission to a nursing home may be one of the most traumatic life transitions. The nurse needs to assist in making the adjustment of the client to the facility as smooth as possible. The client experiencing psychological and emotional difficulty during the admission and transition into any LTC facility needs support from the attending nursing staff. The use of therapeutic communication techniques by the staff in addition to spending adequate time with a transitioning resident can make a difference in the level of anxiety and stress experienced. If indicated, the nurse should initiate a referral for the resident to be seen by mental health services. These services are generally an underused resource for elders.

Accessing community-based LTC services may seem a natural and necessary transition for an elder needing help with either rehabilitation or assistance with other aspects of care. For others, accessing services may create significant emotional turmoil. Once a frail elder can no longer stay in the community environment, the individual and family may decide that a move to another environment that provides needed services is necessary. For those who can afford assisted living, this option may be less emotionally traumatic. Individuals feel they have retained a great deal of autonomy while paying for the services that they can no longer perform, such as food preparation, laundry, housekeeping, and medication management.

An accurate assessment of the client is the critical beginning for the client's experience in the LTC system. During the admission process to an LTC facility, the care provider will complete a battery of paperwork that documents the client's condition and reason for admission. In residential nursing homes, this assessment is important because it provides the basis upon which the care plan is developed and helps set the course for interventions designed to promote the highest level of functioning possible. It is imperative that the admission process not be limited to completing paperwork but includes gaining insight into the client to provide individualized care.

The Minimum Data Set (MDS) for Resident Assessment and Care Screening was developed for use by nursing homes in response to the Nursing Home Reform Legislation of 1987. The MDS provides extensive data about individual residents, but it also makes possible the establishment of a nationwide database regarding nursing home residents. Information requested by the MDS covers the areas of the resident's functional, medical, cognitive, and affective status at the time of admission and periodically thereafter (Sehy & Williams, 1999). This type of information also helps in tracking the improvement or decline of a resident over time, and whether or not quality indicators for care are being met. In the initial or follow-up assessment, the assessment protocol summarizes vulnerable aspects of the client's life that may require special care planning, interventions, and reporting of progress or problems in the resident's chart.

The reliability of the information obtained varies with the knowledge that evaluators are able to obtain about the client.

The latest revision to the MDS system (3.0) (CMS, 2010) has the following broad goals:

- To make the MDS more clinically relevant, while still achieving the federal payment mandates and quality initiatives
- To improve ease of use and efficiency
- To integrate selected standard scales
- To elicit resident voice by introducing interview questions

Other assessment tools are available and can provide more specific or multidimensional information. Tools can help the nurse determine functioning in cognitive, communication, behavioral, and social support domains. Other instruments measure vision, personality, depression, affect, comorbidity, and quality of life (Teresi & Evans, 1997). Examples of individual tools that are readily available in the literature include the Katz Index of Activities of Daily Living (Katz, Downs, Cash, & Grotz, 1970), Older American Resources and Services (Fillenbaum, 1988), the Beck Depression Rating Scale (Beck, Rush, Shaw, & Emery, 1979), and the Arthritis Impact Measurement Scale (Meenan, 1985).

A helpful website with a list of more than 30 assessment tools that can be downloaded for immediate use is http://hartfording.org/Practice/ConsultGeriRN/. For each assessment tool in the *Try This* series from the AACN/Hartford Foundation, explanation of the tool by an expert, validity and reliability information, the tool itself, and how to use it are succinctly provided.

Preservation of Autonomy of the Person

Healthcare professionals dealing with clients in LTC should carefully consider their own position as a moral force. Making decisions with a moral component is a part of everyday practice for most nurses. Understanding the concepts that provide the moral foundation for human existence is important. Those concepts typically include the following: autonomy, nonmaleficence, beneficence, justice, and professional–patient relationships (Beauchamp & Childress, 2009). Autonomy is in the forefront in LTC and the concept is rooted in the idea of self-rule and independent decision making.

Autonomy

The role of the nurse in providing LTC along the continuum of care is to preserve the autonomy of the client. At the same time, the client must be protected from harm. Balancing these issues is not always easy. It is imperative that the care provider not assume that because an individual has lost some physical autonomy, such as requiring personal assistance with daily hygiene, that the individual has given up his or her autonomy or is incapable of making his or her own decisions. Promotion of autonomy is accomplished by allowing the individual to make as many decisions as possible. In decisions that can impact health or health care, the nurse must provide the appropriate information to enable the client to make an informed decision. To more fully understand the concept of autonomy, the caregiver is encouraged to think about autonomy from the client's perspective when making caregiving decisions.

Individual decision making is a complex and multifaceted issue. Loss of decision-making capacity in one area does not indicate loss of all decision-making capacity. Decision-making capacity may fluctuate through the course of an illness, and determining the best approach to preserving safety and autonomy concurrently is at times challenging. At some point after decision-making capacity comes into question, it will be appropriate to consider legal guidelines set in place by the state in which the patient resides. The law in some states defines the line of authority for decision making when competence is in question. In cases where the person has been legally deemed unable to make his own decisions, the designated family member or legal guardian must be informed of all important aspects of the person's life and is responsible for making decisions that are in the person's best interest, that is, on his behalf or at his behest. When a person has lost some degree of autonomy, the nurse must also act in a judicious way that protects the individual from harm or exploitation.

It is also possible for someone who has legally lost autonomy (been declared incompetent) to continue to participate in the decision-making process. For example, a person with early stage dementia may have a legal guardian who is ultimately responsible for decision making in the person's best interest. However, as much as the person is able, the guardian would involve the person in the decision-making process, seeking input and finding out the wishes of the person prior to taking any action. This kind of consideration can contribute significantly to quality of life for the LTC resident.

Decision making or autonomy can be viewed on a continuum. An example of this might be when a person with advanced dementia decides to walk the halls. Autonomous decision making in a small way is appropriate as long as other principles, such as the client's safety and the safety of others, are considered. It is the nurse's responsibility to recognize an individual's capacity for autonomy and preserve that capacity as much as possible (Casada da Rocha, 2009). Sometimes, the nurse must compromise what he or she perceives to be the best treatment

in order to incorporate client preferences. An example would be a client's bathing twice a week as opposed to more frequent bathing. In that case, the nurse might alter other interactions, such as frequency of spot baths or application of lotion to ensure skin integrity, while respecting the autonomy of the client.

Guardianship

One of the ways in which the healthcare system provides for those who are unable to make informed decisions for themselves because of a cognitive or other health problem is to appoint a legal guardian. The responsibility of the guardian is to ensure safety and quality care for the person and to make decisions in the person's best interest. The guardian may be a family member, a friend, or a healthcare professional appointed by the court. In complex cases involving large estates, difficult family relationships, or divorce, the court may choose to appoint a professional guardian or person who will assist in making legal decisions for the incompetent person. The appointment of a guardian by the court usually follows the legal determination of incapacity. The person who has been declared by the court to be an incapacitated person is then no longer able to make any type of contractual decision independently. The guardian of the person is responsible to the court for getting to know the person sufficiently to be able to make decisions in his best interest, to provide documentation to the court as needed on the status of the person, and may be responsible for a variety of tasks ranging from healthcare advocacy to managing finances to ensuring that daily care needs are being met.

Guardianship guidelines vary from state to state and even from county to county within states. There is no established fee for these services, and guardians may be paid a small fee monthly, or a significant hourly fee as a consultant if additional services such as case management are being provided—if there are funds from the estate to cover such costs. These arrangements are generally agreed upon through the court as part of the legal guardian's acceptance of this responsibility.

There is some controversy as to the methods and process used for legal provisions for guardianship and assessment of a person's capacity. A tri-state study (Moye, Butz, Marson, & Wood, 2007) found that the quality of written clinical evidence to establish the need for guardianship was significantly lacking and that key information about the individual's values, preferences, and wishes was rarely documented. Persons were rarely present at the hearing. Functional assessments of persons should be routinely used during the evaluation of the need for guardianship. An assessment template that incorporates six assessment domains of interest to the court is recommended. The areas that should be addressed according to one such model include: medical condition, cognition, functional abilities, values, risk for injury and supervision needed, and ways to enhance capacity (Moye et al., 2007). Continued communication between clinical and legal team members is needed to protect the rights of vulnerable persons.

Nurses and social workers often make excellent guardians, because they are able to professionally address these areas and provide a holistic approach to care for the incapacitated person. Some court systems develop a rapport with certain professionals who act as guardians and will request their appointment in cases such as for older adults with dementia who reside in LTC facilities. To preserve the autonomy of persons as long as possible, guardians should encourage as much participation as possible in decision making, while keeping in mind the goal of safety and quality care for the incapacitated person.

Enablement

The enablement process is defined as a professional intervention aiming to recognize, support, and emphasize the patient's capacity to have control over his or her health and life (Hudson, St. Cyr Tribble, Bravo, & Poitras, 2011). Enablement may even be appropriate for those with cognitive impairment (Dawson, Wells, & Kline, 1993). This perspective focuses on how the disease affects the client's ability to carry out day-to-day activities. The purpose of this intervention is to determine the client's existing abilities and to enhance those abilities. Three areas of human behavior considered by this approach are self-care, social interaction, and interpretive abilities. In the area of self-care, when the client is having difficulty achieving purposeful behaviors, certain nursing interventions have been identified that can assist the caregiver in enhancing the client's abilities. These include object cueing, touch, direct physical assistance, and verbal prompting (Dawson et al., 1993). When a client with dementia loses many of the skills required for daily activity, there is the possibility of retention of some significant skill or pleasure, such as a music-related activity or game playing. The nurse should help preserve those abilities as much as possible by providing opportunities for their expression. Having a time to play cards or a music hour is often very meaningful to residents in LTC.

Advocacy: The Role of the Ombudsman

The LTC ombudsman is an advocate charged with the protection of the rights of all residents in LTC. The purpose of this role is to enhance quality of life for LTC residents and do the following (National Long-Term Care Ombudsman Resource Center, 2008, p. 1):

- Advocate for residents' rights and quality care
- Educate consumers and providers
- Resolve residents' complaints
- Provide information to the public

The LTC ombudsman is a person hired by a state LTC service agency under the auspices of the state or local health department or the statewide aging services. Volunteers who report to the ombudsman supervisor may do many of the actual investigations. The contact information for the ombudsman should be posted conspicuously in each LTC facility. Complaints may come from the LTC resident, concerned family, or caregivers. Findings must be reported to the client and/or family, and the ombudsman is responsible for achieving an equitable settlement between the resident and the LTC facility. The role of the ombudsman is founded in ethical principles and is implemented on behalf of the vulnerable client. (Updates on the organizational activities contacts can be found at http://www.ltcombudsman.org.)

Nursing Care

Nursing care is the primary service provided by residential LTC facilities. The further one progresses along the LTC continuum, the more intense are the nursing care needs. Nursing care in LTC settings is much more complex than it has been in the past and requires greater knowledge and expertise on the part of the nursing staff to manage comorbidities and provide high-quality care to all residents.

Care that nurses provide in LTC facilities should be holistic and multidimensional. Eighty five percent of patients in LTC settings are over age 65 (Mezey, Stierele, Huba, & Esterson, 2007). Because most persons in LTC settings are older, nurses would benefit from education in gerontology. The AACN, with funding from the Hartford Foundation, has released a set of standards outlining geriatric content for inclusion in the baccalaureate educational process for nurses; each program should periodically review and update the curriculum to stay current and prepare expert nurses for practice (Thornlow, Latimer, Kingsborough, & Arietti, 2006).

Pain Management

It is important for the nurse in LTC to adequately assess pain and to provide adequate treatment of that pain (Fink & Gates, 2010). Of particular importance is assessing clients' suffering from the pain associated with arthritis, osteoporosis, or neuralgia. A great deal of information is available on appropriate pain management strategies, and the nurse dealing with such clients should access this body of literature. When implementing pain management strategies in the LTC setting, follow up is critical. Pain relief varies for many reasons, and pain might not be relieved by a method that had previously been successful for the client. When pain is chronic and affects the ability of the client to function, current treatment strategies include routine regular administration of medication to manage the pain. Breakthrough pain, or pain experienced intermittently when a client is on routine pain medication, is then treated with "as-needed" medication. Addiction is not generally considered to be a major problem for elders suffering from chronic pain, but tolerance can become problematic.

For individuals unable to verbally express pain, its presence is noted in other ways. Evidence of pain may include facial expression (grimacing), groaning, body position, bracing, guarding, and rubbing of the painful body part. Alternative methods of dealing with pain should be considered. Massage, heat, cold, and support mechanisms such as knee or back braces may be helpful. The quality of life of the LTC client can be greatly affected by pain. With current advances in pharmacology and treatment, most pain can be managed effectively.

End-of-life care requires an intense management of comfort levels. If the individual is suffering intractable pain, use of palliative sedation may be necessary. Guidelines for such aggressive symptom management must be accessed through a process of evidence-based practice to ensure the most appropriate approach is used (Melnyk & Fineout-Overholt, 2010).

Disease Prevention/Health Promotion

Although it may be impossible to prevent some of the chronic diseases seen in the LTC population, others are certainly preventable. An important preventive health measure is the provision of flu and pneumonia vaccines to LTC residents. A vaccination program in residential facilities is essential and usually mandated by public health guidelines; in such settings, infections such as influenza can spread rapidly and cause deaths among the frail elderly. These types of infections may affect a number of residents at one time, and place a difficult burden on staff to deal with a number of acutely ill clients. Admission of clients to acute care settings in such circumstances is not unreasonable to ensure that all clients receive adequate nursing care during an outbreak of illness.

Certain screenings are recommended for older adults and can be helpful with early identification and treatment initiation. Screenings that are recommended by the U.S. Preventive Services Task Force and *Healthy People 2020* for older adults with chronic illness include: nutrition, tobacco, safety, immunizations, depression, alcohol abuse, lipids, hypertension, osteoporosis, vision and hearing, breast cancer, and colorectal cancer. Each of these screenings is rated as beneficial and supported by at least fair evidence that health outcomes and benefits outweigh the screening risk (Nelson, 2010).

Several key areas are considered standard for health promotion in older adults. These include exercise, not smoking, maintaining a healthy weight, social support, medication adherence, a safe environment, and activities that strengthen cognition and memory (Hardin, 2010). One study of assisted living residents found that "social support is a key variable in bolstering residents' psychological well-being" (Cummings, 2002, p. 300). Thus health promotion, even for those with existing chronic illness, emphasizes the same important strategies that healthcare professionals should encourage in LTC residents.

Cognitive Impairment

Individuals in LTC may suffer cognitive impairment from a variety of pathologic processes. These processes may be either acute or chronic. Individuals with cognitive impairment caused by irreversible causes such as closed head injuries, stroke, or dementia from a number of pathologic processes such as Alzheimer's disease, multi-infarct dementia, or Lewy body disease, often need special assistance to manage activities of daily living. Individuals in LTC who have cognitive impairment caused by an acute condition (delirium) need to receive immediate intervention to reverse the cause of the impairment before permanent disability or death results.

The first and foremost consideration in dealing with cognitively impaired individuals is the determination of whether the cognitive impairment is caused by delirium or dementia. Even an individual who has a diagnosis of dementia may experience a sudden change in cognition with an acute cause. Appropriate assessment of the condition can prevent unnecessary suffering or death.

Delirium is an acute condition brought on by one or more conditions that have altered brain functioning. The chief symptoms include sudden disturbance in consciousness and/or cognition. The underlying condition can be a single factor or a combination of conditions, which include but are not limited to fever, infection, allergic reaction, malnutrition, vitamin deficiency, drug toxicity (over the counter or prescription), drug interactions, food supplement toxicity, hyper- or hypoglycemia, and hypoxia (Tullman, Mion, Fletcher, & Foreman, 2008). The underlying condition can be life threatening and must be corrected or the incident may result in death. If the nurse providing care in the LTC setting determines that a client is suffering from delirium, it may be necessary to arrange transportation to an acute care facility where appropriate emergent care can be provided. In addition to these physiologic processes, cognitive impairment can be brought about by psychosocial factors such as depression, change in health brought on by aging or disease, or change in

location such as a move from a long-time home to live with another family member or a move to an institutionalized setting. The nurse assessing the patient should consider these possibilities in order to provide appropriate interventions.

Because of the physiologic changes that occur with aging, the signs of delirium in a frail elder may develop over a period of days as a subclinical condition worsens to a crisis point. In addition, in a patient who has a complicated medication regimen, symptoms of increased confusion may initially be mild. The astute nurse will make the appropriate observations to detect delirium even when the symptoms are subtle. In a client population with fluctuating cognition, such as at many residential facilities, detection of delirium becomes more challenging.

Dementia differs from delirium in that the condition is chronic and the underlying pathologic process is progressive and irreversible. It is estimated that 13% of individuals older than age 65, and 43% of those 85 and older, suffer from Alzheimer's disease or a related dementia (Alzheimer's Association, 2011). In addition, it is estimated that between 40% and 80% of those living in nursing homes have a cognitive impairment (CDC, 2009). Dementia is defined as the development of multiple cognitive deficits manifested by memory impairment and other problems, such as aphasia (inability to speak), apraxia (loss of ability to use familiar objects or carry out purposeful movements not caused by loss of sensory ability), and agnosia (loss of ability to determine the significance of sensory input, such as recognition of a familiar face or voice) (American Psychological Association, 2000). Primary dementias have no cure, and although a large investment is being made in drugs that could affect the progression of disease, outcomes of pharmacologic interventions have shown varying levels of success.

It is estimated that as much as 80% of dementia care is delivered in the home by a family caregiver (Alzheimer's Association, 2011). In the community LTC setting, the role of the nurse is to support the family caregiver with problem solving or identifying resources such as respite care, adult daycare, or the local chapter of the Alzheimer's Association. The nurse may play a key role in the decision making that takes place when caregiving for a demented loved one is negatively affecting the health of the spousal caregiver (Maas et al., 2004). When caregiving becomes overwhelming at home, the decision to place the individual with dementia in a residential facility is appropriate.

Periodic evaluation of individuals with chronic cognitive changes is necessary so that decline can be detected and care strategies adjusted. Many nurses working in the LTC setting rely on intuitive detection of cognitive changes, but this method can be improved by the inclusion of an objective measure of cognition such as the Mini Mental Status Exam (MMSE) (Folstein, Folstein, & McHugh, 1975), the Dementia Rating Scale (Alexopoulos & Mattis, 1991), or the Blessed Dementia Scale (Blessed, Tomlinson & Roth, 1968). Use of one or more of these instruments can provide data to track changes in cognitive functioning.

Nursing interventions that deal with dementia generally address one or more of three symptom domains: cognitive, functional, and/or behavioral. All clients with dementia demonstrate functional difficulties, whereas only some demonstrate behavioral problems. Dealing with individuals suffering from permanent cognitive impairment takes patience and understanding. It is important that the caregiver not lose sight of the client's perspective. It is more important to validate the client's personhood rather than to insist that he or she achieve "reality orientation." The client may find comfort in some behavior, such as carrying a doll, and this behavior, although not grounded in immediate reality, is grounded in the reality of a universal human behavior regarding caring for others, specifically infants. An evidence-based practice approach should be used in structuring care and the environment in LTC facilities responsible for patients with dementia. This ensures that the patient benefits from the latest research findings regarding best practice in dementia care.

The nurse needs to work closely with the activity director to meet the needs of the clients and to find appropriate and enjoyable activities for those with dementia. The activity director is responsible for providing activities for residents; individuals at different stages of dementia enjoy different types of activities. Those with mild dementia may still enjoy activities requiring personal interaction and following rules such as games or group singing. Those with more advanced dementia may enjoy more isolated activities such as the opportunity to fold laundry or a task related to food preparation.

Many nursing homes and even some assisted-living centers have special care units for dementia clients. The environment in such settings allows for safe wandering. Ideally, the staff has received training specific to caring for clients with dementia. The units are generally set up with consideration given to lighting, color, noise levels, congregate areas, and room setups. Such considerations are used to make the environment more pleasant for the residents. Again, an evidence-based practice approach will ensure that the latest research findings are incorporated into the caring regimen.

CASE STUDY

Mr. Havlin is a 92-year-old man who resides in an Alzheimer's special care unit that is part of a nursing home. Mr. Havlin's prior occupation was as a union laborer, where he worked with his hands to help build bridges and roads. Prior to being diagnosed with dementia, he lived at home with his wife who died recently. The couple had no children and no other close relatives living in the area. Mr. Havlin's neighbors had become concerned when he did not answer the door, had fallen several times at home, and appeared confused when they visited. Eventually, the Area Council on Aging was called in and appointed by the court as Mr. Havlin's guardian because of lack of available family members willing to assume this job.

Mr. Havlin spends much of his time wandering the halls on the Alzheimer's unit and sometimes displays combative, aggressive behavior. The nursing staff members try to get Mr. Havlin more involved in group activities such as playing games and doing art projects, but his behavior becomes agitated at these attempts.

Discussion Questions

1. Is it necessary for Mr. Havlin to be involved in group activities such as games and music therapy? What are the benefits or drawbacks to insisting on his involvement in these types of activities?
2. Is Mr. Havlin's wandering a common problem for persons with dementia? How is this best handled by the nursing staff?
3. Describe what types of therapeutic activities might be most appropriate for Mr. Havlin, considering his occupation and history.

Risk Reduction and Safety

One of the most important functions of the nurse in an LTC setting is to reduce risk and ensure client safety. In a community setting, part of the home assessment includes a thorough examination of the environment to detect possible hazards and correct them. The most obvious hazards include throw rugs, electrical cords strung across traffic areas, stairs (especially those without handrails), loose tiles in the shower, slick flooring, small pets, and similar environmental conditions. In residential settings, the nurse has similar responsibilities to ensure client safety. Facilities should provide a safe environment with adaptations for those with chronic health problems that would place them at higher risk for injuries or falls.

Safe patient handling has become an important issue in best nursing practice. Organized safety programs have been linked to positive outcomes for both patients and staff (Nelson, 2006; Nelson, Collins, Siddharthan, Matz, & Waters, 2008). Researchers found that implementing a safe patient-handling program in an LTC through the VA system resulted in better quality of patient care for residents. Safe-handling programs include four key interventions: appropriate patient-handling equipment and devices, assessment protocols, safe lifting policies, and patient lift teams. Key areas of change for residents after implementation of the program include: improved physical functioning, decreased sedentary states of residents, less deterioration in activities of daily living, decreased fall rate, and increased wakeful states in the mornings (Nelson et al., 2008).

Another important safety consideration is the use of restraints. Falls are a significant problem in LTC, and of persons who fall, 20–30% suffer significant injuries such as hip fractures (Cowley, Deibold, Gross, & Hardin-Fanning, 2006). Originally, restraints were thought to prevent injury to clients and were applied to ensure patient safety through limiting movement. Research has demonstrated, however, that restraints do the opposite and are likely to cause injury (Lekan-Rutledge, 1997). Both physical and chemical restraints in LTC facilities are now strictly regulated. The most current reports regarding restraint use are available online (Agency for Healthcare Research and Quality, 2009; CMS, 2011c).

Exercise has emerged as the "most effective factor in reducing the risk of falls and injuries from falls" (Mitty & Flores, 2007b, p. 349). All LTC facilities should have an exercise plan and program available to residents. The ideal environment for LTC residents is restraint-free, with environmental and staffing accommodations made to meet the needs of each resident and promote optimum physical functioning through exercise, adequate nutrition, and safety.

Palliative and Hospice Care

Palliative care is defined as:

> an approach that improves the quality of life of patients and their families facing the problem associated with life-threatening illness, through the prevention and relief of suffering by means of early identification and impeccable assessment and treatment of pain and other problems, physical, psychosocial and spiritual. (World Health Organization [WHO], 2008, paragraph 1)

The goal of this care is not curative, but centers around comfort. It is both a philosophy of care as well as a treatment system, and not necessarily just for those considered terminally ill. In palliation, physiologic needs are met and aggressive measures are taken for pain relief. A holistic view of the client should be maintained, and the personhood of the client is of primary consideration in this type of nursing care. Palliative care may be used in conjunction with life-prolonging care. For adults, the WHO (2008, paragraph 2) stated that palliative care:

- Provides relief from pain and other distressing symptoms
- Affirms life and regards dying as a normal process
- Intends neither to hasten or postpone death
- Integrates the psychological and spiritual aspects of patient care
- Offers a support system to help patients live as actively as possible until death
- Offers a support system to help the family cope during the patient's illness and in their own bereavement
- Uses a team approach to address the needs of patients and their families, including bereavement counseling, if indicated

- Will enhance quality of life and may also positively influence the course of illness
- Is applicable early in the course of illness, in conjunction with other therapies that are intended to prolong life, such as chemotherapy or radiation therapy, and includes those investigations needed to better understand and manage distressing clinical complications

A person with chronic illness may benefit from palliative care services and yet not qualify for hospice. Hospice is a type of palliative care and is usually delivered in the home by a team of trained professionals who address the needs of the patient and the entire family. Hospice is covered under Medicare Part A, which pays for most of the needed services for the terminally ill. However, Medicare will not pay for curative treatment in hospice. The general requirement for Medicare reimbursement for hospice service is that a physician must certify that the patient probably has 6 months or less to live (CMS, 2007). Determination of the terminal phase of an illness is sometimes difficult, and patients may improve during that 6-month period of time. Patients must be recertified by their physician as terminal in order to continue receiving hospice services. Hospice teams come into nursing homes to augment and oversee comfort care. In the terminal phase of life, appropriate care includes pain relief, comfort, and emotional and spiritual support for the client and family (Tarzian, 2000). The client and family can be referred for grief counseling related to the experience of incurable illness (Ferrell & Coyle, 2010). Death is a natural part of life, and the nurse should be prepared to facilitate the client's end-of-life transition and provide support to the family survivors (DeSpelder & Strickland, 2011). Once hospice services are begun for community-dwelling elders, other LTC services may not be allowed by reimbursement policy.

The End-of-Life Nursing Education Consortium has made enormous strides in providing core information to nurses interested in end-of-life care. This project began in 2000 with a grant from The Robert Wood Johnson Foundation and has provided specialized education and curricula to more than 4,000 nurses representing all 50 states, using a "train-the-trainer" approach (AACN, 2010). During the next decade, it is expected that knowledge on palliative and end-of-life care will continue to increase and that this treatment methodology will advance.

Research in Long-Term Care

The science of caring for those who have chronic illness is changing rapidly. Andersen and Horvath (2004) reported that 85% of seniors and 45% of the working adult population have at least one chronic illness. This growing burden of care for long-term health problems accounts for 78% of the nation's healthcare spending. Research often begins with clinical observations of problems or recurring events that require solutions. A number of nurse researchers have focused research programs dealing with chronic illness and issues related to the nursing home experience (e.g., Cornelia Beck, Kathleen Buckwalter, Jeanne Kaiser-Jones, Meridian Maas, Matty Mezey, and Terri Fulmer). Nurses in a clinical role should take the opportunity to define a problem and propose a solution. A novice researcher may partner with a more experienced researcher to develop an idea into a researchable question. Regional research organizations such as the Southern Nursing Research Society, the Midwest Nursing Research Society, and local chapters of Sigma Theta Tau are available to provide assistance.

As the body of literature grows, more opportunity for implementation of evidence-based practice and translational research exists. One model of evidence-based practice known for its ease of use at the bedside is the PICO method—patient, intervention, compared to, and outcomes. Using the PICO model, questions can be formulated and evidence searched rapidly to find studies that can bring insight into specific problem solving for those in LTC (see http://pubmedhh.nlm.nih.gov/nlm/picostudy/pico3.html for a search engine designed for the PICO question).

OUTCOMES

Simple medical models are rarely sufficient to address desired outcomes for those with complicated chronic medical conditions (Mold, 1995). It is not sufficient to consider the quality of life based on absence of sickness, but one must consider the overall well-being of the client. Outcomes will vary along the LTC continuum. For community-based clients, the overall outcome may be to remain in their homes as long as possible. Interventions to support that outcome may include client and family teaching on medication management, safety issues, or wound care. Rehabilitation may be a desired outcome for a community-based client following hospitalization.

For the resident in an LTC facility, outcomes are different and may include a reduction in the exacerbations of a chronic illness such as congestive heart failure. A client in the rehabilitative area of the facility may determine living independently again to be an outcome. Outcomes for others may be to function at the highest potential within the limitations imposed by the chronic illness. A decrease in pain and/or nausea might be an appropriate outcome for an individual in palliative care. Living each day with optimal quality of life is an outcome for most clients in LTC. Nurses can empower even frail older persons to obtain better outcome by good listening skills, working with them to identify the meaning of frailty to each person, and identifying positive coping and self-care solutions (Hage & Lorensen, 2005).

Evidence-Based Practice Box

The purpose of this study was to "examine the impact of an intervention to improve the health of grandmothers raising grandchildren in parent-absent homes" (p. 379). The authors used a longitudinal, pre- and post-test design with a sample of 529 female caregivers with a mean age of 56.7 years (range 38–83 years). Most subjects in the sample were African Americans of low income. Mental and physical health were measured after the intervention of home visits by RNs and social workers. The results indicated a significant improvement in vitality, physical and emotional effects on role functioning, and mental health. The authors concluded that grandmothers raising their grandchildren may benefit from increased home interventions and that the health of the grandmothers is critical to successful parenting of their grandchildren. Because this presents an increasingly common living arrangement, nurses can play an important role in seeing that grandparents in this situation have the necessary social support to raise healthy grandchildren.

Source: Kelley, S. J., Whitley, D. M., & Campos, P. E. (2010). Grandmothers raising grandchildren: Results of an intervention to improve health outcomes. *Journal of Nursing Scholarship, 42*(4), 379–386.

STUDY QUESTIONS

There are a number of issues in LTC today. What are the most essential issues for the federal government to address first?

Discuss the ethical principle of autonomy when constructing an appropriate plan of care for a LTC recipient.

Discuss the principle of autonomy in relation to the community-dwelling client versus the person in a residential facility.

Analyze nursing interventions that would most likely support the goals of an ideal LTC system.

How is LTC defined?

Describe the major settings in which LTC is provided, giving a specific example of each in your local community.

What are some of the precipitating factors for an individual to access the long-term care system?

What are the major problems facing both caregivers and clients in today's long-term care continuum?

What individuals are considered vulnerable populations?

Internet Resources (Cont.)

Geriatric Nursing Education Project: www.aacn.nche.edu/gnec.htm

Hartford Institute for Geriatric Nursing: http://hartfordign.org/

Leading Age (formerly American Association of Homes and Services for the Aging): http://www.leadingage.org/

Long-term care planning tool from CMS: www.medicare.gov/LTCPlanning/Include/DataSection/Questions/SearchCriteria.asp?version=default&browser=IE%7C6%7CWinXP&language=English&defaultstatus=0&pagelist=Home

Medicare and You, 2012. Centers for Medicare & Medicaid Services publication: www.medicare.gov/Publications/Pubs/pdf/10050.pdf

Long-Term Care Ombudsman: www.ltcombudsman.org

Medicare Hospice Benefits: www.medicare.gov/publications/pubs/pdf/02154.pdf

National Gerontological Nursing Association: http://www.ngna.org/

National Association of Professional Geriatric Care Managers: www.caremanager.org/

National Center for Assisted Living: http://www.ahcancal.org/ncal/Pages/default.aspx

National Hospice and Palliative Care Organization: http://www.nhpco.org

Practicing physician education in geriatrics: www.gericareonline.net

INTERNET RESOURCE

Across the States 2006: Profiles of Long-Term Care and Independent Living: assets.aarp.org/rgcenter/health/d18763_2006_ats.pdf

For a full suite of assignments and additional learning activities, use the access code located in the front of your book and visit this exclusive website: **http://go.jblearning.com/larsen**. If you do not have an access code, you can obtain one at the site.

REFERENCES

Administration on Aging. (2008). The 2005 whitehouse conference on aging. Retrieved September 10, 2011, from http://www.whoa.gov/

Administration on Aging. (2011). A profile of older Americans: 2010. Retrieved September 12, 2011, from: http://www.aoa.gov/AoARoot/Aging_Statistics/Profile/2010/2.aspx

Agency for Healthcare Research and Quality. (2009). Elderly long term care: Use of physical restraints in nursing homes creates substantial adverse consequences for residents. Retrieved September 12, 2011, from: http://www.ahrq.gov/research/mar09/0309RA9.htm

Aging with Dignity. (2010). Five wishes 2010 edition. Retrieved March 29, 2011, from: http://www.agingwithdignity.org/five-wishes.php

Alexopoulos, G. S., & Mattis, S. (1991). Diagnosing cognitive dysfunction in the elderly: Primary screening tests. *Geriatrics, 46*(12), 33–38, 43.

Algase, D., Beck, C., Kolanowski, A., Whall, A., Berent, S., Richards, K., et al. (1996). Need-driven dementia-compromised behavior: An alternative view of disruptive behavior. *American Journal of Alzheimer's' Disease, 11*(6), 10–19.

Alzheimer's Association. (2011). Alzheimer's disease facts and figures. Retrieved September 19, 2011, from www.alz.org/downloads/Facts_Figures_2011.pdf

American Association of Colleges of Nursing. (2010). End of life nursing education consortium (ELNEC) Fact sheet. Retrieved September 12, 2011, from: www.aacn.nche.edu/ELNEC/pdf/FactSheet.pdf

American Association of Colleges of Nursing. (2011). Nursing shortage. Retrieved October 20, 2011, from: www.aacn.nche.edu/media-relations/factsheets/nursing-shortage

American Association of Retired Persons. (2010). Prepare to care: A planning guide for families. Retrieved September 12, 2011, from: http://www.aarp.org/relationships/caregiving/info-04-2010/prepare-to-care.html

American Psychological Association. (2000). *Diagnostic and statistical manual IV-TR.* Arlington, VA: Author.

Andersen, G., & Horvath, J. (2004). The growing burden of chronic disease in America. *Public Health Reports, 119*, 263–270.

Arling, G., Kane, R., L., Mueller, C., Bershadsky, J., & Degenholtz, H. B. (2007). Nursing effort and quality of care for nursing home residents. *The Gerontologist, 47*(1), 672–682.

Beauchamp, T. L., & Childress, J. F. (2009). *Principles of biomedical ethics* (6th ed.). New York: Oxford University Press.

Beck, A. T., Rush, A. J., Shaw, B. F., & Emery, G. (1979). *Cognitive therapy of depression.* New York: Guilford.

Beck, C., Heacock, P., Mercer, S. O., Walls, R. C., Rapp, C. G., & Vogelpohl, T. S. (1997). Improving dressing behavior in cognitively impaired nursing home residents. *Nursing Research, 46*(3), 126–132.

Blessed, B., Tomlinson, B., & Roth, M. (1968). The association between quantitative measures of dementia and of degenerative changes in the cerebral gray matter of elderly subjects. *British Journal of Psychiatry, 114*, 797–811.

Boult, C., & Wieland, G. D. (2010). Comprehensive primary care for older patients with multiple chronic conditions. *Journal of the American Medical Association, 304*(17), 1936–1943.

Casada da Rocha, A. (2009). Towards a comprehensive concept of patient autonomy. *American Journal of Bioethics, 9*(2), 37–38.

Castle, N. G., Engberg, J., & Men, A. (2007). Nursing home staff turnover: Impact on nursing home compare quality measures. *The Gerontologist, 47*(1), 650–661.

Centers for Disease Control and Prevention. (2009). National nursing home survey: 2004 overview. Retrieved September 12, 2011, from: http://www.cdc.gov/nchs/data/series/sr_13/sr13_167.pdf

Centers for Disease Control and Prevention & the Merck Company Foundation. (2007). *The state of aging and health in America, 2007.* Whitehouse Station, NJ: The Merck Company Foundation.

Centers for Medicare & Medicaid Services. (2007). Medicare hospice benefits. Retrieved September 12, 2011, from: www.medicare.gov/publications/pubs/pdf/02154.pdf

Centers for Medicare & Medicaid Services. (2010). State operations manual. Retrieved September 12, 2011, from: http://www.cms.gov/manuals/downloads/som107c01.pdf

Centers for Medicare & Medicaid Services. (2011a). Overview. Retrieved September 19, 2011, from http://www.cms.gov/history

Centers for Medicare & Medicaid Services. (2011b). Nursing home quality indicators. Retrieved September 12, 2011, from: http://www.cms.gov/NursingHomeQualityInits/01_Overview.asp#TopOfPage

Centers for Medicare & Medicaid Services. (2011c). 482.13(e) Standard: Retraint or seclusion. Retrieved September 19, 2011, from http://www/cms.gov/manual/downloads/som107ap_a_hospitals.pdf

Chandra, A., Smith, L. A., & Paul, D. P. (2006). What do consumers and healthcare providers in West Virginia think of long-term care? *Healthcare and Public Policy, 84*(3), 33–38.

Cherry, B., Ashcraft, A., & Owen, D. (2007). Perceptions of job satisfaction and the regulatory environment among nurse aides and charge nurses in long-term care. *Geriatric Nursing, 28*(3), 183–192.

Cowley, J., Diebold, C., Gross, J. C., & Hardin-Fanning, F. (2006). Management of common problems. In K. L. Mauk (Ed.), *Gerontological nursing: Competencies for care* (pp. 475–560). Sudbury, MA: Jones and Bartlett.

Crain, M. (2001). Control beliefs of the frail elderly. *Case Management Journals, 3*(1), 42–46.

Cummings, S. (2002). Predictors of psychological well-being among assisted-living residents. *Health & Social Work, 27*(4), 293–302.

Dawson, P., Wells, D., & Kline, K. (1993). *Enhancing the abilities of persons with Alzheimer's and related dementias: A nursing perspective.* New York: Springer.

DeSpelder, L. A., & Strickland, A.L. (2011). *The last dance: Encountering death and dying* (2nd ed.). New York: McGraw Hill.

Donoghue, C., & Castle, N. G. (2006). Voluntary and involuntary nursing turnover. *Research on Aging, 28*(4), 454–472.

Eakes, G. G. (2004). Chronic sorrow. In S. Peterson & T. Bredow (Eds.), *Middle range theories* (pp. 165–172). Philadelphia: Lippincott Williams & Wilkins.

Elder Abuse Daily. (2010). Elder abuse data and statistics. Retrieved September 19, 2011, from http://www.eadaily.com/15/elder-abuse-statistics/

Feaster, M. (2006). Financing LTC with life insurance. *Provider, 32*(11), 39–40.

Ferrell, B., & Coyle, N. (2010). *Textbook of palliative nursing.* New York: Oxford University Press.

Fillenbaum, G. G. (1988). *Multidimensional functional assessment of older adults: The Duke older Americans resources and services procedures.* Hillsdale, NJ: L. Erlbaum Associates.

Fink, R. M., & Gates, R.A. (2010). Pain assessment. In B. Ferrell & N. Coyle (Eds.), *Oxford Textbook of Palliative Nursing* (3rd ed.). New York: Oxford University Press.

Folstein, M. R., Folstein, S. E., & McHugh, P. R. (1975). Mini-mental state: A practical method for grading the cognitive state of patients for the clinician. *Journal of Psychiatric Research, 12*, 189–198.

Fulmer, T. T. (1999). Elder mistreatment. In J. T. Stone, J. F. Wyman, & S. A. Salisbury (Eds.), *Clinical gerontological nursing: A guide to advanced practice* (2nd ed., pp. 665–674). Philadelphia: Saunders.

Gaugler, J. E., & Teaster, P. (2006). The family caregiving career: Implications for community-based long-term care practice and policy. *Journal of Aging & Social Policy, 18*(3–4), 141–145.

Gift, A. (2004). Unpleasant symptoms. In S. Peterson & T. Bredow (Eds.), *Middle range theories* (pp. 78–89). Philadelphia: Lippincott Williams & Wilkins.

Hage, A. M., & Lorensen, M. (2005). A philosophical analysis of the concept empowerment: the fundament of an education-programme to the frail elderly. *Nursing Philosophy, 6*, 235–246.

Hardin, S. (2010). Promoting quality of life. In K. L. Mauk (Ed.), *Gerontological nursing: Competencies for care* (2nd ed.). Sudbury, MA: Jones & Bartlett.

Harrington, L. (2008). Interview with a quality leader: Peter Buerhaus on workforce issues. *Journal for Healthcare Quality, 30*(6), 31–36.

Harrington, C., Zimmerman, D., Karon, S. L., Robinson, J., & Beutel, P. (2000). Nursing home staffing and its relationship to deficiencies. *The Journals of Gerontology Series B: Psychological Sciences and Social Sciences, 55*, S278–S287.

Harrington, C., Carrillo, H., Blank, B. W., & O'Brian, T. (2010). Nursing facilities, staffing, residents and facility deficiencies, 2004 through 2009. Retrieved September 12, 2011, from: http://www.pascenter.org/nursing_homes/nursing_trends_2009.php

Healthy People, 2020. (2011). Retrieved September 12, 2011, from: www.healthypeople.gov/hp2020

Houser, A., Fox-Grage, W., & Gibson, M. J. (2009). Across the states: Profiles of long-term care and independent living (8th ed.). Retrieved February 25, 2011, from: assets.aarp.org/rgcenter/health/d18763_2006_ats.pdf

Hudson, C., St. Cyr Tribble, D., Bravo, G., & Poitras, M. (2011). Enablement in health care contexts: A concept analysis. *Journal of Evaluation in Clinical Practice, 17*(1), 143–149.

Jonsen, A. R. (2007). A history of bioethics as discipline and discourse. In N. S. Jecker, A. R. Jonsen, & R. A. Pearlman (Eds.), *Bioethics: An introduction to the history, methods, and practice* (pp. 3–16). Sudbury, MA: Jones and Bartlett.

Kalisch, P. A., & Kalisch, B. J. (2004). *American nursing: A history* (4th ed.). Philadelphia: Lippincott Williams & Wilkins.

Kane, R., Freeman, I. C., Caplan, A. L., Aroskar, M. A., & Urv-Wong, E. K. (1990). Everyday autonomy in nursing homes. *Generations, 14*(Suppl.), 69–71.

Katz, S., Downs, T. D., Cash, H. R., & Grotz, R. C. (1970). Progress in development of the index of ADL. *The Gerontologist, 10,* 20–30.

Kelley, S. J., Whitley, D. M., & Campos, P. E. (2010). Grandmothers raising grandchildren: Results of an intervention to improve health outcomes. *Journal of Nursing Scholarship, 42*(4), 379–386.

Kempthorne, D. (2004). State efforts toward creating a national policy on healthy aging and long-term care. *Caring, 23*(1), 52–56.

Kinosian, B., Stallard, E., & Wieland, D. (2007). Projected use of long-term care services by enrolled veterans. *The Gerontologist, 47*(3), 356–364.

Kolcaba, K. (2003). *Comfort theory and practice: A vision for holistic health care and research.* New York: Springer.

Komisar, H. L., Feder, J., & Kasper, J. D. (2005). Unmet long-term care needs: An analysis of Medicare-Medicaid dual eligibles. *Inquiry, 42*(2), 171–182.

Koop, C. E., & Schaeffer, F. (1976). *Whatever happened to the human race?* Old Tappan, NJ: Fleming H. Revell.

Leininger, M. (2002). Culture care theory: A major contribution to advance transcultural nursing and practices. *Journal of Transcultural Nursing, 13*(3), 189–192.

Lekan-Rutledge, D. (1997). Gerontological nursing in long-term care facilities. In M. Matteson, E. McConnell, & A. Linton (Eds.), *Gerontological nursing: Concepts and practice* (2nd ed., pp. 930–960). Philadelphia: Saunders.

Lenz, E. R., Suppe, F., Gift, A. G. Pugh, L. C. & Milligan, R. A. (1995). Collaborative development of middle-range nursing theories: Toward a theory of unpleasant symptoms. *Advances in Nursing Science, 17*(3), 1–13.

Lindbloom, E. J., Brandt, J., Hough, L. D., & Meadows, S. E. (2007). Elder mistreatment in the nursing home: A systematic review. *Journal of the American Medical Director's Association, 8*(9), 610–116.

Lomastro, J. A. (2006). The White House conference on aging: A positive view. *Nursing Homes: Long Term Care Management, 55*(1), 14–16, 18.

Maas, M. L., Reed, D., Park, M., Specht, J. P., Schutte, D., Kelley, L. S., et al. (2004). Outcomes of family involvement in care interventions for caregivers of individuals with dementia. *Nursing Research, 53*(2), 76–86.

McGuire, L. C., Rao, J. K., Anderson, L. A., & Ford, E. S. (2007). Completion of a durable power of attorney for health care: What does cognition have to do with it? *The Gerontologist, 47*(4), 457–467.

Medpac. (2010). Report to the congress: Medicare payment policy. Retrieved September 12, 2011, from: www.medpac.gov/documents/Mar10_EntireReport.pdf

Meenan, R. F. (1985). New approaches to outcome assessment: The AIMS questionnaire for arthritis. *Advances in Internal Medicine, 31,* 167–185.

Melnyk, B. M., & Fineout-Overholt, E. (2010). *Evidence based practice in nursing & healthcare: A guide to best practice* (2nd ed.). Philadelphia: Lippincott Williams & Wilkins.

Mezey, M., Mitty, I., & Ramsey, G. (1997). Assessment of decision making capacity: Nursing's role. *Journal of Gerontological Nursing, 23*(3), 28–34.

Mezey, M., Stierele, L. J., Huba, G. J., & Esterson, J. (2007). Ensuring competence of specialty nurses in care of older adults. *Geriatric Nursing, 28*(6S), 9–14.

Mitty, E., & Flores, S. (2007a). Assisted living nursing practice: The language of dementia: Theories and interventions. *Geriatric Nursing, 28*(5), 283–288.

Mitty, E., & Flores, S. (2007b). Fall prevention in assisted living: Assessment and strategies. *Geriatric Nursing, 28*(6), 349–357.

Mold, J. W. (1995). An alternative conceptualization of health and health care: Its implications for geriatrics and gerontology. *Educational Gerontology, 21,* 85–101.

Moye, J., Butz, S. W., Marson, D. C., & Wood, E. (2007). A conceptual model and assessment template for capacity evaluation in adult guardianship. *The Gerontologist, 47*(5), 591–603.

National Association of Adult Protective Services Administrators. (2005). About NAPSA. Retrieved September 12, 2011, from: www.apsnetwork.org

National Association of Professional Geriatric Care Managers. (2011). What can a PGCM do for me? Retrieved September 12, 2011, from: http://www.caremanager.org/displaycommon.cfm?an=1&subarticlenbr=87

National Center for Assisted Living. (2011). Resident profile. Retrieved September 12, 2011, from: www.ahcancal.org/ncal/resources/Pages/ResidentProfile.aspx

National Center for Elder Abuse. (2011). Definitions of elder abuse. Retrieved September 12, 2011, from: http://www.ncea.aoa.gov/NCEAroot/Main_Site/FAQ/Basics/Definition.aspx

National Center for Health Statistics. (2007). National health interview survey. Retrieved September 12, 2011, from: www.cdc.gov/nchs/nhis.htm

National Institute on Aging. (2007). Growing older in America: The health and retirement study. Retrieved September 12, 2011, from: http://www.nia.nih.gov/ResearchInformation/ExtramuralPrograms/BehavioralAndSocialResearch/HRS.htm

National Institute of Mental Health. (2010). Older adults: Depression and suicide facts. Retrieved September 12, 2011, from: www.nimh.nih.gov/health/publications/older-adults-depression-and-suicide-facts.shtml#how-common

National Long-Term Care Ombudsman Resource Center. (2008). What does an ombudsman do? Retrieved September 12, 2011, from: http://www.ltcombudsman.org/about-ombudsmen#Ombudsman

National PACE Association. (2011). About NPA. Retrieved September 12, 2011, from: http://www.npaonline.org/website/article.asp?id=5

Nelson, A. (Ed.). (2006). *Safe patient handling and movement: A practical guide for health care professionals.* New York: Springer.

Nelson, A., Collins, J., Siddharthan, K., Matz, M., & Waters, T. (2008). Link between safe patient handling and patient outcomes in long-term care. *Rehabilitation Nursing, 33*(1), 33–43.

Nelson, J. M. (2010). Identifying and preventing common risk factors in the elderly. In K. L. Mauk (Ed.), *Gerontological nursing: Competencies for care* (pp. 357–388). Sudbury, MA: Jones & Bartlett.

Peterson, S. J., & Bredow, T. S. (2004). *Middle range theories: Application to nursing research.* Philadelphia: Lippincott Williams & Wilkins.

Remennick, L. I. (2001). All my life is one big nursing home: Russian immigrant women in Israel speak about double caregiver stress. *Women's Studies International Forum, 24*(6), 685–700.

Remsburg, R., & Carson, B. (2006). Rehabilitation. In I. Lubkin & P. Larsen (Eds.), *Chronic illness: Impact and interventions* (pp. 579–616). Sudbury, MA: Jones and Bartlett.

Sehy, Y. B., & Williams, M. P. (1999). Functional Assessment. In W. C. Chenitz, J. Takano Smith, & S. A. Salisbury (Eds.), *Clinical gerontological nursing: A guide to advanced practice* (2nd ed., pp. 175–199). Philadelphia: Saunders.

Sikorska-Simmons, E. (2006). Innovations in long-term care: Organizational culture and work-related attitudes among staff in assisted living. *Journal of Gerontological Nursing, 32*(2), 19–27.

Slaughter, S. E., Eliasziw, M., Morgan, D., & Drummond, N. (2009). Incidence and prevalence of excess disability among nursing home residents with middle-stage dementia: A prospective cohort study of functional transitions. *International Psychogeriatrics, 23*(1), 54–64.

Stewart, M. K., Felix, H., Dockter, N., Perry, D. M., & Morgan, J. R. (2006). Program and policy issues affecting home and community-based long-term care use: Findings from a qualitative study. *Home Health Care Services Quarterly, 25*(3–4), 107–127.

Tarzian, A. J. (2000). Caring for dying patients who have air hunger. *Journal of Nursing Scholarship, 32*(2), 137–143.

Teaster, P. B. (2002). A response to the abuse of vulnerable adults: The 2000 survey of state adult protective services. Washington, DC: The National Center on Elder Abuse.

Teresi, J. A., & Evans, D. A. (1997). Cognitive assessment measures for chronic care populations. In J. A. Teresi, M. P. Lawton, D. Holmes, & M. Ory (Eds.), *Measurement in elderly chronic care populations* (pp. 1–23). New York: Springer.

Thornlow, D., Latimer, D., Kingsborough, J., & Arietti, L. (2006). *Caring for an Aging America: A guide for nursing faculty.* Washington, DC: American Association of Colleges of Nursing.

Tobin, P., & Salisbury, S. (1999). Legal planning issues. In J. T. Stone, J. F. Wyman, & S. A. Salisbury (Eds.), *Clinical gerontological nursing: A guide to advanced practice* (2nd ed., pp. 31–44). Philadelphia: Saunders.

Tullman, D. F., Mion, L. C., Fletcher, K., & Foreman, M. D. (2008). Delirium. Retrieved September 14, 2011, from: http://consultgerirn.org/topics/delirium/want_to_know_more

U.S. Department of Health and Human Services. (1999). Mental Health: A report of the surgeon general. Retrieved September 12, 2011, from: http://www.surgeongeneral.gov/library/mentalhealth/home.html

Varcarolis, E. M., & Halter, M. J. (2010). *Foundation of psychiatric mental health nursing: A clinical approach*. Philadelphia: Saunders.

Wagner, D. L. (2006). Families, work, and an aging population: Developing a formula that works for the workers. *Journal of Aging & Social Policy, 18*(3–4), 115–125.

Willging, P. (2006). Get ready for community-based long-term care. *Long Term Living, 55*(3), 20, 22–23.

World Health Organization. (2008). WHO definition of palliative care. Retrieved September 12, 2011, from: www.who.int/cancer/palliative/definition/en/

CHAPTER 22

Palliative Care

When you do the common things in life in an uncommon way, you will command the attention
of the world.
—George Washington Carver

Barbara M. Raudonis

INTRODUCTION

The aging American population will eventually experience one or more chronic illnesses with which they will live with for years before death (Morrison & Meier, 2004). Four chronic diseases—heart disease, cancer, cerebrovascular disease, and chronic respiratory disease—are the leading causes of death for older adults (Centers for Disease Control and Prevention, 2010). These chronic diseases share protracted illness trajectories that include phases of decline resulting in progressively advanced disease and disability. Individuals who have illness trajectories such as those in chronic disease can benefit from palliative care. In reality many aging adults experience several chronic illnesses simultaneously, which demand complex care and often overwhelm both the elder and their family members.

A conceptual framework published by Nolan and Mock (2004), *A Conceptual Framework: Factors Influencing the Integrity of the Human Person,* addresses the complexity of needs, interventions, and processes needed to provide palliative care. The framework is organized around the core concept of the integrity of the human person and the relationship of the healthcare professional to the patient. It builds on the earlier work of Pellegrino (1990). The framework involves relationships among the following components: *external factors*—the integrity of the health professional, organizational culture, and healthcare resources; *internal factors*—spiritual domain, psychological domain, physical domain, functional domain, and community culture and family. Completing the framework are patient care goals and outcomes of care. Although end of life appears to be a prominent part of the framework, Nolan and Mock (2004) use the Institute of Medicine's (IOM's) definition of end of life that extends further up the illness trajectory to include "the period of time during which an individual copes with declining health from an ultimately terminal illness—from a serious though perhaps chronic illness or from the frailties associated with advanced age even if death is not clearly imminent" (Lunney, Foley, Smith, & Gelband, 2003, p. 22).

The multidimensional nature of the framework provides a structure for future research related to the factors that influence the integrity of the person, patient care goals, and outcomes of care. In essence this framework summarizes the major points about palliative care discussed throughout this chapter. In addition, it provides a foundation to passionately go forward in clinical practice, teaching, and research to build the science and the care to relieve suffering and improve quality of life.

Historical Perspectives

Palliative care grew out of the hospice movement. Hospice is both a philosophy of care and an organized form of healthcare delivery. The Latin origin of the word is *hospes,* which relates to hospitality. During the Middle Ages, pilgrims to the Holy Lands stopped at way stations for food, water, and respite. These way stations (hospices) were also centers of refuge for poor, sick, and dying people.

Dame Cicely Saunders is considered the founder of the modern hospice movement. Educated as a nurse, social worker, and physician, she founded St. Christopher's Hospice in Sydenham England in 1967. St. Christopher's Hospice was the first research and teaching hospice and is known for several innovations including pain and symptom management, a holistic approach to care, home care, family support throughout the illness, and bereavement follow up (Meier, 2010). The services provided by St. Christopher's Hospice evolved over time to meet the needs of patients and families. Service settings include in-patient care, home care, and palliative daycare centers. Based on Saunders's work, palliative care services have spread throughout the United Kingdom and the world (Hansford, 2010). Two years after the opening of St. Christopher's Hospice, Dr. Elisabeth Kubler-Ross's book *On Death and Dying* (1969) was published. One of the outcomes of her seminal work was the identification of the stages of dying. More importantly, her work initiated a national dialogue recognizing the needs of the dying.

Hospice and palliative care is a complex service with the goal of improving the quality of life of terminally ill persons through a variety of programs in an individualized, flexible, and nonmedical environment (Hearn & Myers, 2001). St. Christopher's Hospice continues to serve as a prototype for hospice and palliative care throughout the world. However, Dame Saunders cautions not to clone St. Christopher's but to refine the principles of hospice and palliative care within the cultural context of the needs of the individuals served.

Although Dame Saunders died in 2005, she had already established Cicely Saunders International in 2002. This charity is the only one in the world with the specific mission to promote research and best practice in palliative care. In May 2010 the Cicely Saunders Institute of Palliative Care was officially opened. The institute's new building is located next to King's College Hospital and is a result of the partnership between King's College London and Cicely Saunders International. The Institute of Palliative Care was built to serve as the hub for a network of international research in palliative care to guide clinical practice, education, and policy with the goal of improving palliative care and quality of life for people throughout the world (Cicely Saunders International, 2010; Higginson, 2011).

Florence S. Wald, a nurse and pioneer in the hospice movement in the United States, strengthened her vision for improving the quality of life for terminally ill persons during a visit to St. Christopher's Hospice. She conducted a needs assessment for hospice care in Connecticut. In 1974 the first hospice program in the United States was established in Branford, Connecticut. At that time, the Connecticut Hospice was only a homecare program (no in-patient beds) and became a model of care for the entire United States. As services evolved, in-patient beds were added and Connecticut Hospice became the first independent hospice inpatient facility in the country (Meier, 2010). Wald's work for the next 30 years led the way in translating the English hospice philosophy and models of care into the American hospice movement. She is considered the "mother of hospice and palliative nursing care in the United States" by the Hospice and Palliative Nurses Association (HPNA) and Hospice and Palliative Nurses Foundation (HPNF). She became the first recipient of the Hospice and Palliative Nurses Association Leading the Way Award in January 2004 (HPNA, 2011).

The National Hospice and Palliative Care Organization (NHPCO) (2010) estimated there were 5,000 operational hospice programs throughout the United States in 2009. An estimated 1.56 million patients were served by these programs. These figures illustrate the enormous growth and progress in hospice care in the United States since 1974. The majority of hospice patients, 68.61%, die at their place of residence. This could be their private residence, nursing home, or residential facility (NHPCO, 2010), whereas approximately 50% of the general population die in acute care hospitals (Teno, 2004). In 2009 the median length of stay was 21.1 days while the average length of stay was 69 days (NHPCO, 2010). These numbers suggest that late referrals remain a problem. Noncancer primary diagnoses accounted for 59.9% of hospice admissions in 2009 compared to 40.1% for cancer diagnoses. As evidence of our aging population, 83% of hospice patients were 65 years or older and one third of those were 85 years or older (NHPCO, 2010). Although these numbers portray tremendous growth in the use of hospice services, the patients admitted were 80.5% White/Caucasian. This is not a new finding, but continued evidence that not all those in need of hospice services receive care.

In the 1990s two reports, the *Study to Understand Prognosis and Preferences for Outcomes and Risks of Treatments* (SUPPORT; 1995) and the IOM report, *Approaching Death: Improving Care at the End of Life* (Field & Cassel, 1997) ignited a concern regarding the status of end-of-life care in the United States. As a result improving end-of-life care was placed on the national healthcare agenda.

SUPPORT Study

The landmark SUPPORT study (SUPPORT Principal Investigators, 1995) was funded by the Robert Wood Johnson Foundation for $29 million to study the process of dying in five American major teaching hospitals. The study involved approximately 9,000 participants with diagnoses such as heart failure (HF), chronic obstructive pulmonary disease (COPD), colon and lung cancer, and liver failure. Findings included that more than 50% of patients had serious pain the last 3 days of life. In addition, there was poor communication between doctors and patients about their goals of care. There was substantial emotional suffering of patients, families, and professionals. Thirty-one percent of the families lost most of their life savings. The findings from this study sparked a groundswell of initiatives in research, education, and practice, with the goal of changing the culture of death and dying in the United States.

IOM Report

The second landmark study was the IOM's Committee on Care at the End of Life report, *Approaching Death: Improving Care at the End of Life* (Field & Cassel, 1997). The committee found four broad deficiencies in the care of persons with life-threatening and incurable illnesses. Deficiencies included:

- Too many people suffer needlessly at the end of life both from errors of omission—when caregivers fail to provide palliative and support care known to be effective—and from errors of commission—when caregivers do what is known to be ineffective and even harmful.
- Legal, organizational, and economic obstacles conspire to obstruct reliably excellent care at the end of life.
- The education and training of physicians and other healthcare professionals fail to provide them with the knowledge, skills, and attitudes required to care well for the dying patient.
- Current knowledge and understanding are inadequate to guide and support the consistent practice of evidence-based medicine at the end of life. (pp. 264–265)

Healthcare professionals, patients, families, health plan administrators, agency administrators, and policymakers must work together to change attitudes, policies, and actions in order to surmount the deficiencies in palliative care (Field & Cassel, 1997). The report concluded with optimism that a "vigorous societal commitment . . . would motivate and sustain individual and collective efforts to create a humane care system that people can trust to serve them well as they die" (Field & Cassel, p. 13).

Clinical Practice Guidelines for Palliative Care

The landmark studies—the SUPPORT study and the IOM report—recognized the need to integrate palliative care into health care for all individuals with chronic, debilitating, and life-limiting illnesses. This need resulted in the National Consensus Project for Quality Palliative Care (NCPQPC) and the establishment of the *Clinical Practice Guidelines for Quality Palliative Care* (NCPQPC, 2004).

The first edition of the *Clinical Practice Guidelines* described the core precepts and structures of clinical palliative care programs needed to promote consistent high standards for palliative care. In addition, individual providers, regardless of the care setting, used the guidelines to provide palliative approaches in their daily clinical practice across the healthcare continuum. In 2006 the National Quality Forum (NQF) integrated the *Clinical Practice Guidelines for Quality Palliative Care* into their document *A National Framework for Palliative and Hospice Care Quality Measurement and Reporting* (NCPQPC, 2009). The purpose of the NQF document is to provide a foundational framework for the development of quality measurement and reporting systems and the recommendation of 38 preferred palliative care practices endorsed by the NQF (2006). The *Clinical Practice Guidelines for Quality Palliative Care* was substantially revised in 2009. The rationale for the revision was to: 1) reflect the evolving scientific evidence and clinical practice; 2) ensure that the 38 preferred palliative care practices and the 8 domains from the *Clinical Guidelines* were in agreement; and 3) to provide real-life examples that demonstrate how the theory of the *Clinical Guidelines* were implemented in clinical practice (NCPQPC, 2009). Although both documents operationalize palliative care theory and practice through definitions and recommended practices, each has its own function. The NQF framework is the first step in a process to generate quality measures for palliative care, whereas the guidelines are part of the NCPQPC's ongoing mission to articulate a more expansive vision of quality palliative care.

The National Institutes of Health (NIH) recognized the need to evaluate the current science regarding end-of-life care and convened a State-of-the-Science Conference on Improving End-of-Life Care in December 2004. Historically, this was the first NIH Consensus Conference on End-of-Life Care. The document produced from this conference provides only a snapshot of the medical knowledge and evidence available up to that 2004 meeting. Palliative care research and clinical practice continue to evolve, requiring one to read the literature on a regular basis to keep current.

Clinical Specialty of Palliative Care

Palliative care is the broad term used to describe the care provided by an interdisciplinary team consisting of physicians, nurses, social workers, chaplains, and other healthcare professionals. Palliative medicine is a medical specialty practiced by physicians (Derek, Hanks, Cherny, & Calman, 2004).

Palliative Medicine

On October 6, 2006, the American Board of Medical Specialties (ABMS) announced the addition of a new subspecialty certificate in Hospice and Palliative Medicine. Historically, this was the first time that 10 ABMS Member

Boards collaborated in the offering of certification in one specific area. The first certification examination was offered in October 2008 (ABMS, 2006). This recognition as a subspecialty was the result of the diligent collaboration of the American Academy of Hospice and Palliative Medicine (AAHPM) and the American Board of Hospice and Palliative Medicine (ABHPM). The United States joined members of the international community such as Great Britain, Ireland, Australia, and Canada in formally recognizing palliative medicine as a subspecialty (von Gunten & Lupu, 2004). Palliative medicine is defined as "a sub-speciality that focuses on relieving suffering and improving quality of life for patients with serious illness and their families" (Gelfman & Morrison, 2008, p. 36).

The AAHPM is the professional organization for physicians specializing in hospice and palliative medicine. The academy's purpose is succinctly summarized in the organization's tagline "Physicians caring for patients with serious illness" (AAHPM, 2011). The AAHPM celebrated its 20th anniversary in 2008 and has grown to nearly 4,000 members, which include physicians and other medical professionals.

Palliative Care Nursing

Palliative care nursing parallels the continuing development of the art and science of palliative care. Individuals and families experiencing life-limiting progressive illness are the focus of the nurse's evidenced-based physical, emotional, psychosocial, and spiritual or existential care (HPNA & American Nurses Association, 2007). Coyle (2010) describes the distinctive features of palliative care nursing as "a whole person" philosophy of care. This care is provided across the lifespan, in different care settings, and throughout the illness trajectory, the patient's death, and the family's bereavement. A nurse's individual relationship with the patient and family is a critical part of the healing relationship. This healing relationship together with scientific knowledge (effective pain and symptom management) and clinical skills (addressing the emotional, psychosocial, spiritual needs, and cultural values) is the essence of palliative care nursing, setting the specialty apart from other nursing specialty areas (Coyle, 2010, pp. 5–6). As a philosophy of care and therapeutic approach, palliative care can be practiced by all nurses (Coyle, 2010).

Professional Associations Related to Hospice and Palliative Nursing

The Alliance for Excellence in Hospice and Palliative Nursing (AEHPN) includes the National Board for Certification of Hospice and Palliative Nurses (NBCHPN), the HPNA and the HPNF. The mission of the alliance is to "be the unified voice of professional membership, certification, research and education to advance quality palliative care for the benefit of the public at large" (AEHPN, 2011).

The NBCHPN offers four certification examinations: the advanced practice nurse (APN), the registered nurse (RN), licensed practical/vocational nurse (LPN/LVN), and nursing assistant (NA). Role-delineation studies were conducted to support the original certification examinations for each of the respective levels of nursing practice. The role delineation studies are repeated periodically to ensure that the certification examinations match the reality of clinical practice. Hospice and palliative nursing is the only nursing specialty that offers certification at all levels of practice.

The first hospice nursing organization, the Hospice Nurses Association, was formed in 1987 to serve the networking and support needs of nurses caring for terminally patients and their families who were receiving hospice care. In 1998 the name of the organization was changed to the Hospice and Palliative Nurses Association (HPNA) to reflect the needs of nurses working in palliative care settings outside of the realm of hospice agencies. HPNA is now the largest professional nursing organization dedicated to the care of those with life-threatening and terminal illness.

The HPNF was incorporated in 1998 to: 1) support research and education in end-of-life care; and 2) to strive to meet the strategic goals of the HPNA. The foundation believes that evidenced-based practice is the key to quality care for people with life-limiting and terminal illness. HPNF is a source for funding research and supporting education related to hospice and palliative care to both individuals and groups. The 2008 HPNA Research Committee was given the charge to develop a research agenda that could guide nurse researchers in developing programs of research in palliative nursing and the HPNF in funding those programs (D. J. Sutermaster, personal communication, January 30, 2008). The 2009–2011 HPNA Research Agenda is the first such agenda for the organization. It focuses on the symptoms of dyspnea, fatigue, and constipation with the purposes of 1) providing a focus for graduate students, junior, and established researchers; 2) guide HPNA and HPNF research funding; and 3) illustrate to other stakeholders the importance of these research foci (Campbell et al., 2009). HPNA expects that the research agenda will be revised regularly to reflect needed research to support evidence-based practice in end-of-life care.

Differentiating Hospice Care and Palliative Care

It is critical to differentiate between hospice care and palliative care in the context of clinical practice. The terms *hospice* and *palliative* care are frequently used interchangeably. Palliative care is a broader concept and includes the entire continuum of care. Hospice care is always palliative care, but not all palliative care is hospice care.

CASE STUDY

Mr. James is an 80-year-old widower who resides alone in his first-floor apartment. He has a history of cardiac disease requiring a pacemaker and medication for hypertension. Mr. James was diagnosed with congestive heart failure (CHF) 4 years ago after increasing episodes of fatigue and dyspnea. He was recently discharged from the hospital after an episode of extreme shortness of breath and fluid retention. His daughter is visiting from out of town and brought him to his post-discharge appointment with his geriatric nurse practitioner (GNP). His recent hospitalization occurred because of his most severe exacerbation of his symptoms to date. His cardiologist changed his CHF classification to the New York Heart Association Functional Class III. His GNP reviews his medical record, medication profile, and family care conference notes. An advance directive has been completed and is now part of his medical record. His daughter is the designated healthcare power of attorney.

Mr. James's daughter is very concerned about her father's physical and emotional health. He seems depressed and "ready to go home to be with his wife". The daughter suggested that Mr. James consider moving so that the family could take care of him. Mr. James wants to remain in his own apartment and manage his symptoms at home rather than in the hospital. His GNP realizes that this is an opportunity to discuss Mr. James's future, his options, and goals of care. Available treatment options include medication changes, antidepressants, home oxygen therapy, nutrition, physical therapy, home health care, and support groups for persons with heart failure (some are online). After the discussion with Mr. James and his daughter, the GNP will write up the plan chosen by Mr. James and document it in his medical chart to maintain continuity of care with all of his healthcare providers.

Discussion Questions

1. Would you describe this situation as palliative care? If so, why? If not, why not?
2. What is your recommended plan of care for Mr. James?
3. Identify some examples of when Mr. James might be transitioning from palliative care to hospice care?
4. Why is it important that Mr. James's daughter, his designated healthcare power of attorney, be involved in the discussion regarding his future healthcare goals of care?
5. How would you respond to Mr. James when he stated, "I want to go home and be with my wife"?
6. Based on this case study how would you describe the difference between palliative care and hospice care?

Hospice is a specific type of palliative care, and in the United States it is generally considered a philosophy or program of care rather than a building of bricks and mortar. Hospice programs provide state-of-the-art palliative care and supportive services to dying persons and their families. This comprehensive care is available 24 hours a day, every day of the year in community-based settings, patients' homes, and facility-based care settings. A medically directed interdisciplinary team (clients, family members, professionals, and volunteers) provides physical, psychosocial, and spiritual care during the final phase of an illness, the process of imminently dying, and the period of bereavement (NCPQPC, 2009). In hospice care the dying person and the family are the unit of care. Client and family values direct the care. However, the current Medicare hospice benefit eligibility criteria for hospice services include a terminal diagnosis and a 6-month prognosis. In addition, it requires that clients discontinue curative or life-prolonging treatments to access comprehensive hospice care (Lynn, 2001). There are three outcomes of hospice care: self-determined life closure; safe and comfortable dying, and effective grieving (National Hospice Organization Standards and Accreditation Committee, 1997). Humane, holistic, comprehensive plans of care involving an interdisciplinary healthcare team are critical to maintain quality of life for the person and family making the transition to end of life. One of the first definitions of palliative care accepted throughout the world was developed by the World Health Organization (WHO, 1990). Subsequent definitions have been developed or refined by the NHPCO, IOM, and other professionals providing palliative care (**Table 22-1**). As the number of palliative care programs continues to grow,

differentiating between hospice and palliative care is necessary for consumers and healthcare providers.

Although it appears that hospice and palliative care have much in common, there are two major distinctions. First, palliative care permits life-prolonging therapies. Secondly, palliative care is integrated throughout the course of a chronic, progressive, and incurable disease, from diagnosis through death, rather than only during the final 6 months of life. The chronic illness experience of clients and their families demonstrates the need for comprehensive palliative care earlier in the disease trajectory (NCPQPC, 2009).

In response to the need for broadening the scope of palliative care, the *Clinical Practice Guidelines for Quality Palliative Care* (NCPQPC, 2009) describe palliative care as appropriate from the time of a life-threatening or debilitating illness through cure or until death as well as into the family's period of bereavement.

Palliative Care and Chronic Illness

According to Curtin and Lubkin (1995), chronic illness is never completely cured, and it involves the "total human environment for supportive care and self-care, maintenance of function and prevention of further disability" (pp. 6–7). Symptoms may increase or decrease during phases of stability, exacerbation, remission, and eventually death (Corbin, 2001). The Last Acts Palliative Care Task Force developed five palliative care precepts or principles of care (see **Table 22-2**). Integration of these precepts into clinical practice enables clinicians to provide a continuum of care otherwise unavailable to clients with advancing illness and their families (Cumming & Okun, 2004). The meaning of these precepts are integrated into the eight domains of palliative care described in the

---

Table 22-1 Definitions of Palliative Care with Distinctions from Hospice Care

World Health Organization (WHO)

The active total care of clients whose disease is not responsive to curative treatment. Control of pain, of other symptoms, and of psychological, social, and spiritual problems is paramount. The goal of palliative care is achievement of the best quality of life for clients and families. It affirms life and regards dying as a normal process. Palliative care neither hastens nor postpones death. It emphasizes relief from spiritual aspects of client care and offers a support system to help the family cope during the client's illness and in their own bereavement.

National Hospice and Palliative Care Organization (NHPCO)

The treatment that enhances comfort and improves the quality of an individual's life during the last phase of life. No specific therapy is excluded from consideration. The test of palliative care lies in the agreement between the individual, physician(s), primary caregiver, and the hospice team that the expected outcome is relief from distressing symptoms, the easing of pain, and/or enhancing the quality of life. The decision to intervene with active palliative care is based on an ability to meet the stated goals rather than affect the underlying disease. An individual's needs must continue to be assessed and all treatment options explored and evaluated in the context of the individual's values and symptoms. The individual's choices and decisions regarding care are paramount and must be followed.

Institute of Medicine (IOM)

Palliative care seeks to prevent, relieve, reduce, or soothe the symptoms of disease or disorder without effecting a cure (Field & Cassel, 1997).

Distinctions Between Hospice and Palliative Care

The Center to Advance Palliative Care (CAPC) developed a website for patients and their families (www.getpalliativecare.org). The website states that: Palliative care is not the same as hospice care. Palliative care may be provided at any time during a person's illness, even from the time of diagnosis. And, it may be given at the same time as curative treatment. Hospice care always provides palliative care. However, it is focused on terminally ill patients—people who no longer seek treatments to cure them and who are expected to live for about 6 months or less.

Sources: Center to Advance Palliative Care. Resources for patients and families. Retrieved February 1, 2008, from: http://getpalliativecare.org; Field, M. J., & Cassel, C.K. (Eds.). (1997). *Approaching death: Improving care at the end of life.* Committee on Care at the End of Life, Division of Health Care Services, Institute of Medicine. Washington, DC: National Academies Press; National Hospice and Palliative Care Organization (NHPCO). Retrieved January 28, 2008, from: http://www.nhpco.org; World Health Organization. (1990). Cancer pain relief and palliative care. *WHO Technical Report Series 804* (p.11). Geneva, Switzerland: Author.

Clinical Practice Guidelines for Quality Palliative Care (NCPQPC, 2009).

The SUPPORT study (1995) findings identified several problems related to palliative care. Patient suffering included dying in pain with a severe symptom burden. Poor communication among patients, families, and their physicians led to undesired resuscitation efforts and extensive use of hospital resources.

Communication is a core skill of palliative care. However, many clinicians are uncomfortable sharing bad news and poor prognoses. Some

Table 22-2 Precepts of Palliative Care
1. Respecting patient goals, preferences, and choices
2. Providing comprehensive caring
3. Utilizing the strengths of interdisciplinary resources
4. Acknowledging and addressing caregiver concerns
5. Building systems and mechanisms of support

Source: Lomax, K. J., & Scanlon, C. (1997). *Precepts of palliative care.* Princeton, NJ: The Robert Wood Johnson Foundation.

studies suggest that "patient-centered" interviews are associated with improved levels of satisfaction on the part of patients and their families (Dowsett et al., 2000; Steinhauser, Christakis, Clipp, McNeilly, & Tulsky, 2000).

The IOM study, *Approaching Death: Improving Care at the End of Life* (Field & Cassel, 1997), revealed a critical need for improvement in the education and training of healthcare professionals in palliative and end-of-life care. Healthcare professionals have traditionally received inadequate education and training in the safe and effective management of pain and other symptoms. They also lack the skills and confidence to address the psychological, social, and spiritual aspects of care (Sullivan, Lakoma, & Block, 2003).

Nursing curricula and textbooks are deficient in palliative and end-of-life content and clinical learning opportunities. If nurses are not taught that their professional role includes providing quality palliative and end-of-life care, then they cannot practice it (Ferrell, Virani, & Grant, 1999). In response to these identified needs, resources for teaching palliative care nursing to students and practicing nurses have been and continue to be developed and disseminated. Essential

nursing competencies in end-of-life care were proposed and disseminated by the American Association of Colleges of Nursing (AACN, 2004) in the document, "Peaceful Death." Matzo and Sherman (2001, 2006, 2010) used the AACN competencies as the framework for their nursing textbook entitled Palliative Care Nursing: Quality Care at the End of Life. The third edition (Matzo & Sherman, 2010) addresses both the undergraduate and graduate AACN end-of-life nursing competencies. Ferrell and Coyle (2001, 2006) wrote a comprehensive volume—*Textbook of Palliative Nursing*—the third edition of which has been renamed as *Oxford Textbook of Palliative Nursing* to recognize it as a leading resource in the field of palliative nursing. An indication that the science of palliative care and palliative care nursing continues to grow is that these two textbooks are both in their third editions. Recognizing the special needs of older adults, Matzo and Sherman also authored *Gerontologic Palliative Care Nursing* (2004). Morrison and Meier, two expert palliative care physicians, authored the textbook, *Geriatric Palliative Care* (2003). Experienced clinicians and researchers continue to share their knowledge, skills, and passion for palliative care through diverse publications, websites, conferences, and now social media such as Facebook and Twitter.

Palliative care seeks to treat, reduce, or prevent symptoms of diseases, relieve suffering, and improve the patient and family's quality of life without affecting a cure. It is not restricted to dying hospice patients (Field & Cassel, 1997). The principles of palliative care extend to broader populations that could benefit from holistic, comprehensive plans of care involving interdisciplinary healthcare teams from the time of diagnosis and throughout the disease processes and illness trajectory.

According to von Gunten and colleagues (2001), palliative care is interdisciplinary care that focuses on relief of suffering and improving quality of life. This simple definition illustrates the fit between chronic illness and palliative care. Based on the preceding description, it is clear that persons with chronic illness would benefit from palliative care.

PROBLEMS AND BARRIERS RELATED TO PALLIATIVE CARE

Barriers to palliative care exist for numerous reasons. The major underlying resistance to palliative care stems from a medical philosophy that emphasizes cure and prolongation of life over quality of life and relief of suffering (Morrison & Meier, 2004). Insurance reimbursement also forces consumer choice between cure and comfort care. Regular Medicare reimburses for curative treatment only, leaving the Medicare hospice benefit to cover comfort care (Fisher et al., 2003).

Prognostication in chronic, debilitating, and life-threatening illness presents a major challenge for healthcare professionals and is a barrier to adequate palliative care (Christakis & Lamont, 2000). Our current healthcare system forces patients and families to choose between curative treatment and comfort care. However, there is growing recognition that palliative care is needed from diagnosis through the process of dying (Foley, 2001). To reiterate, palliative care can be defined as: interdisciplinary care focused on the relief of suffering and improving quality of life; it removes any burden of prognostication and the requirement of a terminal diagnosis (von Gunten & Romer, 1999).

The public's lack of understanding related to the options available to dying patients and their families results in delayed access to hospice and palliative care services (Field & Cassel, 1997). Surveys consistently indicate patients prefer to die at home. In 2009, 68.6% of all hospice patients died at a place they called "home"— 40.1% died in their private residence, 18.9% died in nursing homes, 9.6% died in residential facilities, and 21.2% died in hospice in-patient units (NHPCO, 2010). Consumers' and communities' lack of understanding of what comprehensive palliative care programs offer and poor communication about patient and family preferences and denial of death all impede timely referrals to palliative care services (End-of-Life Nursing Education Consortium [ELNEC], 2009a).

Family Caregiving: Burden

In palliative care, the client and family are the unit of care. Family caregivers provide supportive care throughout the chronic illness trajectory, in all care settings, and for all types of needs (McMillan, 2004). The caregiver's burden is increasing significantly as more complex health care moves into the home setting. Evidence is growing that extended service as a caregiver can negatively impact the physical, social, and emotional well-being of caregivers (Pinquart & Sorenson, 2003). Some caregivers experience sustained stress related to highly stressful times of caregiving, and this negatively impacts their bereavement process (Schulz et al., 2003; Schulz, Newsom, Fleissner, DeCamp, & Nieboer, 1997).

Successful intervention studies have been carried out with caregivers of clients with Alzheimer's disease, but little has been done with caregivers of hospice and palliative care clients. The NIH (2004) consensus statement on improving end-of-life care concluded that more randomized clinical trials examining decreasing caregiver burden are needed. Studies are needed to determine which caregivers are at greatest risk for distress and specific interventions that are most likely to relieve the distress (see Chapter 10: Family Caregiving).

Although these barriers seem overwhelming, progress has been made since the release of the two seminal reports (Field & Cassel, 1997; SUPPORT Principal Investigators, 1995) brought the unfavorable conditions of dying persons in the United States to the forefront of the national healthcare agenda.

INTERVENTIONS

The IOM report (Field & Cassel, 1997) made seven recommendations (see **Table 22-3**) to resolve the four identified areas of deficiency in palliative and end-of-life care. Change is occurring in part because of the increased involvement of 21st-century healthcare consumers in the issues related to quality of care, quality of life, advance care planning, and the burdens of caregiving (Berry, 2004).

Approximately 100 articles have been published based on the findings of the SUPPORT study (1995). Implications of the data for future reform suggest that improved individual, patient-level decision making may not be the most effective strategy for improving end-of-life care. The SUPPORT investigators recommended

---

Table 22-3   Recommendations from the IOM Committee on Care at the End of Life

1. People with advanced, potentially fatal illnesses and those close to them should be able to expect and receive reliable, skillful, and supportive care.
2. Physicians, nurses, social workers, and other health professionals must commit themselves to improving care for dying patients and to using existing knowledge effectively to prevent and relieve pain and other symptoms.
3. Because many deficiencies in care reflect system problems, policymakers, consumer groups, and purchasers of health care should work with healthcare providers and researchers to:
   a. Strengthen methods for measuring the quality of life and other outcomes of care for dying patients and those close to them
   b. Develop better tools and strategies for improving the quality of care and holding healthcare organizations accountable for care at the end of life
   c. Revise mechanisms for financing care so that they encourage rather than impede good end-of-life care and sustain rather than frustrate coordinated systems of excellent care
   d. Reform drug prescription laws, burdensome regulations, and state medical board policies and practices that impede effective use of opioids to relieve pain and suffering
4. Educators and other healthcare professionals should initiate changes in undergraduate, graduate, and continuing education to ensure that practitioners have the relevant attitudes, knowledge, and skills to care well for dying patients.
5. Palliative care should become, if not a medical specialty, at least a defined area of expertise, education, and research.
6. The nation's research establishment should define and implement priorities for strengthening the knowledge base for end-of-life care.
7. A continuing public discussion is essential to develop a better understanding of the modern experience of dying, the options available to dying patients and families, and the obligations of communities to those approaching death.

Source: Field, M. J., & Cassel, C. K. (Eds.). (1997). *Approaching death: Improving care at the end of life.* Committee on Care at the End of Life, Division of Health Care Services, Institute of Medicine (pp. 270–271). Washington, DC: National Academies Press.

system-level innovations and quality improvement in routine care as potentially effective strategies for change (Lynn et al., 2000; Lynn, Schuster, Wilkinson, & Simon, 2008).

Interventions for palliative care must relate to the domains of its science and practice. Researchers (Emanuel & Emanuel, 1998; Steinhauser et al., 2000; Teno, 2001) and professional organizations such as the NHPCO (2006) and the American Geriatrics Society (Lynn, 1997) have published standards of care as well as philosophical or conceptual frameworks describing proposed domains of end-of-life care (Ferrell, 2004).

Recognizing a need for clarity in the definitions of key concepts or domains of end-of-life care and a framework for advancing research and practice, the NCPQPC (2009) developed the following domains:

Domain 1: Structure and processes of care
Domain 2: Physical aspects of care
Domain 3: Psychological and psychiatric aspects of care
Domain 4: Social aspects of care
Domain 5: Spiritual, religious, and existential aspects of care
Domain 6: Cultural aspects of care
Domain 7: Care of the imminently dying patient
Domain 8: Ethical and legal aspects of care

As described earlier in this chapter, the second edition of the clinical guidelines was released in 2009 and will continue to be revised to reflect changes over time in the professional practice, education, evidence base, and healthcare system related to palliative care.

Determining Goals of Care

The domains identified by the NCPQPC guide decision making regarding research, practice, and policy. Each domain is an area for an intervention for improving end-of-life care and meeting the needs of palliative care patients and families. Palliative care interventions logically flow from goals of care. Therefore, the first step in palliative care is to establish the goals of care (Morrison & Meier, 2004). In the context of chronic, debilitating, and life-threatening illness, realistic and attainable goals of care that relieve pain and other symptoms, improve quality of life, limit the burden of care, enhance personal relationships, and provide a sense of control are crucial to the dying person and their families (Steinhauser et al., 2000).

Healthcare professionals must work with clients and their families to establish appropriate goals of care (Vollrath & von Gunten, 2007). Using open-ended and probing questions may be helpful when interviewing the client (Morrison & Meier, 2004). Examples of possible questions are: "What makes life worth living for you?" "Given the severity of your illness, what are the most important things for you to achieve?" "What are your most important hopes?" "What are your biggest fears?" and "What would you consider to be a fate worse than death?" (Quill, 2000).

Goals of care are dynamic across the trajectory of a disease (EPEC Project, 2004; Quill, 2000). Meier, Back, and Morrison (2001) describe some of the warning signs of ineffective or contradictory goals as: frequent or lengthy hospitalizations, physician feelings of frustration, anger or powerlessness, and feelings of caregiver burden.

Assessment and Treatment of Symptoms

A core principle of palliative care is comprehensive care that includes the relief of pain and other symptoms (Steinhauser et al., 2000). Effective symptom management begins with a thorough assessment. Research findings support the practice of routine and standardized symptom assessment with validated instruments (Morrison & Meier, 2004). Benefits attributed to routine assessments include identification of overlooked or unreported symptoms (Bookbinder et al., 1996; Manfredi et al., 2000). Dissemination and increased use of the same validated instruments will facilitate the comparison of findings across practice settings and research studies. The Center to Advance Palliative Care (CAPC) (www.capc.org) and Brown University's Center for Gerontology and Health Care Research provide access to clinically useful instruments through their respective websites. Brown's website features a tool kit of instruments to measure end-of-life care (www.chcr.brown.edu/pcoc/toolkit.htm).

The nursing assessment of clients who are receiving palliative care is the same as a standard nursing assessment. However, the palliative care assessment focuses on enhancing the client's quality of life. Ferrell's (1995) quality-of-life framework is useful in organizing the assessment according to four domains: physical, psychological, social, and spiritual well-being. Based on the changing needs of clients and families across the trajectory of the chronic illness, quality of life should be assessed four times: 1) at the time of diagnosis; 2) treatment, post-treatment; 3) long-term survival or terminal phase; and 4) active dying. A comprehensive assessment serves as the foundation for goal setting, developing a plan of care, implementing interventions, and evaluating the outcomes and effectiveness of care (Glass, Cluxton, & Rancour, 2001).

The prevalence and symptom burden for clients at the end of life is high. According to the NIH *National Institutes of Health State-of-the Conference Statement: Improving End-of-Life Care* (2004), assessment and management of symptoms have been studied most thoroughly in clients with cancer. Clients with other life-limiting illnesses, such as CHF, have their own challenges. Regardless of the diagnosis, there are symptoms common to advanced disease. These common symptoms include anorexia and cachexia, anxiety, constipation, depression, delirium, dyspnea, nausea, and pain (Morrison & Meier, 2004). It is beyond the scope of this chapter to describe in detail the assessment and management recommendations for these symptoms; however, there are numerous resources in the literature with specific protocols and interventions, including the AGS Panel on Persistent Pain in Older Persons (2002); Block (2000); Casarett and Inouye (2001); Luce and Luce (2001); and Strasser and Bruera (2002).

Palliative care is needed across the lifespan, and assessments and interventions should be tailored to the specific population served. Often the literature categorizes adults as a homogenous group needing palliative care. Experts in gerontology, however, are calling for recognition of the unique palliative care needs of older adults (Cassel, 2003). Amella (2003) described the common goal of helping clients experience the best quality of life as the touchstone for collaboration between geriatric and palliative care nurse specialists. Symptoms of illness and dying may appear differently, for longer periods, and in greater numbers in older adults (Amella, 2003). Pain, confusion, dyspnea, fatigue, satiety and anorexia, gastrointestinal distress, infection and fever, and fears and depression are symptoms that can present differently in older adults.

At the other end of the lifespan, initiatives are underway that address palliative care in children. In 2003, the IOM released its report, *When*

Table 22-4   Four Basic Challenges to Improve Pediatric Palliative Care
1. Children should have care that is focused on their special needs and the needs of their families.
2. Health plans should make it easier for children and families to get palliative care.
3. Healthcare professionals should be trained to give palliative care to children.
4. Researchers should find out more about what care works best for children.
Source: Field, M. J., & Behrman, R. E. (Eds.). (2003). *When children die: Improving palliative and end-of-life care for children and their families.* Washington, DC: National Academies Press.

Children Die: Improving Palliative and End-of-Life Care for Children and Their Families (Field & Behrman, 2003). The report identified challenges that can be used to focus efforts and resources to improve palliative care for children and their families (see **Table 22-4**). Many palliative care textbooks are now including chapters addressing pediatric palliative care (Ferrell & Coyle, 2006, 2010).

Advance Directives

Following the establishment of the goals of care, the next logical intervention is the completion of advance directives. Goals of care reflect the values, beliefs, and culture of the person with a serious, life-threatening illness. Numerous studies (Miles, Koepp, & Weber, 1996) report that most people do not have advance directives and that the documents that do exist are ineffective in improving communication between clients and their physicians (Morrison & Meier, 2004). Other authors report that advance directives are ineffective related to the decision making relative to cardiopulmonary resuscitation (Teno et al., 1997). Morrison and Meier (2004) suggest that as the number of advance directives increase, more consumers and healthcare professionals will become familiar with the documents, thus improving their effectiveness.

However, current literature suggests that the focus of advance-care planning should shift to determine an acceptable quality of life and goals of care (Fried, Bradley, Towle, & Allore, 2002; Meier & Morrison, 2002). This type of discussion is the crucial element, not the mere completion of the forms. Consumers and healthcare professionals can use a variety of resources such as the *Caring Conversations Program* developed through the Center for Practical Bioethics (2011). Workbooks can be purchased that help families discuss their values and wishes regarding medical treatment if they cannot speak for themselves. It is also important to be aware of each state's required documents and process for the completion of advance directives. The process and forms vary from state to state. The names of the documents may also vary. The basic two forms are: 1) power of attorney for health care (this document appoints an agent or proxy who becomes the decision maker when the client can no longer do so) and 2) directive to physician (living will; this document gives direction to a physician regarding what type of care/procedures are wanted or not wanted—for example, artificial nutrition, hydration, or mechanical ventilation—if the individual cannot speak for him- or herself).

Psychosocial, Spiritual, and Bereavement Needs

Psychosocial, spiritual, and bereavement care are key components of palliative care. Professional and accrediting bodies such as The

Joint Commission require documentation of spiritual assessments of patients. Members of interdisciplinary palliative care teams assess and intervene to meet the spiritual and psychosocial needs of clients and their families. Bereavement support is part of the follow up after an individual dies. Research demonstrates that family members with spiritual and psychological distress are more likely to experience an extended or complicated grief and bereavement process (McClain, Rosenfield, & Breitbart, 2003).

The act of acknowledging spiritual distress can be an intervention. However, a common language and mutual comfort must be present for a meaningful exchange to occur (Chochinov, 2004). Helping clients die with dignity is a basic tenet of palliative care. Empirical work with dying clients found that the paradigm of dignity, which includes matters of spirituality, meaning, purpose, and other psychosocial issues related to dying, included acceptable language and topics for discussion (Chochinov et al., 2004). This work is adding to the growing empirical evidence that palliative care is more than symptom management and must include the spiritual, psychosocial, and existential concerns. It must be person centered and maintain a person's dignity through his or her last breath of life.

Chochinov and associates developed a dignity-conserving model and interventions based on the analysis of 50 qualitative interviews of patients with advanced cancer. The interviews were conducted in order to understand the patients' perceptions of dignity. The dignity-conserving model of care consists of three areas of influence on a person's perception of dignity: 1) influences stemming directly from the illness, 2) influences from the person's psychological and spiritual resources or self (dignity-conserving repertoire), and 3) environmental influences (social dignity inventory) (Chochinov, 2011, p. 354). The model serves as the basis for the psychotherapeutic intervention, *dignity therapy*. In dignity therapy, dying patients are interviewed about aspects of their life that they would like recorded and remembered. The interviews are transcribed and edited to read "like well-honed narratives." The narratives are returned to the patient and ultimately given to the patient's loved ones. Chochinov reported that 76% of the 100 patients in a clinical trial of the dignity therapy intervention reported a sense of heightened dignity, and 91% were satisfied with the intervention (Chochinov et al., 2005). Ninety-five percent of the family members of the dignity therapy participants reported that they would recommend dignity therapy for other patients and families faced with a terminal illness; 77% would continue to use the recorded narratives as a source of remembrance and comfort (McClement et al., 2007). These researchers acknowledge that dignity-conserving care must be validated in diverse populations. However, they urge that the concept of "conserving dignity in end-of-life care should become part of the palliative care lexicon and the overarching standard of care for all patients nearing death" (Chochinov, 2011, p. 359).

Culture and Palliative Care

Culture is a defining component of the human experience. Each individual's culture provides the sense of security, belonging, and guidelines regarding how to live and die (ELNEC, 2009b). Cultural diversity refers to differences between people based on shared teachings, beliefs, customs, language, and so forth, which influence an individual's and family's response to illness, treatment, death, and bereavement (Showalter, 1998). Despite the enormous differences among individuals, an understanding of common cultural characteristics is helpful in providing culturally sensitive and effective care (Kemp, 1999). It is beyond the scope of this chapter to describe all the cultural perspectives of individual populations regarding dying, death, and bereavement. However, it is important to be aware of the principles of culturally sensitive care to provide quality palliative care for clients and their families. **Table 22-5** outlines 10 principles of

Table 22-5 **Principles of Culturally Sensitive Care**
Healthcare providers should:
1. Be knowledgeable about cultural values and attitudes
2. Attend to diverse communication styles
3. Ask the patient for his/her preferences for decision making early in the care process
4. Recognize cultural differences and varying comfort levels with regard to personal space, eye contact, touch, time orientation, learning styles, and conversation styles
5. Use a cultural guide from the palliative care patient's ethnic or religious background
6. Get to know the community, its people, and its resources available for social support
7. Create a culturally friendly physical environment (e.g., decorate facilities with artwork or pictures valued by the cultural groups to whom care is most commonly provided)
8. Determine the acceptability of patients being physically examined by a practitioner of a different gender
9. Advocate for availability of services, accessibility in terms of cost and location, and acceptability of services that are compatible with cultural values and practices of the person served
10. Conduct a self-assessment of the healthcare provider's own beliefs about illness and death

Source: Adapted from Council on Social Work Education (CSWE) Faculty Development Institute, 2001 as cited in Sherman, D. W. (2004). Cultural and spiritual backgrounds of older adults. In M. L. Matzo & D. W. Sherman (Eds.), *Gerontologic palliative care nursing* (p. 11). St. Louis: Mosby.

culturally sensitive care originally developed by the Council on Social Work Education (CSWE) Faculty Development Institute in 2001, as cited in Sherman (2004).

An example of the cultural beliefs of Hispanic Americans (Latinos) that may impact palliative care for this population follows. Hispanics from Mexico, Puerto Rico, and Central and South America all have distinct cultures. However, many non-Hispanics use the frequently shared language (Spanish) or religion (Catholicism) to group these clients together.

Sullivan (2001) identified Latino views regarding end-of-life care using focus groups as the method of data collection. The focus groups were conducted in Latino communities. The Latino participants believed that they could not communicate effectively with healthcare providers because of language barriers, and they did not understand the concept of informed consent even with the use of interpreters. Latinos believe it is the responsibility of the family to care for their relatives and not send them away to nursing homes. Consequently, these participants did not want to die in nursing homes. Most of the participants were unaware of hospice services or had inaccurate information. Religious beliefs, primarily reliance on God, and fatalism were critical components of their decision making regarding end-of-life care. Racial discrimination and cultural insensitivity were perceived by many of the participants.

Several beliefs in the Hispanic culture can influence the experience of palliative care for individuals. Many Hispanic families will assume the responsibility of caring for their dying member at home based on their belief in strong family support, including extended family members. The dying member is protected from the prognosis. A major challenge to thorough pain assessment in palliative care is the reluctance of Hispanics to acknowledge, report, or describe pain. Stoicism is highly regarded. However, moaning is acceptable but cannot serve as a valid indicator of the severity of pain (Kemp, 1999). Although death is an adversity, funerals are an integral part of family life, lasting several days. They hold a belief in the afterlife. The Day of the Dead is celebrated in November on the same day that All Souls Day is celebrated in the Catholic religion. Day of the Dead is a day of celebration with special foods and decorating of the graves.

Education for Healthcare Professionals

The AACN and City of Hope National Medical Center received major funding from the Robert Wood Johnson Foundation for the development and dissemination of the ELNEC Curriculum (2011). Versions for baccalaureate, graduate, continuing education/in-service, pediatric, oncology, and geriatric nurses and nurse educators have been developed with Train-the-Trainer methodology utilized. A quarterly newsletter "ELNEC Connections" is sent to all ELNEC trainers. The newsletter provides updates, ongoing resources, and project ideas from the ELNEC staff as well as trainers throughout the country. Collegial sharing is in the spirit of improving and disseminating the science and art of palliative care nursing. One of the outcomes of the project was the award-winning series of palliative care articles that ran every other month in the *American Journal of Nursing* from August 2004 through December 2006, which included 17 articles. ELNEC celebrated its 10th anniversary with its 78th national ELNEC Summit in January 2011.

Physicians have a parallel program to ELNEC: The EPEC Project, Education on Palliative and End-of-Life Care. However, the mission of EPEC is to educate *all* healthcare professionals on the essential clinical competencies in palliative care. Conferences using the Train-the-Trainer methodology are also used. In addition, the entire curriculum is available online (see www.epec.net). Another useful resource for healthcare professionals is the End of Life/Palliative Education Resource Center (www.eperc.mcw.edu). Its purpose is advancing end-of-life care through an online community of educational scholars. Case studies, presentations, and articles are a few of the resources available. At this website there is access to a palliative care blog: *Pallimed: A Hospice and Palliative Medicine Blog* (www.pallimed.org). The site has a main page for discussion and posts, an arts page (i.e., book reviews related to hospice and palliative medicine topics) and a page of case studies for discussion.

Research

The continued evolution of palliative care to meet the needs of an aging population rests in part on research. These needs include interventions to manage the symptoms and distress of chronic illness. However, the knowledge base to support symptom management, communication, and decision-making skills and models for the delivery of palliative care are inadequate. The National Palliative Care Research Center (NPCRC; see www.npcrc.org) was developed in direct response to this need, consistent recommendations from multiple IOM reports, and the National Institutes of Health State-of-the Conference Statement: Improving End-of-Life Care (2004)—which called for the development of a prioritized research agenda, researchers committed to palliative care research, and a developing new generation of palliative care researchers. NPCRC's initial funding of research grant proposals occurred in 2007. The NPCRC is located in New York City and receives direction and technical assistance from the Mount Sinai School of Medicine. It also works closely with the CAPC (www.capc.org).

The NHPCO developed a Research Agenda in 2004 to guide researchers in developing the scientific knowledge to support hospice and palliative care. The broad topics include improving access to hospice and palliative care, improving the quality of hospice and palliative care, and improving the conduct of research in hospice and palliative care. According to the NHPCO strategic plan for 2010–2012, one of its objectives is to update the 2004 agenda by defining and disseminating a comprehensive research agenda for end-of-life care that will guide future doctoral dissertations, academic, and other formal types of research (NHPCO, 2010).

Goldstein and Morrison (2005) called for a new research agenda for geriatric palliative care. Their premise, based on the NIH (2004) and IOM (Field & Cassel, 1997; Cleeland, 2001) reports, was that the evidence base for palliative care in older adults is sparse. Adults 75 years or older with comorbidities and noncancer diagnoses have repeatedly been excluded from palliative care research. Their proposed research agenda for palliative care in geriatrics includes the following: 1) establishing the prevalence of symptoms in patients with chronic disease, 2) evaluating the association between symptom treatment and outcomes, 3) increasing the evidence base for symptom treatment, 4) understanding patients' psychological/spiritual well-being and quality of life, 5) elucidating sources of caregiver burden; 6) reevaluating service delivery, 7) adapting research methodologies specifically for palliative care, and 8) increasing the number of geriatricians trained in palliative care research (Goldstein & Morrison, 2005, p. 1594).

As we build the science supporting the practice of palliative care, the question becomes whether the research, education, and clinical interventions already funded to improve care for individuals with life-limiting or terminal illnesses were effective. Measuring the effectiveness of palliative care is a challenge that requires both prospective and retrospective studies (Steinhauser, 2004). Four challenges exist related to outcome measurement in palliative care:

- End of life is a complex multidimensional experience in which understanding of the interrelatedness of domains is unclear.
- The period "end of life" is ill-defined.
- Both patient and family are the unit of care, yet little is known about the correlations between the trajectories of their experiences.
- Patients, the primary focus of care, are often unable to communicate in their last days or weeks, rendering their subjective experience unable to be evaluated. (Steinhauser, 2004, p. 33)

Palliative Care and Genomics

The sequence of the human genome was completed in April 2003. Advances in technology now allow the exploration of genetic material ranging from genetic screening to genomic-based therapies (Conley & Tinkle, 2007). The genetic risk for many diseases, such as Huntington's disease, can be determined, but there is no cure yet available (Heitkemper & Bond, 2003). How does this apply to hospice and palliative care? This discussion focuses on three connections between palliative care and genomics: pharmacogenomics, family history, and nurse competencies in genetics and genomics. See **Table 22-6** for definitions of terms used in this section.

Pharmacogenetics (role of inheritance in the individual variation in drug response) has converged with knowledge from the sequencing of the human genome resulting in pharmacogenomics (effect of DNA sequencing on the effect of a drug; science combining pharmacology and genomics) (Weinshilboum, 2003). Medications are a major intervention for symptom management in palliative care. It is important that physicians and nurses,

including those in palliative, care understand the impact of genotypic variation on the therapeutic effect and adverse effects of medications. The cytochrome P450 system is an example. A specific cytochrome enzyme, CYP2D6, converts codeine to morphine. Genotypic variants of the CYP2D6 enzyme in 5–10% of the population results in too little or no CYP2D6 enzyme produced. Therefore, these individuals cannot change codeine into morphine and have little or no analgesic relief with codeine or codeine-derivative medications (e.g., hydrocodone, oxycodone, ethylmorphine, and dihydrocodeine) (Howe & Eggert, 2007; Meyer, 2000; Prows, 2004).

Scientists discovered genetic variations in the gene that plays a major role in an individual's initial sensitivity to warfarin treatment (Schwarz et al., 2008). Members of the NIH Pharmacogenetics Research Network found that these variations explain why some patients require a higher or lower dose to reach the therapeutic benefit of the drug. The U.S. Food and Drug Administration (FDA) now recommends genetic testing to assist in the quick and precise determination of optimal warfarin doses. These are just two examples that illustrate the impact of pharmacogenomics in providing safe and effective care regardless of the trajectory of illness.

In palliative care, the client and the family are the unit of care. However, what is the impact of a family's health history? Is the client who is receiving palliative care worried about an illness that may be transmitted to other family members? Are family members concerned that they may be carriers of an incurable disease? The U.S. Surgeon General spearheaded the Family History Initiative. Family history is the best inexpensive, noninvasive genetic test available (http://familyhistory.hhs.gov). Many diseases "run in families." Detailed family histories allow

---

Table 22-6   Definition of Terms Related to Genetics and Genomics

Allele—An alternative form of a gene

Genetics—The study of individual genes and their impact on relatively rare single gene disorders (Guttmacher & Collins, 2002)

Genomics—The study of the functions and interactions of all the genes in the genome, including their interactions with environmental factors (Guttmacher & Collins, 2002)

Genotype—A person's genetic makeup as reflected by his or her DNA sequence

Pharmacogenetics—The study of genetic factors that influence an organism's reaction to a drug (Howe & Eggert, 2007)

Pharmacogenomics—The study of how an individual's genetic inheritance affects the body's response to drugs (Howe & Eggert, 2007)

Phenotype—The clinical presentation or expression of a specific gene or genes, environmental factors, or both (Guttmacher & Collins, 2002)

individuals at risk to be identified and to implement disease-prevention strategies. Patterns of inheritance may be sources of guilt in persons with advanced disease or concerns of bereaved individuals. The current palliative literature does not yet discuss these types of concerns.

What is the role of palliative care for individuals diagnosed with genetic diseases? How can palliative care providers help those diagnosed with the genotype for a terminal disease that is not yet expressed? Huntington's disease is such an example. These individuals would benefit from the support of palliative care. The HPNA along with 48 other professional nursing organizations have endorsed the Genetic and Genomic Nursing Competencies (http://www .genome.gov/pages/careers/healthprofessionale-ducation/geneticscompetency.pdf). Regardless of specialty and setting, all nurses need to understand that all diseases have a genetic and genomic component. Patients and their families may turn to the nurse seeking genetic and genomic information involved in the prevention, screening, diagnostics, prognostics, and selection of and effectiveness of treatment. Within the context of hospice and palliative care, requests for this information may occur during bereavement and thus add another layer of complexity to the grief process. The following are two examples of the competencies relevant to the preceding discussion:

1. *Domain: Professional Responsibility.* Incorporate genetic and genomic technologies and information into RN practice
2. *Domain: Professional Practice.* Demonstrates an understanding of genetics/genomics to health, prevention, selection of treatment, monitoring of treatment effectiveness. (Consensus Panel, 2006)

It may seem strange to some readers to find a section of this chapter on genomics and palliative care, but palliative care is not practiced in a vacuum. Nurses must be aware of the advances in science that impact the health of clients and their families prior to interacting with them. The advances in the science of comfort and the art of caring must converge to improve the quality of life for those with life-limiting or terminal illness.

OUTCOMES

Outcomes research in palliative care continues to develop. There is consensus about the broad domains related to end of life: physical or psychosocial symptoms, social relationships, spiritual or philosophical beliefs, hopes, expectation and meaning, satisfaction, economic considerations, and caregiver and family experiences. Quality of life is also considered an outcome, but quality of life needs a clearer definition and consistent measurement in order to strengthen the relationship.

The CAPC has identified major outcomes of palliative care (www.capc.org), including: 1) relief of pain and other distressing symptoms; 2) clear communication and decision making regarding goals of care and development of treatment plans; 3) completion of life-prolonging or curative treatments; and 4) increased patient and family satisfaction. The next steps in palliative care are to develop the science, the care delivery systems, and the instruments to deliver and evaluate the outcomes of quality palliative care.

Morrison (2005) eloquently described the progress of the palliative care movement in the United States as well as the next steps that need to be taken to continue to meet the needs of an aging population:

> As we look at the growth and development of the field of palliative care in the United States, we have moved from recognition of a public health crisis (poor quality of life for clients with serious illness and their families), to identifying the system and care gaps that result in this compromised quality of life (inadequate assessment and treatment of pain and other symptoms, disjointed and unclear goals of care, poor transition management), to developing interventions (palliative care education at all levels of professional training, creation of hospital-based palliative care teams) to address these care and system gaps. What is now needed is comprehensive and rigorous research to evaluate the effect of well-delineated and generalizable palliative care structures and process on important clinical and utilization outcomes to guide the further development of the field. (p. 14)

Evidence-Based Practice Box

Metastatic non-small cell lung cancer is a debilitating disease with a high symptom burden, poor quality of life, and a prognosis of death within a year of diagnosis. The purpose of this study was to examine the effect of early palliative care given simultaneously with standard oncologic care on patient-reported outcomes among patients with metastatic non-small cell lung cancer in an ambulatory care setting. A randomly assigned sample of 151 patients (power of 80% and effect size of 0.5 SD required 120

patients; to account for loss of any participants, an additional 30 were enrolled in the study). Patient-reported measures included health-related quality of life as measured by the Functional Assessment of Cancer Therapy-Lung (FACT-L) Scale. This scale assesses multiple dimensions of quality of life including physical, functional, emotional, and social well-being. Mood was measured with the Hospital Anxiety and Depression Scale (HADS) and the Patient Health Questionnaire 9 (PHQ-9). The patients' use of health services and end-of-life care were collected from the electronic medical record.

The patients receiving early palliative care met with a member of the palliative care team within 3 weeks of enrollment in the study and at least monthly in the outpatient setting until death. Guidelines for the palliative care visits were adopted from the NCPQPC and were part of the study protocol. Standard care patients did not meet with members of the palliative care team unless specifically requested by the patient, family, or oncologist. All participants in the study continued to receive routine oncologic care.

These two groups were well matched, and there were no significant differences in their demographic characteristics. Participants receiving early palliative care had an average of four visits within the first 12 weeks of the study. Comparing the quality of life scores at 12 weeks found that the patients assigned to early palliative care had significantly higher scores than the standard care group. Depression scores in the palliative care group were also significantly lower at 12 weeks. Patients assigned to the standard care only group received more aggressive end-of-life care and had less documentation regarding their resuscitation preferences in their electronic medical records.

This study clearly demonstrated the effect of palliative care when provided from the time of diagnosis through death for advanced lung cancer: prolonged survival by 2 months and improved quality of life and mood. The authors of the study hypothesized that improvements in quality of life and mood may account for the increased survival, a benefit of early palliative care.

Source: Temel, J. S., Greer, J. A., Muzikansky, A., Gallaher, E. R., Admane, S., Jackson, V. A., et al. (2010). Early palliative care for patients with metastatic non-small cell lung cancer. *New England Journal of Medicine, 363,* 733–742.

STUDY QUESTIONS

www

Discuss the differences in the definitions of palliative care listed in Table 22-1.

Describe how the goals of care might differ for an 85-year-old man diagnosed

Study Questions (Cont.)

www

with heart failure (HF) at the time of diagnosis and goals of care in an advanced stage of the illness.

Explain the following statement: Hospice care is palliative care but not all palliative care is hospice care.

List the domains of end-of-life care developed by the NCPQPC.

Identify barriers to palliative care for an individual with a serious, life-limiting illness.

Identify the components of Ferrell's framework/model for quality of life.

What is your vision of palliative care?

Discuss how stoicism may impact palliative care for a Latino grandmother?

List three online resources to use to continue your education in palliative care.

Go online and find support information appropriate for the family caregiver of a palliative care patient.

Describe how you could you use Nolan and Mock's (2004) *Integrity of the Person: A Conceptual Framework for End-of-Life Care* as an organizing framework in your clinical practice.

Identify two nurse competencies in genetics and genomics.

Discuss how pharmacogenomics can help relieve the pain for future patients receiving hospice care.

How would palliative care assist a man diagnosed with Huntington's disease?

Discuss your vision for integrating genomics into palliative care.

INTERNET RESOURCES

WWW

American Association of Colleges of Nursing,
   End-of-Life Care: www.aacn.nche.edu/elnec
American Pain Society: www.ampainsoc.org
Edmonton Regional Palliative Care Program:
   www.palliative.org
Education in Palliative and End-of-Life Care:
   www.epec.net
Hospice and Palliative Nurses Association: www.
   hpna.org
HPNA Research Agenda: www.hpna.org/PicView.
   aspx?ID=828
National Consensus Project: www.nationalconsen-
   susproject.org
National Consensus Project for Quality Palliative
   Care: www.nationalconsensusproject.org
National Guideline Clearing House: www.guide-
   line.gov
National Hospice and Palliative Care Organization:
   www.nhpco.org
National Palliative Care Research Center: www.
   npcrc.org
Oncology Nursing Society: www.ons.org
Pain Resource Center: prc.coh.org
Palliative Care: www.getpalliativecare.org
Palliative Care Framework: www.nhpco.org/i4a/
   pages/index.cfm?pageID=5122
Toolkit of Instruments to Measure End of Life
   Care (TIME): www.chcr.brown.edu/pcoc/
   toolkit.htm

For a full suite of assignments
and additional learning activities,   WWW
use the access code located in
the front of your book and visit this exclusive
website: **http://go.jblearning.com/larsen**. If
you do not have an access code, you can
obtain one at the site.

REFERENCES

AGS Panel on Persistent Pain in Older Persons. (2002).
   The management of persistent pain in older persons.
   *Journal of the American Geriatrics Society,
   50*(Suppl.), S205–S224.

Alliance for Excellence in Hospice and Palliative
   Nursing. (2011). *Mission statement.* Retrieved
   September 16, 2011, from: http://www.hpna.org/
   DisplayPage.aspx?Title=Mission%20of%20HPNA
Amella, E. J. (2003). Geriatrics and palliative care:
   Collaboration for quality of life until death. *Journal
   of Hospice and Palliative Nursing, 5*(1), 40–48.
American Academy of Hospice and Palliative Medicine.
   (2011). *About AAHPM.* Retrieved September 16,
   2011, from http://www.aahpm.org/about/default/
   index.html
American Association of Colleges of Nursing. (2004).
   *Peaceful death: Recommended competencies and
   curricular guidelines for end-of-life nursing care.*
   Retrieved September 16, 2011, from: http://www.
   aacn.nche.edu/publications/deathfin.htm
American Board of Medical Specialties. (2006). *News
   Release: ABMS Establishes New Subspecialty
   Certificate in Hospice and Palliative Care.* Retrieved
   September 16, 2011, from: http://www.abms.org/News_
   and_Events/downloads/NewSubcertPalliativeMed.pdf
Berry, P. H. (2004). Promoting quality of life during the
   dying process. In M. L. Matzo & D. W. Sherman
   (Eds.), *Gerontologic palliative care nursing* (pp. 1–2).
   St. Louis: Mosby.
Block, S. D. (2000). Assessing and managing depression
   in the terminally ill patient. *Annals of Internal
   Medicine, 132*(3), 209–218.
Bookbinder, M., Coyle, N., Kiss, M., Goldstein, M. L.,
   Holritz, K., Thaler, H., et al. (1996). Implementing
   national standards for cancer pain management:
   Program model and evaluation. *Journal of Pain and
   Symptom Management, 12,* 334–347.
Campbell, M. L., Happ, M. B., Hultman, T., Kirchoff, K. T.,
   Mahon, M. M., McMillan, S., & Raudonis, B. (2009).
   The HPNA Research Agenda for 2009-2012. *Journal
   of Hospice and Palliative Nursing, 11*(1), 10–18.
Casarett, D. J., & Inouye. S. K. (2001). Diagnosis and
   management of delirium near the end of life. *Annals
   of Internal Medicine, 135,* 32–40.
Cassel, C. K. (2003). Foreword. In R. S. Morrison &
   D. E. Meier (Eds.), *Geriatric palliative medicine*
   (pp. vii–ix). Oxford, UK: Oxford University Press.
Center for Practical Bioethics. (2011). *Caring conversations.* Retrieved September 16, 2011, from: http://
   practicalbioethics.org/about/model-and-methodol-
   ogy/making-your-wishes-known-for-end-of-life-care/
Center to Advance Palliative Care (CAPC). (2011).
   Improving clinical outcomes. Retrieved September

26, 2011, from www.eapc.org/building-a-hospital-based-palliative-care-program/case/outcomes

Center to Advance Palliative Care. Resources for patients and families. Retrieved February 1, 2008, from: http://getpalliativecare.org;

Centers for Disease Control and Prevention, National Center for Health Statistics. (2010). *National vital statistics report, 58*(19).

Chochinov, H. M. (2004). Interventions to enhance the spiritual aspects of dying. *National Institutes of Health state-of-the science conference on improving end-of-life care program & abstracts.* Bethesda, MD: U.S. Department of Health and Human Services, National Institutes of Health.

Chochinov, H. M., Hack, T., Hassard, T., Kristjanson, L. J., McClement, S., & Harlos, M. (2004). Dignity and psychotherapeutic considerations in end-of-life care. *Journal of Palliative Care, 20*(3), 134–142.

Chochinov, H. M. (2011). Dignity-conserving care—a new model for palliative care: Helping the patient feel valued. In S. J. McPhee, M. A. Winker, M. W. Rabow, S. Z. Pantilat, & A. J. Markowitz (Eds.), *Care at the close of life: Evidence and experience* (pp. 353–362). New York: McGraw.

Chochinov, H. M., Hack, T., Hassard, T. Kristjanson, L. J., McClement, S., Harlos, M. (2005). Dignity therapy: A novel psychotherapeutic intervention for patients near the end of life. *Journal of Clinical Oncology, 23*(24), 5520–5525.

Christakis, N., & Lamont, E. B. (2000). Extend and determinants of error in doctors' prognoses in terminally ill patients: Prospective cohort study. *British Medical Journal, 320*, 469–473.

Cicely Saunders International. (2010). Cicely Saunders Institute. Retrieved December 18, 2010, from: http://www.cicelysaundersfoundation.org

Cleeland, C. S. (2001). Cross-cutting research issues. A research agenda for reducing distress of patients with cancer. In K. Foley & H. Gelband (Eds.), *Improving Palliative Care for Cancer* (pp. 233–274). Washington, DC: National Institute of Medicine.

Conley, Y. P., & Tinkle, M. B. (2007). The future of genomic nursing research. *Journal of Nursing Scholarship, 39*(2), 17–24.

Consensus Panel. (2006). *Essential nursing competencies and curricula guidelines for genetics and genomics.* Washington, DC: American Nurses Association.

Corbin, J. (2001). Introduction and overview: Chronic illness and nursing. In R. Hyman & J. Corbin (Eds.), *Chronic illness: Research and theory for nursing practice* (pp. 1–15). New York: Springer.

Coyle, N. (2010). Introduction to palliative nursing care. In B. R. Ferrell & N. Coyle (Eds.), *Textbook of palliative nursing* (3rd ed., pp. 3–11). Oxford, UK: Oxford University Press.

Cumming, K. T., & Okun, S. N. (2004). Community-based palliative care for older adults. In M. L. Matzo, & D. W. Sherman (Eds.), *Gerontologic palliative care nursing* (pp. 52–65). St. Louis: Mosby.

Curtin, M., & Lubkin, I. (1995). What is chronicity? In I. Lubkin (Ed.), *Chronic illness: Impact and interventions* (3rd ed., pp. 3–25). Sudbury, MA: Jones and Bartlett.

Derek, D., Hanks, G., Cherny, N., & Calman, K. (2004). Introduction. In D. Doyle, G. Hanks, N. Cherny, & K. Calman (Eds.), *Oxford textbook of palliative medicine* (3rd ed., pp. 1–4). Oxford, UK: Oxford University Press.

Dowsett, S. M., Saul, J. L., Buttow, P. N., Dunn, S. M., Boyer, M. J., Findlow, R., & Dunsmore, J. (2000). Communication styles in the cancer consultation: Preferences for a patient-centered approach. *Psychooncology, 9*, 147–156.

Emanuel, E. J., & Emanuel, L. L. (1998). The promise of a good death. *Lancet, 351*(Suppl. 2), SII21–SII29.

End of Life Nursing Education Consortium. (2009a). *Module 1: Nursing at the end of life.* American Association of Colleges of Nursing and City of Hope National Medical Center. Washington, DC: Author.

End of Life Nursing Education Consortium. (2009b). *Module 5: Cultural considerations in EOL care.* American Association of Colleges of Nursing and City of Hope National Medical Center. Washington, DC: Author.

End of Life Nursing Education Consortium. (2011). Retrieved September 26, 2011, from www.aacn.nche.edu/elnec/factsheet.htm

EPEC Project. (2004). Education on palliative and end-of-life care. Retrieved September 16, 2011, from: www.epec.net

Ferrell, B. R. (1995). The impact of pain on quality of life: A decade of research. *Nursing Clinics of North America, 30*, 609–624.

Ferrell, B. R. (2004). Overview of the domains of variables relevant to end-of-life care. *National Institutes of Health state-of–the science conference on improving end-of-life care program & abstracts.* Bethesda, MD: U.S. Department of Health and Human Services, National Institutes of Health.

Ferrell, B. R., & Coyle, N. (Eds.). (2001). *Textbook of palliative nursing.* New York: Oxford University Press.

Ferrell, B. R., & Coyle, N. (Eds.). (2006). *Textbook of palliative nursing* (2nd ed.). New York: Oxford University Press.

Ferrell, B. R., & Coyle, N. (Eds.). (2010). *Oxford textbook of palliative nursing* (3rd ed.). New York: Oxford University Press.

Ferrell, B., Virani, R., & Grant, M. (1999). Analysis of end-of-life content in nursing textbooks. *Oncology Nursing Forum, 26*(5), 869–876.

Field, M. J., & Behrman, R. E. (Eds.). (2003). *When children die: Improving palliative and end-of-life care for children and their families.* Washington, DC: National Academies Press.

Field, M. J., & Cassel, C. K. (Eds.). (1997). *Approaching death: Improving care at the end of life.* Committee on Care at the End of Life, Division of Health Care Services, Institute of Medicine. Washington, DC: National Academies Press.

Fisher, E. S., Wennberg, D. E., Stukel, T. A., Gottlieb, D. J., Lucas, F. L., & Pinder, E. L. (2003). The implications of regional variations in Medicare spending: Health outcomes and satisfaction with care. *Annals of Internal Medicine, 138*, 288–298.

Foley, K. (2001). Preface. In K. M. Foley & H. Gelband (Eds.), *Improving palliative care for cancer* (pp. xi–xii). Washington, DC: National Academies Press.

Fried, T. R., Bradley, E. H., Towle, V. R., & Allore, H. (2002). Understanding the treatment preferences of seriously ill patients. *New England Journal of Medicine, 346*, 1061–1066.

Gelfman, L. A., & Morrison, R. S. (2008). Research funding for palliative medicine. *Journal of Palliative Medicine, 11,* 36–43.

Glass, E., Cluxton, D., & Rancour, P. (2001). Principles of patient and family assessment. In B. R. Ferrell & N. Coyle (Eds.), *Textbook of palliative nursing.* New York: Oxford University Press.

Goldstein, N. E., & Morrison, R. S. (2005). The intersection between geriatrics and palliative care: A call for a new research agenda. *Journal of the American Geriatrics Society, 53,* 1593–1598.

Guttmacher, A., & Collins, F. (2002). Genomic medicine: A primer. *New England Journal of Medicine, 347,* 1512–1520.

Hansford, P. (2010). Palliative care in the United Kingdom. In B. R. Ferrell & N. Coyle (Eds.), *Oxford textbook of palliative nursing* (3rd ed., pp. 1265–1274). Oxford, UK: Oxford University Press.

Hearn, J., & Myers, K. (2001). *Palliative day care in practice.* New York: Oxford University Press.

Heitkemper, M. M., & Bond, E. F. (2003). State of nursing science: On the edge. *Biological Research for Nursing, 4*(3), 151–162; Discussion 163–164, 170.

Higginson, I. J. (2011). Forward. In S. J. McPhee, M. A. Winker, M. W. Rabow, S. Z. Pantilat, & A. J. Markowitz (Eds.), *Care at the close of life: Evidence and experience.* New York: McGraw Hill.

Hospice and Palliative Nurses Association & American Nurses Association. (2007). *Scope and standards of hospice and palliative nursing practice.* Washington, DC: Author.

Hospice and Palliative Nurses Association. (2011). Leading the way. Retrieved September 26, 2011 from http://www.hpna.org/Displaypage.aspx?Title=LeadingtheWay

Howe, L. A., & Eggert, J. (2007). Influence of pharmacogenomics on disease and symptom management. Retrieved September 16, 2011, from: journal.hsmc.org/ijnidd

Kemp, C. (1999). *Terminal illness: A guide to nursing care* (2nd ed.). Philadelphia: Lippincott.

Kubler-Ross, E. (1969). *On death and dying.* New York: Macmillan.

Lomax, K. K., & Scanlon, C. (1997). *Precepts of palliative care* (Last Acts Task Force on Palliative Care). Princeton, NJ: The Robert Wood Johnson Foundation/ Last Acts.

Luce, J. M., & Luce, J. A. (2001). Perspective on care at the close of life: Management of dyspnea in patients with far-advanced lung disease: "Once I lose it, it's kind of hard to catch it…" *JAMA, 285*, 1331–1337.

Lunney, J. R., Foley, K. M., Smith, T. J., & Gelband, H. (2003). *Describing death in America: What we need to know.* Washington, DC: National Academies Press.

Lynn, J. (1997). Measuring quality of care at the end of life: A statement of principles. *Journal of the American Geriatrics Society, 45*, 526–527.

Lynn, J. (2001). Serving patients who may die soon and their families: The role of hospice and other services. *JAMA, 285*, 925–932.

Lynn, J., Arkes, H. R., Stevens, M., Cohn, F., Koenig, B., Fox, E., et al. (2000). Rethinking fundamental assumptions: SUPPORT's implications for future reform. *Journal of the American Geriatrics Society, 48*(5), S214–S221.

Lynn, J., Schuster, J. L., Wilkinson, A., & Simon, L. N. (2008). *Improving care for the end of life: A sourcebook for health care managers and clinicians* (2nd ed.). Oxford, UK: Oxford University Press.

Manfredi, P. L., Morrison, R. S., Morris, J., Goldhirsch, S. L., Carter, J. M., & Meier, D. E. (2000). Palliative care consultations: How do they impact the care of hospitalized patients? *Journal of Pain and Symptom Management, 20,* 166–173.

Matzo, M. L., & Sherman, D. W. (Eds.). (2001). *Palliative care nursing: Quality care at the end of life.* New York: Springer.

Matzo, M. L., & Sherman, D. W. (Eds.). (2004). *Gerontologic palliative care nursing.* St. Louis: Mosby.

Matzo, M. L., & Sherman, D. W. (2006). *Palliative care nursing: Quality care at the end of life* (2nd ed.). New York: Springer.

Matzo, M. L., & Sherman, D. W. (2010). *Palliative care nursing: Quality care at the end of life* (3rd ed.). New York: Springer.

McClain, C. S., Rosenfield, B., & Breitbart, W. (2003). Effect of spiritual well-being on end-of-life despair in terminally ill cancer patients. *Lancet, 361,* 1603–1607.

McClement, S., Chochinov, H. M., Hack, T., Hassard, T., Kristanson, L. J., & Harlos, M. (2007). Dignity therapy: Family member perspectives. *Journal of Palliative Medicine, 10(*5), 1076–1082.

McMillan, S. C. (2004). Interventions to facilitate family caregiving. *National Institutes of Health state-of–the science conference on improving end-of-life care program & abstracts.* Bethesda, MD: U.S. Department of Health and Human Services, National Institutes of Health.

Meier, D. E. (2010). The development, status, and future of palliative care. In D. E. Meier, S. L. Isaacs, & R. G. Hughes (Eds.), *Palliative care: Transforming the care of serious illness* (pp. 4–76). San Francisco, CA: Jossey-Bass.

Meier, D. E., Back, A. L., & Morrison, R. S. (2001). The inner life of physicians and care of the seriously ill. *JAMA, 286,* 3007–3014.

Meier, D. E., & Morrison, R. S. (2002). Autonomy reconsidered. *New England Journal of Medicine, 346,* 1087–1089.

Meyer, U. A. (2000). Pharmacogenetics and adverse drug reaction. *Lancet, 356(b),* 1667–1671.

Miles, S. H., Koepp, R., & Weber, E. P. (1996). Advance end-of-life treatment planning: A research review. *Archives of Internal Medicine, 156,* 1062–1068.

Morrison, R. S. (2005). Palliative care outcomes research: The next steps. *Journal of Palliative Medicine, 8*(1), 13–16.

Morrison, R. S., & Meier, D. E. (Eds.). (2003). *Geriatric palliative care.* New York: Oxford University Press.

Morrison, R. S., & Meier, D. E. (2004). Palliative care. *New England Journal of Medicine, 350,* 2582–2590.

National Consensus Project for Quality Palliative Care. (2004). *Clinical practice guidelines for quality palliative care.* Retrieved September 24, 2007, from: www.nationalconsensusproject.org

National Consensus Project for Quality Palliative Care. (2009). *Clinical practice guidelines for quality palliative care* (2nd ed.). Retrieved September 16, 2011, from: www.nationalconsensusproject.org/guideline .pdf

National Hospice and Palliative Care Organization (NHPCO). Retrieved January 28, 2008, from: http://www.nhpco.org

National Hospice and Palliative Care Organization. (2004). *Research agenda.* Arlington, VA: Author. Retrieved September 16, 2011, from: www.NHPCO.org/files/public/2004_Research_Agenda_May04.doc

National Hospice and Palliative Care Organization. (2006). *Standards of practice for hospice programs.* Arlington, VA: Author.

National Hospice and Palliative Care Organization. (2010). *NHPCO facts & figures: Hospice care in America.* Retrieved September 16, 2011, from: http://www.nhpco.org/files/public/Statistics_Research/Hospice_Facts_Figures_Oct-2010.pdf

National Hospice Organization Standards and Accreditation Committee. (1997). *A pathway for patients and families facing terminal illness.* Arlington, VA: Author.

National Institutes of Health. (2004). *National Institutes of Health State-of-the Conference Statement: Improving End-of-Life Care.* Washington, DC: Author.

National Quality Forum. (2006). A National Framework for Palliative and Hospice Care Quality Measurement and Reporting. Washington, DC: Author.

Nolan, M. T., & Mock, V. (2004). A conceptual framework for end-of-life care: A reconsideration of factors influencing the integrity of the human person. *Journal of Professional Nursing, 20*(6), 351–360.

Pellegrino, E. (1990). The relationship of autonomy and integrity in medical ethics. *Bulletin of PAHO, 24,* 361–371.

Pinquart, M., & Sorenson, D. (2003). Differences between caregivers and noncaregivers in psychological health and physical health: A meta-analysis. *Psychology and Aging, 18*(2), 250–257.

Prows, C. A. (2004). Medication selection by genotype. *American Journal of Nursing, 104*(5), 60–70.

Quill, T. E. (2000). Perspectives on care at the end of life: Initiating end-of-life discussions with seriously ill patients: addressing the "elephant in the room." *JAMA, 284,* 2502–2507.

Schulz, R., Mendelsohn, A. B., Haley, W. E., Mahoney, D., Allen, R., Zhang, S., et al. (2003). End of life care and the effects of bereavement among family caregivers of persons with dementia, *New England Journal of Medicine, 349,* 1936–1942.

Schulz, R. Newsom, J. T., Fleissner, K., DeCamp, A. R., & Nieboer, A. P. (1997). The effects of bereavement after family caregiving. *Aging and Mental Health. 1,* 269–282.

Schwarz, U. I., Ritchie, M. D., Bradford, Y., Li, C., Dudek, S. M., Fry-Anderson, A., et al. (2008). Genetic determinants of response to warfarin during initial anticoagulation. *New England Journal of Medicine, 358,* 999–1008.

Sherman, D. W. (2004). Cultural and spiritual backgrounds of older adults. In M. L. Matzo & D. W. Sherman (Eds.), *Gerontologic palliative care nursing* (p. 11). St. Louis: Mosby.

Showalter, S. (1998). Looking through different eyes: Beyond cultural diversity. In K. Doka & J. Davidson (Eds.), *Living with grief when illness is prolonged* (pp. 71–82). Washington, DC: Hospice Foundation of America.

Steinhauser, K. E. (2004). Measuring outcomes prospectively. *National Institutes of Health state-of-the-science conference on improving end-of-life care program & abstracts.* Bethesda, MD: U.S. Department of Health and Human Services, National Institutes of Health.

Steinhauser, K. E., Christakis, N. A., Clipp, E. C., McNeilly, L., & Tulsky, J. A. (2000). Factors considered important at the end of life by patients, family, physicians, and other care providers. *JAMA, 284,* 2476–2482.

Strasser, F., & Bruera, E. D. (2002). Update on anorexia and cachexia. *Hematology and Oncology Clinics of North America, 16,* 589–617.

Sullivan, A. M., Lakoma, M. D., & Block, S. D. (2003). The status of medical education in end-of-life care: A national report. *Journal of General Internal Medicine, 18,* 685–695.

Sullivan, M. C. (2001). Lost in translation: How Latinos view end-of-life care. *Plastic Surgery Nursing, 21*(2), 90–91.

SUPPORT Principal Investigators. (1995). A controlled trial to improve care for seriously ill, hospitalized patients: The study to understand prognoses and preferences for outcomes and risks of treatments (SUPPORT). *JAMA, 274,* 1591–1598.

Temel, J. S., Greer, J. A., Muzikansky, A., Gallaher, E. R., Admane, S., Jackson, V. A., et al. (2010). Early palliative care for patients with metastatic non-small cell lung cancer. *New England Journal of Medicine, 363,* 733–742.

Teno, J. (2001). Quality of care and quality indicators for lives ended by cancer. In K. M. Foley & H. Gelband (Eds.), *Improving palliative care for cancer.* Washington, DC: National Academies Press.

Teno, J. M. (2004). *Brown atlas of dying.* Brown University Center for Gerontology and Health Care Research. Retrieved September 16, 2011, from: www.chcr.brown.edu/dying

Teno, J., Lynn, J., Wenger, N., Phillips, R. S., Murphy, D. P., Connors, A. F., et al. (1997). Advance directives for seriously ill hospitalized patients: Effectiveness with the patient self-determination act and the

SUPPORT intervention. *Journal of the American Geriatrics Society, 45*, 500–507.

Vollrath, A. M., & von Gunten, C. F. (2007). Negotiating goals of care: Changing goals along the trajectory of illness. In L. L. Emanuel & S. L. Librach (Eds.), *Palliative care: Core skills and clinical competencies* (pp. 70–82). Philadelphia: Saunders/Elsevier.

von Gunten, C. F., Ferris, F. D., Portenoy, R. K., & Glajchen, M. (Eds.). (2001). *Manual: How to establish a palliative care program*. New York: NY: Center to Advance Palliative Care.

von Gunten, C. F., & Lupu, D. (2004). Recognizing palliative medicine as a subspecialty: What does it mean for oncology? *The Journal of Supportive Oncology, 2*(2), 166–174.

von Gunten, C., & Romer, A. L. (1999). Designing and sustaining a palliative care and home hospice program: An interview with Charles von Gunten. *Innovations in end-of-life care, 1*(5).

Weinshilboum, R. (2003). Inheritance and drug response. *New England Journal of Medicine, 348(*5), 529–537.

World Health Organization. (1990*). Cancer pain relief and palliative care* (Technical Report Series 804) (p. 11). Geneva, Switzerland: World Health Organization.

CHAPTER 23

Health Policy

The purpose of the healthcare system must be to continuously reduce the impact and burden of illness, injury, and disability and to improve the health and functioning of the people of the United States.

—The President's Advisory Commission on Consumer Protection and Quality in the Health Care Industry: Final Report, 1998

Anne Deutsch and Betty Smith-Campbell

INTRODUCTION

For individuals with chronic illness, access to high-quality healthcare services that are safe, effective, patient centered, timely, efficient (affordable), and equitable is critical. Although many Americans receive high-quality healthcare services, others receive care that is substandard (The President's Advisory Commission on Consumer Protection and Quality in the Health Care Industry, 1998). Much of the work that healthcare professionals perform and experience as they deliver care to patients is influenced by laws, regulations, and other policies. For example, policy affects the availability of affordable health insurance for individuals and families, coverage of home health care, outpatient therapy, and durable medical equipment. Further, changes in health policy can positively or negatively affect access to the healthcare delivery system and the quality of care delivered.

Increasingly, nurses are expected to have knowledge of key health policy issues and the policy development process. This knowledge is fundamental for nurses who want to improve the healthcare delivery system by influencing the policymaking process. To have an impact on patient care and nursing practice, nurses should be able to: 1) assess and understand current health policies, 2) identify the strengths and limitations of healthcare policies, and then 3) act to influence changes in health policy to improve care for patients with chronic illnesses and conditions and their caregivers.

Health Policy Defined

Policy has been defined as the "choices society, segments of society, or organizations make regarding its goals and priorities and the ways it will allocate its resources to attain those goals" (Mason, Leavitt, & Chaffee, 2007, p. 3). Policy is never static; it is continuously influenced by cultural, political, and financial factors in the environment (Chopoorian, 1986). The U.S. healthcare delivery system is influenced by a complex mix of private- and public-sector policies. Private-sector policies are decisions made by executives at private entities, such as private insurance companies and pharmaceutical companies, whereas public health policy decisions are made within any of the three branches of government (the executive, legislative, or judicial branches) and at any level of government (federal, state, or local) (Longest, 2006). Examples of federal legislation include Medicare's prescription drug program and funding to the National Institutes of Health to support research related to chronic diseases such as Alzheimer's disease, stroke, arthritis, and diabetes. Local government examples include city or county governments restricting smoking in public buildings. State and local boards of health have policies that monitor water quality and provide minimum safety requirements for nursing homes and daycare centers.

Health is determined by many factors, including our genetic makeup, our physical environment, our employment and home situations, our social environment, our behaviors, and access to healthcare services and the delivery of healthcare services. This chapter focuses primarily on health policy related to the access to and delivery of healthcare services.

Major Stakeholders in the U.S. Healthcare Industry

An important feature of the U.S. healthcare delivery system is its large and diverse collection of stakeholders (Kovner & Knickman, 2008; Sultz & Young, 2009). Health policies can affect individuals with a common characteristic (e.g., nurses, the elderly, the disabled, the poor) or certain types of organizations (e.g., hospitals, skilled nursing facilities [SNFs], health plans, biotechnology companies, or employers). A stakeholder group's interest level and its support for or opposition to health policy changes vary by issue, and it is not uncommon for some stakeholder groups to agree on one issue, but disagree on another issue (Kovner &

Knickman, 2008; Sultz & Young, 2009). For most stakeholder groups, their perspective on key issues can be anticipated. For example, a key stakeholder group is *patients*, who tend to favor comprehensive insurance coverage, high-quality healthcare delivery, and low out-of-pocket expenses and tend to oppose limited access to care and increased patient payments. A second key stakeholder group is *providers*, including individuals and entities, who tend to favor maintaining income, autonomy, and comprehensive coverage and tend to oppose limits on provider payments. Another key stakeholder group is *taxpayers*, who tend to favor limits on provider payments and tend to oppose higher taxes. *Regulators* (government) are also a stakeholder group and tend to favor disclosure and reporting by providers, cost containment, access to care, and high-quality health care, and tend to oppose provider autonomy. Another key stakeholder group is *employers*, who tend to favor cost containment, administrative simplification, and the elimination of cost shifting, and tend to oppose government regulation. *Pharmaceutical manufacturers, biotechnology companies, assistive technology vendors,* and *suppliers* tend to favor comprehensive coverage and tend to oppose limits on provider payments, and *private insurance companies* tend to favor business autonomy. *Consumer organizations*, such as the American Stroke Association and the Paralyzed Veterans Association, favor securing money for research and public education.

PROBLEMS AND KEY ISSUES _____

U.S. Health Care: A Fragmented System of Care

The United States does not have a national healthcare system or health insurance system.

The prevailing value of individual choice over government care and a strong cultural belief that if one works hard enough, one should be able to support one's self and one's family imply that one should then be able to afford health care (Bellah, Madsen, Sullivan, Swidler, & Tipton, 1985). In addition, current health policy is guided by society's value that a competitive market is the best way to provide healthcare services. Policymakers, with the approval of society, have agreed that some segments of the population need assistance, such as the elderly, the very poor, and the disabled. This has led to separate programs for the elderly and disabled (Medicare), the poor (Medicaid), and uninsured children (SCHIP—State Children's Health Insurance Program). Policymakers have also agreed to reward, through healthcare coverage, those who have provided service to the nation (military and veterans), leading to another separate healthcare system (Veterans Affairs). The mix of privately and publicly funded healthcare coverage has given us a fragmented and complex healthcare system. To better understand this system, an overview of health insurance, including privately and publicly funded options, is discussed.

Health Insurance

Most Americans under the age of 65 have private health insurance coverage through an employer, and almost all older adults receive coverage through Medicare. Medicaid and SCHIP provide insurance for millions of non-elderly, low-income people and children. However, program limits and gaps in employer coverage have resulted in many people not having health insurance. In 2010, 22.7% of individuals under 65 (60.2 million people) were uninsured for part of the past year, and this rate increased for adults 18 to 65 years of age

to 26.8% (51 million) (Martinez & Cohen, 2010). More recently, an estimated 26 million adult workers who lost their jobs between 2007 and 2010 reported that they bought or tried to buy a health plan in the individual market; more than one third (35%), or 9 million people, were turned down or charged a higher price because of a health problem. It can be assumed that many of these health problems were chronic conditions (Collins, Doty, Robertson, & Garber, 2011). The Affordable Care Act of 2010 seeks to eliminate the increasing gap in health insurance coverage by making affordable coverage more accessible, including an expansion of the Medicaid program and a requirement that individuals obtain health insurance. Starting in 2014 no one will be charged a higher premium or denied coverage because of a preexisting health condition.

Health insurance coverage does not always ensure access to care. As of 2007, there were an estimated 25 million underinsured adults in the United States, 60% more than the 16 million who were underinsured in 2003 (Schoen, Collins, Kriss, & Doty, 2008). There are often limitations on coverage for special services, such as behavioral health care, preventive care, long-term care, catastrophic illnesses or accidents, and psychiatric care. Also, exclusions or waiting periods for illnesses or conditions may exist at the time the person enrolls in the health plan. Most health insurance plans also include copayments or deductibles to discourage overuse of services and to reduce premium costs. Copayments and high deductibles can discourage some patients from seeking preventive care (e.g., immunizations, mammograms) and essential care for the management of a chronic condition. This is particularly a problem for people with a low income. Rising costs have become a major problem for insured people with chronic conditions. Nearly 40% of nonelderly adults with three or more chronic conditions had out-of-pocket expenses and premiums exceeding 5% of their income compared with 14% of those who had no chronic conditions (Cunningham, 2009).

Traditional or Conventional Health Insurance

In the 1970s, the most common type of health insurance was a traditional fee-for-service (FFS) plan. Traditional health insurance plans generally allowed the insured person to choose a healthcare provider, and the healthcare provider made most healthcare decisions with minimal oversight by the insurance company. The covered services included acute care services, such as hospitalization, medication, and medical equipment, with little or no emphasis on prevention, health maintenance, or supportive healthcare services. This type of coverage typically included acute care services and limited the services needed to prevent chronic conditions and long-term care services. The number of traditional or conventional plans have declined dramatically from 73% in 1988 to just 1% in 2010 (Kaiser Family Foundation [KFF] & Health Research and Education Trust [HRET], 2010).

A major problem with the traditional FFS plans has been the lack of control on service use that led to high costs. Healthcare providers have few incentives to control costs. Therefore, insurance premiums increased to cover the rising costs of services. Rising insurance costs have become a major issue for employers, who pay for some of the insurance premiums on behalf of employees. As the cost of providing insurance continues to rise above inflation, employers often look for less costly options to provide coverage for their

employees. One solution for employers has been to select managed care organizations (MCOs) for health insurance plans.

Managed Care Organizations

MCO generally refers to any non–FFS plan that attempts to contain costs and manage the delivery of care (KFF, 2004). Types of MCOs include health maintenance organizations (HMOs), preferred provider organizations (PPOs), and point of service (POS) plans. The percentage of persons with MCOs has risen dramatically from 27% in 1988 to 85% in 2010 (KFF & HRET, 2010). With the increase of MCOs in the 1990s, many were hopeful that there would be a system to promote health and assist in preventing disease, and reduce costs. MCOs could help eliminate inappropriate overutilization of services and also offer advantages in setting standard protocols by providing preventive healthcare services. Most experts agree that the main system change MCOs, especially HMOs, have emphasized is that of controlling costs. Average family annual premiums in 2010 were: MCO—$4,357 per employee and $9,768 per employer; PPO—$3,823 per employee and $10,210 per employer; POS—$5,195 per employee and $8,018 per employer.

Consumer-Directed Health Plans

Politicians and employers have been advocating health savings accounts (HSAs), which are a component of consumer-directed health plans (CDHPs) or high-deductible health plans with savings options (HDHP/SO). The majority of covered workers (58%) in 2010 were enrolled in an HDHP/SO (KFF & KRET, 2010). HSAs have lower premiums, but higher deductibles and out-of-pocket spending limits. In 2010, the average family HDHP deduction was $3,577 (Claxton et al., 2010).

HDHP/SOs are insurance plans where financial incentives or disincentives are provided to the consumer or person to become more involved with purchasing their healthcare services. To enroll in an HSA, a consumer must be in an HDHP that meets certain requirements. For 2011, the U.S. Department of the Treasury (2010) defined a high-deductible health plan with an annual deductible that is not less than $1,200 for an individual or $2,400 for family coverage. Annual out-of-pocket expenses (deductibles, copayments, and other amounts, but not premiums) cannot exceed $5,950 for self-only coverage or $11,900 for family coverage. Supporters of these plans believe they will help individuals become more aware of their healthcare needs and, therefore, influence their decisions related to cost and quality of services. Opponents are concerned that individuals will not seek out preventive or needed healthcare services because of high cost. Research studies found enrollees of CDHPs are less satisfied with their plans; spend significantly more of their income on out-of-pocket expenses; and often avoid, skip, or delay health care because of costs. People in these healthcare plans were also more aware of the cost of their care and considered the cost of care when deciding to use healthcare services when compared to enrollees of other plans (Fronstin & Collins, 2006). The results of these and other studies suggest that CDHPs/HSAs negatively affect people with low incomes and those with chronic illnesses.

Medicare

Medicare was implemented in 1965 through Title XVIII of the Social Security Act—Health Insurance for the Aged and Disabled (Pulcine & Hart, 2007). In 2010, Medicare provided health insurance coverage to 47 million people, of which 39 million were age 65 or older and 8 million people with permanent disabilities who were younger than 65. With federal government spending estimated to be $3.6 trillion in 2010, the Medicare program accounted for 12% of the federal budget and 23% of the national health expenditures (KFF, 2010; Medicare Payment Advisory Commission, 2010). Medicare includes four parts:

- *Part A: Hospital Insurance.* The hospital insurance component includes coverage for inpatient hospital services, home health care (skilled care only), hospice care, and short-term stays in SNFs. Most Medicare beneficiaries do not pay a monthly premium for the hospital insurance plan but are responsible for a deductible ($1,100 in 2010) for a hospital stay, a co-insurance for an extended hospital stay ($275 per day for days 61 to 90 in 2010) and co-insurance for extended SNF stays ($137.50 per day for days 21 to 100 in 2010). Medicare Part A is financed through the Hospital Insurance Trust Fund by taxes paid by employers and their employees.
- *Part B: Supplemental Medical Insurance.* The supplementary medical insurance program covers physician, outpatient, home health, and preventive services. It is financed through the Supplementary Medical Insurance Trust Fund by federal taxes and monthly premiums paid by beneficiaries (typically $110.50 in 2010).
- *Part C: Medicare Advantage.* The Medicare Advantage program allows beneficiaries to enroll in private health plans. Plans include

PPOs, provider-sponsored organization (PSOs), private FFS plans, high-deductible plans linked to medical savings accounts, and special needs programs (SNPs) for individuals who are dually eligible for Medicare and Medicaid. Medicare Advantage covers hospital and physician care, often includes prescription drug coverage, and is an alternative to Part A, Part B, and Part D coverage. The plans receive payments from Medicare Advantage to provide Medicare-covered benefits; it is not separately financed from Parts A, B, and D. Medicare Advantage enrollees generally pay the monthly Part B premium and often pay an additional premium directly to their plan (average was $56 per month in 2010).

• *Part D: Prescription Drug Benefit.* The prescription drug benefit provides coverage for outpatient prescription drugs offered through private companies. Coverage varies depending on the plan chosen. The prescription drug benefit is financed through taxes, beneficiary premiums, and state payments for individuals with both Medicare and Medicaid coverage.

Medicare services seem comprehensive and clearly defined; yet, as with all health insurance programs, when assessing how a policy is implemented, either through specific laws or administrative regulatory policy, services are often found to be neither comprehensive nor clearly defined. For example, to receive home health care through Medicare, an individual must meet each of the following requirements: 1) be confined to his or her home; 2) have a physician prescribe treatment; 3) need intermittent skilled nursing care, physical therapy, or speech therapy; and 4) receive services from a certified home health agency participating in Medicare. Therefore, if a nurse practitioner's client with diabetes and congestive heart failure needed skilled nursing care for leg ulcers, the client would first have to be referred by a physician. Second, if the client could leave his or her home to obtain groceries from the store across the street but could not physically tolerate the half-hour bus ride to the practitioner's office, the client would not be eligible to receive home health services through Medicare. It is important to note, especially for those with chronic illness and disabilities, that Medicare does not cover nursing home care.

Medicaid

Medicaid was an amendment to Title XIX of the Social Security Act in 1965 and was implemented in 1966. Medicaid was established to provide health insurance to low-income families with dependents. Individual states define the program, and it is jointly funded by federal and state governments. Medicaid covers a wide range of health and long-term care services, but because coverage by Medicaid is administered at the state level, coverage varies from state to state, and there are vast differences regarding who is eligible (Rowland & Tallon, 2004). In most states, adults who are not pregnant are usually not covered. To receive matching federal dollars, the state program must offer certain basic medical services, such as inpatient and outpatient hospital care and physician and family nurse practitioner services. Medicaid managed care and non–managed care options are available. Some states require enrollment in a managed care plan. Covered services include long-term care, mental health care, and services and supports needed by individuals with disabilities. Medicaid covers comprehensive services for children. Medicaid is the largest funding source for coverage of long-term care, covering approximately 70% of all nursing home residents (The Kaiser Commission on Medicaid and the Uninsured [KCMU], 2010). Medicaid will cover services such as prescription drugs, eyeglasses, and hearing aids. Medicaid also covers those with disabilities and the elderly who are enrolled in Medicare, known as "dual eligibles," but have incomes below a certain level. This limited coverage for low-income Medicare beneficiaries assists with premiums, deductibles, and coinsurance.

In 2007, Medicaid covered 59.4 million people (U.S. Department of Health and Human Services [USDHHS], 2011). Medicaid spending was approximately $339 billion in 2008. The Affordable Care Act is expected to provide coverage for an additional 16 million people by 2014 with eligibility reform, simplified enrollment, improved access to care, and changes in financing (KCMU, 2010). By 2014, Medicaid is anticipated to include the majority of people younger than 65 with income up to 133% of the poverty level (KCMU, 2010).

SCHIP: State Children's Health Insurance Program

The Balanced Budget Act (BBA) of 1997 expanded health insurance coverage to children through SCHIP. SCHIP was created to help states cover uninsured children who do not meet Medicaid eligibility requirements (KCMU, 2007). Similar to Medicaid, SCHIP is administered through states, and the type of program offered varies by state. As employer insurance coverage has declined, the rate of children who are uninsured has risen. Without health insurance, children often do not receive care to prevent chronic conditions or illnesses such as complications from diseases that could have been prevented by immunizations (e.g., hepatitis) or disabilities created because of lack of treatment (e.g., hearing loss from otitis media). Early in 2009, President Obama signed into law the Children's Health Insurance Program Reauthorization Act of 2009 (CHIPRA) (Garner, 2009). CHIPRA provides additional resources to states to cover more children and women and expands the option for states to include low-income adults.

Costs, Access, and Quality

Costs

The increasing cost of delivering health care has been a challenge for policymakers for several decades. The national health expenditures represented 5.1% of U.S. gross domestic product (GDP) in 1960. In 2009, the percentage of GDP rose to 17.3% from 16.2% in 2008—the largest 1-year increase since 1960 (Truffer et al., 2010). It is expected to be 19.3% of the GDP in 2012, which is almost one fifth of our GDP, and public spending is projected to account for more than half of all U.S. healthcare spending. The rising costs are attributed to many factors, including population growth, advances in healthcare technology, increased utilization of services, increasing labor costs, and increases in the costs of pharmaceuticals and malpractice insurance. While almost everyone agrees that rising healthcare costs are a problem, the development of policies aimed at controlling costs is challenging, because one or more stakeholder groups may receive less money, and access to care may become more limited. Issues that have been proposed to control costs include: managed care, use of information technology, evidence-based care, management initiatives, controlling prescription drug costs, Medicare and Medicaid reform, using competition, fraud prevention and detection, and price controls.

Access to Care

There are many reasons why individuals do not have equal access to healthcare services. The most common reason for reduced access to necessary health services is the inability to pay for care (Sultz & Young, 2009). A growing number of people have no health insurance or are underinsured, and when individuals and families are either uninsured or underinsured, they are: less likely to have a usual source of care outside the emergency room; often go without screenings and preventive care; often delay or forgo needed medical care; are sicker and die earlier than those who have insurance; and pay more for their care. This lack of access places a higher burden on those with chronic illness. In Great Britain, Canada, and The Netherlands, individuals state they rarely forgo needed medical care because of cost; yet in the United States, 54% of those with chronic diseases "had skipped medications, not seen a doctor when sick, or foregone recommended care in the past year because of costs" (Schoen, Osborn, How, Doty & Peugh, 2009). More than 84% of individuals who are considered high users of the emergency room have chronic conditions (Peppe, Mays, Chang, Becker, & DiJulio, 2007). The Affordable Care Act seeks to address the issue of uninsurance, with some provisions already implemented and more significant ones due for implementation in 2014.

There are many other individuals with limited access to care, particularly specialty care, because healthcare personnel and facilities are not close to where they live (e.g., rural locations), culturally acceptable, or capable of providing the type of care needed (Sultz & Young, 2009).

Quality and Quality Measures

The Institute of Medicine (IOM) has defined quality as the "degree to which health services for individuals and populations increase the likelihood of desired health outcomes and are consistent with current professional knowledge" (2006, p. 468), and the only way to know if healthcare quality is improving is to document performance using measures of quality. The term *quality measure* has been defined as the "quantification of the degree to which a desired health care process or outcome is achieved or the extent that a desirable structure to support health care delivery is in place" (p. 42).

Quality measures (also known as quality indicators, performance measures, and performance indicators) evaluate healthcare performance in a manner that permits comparisons across facilities and across time. Uses of quality measures are public reporting, quality improvement, and pay-for-performance activities (IOM, 2006). The Centers for Medicare & Medicaid Services (CMS) and private-sector payers have been leaders in using quality measures for public reporting and pay for performance. Proponents of public reporting of quality information argue that it helps patients, referring physicians, and purchasers of health care make better, more informed choices about providers who offer the best care. Another use of quality measures is rewarding providers that demonstrate better quality of care based on performance data (i.e., pay-for-performance programs). The Affordable Care Act expands the development of quality measures and pay-for-performance programs in post-acute care settings.

Quality measures can include structure measures, process measures, and outcome measures (Donabedian, 2005). *Structure measures* document whether a particular mechanism or system is in place, *process measures* track performance of a particular action, and *outcome measures* document the end results of care, such as morbidity and mortality resulting from a disease. The IOM identified the six aims of healthcare delivery as care that is safe, effective, patient centered, timely, efficient, and equitable. *Safe care* is the avoidance of injuries to patients as a result of care that is intended to help. *Effective care* means that services are based on scientific knowledge and provided to all who could benefit and not providing services to those who would not likely to benefit. *Patient-centered care* refers to care that is respectful of and responsive to individual patient preferences, needs, and values, and *timely care* is provided in a way that reduces wait times. *Efficient care* avoids waste, including waste of equipment, supplies, ideas, and energy; and *equitable care* refers to care that does not vary in quality because of personal characteristics (e.g., gender, ethnicity, geographic location, and socioeconomic status).

In the book *Crossing the Quality Chasm*, the IOM (2001) proposed 10 rules for redesigning healthcare processes to improve care:

1. *Care based on continuous healing relationships*. Care should be available 24 hours a day, 7 days a week, and access to care should occur over the Internet, by telephone, and by other means as well as face-to-face.
2. *Customization based on patient needs and values*. The system should meet the most common types of patient needs and have the ability to respond to patient choices and preferences.
3. *The patient as the source of control*. Patients should be given the necessary information and the opportunity to be involved in shared decision making.
4. *Shared knowledge and the free flow of information*. Patients should have access to

their own medical information and clinical knowledge.
5. *Evidence-based decision making*. Patients should receive care based on the best scientific knowledge.
6. *Safety*. Patients should be safe from injury that is caused by the healthcare delivery system.
7. *Transparency*. The system should make information available to patients and their families that allows them to make informed decisions when selecting a health plan, hospital, or clinician.
8. *Anticipation of needs*. The system should anticipate patients' needs.
9. *Continuous decrease in waste*. The health system should not waste resources, including patients' time.
10. *Cooperation among clinicians*. Clinicians and institutions should actively collaborate and communicate to foster greater coordination of care and integration.

The Affordable Care Act includes several initiatives that focus on improving the coordination of healthcare services. Care coordination is a critical component of high-quality care for individuals with chronic illness, who may be seeing more than one health professional and may have multiple hospitalizations. One initiative is the Accountable Care Organization, which is defined as a network of healthcare providers that provide a full continuum of healthcare services. Proposed accountable care organization pilot programs in Medicare and Medicaid focus on improving quality and reducing costs by offering financial incentives to these goals. A second initiative, medical homes, involves healthcare settings that offer comprehensive primary care services, as well as nonemergent primary, secondary, and tertiary care. The medical home primary care provider directs and coordinates care for patients.

INTERVENTIONS: POLITICS, A CARING ACTION

Public policy has greatly influenced the U.S. healthcare system. Basic health services are provided to the majority of U.S. elderly and the severely disabled, but, as discussed, the health system is fragmented and complex. Initiating changes in current policies can benefit individuals with chronic illness, but to do so requires political action.

To influence and change policy requires more than a one-time intervention; it requires continued action (Smith-Campbell, 1999). Being active in politics allows nurses the ability to shape policy that influences the care individuals with chronic illness receive and gives nurses an opportunity to partner with clients to meet common goals. Helping individuals with chronic conditions and their families understand the political process and the power of politics can empower them to work to improve the healthcare system.

As healthcare providers for individuals with chronic illness, it is imperative that we recognize the need to intervene on policy issues for our patients/clients—because it does affect their health. Can an individual with a chronic illness get health insurance—even if they can pay for it? Will their health insurance cover their medications? Will Medicare or Medicaid provide needed healthcare services for those with chronic illnesses? Does the public health system have enough funding to educate the public on ways to prevent chronic illnesses? These are just a few policy issues affecting those with chronic

illness for whom interventions may be required. Such interventions involve influencing policy or becoming politically active.

Stages of Influencing Policy

Health policy making can be separated into three phases (see **Figure 23-1**): 1) policy formulation (agenda setting and legislation), 2) policy implementation, and 3) policy modification (Longest, 2006). At each phase, a person can take on an important role in the development of policy, which can have a significant impact on healthcare delivery.

Policy Formulation: Agenda Setting

Policy formulation begins with agenda setting, which refers to the identification of problems and possible solutions. Most national policy agenda setting begins with Congressional members or comes from the office of the U.S. President. The personal values and beliefs of public officials and the values and desires of their constituents influence governmental officials in determining new agenda items or attempting to change agenda items. Agendas may be pushed to the forefront at local, state, or national levels, because of a single injustice or tragedy. Before the organization Mothers Against Drunk Driving (MADD) existed, most of the American populace viewed drinking and driving as normal; yet, drunk drivers were causing death and disabling individuals across the nation. Because one mother felt passionate about the injustice of her child being killed by a drunk driver, a new advocacy organization was formed and MADD chapters that fight drinking and driving now exist across the nation. Policies, as well as national values, have changed regarding drinking and driving, all because one woman

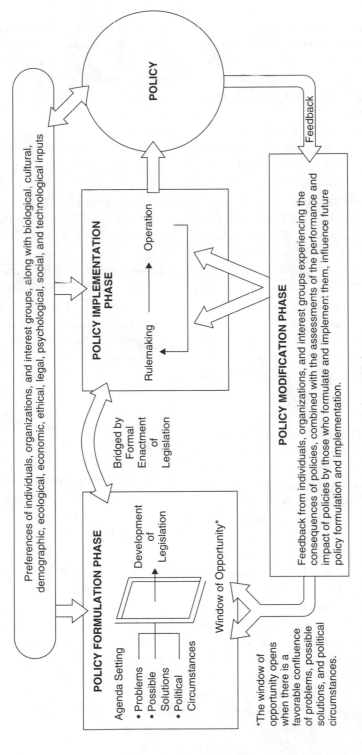

FIGURE 23-1   A Model of the Public Policymaking Process in the United States.

Source: Longest, B. B. (2006). *Health Policymaking in the United States* (4th ed.). Chicago, IL: Health Administration Press.

became passionate about an injustice (Dodd, 2004). MADD was successful because the political climate was ripe for change.

As conditions in society change or there is a shift in values and beliefs, new agenda items take on more importance. Recently such issues have been and continue to be: affordable health insurance, the war on terror, and illegal immunization. Agenda setting can also be influenced by other factors such as publication of research findings. Based on an IOM report on errors in the healthcare system, patients, families, and legislators continue to ask questions about the safety of healthcare delivery (Kohn, Corrigan, & Donaldson, 2000). This report continues to impact health care through new and modified Medicare policies. Once an agenda becomes recognized, governmental officials legislate programs and develop and/or change policy to address problems identified in agenda setting. However, only a small number of issues reach policy formulation.

Policy Formulation: Legislation

The legislative process begins with proposals, such as bills, which are drafted by senators or representatives and their staff members, by members of the executive branch, by political or special interest groups, or by individual citizens. Only members of Congress can officially sponsor a bill. On occasion, bills that are identical are introduced simultaneously in the Senate and the House of Representatives for consideration. Each bill is assigned to the appropriate committee(s) based on the content of the bill and the jurisdiction of the committees and subcommittees. Hearings are held, and the bill is marked up.

Once the bill is approved by the full committee, the House or Senate receives the bill and places it on the legislative calendar for floor action. The bill may be amended further during debate on the floor. If the bill passes either the

House or the Senate, it is then sent to the other chamber of Congress, where the process is repeated. If the second chamber passes the bill, any differences between the Senate and House versions must be resolved before the bill is sent to the White House for presidential action. The president then has the option to sign the bill to make it a law or to veto the bill and return it to Congress with an explanation for the rejection. A presidential veto may be overridden by a two-thirds vote in both houses of Congress. If the president does not sign or veto the bill after 10 days, the bill automatically becomes law. The process is similar at the state level, with the endpoint being the governor of the state.

There are many ways to influence the process of legislation. This can be done directly with legislators themselves, but other players may impact the legislative process. These groups include legislative staff persons, interest groups, research, media, and constituents (Hanley & Falk, 2007). The key players not only influence the form of the final bill but can also have an impact on the bill's continuation or abandonment at any time during the process. Broad language is used to write laws for flexibility and adaptability of their application over time.

Once a bill becomes law, it is the responsibility of administrative agencies to write regulations based on the approved law.

Policy Implementation

After a law is enacted, policy implementation begins. Policy implementation includes rule making and policy operation, and becomes the responsibility of the executive branch of the government. Cabinet departments such as the USDHHS and its agencies, such as the Centers for Disease Control and Prevention (CDC) and the CMS, oversee the implementation of the law. Oversight of the implementation is the responsibility of agencies such as the Congressional Budget Office, the Government Accountability Office, the Congressional Research Office, and the Office of Technology and Assessment. Laws are often vague on implementation details, so the entity responsible for implementing the law publishes a "Notice of Proposed Rule Making" and a "Final Rule" in the *Federal Register* provide the details. Any person may comment on the proposed rules/regulations. This is an important and potentially powerful way for stakeholders to influence the regulations that direct policy implementation. The administrative agency reviews the comments based on the proposed rule making and may make changes to the final rules and regulations. Once approved by an executive level agency, the regulations go into effect. After regulations are approved, programs are then established or past programs are modified, based on the new regulations.

Policy Modification

In the policy modification phase, prior decisions are reviewed and in some cases, the decisions are modified once the outcomes, perceptions, and consequences of existing policies are discovered. Modifications to any legislation begin at the agenda-setting stage. For example, national and state policies have attempted to deinstitutionalize individuals with mental illness. Although the program goals to decrease the number of individuals that are institutionalized have been successful, the problem of inadequate community services has led many with chronic mental illness to become homeless or housed within the criminal justice system.

Nursing Interventions—Action Steps

To affect public policy, nurses need to learn the skills necessary to influence policymakers at all stages of policy development. These skills can also be taught to individuals with chronic conditions and their families so they, too, can influence the system. Vance (1985) identified communication, collectivity, and collegiality as the three components of political influence.

Communication

Skillful communication can be influential in the political process. Nurses usually are expert one-to-one communicators, but to affect policy, nurses must broaden their communication skills. The first step of communication is listening and learning. It is essential to learn about the political process. Knowing how a bill becomes law is one way of learning about the political process. It is also important to identify the key players at different steps in the process. Knowing when a bill is in committee and knowing the chairperson and committee membership is important information that can help one attempt to apply influence. In addition to directly trying to influence public policymakers, indirect influence is also a strategy. Communicating with Congressional/executive staff members, the media, and constituents also can influence policymakers. Knowing who one is trying to influence and how one wants to influence their actions are key factors. Once these details are determined, there are several communication strategies that one can use:

- Send a message and/or position statement by email, fax, or letter. In small states, it may be possible to contact legislators directly; in larger states or at the national level either talk with a staff person or leave a short message. Email, fax, or phone calls are probably the best ways to communicate with legislators. In addition, many elected or policy leaders have their own website where there is usually a mechanism to send a message (**Table 23-1**).

- Write letters to newspaper editors; talk on the radio/TV.
- Visit legislators and/or their staff (**Table 23-2**).
- Testify at public hearings.
- Vote and get others to vote.

Collectivity

Collectivity is critical to the development of political influence and is built on a foundation of networking, coalition building, and collaboration (Vance, 1985). One of the first steps in advocacy is finding mentors who can assist in developing

needed skills (Leavitt, Chaffee, & Vance, 2007). Mentors can assist in learning about the policy process as well as provide access to key stakeholders. Working to change policy at any level of government requires group action and collaboration. The American Nurses Association, which speaks for more than 2.8 million nurses, has testified on many key issues relevant to nursing and the patients they serve, including healthcare

---

Table 23-1   Guidelines for Writing an Email, Letter, or Fax to Policymakers and Their Staff

Writing to a policymaker is one of the easiest and most effective ways for individuals and groups to correspond with policymakers.

1. Be professional. Use the proper forms of address when writing to any policymaker. Use a polite tone and present your message clearly, concisely, and with respect.
2. State who you are and why you are writing.
3. Be concise and informed.
4. Personalize your letter by including a description of a personal experience or patient story.
5. Be accurate and clear.
6. Be modest with the request.
7. Offer your assistance as a resource.
8. Express thanks for their time and consideration.
9. Ask for a response.
10. If you do not get a response in about 1 month, follow up with the policymaker.

Source: Adapted from Association of Rehabilitation Nurses. (2011). Health policy toolkit. Retrieved September 16, 2011, from: http://www.rehabnurse.org/advocacy/content/toolkit.html

---

Table 23-2   Guidelines for Meeting with Policymakers and Their Staff

1. Be prepared and be on time for your appointment. Always introduce yourself, even if this is your third or fourth meeting. State that you are a registered nurse, or if a client is speaking, have that person share the nature of the chronic condition he or she or the family member has.
2. Thank the legislator for seeing you and then briefly and clearly identify the issue you want to discuss. If it is a specific bill, state its number, its title, your position, and what you want the legislator to do.
3. Provide a real-life example or personal story to illustrate your position.
4. Listen to the policymaker's/staffer's comments and respond to any questions.
5. Ask the policymaker's/staffer's position on the issue.
6. Bring written materials on the issue that can be left with policymakers.
7. Leave your contact information, such as a business card.
8. Summarize your requests of the policymaker.
9. Follow up your visit with a thank-you note.
10. Summarize your meeting in writing and share with the organization(s) with which you are working.

Source: Adapted from Association of Rehabilitation Nurses. (2011). Health policy toolkit. Retrieved September 16, 2011, from: http://www.rehabnurse.org/advocacy/content/toolkit.html

reform, Medicare funding, and funding for nursing education programs.

National and state professional and community organizations also work for policy initiatives that impact their organizations or members of their organizations. The American Heart Association has specific legislative goals related to heart disease and stroke. It works with individuals and groups in policy initiatives, including help in finding local legislators, how and when to write legislators, as well as keeping the public informed about policy issues that impact their stated goals. Professional and community organizations, especially at the local level, can provide great mentoring opportunities. These organizations are often looking for individuals to help with their advocacy strategies and may often help in the development of those skills.

Networking is key, because sometimes success comes down to having just one important personal connection (Leavitt, Cohen, & Mason, 2007). Networking with client groups can also be helpful. Having clients communicate with legislators about how they or their families have been or will be affected by legislation is an important strategy to influence policymakers. Working with groups that have been active in advocacy can provide a novice political advocate needed assistance and support. Advocacy groups such as the American Association of People with Disabilities (2007) can help professionals or families of individuals with disabilities provide testimony at public hearings.

Collegiality

Central to the political process is collegiality—a spirit of cooperation and solidarity with associates (Vance, 1985). To be a political activist and risk taker requires support from colleagues. It is helpful to work with others with an attitude of mutual respect and shared convictions. Sometimes diverse groups (i.e., stakeholders) can work together on a mutual issue, even if they are opponents on other issues. Disassociating the emotional context of working with opponents is key. Politics is neither negative nor positive, but each side often has different values and beliefs. Working in solidarity with a group provides support during conflict and can assist in an important factor in political influencing—not taking it personally. Influencing policy changes requires patience, perseverance, and compromise. Working with those who share similar values, beliefs, and convictions will be of great assistance when working for change.

The strategies discussed in this section emphasize influencing policy at the national level. These same strategies can also be used to influence local and state policy, as well as policymakers in work and community organizations. It is vital that nurses become political, or they risk being excluded from important decisions that affect nursing practice or the care provided to their patients with chronic illness.

Becoming a political person can be an overwhelming experience as you realize you cannot change a whole system alone. As a beginning political advocate—start by voting. Next, choose an issue about which you feel passionate (e.g., the inability of your clients with chronic illness to get long-term home care). Educate yourself on the issue, and join others who are interested in the issue. Communicate your position to the key players. Know that your cause is just, and be proud of the political influence you, your clients, and your colleagues can accomplish.

CASE STUDY

As a nurse who works in a heart failure clinic, you recognize the importance of preventing and reducing heart disease. Lately you have seen younger patients being diagnosed with heart failure related to lifestyle behaviors such as obesity and smoking. You have also noted that many of these individuals have not sought out health care prior to their diagnosis of heart failure because they lack health insurance.

Discussion Questions

1. What national and statewide advocacy organization might be able to mentor/assist you in advocacy efforts to reduce heart disease and stroke risks?
2. If your state had a bill pending to ban smoking in all public buildings, who would you contact to support passage of the bill?
3. Who are the potential stakeholders related to a statewide smoking ban and what strategies would you utilize to influence them?

OUTCOMES

Through public policy, society has made choices to assist many Americans. There are policies to care for the elderly and severely disabled through Medicare and provide health insurance to the poor through Medicaid. Society's belief in the market system and individual rights has left many with inadequate or absent health insurance. The U.S. healthcare system is complex, fragmented, and difficult to navigate, especially for vulnerable populations such as the individual with chronic illness, the individual with disabilities, and the elderly. Changes are expected with the implementation of the Affordable Care Act, but many details remain unclear as key issues are debated by policymakers and the public. The profession of nursing and individuals with chronic illness and their families can influence change through political action.

Evidence-Based Practice Box

The evidence clearly shows that health policy impacts the health of individuals. Policies related to insurance are associated with the health of individuals:

*   The treatment and control of hypertension and hypercholesterolemia are lower among uninsured adults when compared to insured individuals (Brooks et al., 2010).
*   Medicare beneficiaries who qualify for Medicare as a result of disabilities, when compared with the beneficiaries who qualify because of age, reported more problems with accessing care and finding affordable care. The beneficiaries who were disabled reported a

higher rate of health consequences as a result of delayed or missed care because of cost concerns, including a worsening in the primary disability or existing medical condition, more problems that require medical attention, a higher level of a significant amount of stress or anxiety and a higher level of a significant amount of physical pain (Cubanski & Neuman, 2010).

- Using the 2002–2004 Medical Expenditure Panel Survey, researchers found that among 92 million adults with chronic conditions, 21% experienced at least 1 month uninsured during the average year. The gaps in health insurance coverage were associated with significantly higher levels of access problems, fewer ambulatory visits, and higher out-of-pocket costs (Gulley, Rasch, & Chan, 2010).

STUDY QUESTIONS

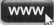

Describe the trends of chronic illness and how these trends are significant in relation to health policy.

Differentiate between Medicare and Medicaid.

Identify the major social issues affecting health policy for the individual with chronic illness.

How does the current U.S. healthcare system affect those with chronic illness?

Explain how a bill becomes law.

Identify the three components of political influence, and explain each.

What are the first steps in which you can engage to become politically active?

INTERNET RESOURCES

- How to find and communicate with legislators and stakeholders:

Federal Legislative link site: http://thomas.loc.gov
Leading Age (formerly AAHSA): www.leadingage.org

Policy/political resources:

- Health System Change policy analysis site: http://www.hschange.com
- Summary of national political news: www.politicalwire.com
- State policy and politics: www.stateline.org/live

Government websites:

- Centers for Medicare & Medicaid Services (CMS): www.cms.gov
- Department of Veterans Affairs: www.va.gov
- U.S. House of Representatives and U.S. Senate: www.house.gov

Advocacy or other relevant websites:

- American Association of People with Disabilities: www.aapd.com
- American Heart Association: http://www.heart.org/HEARTORG/Advocate/Advocate_UCM_001133_SubHome Page.jsp
- American Nurses Association-government affairs: http://www.nursingworld.org/MainMenuCategories/ANAPoliticalPower.aspx
- Consortium for Citizens with Disabilities: www.c-c-d.org
- Families USA: www.familiesusa.org
- National Alliance for Caregiving: www.caregiving.org

(continues)

> ### Internet Resources (Cont.)
>
> - National Citizen's Coalition for Nursing Home Reform: www.nccnhr.org
> - National Respite Coalition: http://www.archrespite.org
> - Partnership to fight chronic disease: www.fightchronicdisease.org
> - Preventing Chronic Disease Journal: www.cdc.gov/pcd
> - United Cerebral Palsy: www.ucp.org
> - WHO—World Health Organization-Chronic Disease and Health Promotion: www.who.int/chp/en

For a full suite of assignments and additional learning activities, use the access code located in the front of your book and visit this exclusive website: **http://go.jblearning.com/larsen**. If you do not have an access code, you can obtain one at the site.

REFERENCES

American Association of People with Disabilities. (2007). AAPD policy positions & activities. Retrieved September 16, 2011, from: http://www.aapd.com/site/c.pvI1IkNWJqE/b.5606943/k.669B/AAPD_Policy_Positions.htm

Association of Rehabilitation Nurses. (2011). Health policy toolkit. Retrieved September 16, 2011, from: http://www.rehabnurse.org/advocacy/content/toolkit.html

Bellah, R. N., Madsen, R., Sullivan, W. M., Swidler, A., & Tipton, S. M. (1985). *Habits of the heart: Individualism and commitment in American life*. New York: Harper & Row.

Brooks, E. L., Preis, S. R., Hwang, S. J., Murabito, J. M., Benjamin, E. J., Kelly-Hayes, M., et al. (2010). Health insurance and cardiovascular disease risk factors. *American Journal of Medicine, 123*(8), 741–747.

Chopoorian, T. J. (1986). Reconceptualizing the environment. In P. Moccia (Ed.), *New approaches to theory development* (pp. 39–54). New York: National League for Nursing.

Claxton, G., DiJulio, B., Whitmore, H., Pickreign, J., McHugh, M., Osei-Anto, A., & Finder, B. (2010). Health benefits in 2010: Premiums rise modestly, workers pay more toward coverage. *Health Affairs, 29*, 1942–1950.

Collins, S. R., Doty, M. M., Robertson, R., & Garber, T. (2011, March). *Health insurance, and how health reform will bring relief findings from the Commonwealth Fund Biennial Health Insurance Survey of 2010*. Retrieved September 16, 2011, from: http://www.commonwealthfund.org/~/media/Files/Publications/Fund%20Report/2011/Mar/1486_Collins_help_on_the_horizon_2010_biennial_survey_report_FINAL_v2.pdf

Cubanski, J., & Neuman, P. (2010). Medicare doesn't work as well for younger, disabled beneficiaries as it does for older enrollees. *Health Affairs, 29*(9), 1–9.

Cunningham, P. (2009). *Chronic burdens: The persistently high out-of-pocket health care expenses faced by many Americans with chronic conditions, The Commonwealth Fund*. Retrieved September 16, 2011, from: http://www.commonwealthfund.org/~/media/Files/Publications/Issue%20Brief/2009/Jul/Chronic%20Burdens/1303_Cunningham_chronic_burdens_high_OOP_expenses_chronic_conditions_ib.pdf

Dodd, C. J. (2004). Making the political process work. In C. Harrington & C. L. Estes (Eds.), *Health policy crisis and reform in the U.S. health care delivery system* (4th ed., pp. 18–28). Sudbury, MA: Jones and Bartlett.

Donabedian, A. (2005). Evaluating the quality of medical care. *Milbank Quarterly, 83*(4), 691–729.

Fronstin, P., & Collins, S. R. (2006). The 2nd annual EBRI/commonwealth fund consumerism in health care survey, 2006: Early experience with high-deductible and consumer-driven health plans. Retrieved September 16, 2011, from: http://www.commonwealthfund.org/Publications/Issue-Briefs/2006/Dec/The-2nd-Annual-EBRI-Commonwealth-Fund-Consumerism-in-Health-Care-Survey–2006–Early-Experience-With.aspx

Garner, J. (2009, April 17). *Centers for Medicaid & State Operations*. Retrieved September 16, 2011, from: http://www.cms.gov/SMDL/downloads/SHO041709.pdf

Gulley, S. P., Rasch, E. K., & Chan, L. (2010). Ongoing coverage for ongoing care: Access, utilization, and out-of-pocket spending among uninsured working-aged adults with chronic health care needs. *American Journal of Public Health, 101*(2), 368–375.

Hanley, B., & Falk, N. L. (2007). Policy development and analysis: Understanding the process. In D. J. Mason, J. K. Leavitt, & M. W. Chaffee (Eds.), *Policy & politics in nursing and health care* (5th ed., pp. 75–93). St. Louis: Saunders Elsevier.

Institute of Medicine. (2001). *Crossing the quality chasm: A new health system for the 21st century*. Washington, DC: The National Academies Press.

Institute of Medicine. (2006). *Performance measurement: Accelerating improvement*. Washington, DC: The National Academies Press.

Kaiser Commission on Medicaid and the Uninsured. (2007). Health coverage of children: The role of Medicaid and SCHIP. Retrieved September 16, 2011, from: www.kff.org/uninsured/upload/7698.pdf

Kaiser Commission on Medicaid and the Uninsured. (2010). *Medicaid: A primer*. Menlo Park, CA: The Henry J. Kaiser Family Foundation. Retrieved September 16, 2011, from: http://www.kff.org/medicaid/7334.cfm

Kaiser Family Foundation. (2004). Trends and indicators in the changing healthcare marketplace, 2004 update. Retrieved September 16, 2011, from: http://www.kff.org/insurance/7031/loader.cfm?url=/commonspot/security/getfile.cfm&PageID=36091

Kaiser Family Foundation, Health Research and Education Trust. (2010). Employer health benefits 2010 annual survey. Retrieved September 16, 2011, from: http://ehbs.kff.org

Kaiser Family Foundation. (2010). *Medicare: A primer*. Menlo Park, CA: Author. Retrieved September 16, 2011, from: http://www.kff.org/medicare/7615.cfm

Kohn, L. T., Corrigan, J. M., & Donaldson, M. S. (2000). *To err is human: Building a safer health system*. Washington, DC: National Academies Press.

Kovner, A. R., & Knickman, J. R. (Eds.). (2008). *Health care delivery in the United States* (9th ed.). New York: Springer.

Leavitt, J. K., Chaffee, M. W., & Vance, C. (2007). Learning the ropes of policy, politics, and advocacy. In D. J. Mason, J. K. Leavitt, & M. W. Chaffee (Eds.), *Policy & politics in nursing and health care* (pp. 34–36). St. Louis, MO: Elsevier.

Leavitt, J. K., Cohen, S. S., & Mason, D. J. (2007). Policy analysis and strategies. In D. J. Mason, J. K. Leavitt, & M. W. Chaffee (Eds.), *Policy & politics in nursing and health care* (pp. 94–109). St. Louis, MO: Elsevier.

Longest, B. B. (2006). *Health policymaking in the United States* (4th ed.). Chicago, IL: Health Admini-stration Press.

Martinez, M. E., & Cohen, R. A. (2010, December). Health insurance coverage: Early release of estimates from the National Health Interview Survey, January–June 2010. National Center for Health Statistics. Retrieved September 16, 2011, from: ://www.cdc.gov/nchs/data/nhis/earlyrelease/insur201012.pdf

Mason, D. J., Leavitt, J. K., & Chaffee, M. W. (2007). Policy and politics: A framework for action. In D. J. Mason, J. K. Leavitt, & M. W. Chaffee (Eds.), *Policy & politics in nursing and health care* (5th ed.). St. Louis: Saunders Elsevier.

Medicare Payment Advisory Commission. (2010). *Data Book: Healthcare Spending and the Medicare Program*. Washington, DC: Author.

Peppe, E. M., Mays, J. W., Chang, H. C., Becker, E., & DiJulio, B. (2007). Characteristics of frequent emergency department users. Retrieved September 16, 2011, from: http://www.kff.org/insurance/7696.cfm

The President's Advisory Commission on Consumer Protection and Quality in the Health Care Industry. (1998). *Quality first: Better health care for all Americans*. Washington, DC: Author.

Pulcine, J. A., & Hart, M. A. (2007). Financing health care in the United States. In D. J. Mason, J. K., Leavitt, & M. W. Chaffee (Eds.), *Policy & politics in nursing and health care* (5th ed., pp. 384–408). St. Louis: Saunders Elsevier.

Rowland, D., & Tallon, J. R. (2004). Medicaid: Lessons from a decade. In C. Harrington & C. L. Estes (Eds.), *Health policy crisis and reform in the U.S. health care delivery system* (4th ed.). Sudbury, MA: Jones and Bartlett.

Schoen, C., Collins, S. R., Kriss, J. L., & Doty, M. M. (2008). How many are underinsured? Trends among U.S. Adults, 2003 and 2007. *Health Affairs Web Exclusive*, w298–w309.

Schoen, C., Osborn, R., How, S. K. H. Doty, M. M., & Peugh, J. (2009). In chronic condition: Experiences of patients with complex health care needs, in eight countries, 2008. *Health Affairs, 28,* w1–w16.

Smith-Campbell, B. (1999). A case study on expanding the concept of caring from individuals to communities. *Public Health Nursing, 16,* 405–411.

Sultz, H. A., & Young, K. M. (2009). *Health Care USA* (6th ed.). Sudbury, MA: Jones and Bartlett.

Truffer, C. J., Keehan, S., Smith, S., Cylus, J., Sisko, A., Poisal, J. A., et al. (2010). Health spending projections through 2019: The recession's impact continues. *Health Affairs, 29,* 522–529.

U.S. Department of Health and Human Services. (2011). *2010 CMS statistics.* Retrieved February 15, 2011, from: http://www.cms.gov/ResearchGenInfo/02_CMSStatistics.asp#TopOfPage

U.S. Department of the Treasury. (2010). Health Savings Accounts—2011 Indexed Amounts. http://www.treasury.gov/resource-center/tax-policy/Pages/HSA-2011-indexed-amounts.aspx

Vance, C. (1985). Politics: A humanistic process. In D. J. Mason, S. W. Talbott, & J. K. Leavitt (Eds.), *Policy and politics for nurses* (pp. 104–118). Philadelphia: Saunders.

CHAPTER 24

Rehabilitation

Kristen L. Mauk

INTRODUCTION

"Rehabilitation refers to services and programs designed to assist individuals who have experienced a trauma or illness that results in impairment that creates a loss of function (physical, psychological, social, or vocational)" (Remsburg & Carson, 2006, p. 579). Rehabilitation is also an approach to care in which persons with chronic illness and disability are "made able" again (Pryor, 2002).

Rehabilitation assists individuals with long-term health alterations to regain independence and adapt to changes that have occurred as a result of deviations in their health status. A popular rehabilitation saying is that "rehabilitation begins day one" and thus should be considered as part of the overall plan of care for most acute illness episodes and throughout the duration of most chronic illnesses.

The primary goal of rehabilitation is to achieve the highest level of independence possible for the client. This goal is highly individualized. For example, a person with a mild stroke may have the goal to walk again and resume gainful employment at the same job he held previously. Another person with a high-level spinal injury may realistically have a different goal of being able to be mobile independently with the use of a mechanically adapted wheelchair such as a Sip-N-Puff chair. Both persons have achievable goals that are based upon their capacity and functional limitations that have resulted from illness or injury.

The goals of rehabilitation may be summarized with a few concepts: restoring or maximizing the level of function, facilitating independence, preventing complications, and promoting quality of life. Rehabilitation typically involves an interdisciplinary team of professionals working toward a common goal. The client and family are considered the most important team members. Professional team members may include physicians, nurses, therapists, social workers, vocational counselors, nutritionists, orthotists, prosthetists, and chaplains. Additional professionals may be consulted to help meet the unique needs of the individual.

Rehabilitation is commonly associated with certain disorders or illnesses in which therapeutic interventions have been shown to be effective. These include health alterations such as stroke, spinal cord injury, traumatic or other brain injury; neurologic diseases such as Parkinson's disease, multiple sclerosis (MS), Guillain-Barré syndrome; orthopedic problems such as arthritis, fractures, or joint replacements; and less commonly, burns, cancer, or respiratory disorders. In each of these conditions, persons can be assisted to regain maximal functioning that may have been altered because of a disease process, injury, or congenital defect.

One of the foci of the rehabilitation process is community reintegration or re-entry, sometimes referred to as resocialization. This is a process by which individuals are reintegrated into society after a life-altering health condition or situation changes their previous roles and abilities. Within a rehabilitation setting, reintegration is an ongoing goal. Rehabilitation professionals work with disabled clients or individuals with chronic illness and their families to help them re-enter their communities; they may have to accomplish significant adjustments to adapt to changes that have occurred in every area of their lives. Often this process involves the client re-learning how to do self-care with activities of daily living (ADLs) such as bathing, grooming, toileting, eating, and dressing. Rehabilitation is a hopeful process that encourages individuals to maximize their strengths while making positive adaptations to their limitations.

Definitions

Rehabilitation

Rehabilitation refers to services and programs designed to assist individuals who have experienced a trauma or illness that results in impairment that creates a loss of function (physical, psychological, social, or vocational) (Remsburg & Carson, 2006). Common themes among these definitions should be considered. Concepts include the complex, dynamic interactions among the individual, the disease or health condition, and the environment. Most definitions of rehabilitation include assisting an individual with a limitation to attain his or her maximal

independence and function. The Institute of Medicine (IOM) has defined rehabilitation as "the process by which physical, sensory or mental capacities are restored or developed. . . . Rehabilitation strives to reverse what has been called the disabling process, and may therefore be called the enabling process" (Brandt & Pope, 1997, pp. 12–13).

Rehabilitation Nursing

Rehabilitation is a continuous process, and clients rehabilitate themselves through the influence of the comprehensive approach to care provided by the rehabilitation nurse. Rehabilitation nurses are leaders who specialize in assisting individuals affected by chronic illness and disability to maximize their health through health restoration, maintenance, and promotion (Association of Rehabilitation Nurses [ARN], 2007). The ARN (2008) defines rehabilitation nursing as "the diagnosis and treatment of human responses of individuals and groups to actual or potential health problems related to altered functional ability and lifestyle" (p. 13).

General information for rehabilitation nurses and advanced rehabilitation nurses is included in the *Standards and Scope of Rehabilitation Nursing Practice* (ARN, 2008) and *Scope and Standards of Advanced Clinical Practice in Rehabilitation Nursing* (1996). Because of the growth of the specialty of rehabilitation nursing, there are many subspecialties associated with this field. The ARN has developed role descriptions of each of the emerging areas where rehabilitation nurses work.

Restorative Care

"The purpose of restorative care is to actively assist individuals in long-term care settings to maintain their highest level of function and to assist residents in retaining the gains made during formal therapy" (Remsburg & Carson, 2006, p. 580). Restorative care differs from rehabilitation in that it does not include activities directed by therapists but emphasizes nursing interventions that promote adaptation, comfort, and safety within a long-term care setting. Restorative care focuses on maximizing an individual's abilities, helping to rebuild self-esteem and to achieve appropriate goals (Nadash & Feldman, 2003; Resnick & Fleishall, 2002; Resnick & Remsburg, 2004). Restorative care often focuses on assisting individuals with ADLs as well as walking and mobility exercises, transferring, amputation/prosthesis care, and communication. Self-care skills, such as management of one's diabetes, ostomy care, or medication set-up and administration, are also emphasized (Remsburg, 2004). Restorative care, although conceptually similar to rehabilitation, is most appropriate for those individuals who either have already reached their maximal functional level and need to maintain that function, or for those who are not appropriate candidates for intensive rehabilitation services.

Vocational Rehabilitation

Vocational rehabilitation assists the disabled individual to return to gainful employment and focus on financial independence through programs specifically designed for this purpose (Kielhofner et al., 2004; Lysaght, 2004; O'Neill, Zuger, Fields, Fraser, & Pruce, 2004; Targett, Wehman, & Young, 2004). The federal government requires each state to have an office of vocational rehabilitation to provide these services for people with disabilities, and provides funding and support to integrate clients into the work community (Parker & Neal-Boylan, 2007).

Rehabilitation Models and Classification Systems

Models are used to help explain, guide, or direct practice or processes. Rehabilitation models can aid in understanding how chronic conditions and disability develop and progress, or how they can be managed. There are several major classification systems used to document rehabilitation processes and outcomes (Brandt & Pope, 1997; World Health Organization [WHO], 1980; WHO, 2002). These include the Functional Limitations System (FLS), the Enabling–Disabling Model, and the WHO International Classification of Functioning, Disability, and Health (ICF).

The IOM recommends the use of the Enabling–Disabling Process Model, whereas the WHO recommends the use of the ICF to help standardize and effectively communicate information about diagnoses, care, and treatment. The model used may depend largely on the facility and its preferences and choices. The use of standard terminology within these models can help facilitate communication, but rehabilitation professionals must be thoroughly familiar with the chosen model and understand the terminology within it.

The Enabling–Disabling Process

The Enabling–Disabling Process was developed at the IOM in 1997 as a framework for professional rehabilitation practice. It emphasizes the uniqueness of each individual client by revising the original Disability in America model generated by the IOM (Pope & Tarlov, 1991). A committee of professionals enhanced the 1991 IOM model "to show more clearly how biological, environmental (physical and social), and lifestyle/behavioral factors are involved in reversing the disabling process, i.e., rehabilitation, or the enabling process" (Brandt & Pope, 1997, p. 13). In the new Enabling–Disabling Process, "disability does not appear in this model since it is not inherent in the individual but, rather, a function of the interaction of the individual and the environment" (Brandt & Pope, 1997, p. 11). Disability is seen as a product of the interaction of an individual with the environment. The model posits that rehabilitation depends largely upon the individual and his or her unique characteristics, and that the disabling process may even be reversed with appropriate rehabilitation interventions (Lutz & Bowers, 2003). The basic concepts of the model include pathology, impairment, functional limitation, disability, and society limitation (Brandt & Pope, 1997). **Table 24-1** provides a summary of the concepts of the Enabling–Disabling Process.

Enabling America (Brandt & Pope, 1997) urged rehabilitation professionals to adopt a framework that better described the rehabilitation process. Since its introduction, however, the Enabling–Disabling Model has not received the recognition or use within healthcare professions that was probably hoped for by the IOM. A search of several notable scholarly databases over the last 10 years revealed few articles written by rehabilitation professionals in healthcare professions that mentioned this process or used it as a framework for research.

International Classification of Functioning, Disability, and Health

In 1980, the WHO developed a classification system that was widely used for years internationally. The WHO originally defined impairment as a loss related to structure and function;

a disability was related to a loss of ability to perform an activity, and a handicap was a disadvantage for a person related to the environment.

The ICF is the WHO's framework for measuring health and disability at both individual and population levels: "ICF is a classification of health and health related domains that describe body functions and structures, activities and participation. The domains are classified from body, individual and societal perspectives" (WHO, 2007, p. 1). The ICF provides a shift in viewing disability as gradually becoming a part of the majority of person's lives over time. It provides a holistic look at the process of disability related to health, considering all aspects, not just the medical or physical (WHO, 2007). The four major sections of the classification document are body functions (by system and including mental health), body structures (by system), activities and participation (such as learning, communication, self-care, community involvement), and environmental factors (such as products, technology, attitudes, service, and policy) (WHO, 2007). **Table 24-2** provides an overview of ICF.

Other models that can guide rehabilitation practice have emerged from rehabilitation nurse scientists. These middle-range theories are not classification systems for general rehabilitation, but provide insight and direction about specific processes or phenomena. An example of an area in which several new frameworks or models have arisen is in stroke rehabilitation and recovery. Secrest and colleagues (Secrest & Zeller, 2007; Secrest & Thomas, 1999) have explored the relationship of continuity and discontinuity following stroke. They continue to publish about the relationship of this phenomenon with

Table 24-1   Concepts of the Enabling–Disabling Process

Pathophysiology	Impairment	Functional Limitation	Disability	Societal Limitation
Interruption of or interference with normal physiologic and developmental processes or structures	Loss and/ or abnormality of cognition, and emotional, physiologic, or anatomic structure or function, including all losses or abnormalities, not just those attributable to the initial pathophysiology	Restriction or lack of ability to perform an action in the manner or within a range consistent with the purpose of an organ or organ system	Inability or limitation in performing tasks, activities, and roles to levels expected within physical and social contexts	Restriction, attributable to social policy or barriers (structural or attitudinal), that limits fulfillment of roles or denies access to services and opportunities that are associated with full participation in society

Level of Impact				
Cells and Tissues	**Organs and Organ Systems**	**Function of the Organ and Organ System**	**Individual**	**Society**
Structural or functional	Structural or functional	Action or activity performance or organ or organ system	Task performance by person in physical, social contexts	Societal attributes relevant to individuals with disabilities

Patient Examples				
Lacunar infarct of the cerebellum (right hemisphere) related to microvascular changes associated with chronic hypertension	Neuromotor function of the brain	Left hemiparesis or difficulty with spatial–perceptual tasks, difficulty sequencing, memory deficits	Deficits in ambulation, self-care, shopping, work	Lack of adaptations in the work environment that would enable the person to continue employment

Source: Whyte, J. (1998). Enabling America: A report from the Institute of Medicine on rehabilitation science and engineering. *Archives of Physical Medicine and Rehabilitation, 79*(11), 1477–1480. Reprinted with permission from Elsevier.

functional ability, depression, and quality of life. Their work resulted in the development of a tool to measure themes common to the post-stroke experience such as control, connection with others, and independence (Secrest & Zeller, 2003).

Mauk (Easton, 2001; Mauk, 2006) developed a model from grounded theory that

Table 24-2   Concepts of the International Classification of Functioning, Disability, and Health

Major Concepts

Health Condition	Impairment	Activity Limitation	Participation Restriction
Diseases, disorders, and injuries, e.g., leprosy, diabetes, spinal cord injury	Problems in body function or structure such as a significant deviation or loss, e.g., anxiety, paralysis, loss of sensation of extremities	Problems in body function or structure such as a significant deviation or loss, e.g., anxiety, paralysis, loss of sensation of extremities	Problems an individual may experience in involvement in life situations, e.g., unable to attend social events, unable to use public transportation to get to church, unable to perform job functions

Example

Spinal cord injury	Paralysis	Incapable of using public transportation	Unable to attend religious activities

Source: World Health Organization. (2002). *Towards a common language for functioning, disability and health ICF*. Retrieved September 21, 2011, from: www.who.int/classifications/icf/training/icfbeginnersguide.pdf.

identified six phases of post-stroke recovery that may help guide practice and interventions. She found that stroke survivors journey through a predictable pattern, with certain variables influencing the ease of adaptation after stroke. Other rehabilitation nurse scientists have explored the experience of caregivers of stroke survivors (Hartke & King, 2002; Pierce, Steiner, Govani, et al., 2004; Pierce, Steiner, Hicks, & Holzaepfel, 2006). Each of these examples suggest that although large, general models and classification systems are necessary and helpful, more manageable models, frameworks, and instruments are also needed to better reflect the unique experiences in rehabilitation and to guide practice.

Historical Perspectives

Rehabilitation as a specialty within medicine, and later nursing, was slow to develop (see **Table 24-3**). A general apathy toward the poor,

disabled, disenfranchised, and elderly prevailed in European countries and the United States. England was the first developed country to pass legislation in The Poor Relief Act of 1662 to provide assistance to the poor and disabled (Edwards, 2007).

There was some interest in rehabilitation in the 1800s, mainly with regard to helping "crippled" children (Edwards, 1992). In the first half of the 1900s, society began to focus more on the needs of persons with physical limitations. Susan Tracy, a nurse and teacher, helped to develop the discipline of occupational therapy. The first medical social service department was established at Bellevue Hospital in New York City, and Lillian Wald began the first visiting nursing service (Easton, 1999).

The World Wars provided an impetus for the growth of rehabilitation. The number of American soldiers wounded in World War I led to the establishment of a national rehabilitation

Table 24-3   Historical Events and Legislative Initiatives Affecting Rehabilitation

Date	Event/Initiative	Purpose
1910	"Studies of Invalid Occupation"	Published by nurse Susan Tracy; beginning of occupational therapy
1917	American Red Cross Institute for Crippled and Disabled Men personnel	Created to provide vocational training for wounded military
1918	Smith-Sears Legislation (PL 65-178)	Authorized Federal Board for Vocational Education to administer a national vocational rehabilitation service to disabled veterans of World War I
1920	Smith-Fess Legislation (PL 66-236)	Provided vocational rehabilitation services to people disabled in industry and otherwise
1930	Veteran's Administration (VA)	Created by Executive Order 5398 to care for those with service-related disabilities, signed by President Herbert Hoover. At this time there were 54 hospitals and 4.7 million living veterans.
1935	Social Security Act (PL 74-271)	Provided permanent authorization for the civilian vocational rehabilitation program
1938	American Academy of Physical Medicine	Organization formed; physical medicine and rehabilitation emerges as a specialty
1941	First comprehensive book on physical medicine and rehabilitation	*Krusen's Handbook of Physical Medicine and Rehabilitation*, written by Frank Krusen, MD
1942	Sister Kenny Institute	Institute and Sister Kenny's research led to the development of the profession of physical therapy and provided support for physiatry as a specialty
1943	Welsh-Clark Legislation (PL 78-16)	Provided vocational rehabilitation for disabled veterans of World War II
1943	United Nations Rehabilitation Administration	Organization established with representatives from 44 countries to plan care for disabled WWII veterans
1946	Department of Medicine and Surgery	A department within the VA established to provide medical care for veterans; succeeded in 1989 by the Veterans Health Services and Research Administration, renamed the Veterans Health Administration in 1991
1947	Bellevue Medical Rehabilitation Services	First U.S. rehabilitation program, established by Howard Rusk, MD
1947	American Board of Physical Medicine and Rehabilitation	Board formed, and rehabilitation becomes a board-certified specialty

(continues)

Table 24-3   Historical Events and Legislative Initiatives Affecting Rehabilitation (Continued)

Date	Event/Initiative	Purpose
1954	Hill-Burton Act (PL 83-565)	Provided greater financial support, research and demonstration grants, state agency expansion, and grants to expand rehabilitation facilities
1958	Rehabilitation Medicine	H. Rusk and colleagues publish a rehabilitation text
1965	Vocational Rehabilitation Act (PL 89-333)	Expanded and improved vocational rehabilitation services
1973	Rehabilitation Act (PL 93-112)	Expanded services to the more severely handicapped by giving them priority; affirmative action in employment and nondiscrimination in facilities
1974	Association of Rehabilitation Nurses	Organization formed; rehabilitation nursing emerges as a specialty
1975	Education for All Handicapped Act (PL 94-142)	Provided for a free appropriate education for handicapped children in the least restrictive setting possible
1975	National Housing Act Amendments (PL 94-173)	Provided for the removal of barriers in federally supported housing; established Office of Independent Living for disabled people in Department of Housing and Urban Development
1975	*Rehabilitation Nursing*	First issue published
1981	*Rehabilitation Nursing: Concepts and Practice—A Core Curriculum*	First core curriculum of rehabilitation nursing published
1982	Tax Equity and Fiscal Responsibility Act (TEFRA)	Originally designed to be a bridge from the old fee-for-service system to the DRG system; free-standing rehabilitation hospitals reimbursed based on reasonable costs (with limits)
1984	Diagnosis-Related Groupings (DRGs)	Established to decrease Medicare payments through the establishment of a prospective payment system for acute care
1989	Omnibus Budget Reconciliation Act (OBRA)	Contained legislation on nursing home reform; required standards for nursing assistant education and certification; required Health Care Financing Administration (HCFA) to develop a standardized assessment instrument and move from a fee-for-service system to a prospective payment system
1989	Department of Veterans Affairs	VA becomes the 14th department in the President's Cabinet.
1990	Americans with Disabilities Act (PL 101-336)	Established a clear discrimination on the basis of disability
1997	Balanced Budget Act (BBA)	Enacted to restructure Medicare Part A reimbursement methods; mandated a prospective payment reimbursement system for rehabilitation hospitals and units

Table 24-3 Historical Events and Legislative Initiatives Affecting Rehabilitation (Continued)

Date	Event/Initiative	Purpose
1999	Balanced Budget Act Amendment	Provided adjustments to PPS for skilled nursing facilities
2001	PPS for Inpatient Rehabilitation Facilities	PPS mandated by the 1997 BBA phase-in begins
2001	New Freedom Initiative	President George W. Bush launches a nationwide effort to remove barriers to community living for people of all ages with disabilities and long-term illnesses; goals of the initiative include increasing access to assistive technologies, expanding educational opportunities, and promoting full access to community life.
2003	PPS for Inpatient Rehabilitation Facilities	Phase-in complete; case-mix groups (CMGs) are used as the basis for reimbursement.
2004	CMS modifies criteria used to classify inpatient rehabilitation facilities (IRF)	Phase-in begins for "75% rule." By 2007, 75% of population treated in the facility must match one or more specified medical conditions.

Sources: Adapted from Larsen, P. (1998). "Rehabilitation." In I. Lubkin & P. Larsen (Eds.), *Chronic illness: Impact and interventions* (4th ed., p. 534); Easton, K. (1999). *Gerontological rehabilitation nursing* (pp. 32, 41). Philadelphia: W.B. Saunders; Kelly, P. (1999). Reimbursement mechanisms. In A. S. Luggen & S. Meiner (Eds.), *NGNA core curriculum for gerontological nursing* (pp. 185–186). St. Louis: Mosby; Blake, D., & Scott, D. (1996). Employment of persons with disabilities. *Physical Medicine and Rehabilitation* (p. 182). Philadelphia: W.B. Saunders; Department of Veterans Affairs. (2000). Facts about the Department of Veterans Affairs. Retrieved from: http://www.va.gov/vetdata/Quick_Facts.asp

program for veterans. It is interesting to note that rehabilitation services at this time were not generally available to the public. With the discovery of sulfa drugs and antibiotics, those injured in World War II had a much greater chance of survival. So, the numerous veterans of World War II coming home with multiple trauma, amputations, traumatic brain injuries, and spinal cord injuries necessitated a more comprehensive rehabilitation program. During this time, Dr. Howard Rusk (1965) emerged as both a pioneer and champion for rehabilitation, believing that these therapeutic services should be available not just to veterans, but to the entire world population. He demonstrated to the military powers through his personal assistance with the rehabilitation of those whom other medical professionals deemed a lost cause, that rather than convalescence, rehabilitation could promote recovery (Kottke, Stillwell, & Lehmann, 1982). Rusk showed that disabled persons could still be productive members of society and enjoy a good quality of life. As technology continued to explode in the 1940s, the number of civilians with industry and motor vehicle injuries increased, leading to a need for rehabilitation to address continuing disability. In 1947, Dr. Rusk established the first hospital-based medical rehabilitation services for civilians (Edwards, 2007).

The American Academy of Physical Medicine and Rehabilitation was established in 1938, and rehabilitation medicine was recognized as a board-certified medical specialty in 1947. In 1974, the ARN was created, recognizing rehabilitation as a nursing specialty.

As societies continue to pursue medical and technologic advances that allow persons with extreme levels of physical disability to live longer, rehabilitation has become a specialty in demand. In the civilian population, more persons are living with disabilities, as first responders are better equipped to aid survival of serious injury. However, the need to address continuing adjustment to disability remains. In addition, as life expectancy in developed countries increases, chronic illness rates also rise, providing additional opportunities for rehabilitation professionals to enhance quality of life for those aging with disability or acquiring it with age.

For soldiers, the types of weapons used in the wars in Iraq and Afghanistan have resulted in polytraumatic injuries never seen before. Rehabilitation professionals are being called upon to address multiple injuries that may include a combination of multiple traumatic amputations, burns, internal organ and soft-tissue damage from explosive forces, brain and spinal injuries, as well as post-traumatic stress.

Public Policy and Rehabilitation

There are several ways in which rehabilitation services may be paid for. These include Medicare, Medicaid, workers' compensation, private insurance, and social security disability benefits. Rehabilitation professionals should be familiar with these types of reimbursement and what is covered under the client's insurance provider. Case managers and social workers are team members who may be excellent resources regarding payment for rehabilitation.

Medicare

Medicare is a federal social insurance program that provides care for persons over the age of 65 and for certain younger persons with disabilities. The coverage and costs for Medicare change each year, so clients need to be aware of significant changes annually. Medicare Part A is the hospital insurance, providing funds for hospital care, skilled nursing, hospice, and home health care. Medicare Part B covers medically necessary services as well as some preventive services, with a monthly charge. Part B covers 80% of the costs of physician services, and other services including physical and occupational therapy, durable medical equipment, cardiac rehabilitation, pulmonary rehabilitation (for those with moderate to severe chronic obstructive pulmonary disease [COPD] within certain parameters), and prosthetics and orthotics (Centers for Medicare & Medicaid Services [CMS], 2011b). Many services that a rehabilitation client may need are not covered under Medicare. For example, Medicare has limited coverage for eye or hearing exams in special cases, but it does not cover routine foot care or nursing home care. Medicare Part C, referred to as the Medicare Advantage Plan, is a combination of Parts A and B, and functions much like a preferred provider organization or health maintenance organization using managed care (Doherty, 2004; Emmer & Allendorf, 2004; Stuart, 2006). Medicare Part D (CMS, 2011b) is a prescription drug plan in which private companies issue plans through Medicare. Part D is available for anyone with Medicare regardless of income. Costs vary greatly within this plan and clients would be wise to compare and review various plans each year prior to re-enrollment or plan changes.

The major changes in Medicare for 2011 were summarized in the CMS (2011b) publication *Medicare and You* and include: 1) no coinsurance or deductible for most preventive services, 2) a paid yearly wellness exam, 3) having to use certain suppliers for durable medical equipment, and 4) specific dates for making changes to health and prescription drug coverage.

Rehabilitation facilities and hospitals, collectively called inpatient rehabilitation facilities (IRFs), currently receive reimbursement using a Prospective Payment System (PPS) through the Social Security Act (CMS, 2011a). The IRF PPS uses information from the Uniform Data System for Medical Rehabilitation (UDSMR), better known as the Functional Independence Measure (FIM) tool, "to classify patients into distinct groups based on clinical characteristics and expected resource needs. Separate payments are calculated for each group, including the application of case and facility level adjustments" (CMS, 2011a, paragraph 2). Codes are assigned to case-mix groups (CMGs), and Medicare pays a specific amount per discharge.

Since 2004, Medicare has been phasing in new rules for IRFs. The case-mix classifications for 2008 used the same as those for 2007. Common medical conditions covered under the IRF rule include stroke, brain injury, spinal cord injury, amputation, multiple trauma, neurologic disorders, cardiac and pulmonary conditions, osteoarthritis, rheumatoid arthritis, pain syndrome, and certain joint replacements (Federal Register, 2007).

Medicare limits the amount it pays for physical, occupational, and speech therapy services. There is a deductible for Part B Medicare, after which Medicare pays 80% and the individual pays 20% up to the set limits for medically necessary therapies. There are some allowable exceptions to this rule, and appropriate documentation by the provider is essential.

Medicaid

Medicaid is a state-run program in concert with the federal government that is the largest source of medical care payments for persons with low income and limited resources. In 2007, President Bush introduced a plan to place new restrictions on the rehabilitative services (called the rehab option) allowed through Medicaid to save the federal budget $2.29 billion over 5 years. Nearly 75% of persons receiving rehab services under Medicaid were those with mental health needs, and they were responsible for 79% of the rehab option spending (Kaiser Commission, 2007). Currently 47 states provide some type of mental or physical health services under the rehab option.

Establishing Medicaid is a complex process that varies among states (Santerre, 2002). Although each state sets standards for its own programs, the federal government provides broad guidelines for those who may qualify under categorically needy, medically needy, and special groups (such as some persons with disabilities). States must provide long-term care for persons who are Medicaid eligible. State Medicaid programs offer a variety of services within a variety of settings. Services that are provided relative to rehabilitation for the categorically needy include: hospitalization, lab and X-rays, nursing facilities for those age 21 and older, physician and some nurse practitioner services, medical-surgical dental needs, and home health (CMS, 2005).

Workers' Compensation

Workers' compensation is a state income-support program. To be eligible, the injury or condition must be work related. Benefits are usually calculated as a percentage of the employee's weekly earnings at the time the injury occurred. There are restrictions placed by each state on the maximum amount of benefits, often two-thirds of the gross salary (Deutsch & Dean-Baar, 2007). The types of benefits may range from temporary partial or total disability to permanent partial or total disability, or death. Some states have a maximum benefit period and some may require a waiting period. Disabled workers may be compensated through spousal benefits (in case of death), medical and rehabilitation expense coverage, and lost wages (Kiselica, Sibson, & Green-McKenzie, 2004). Current workers' compensation programs are more restrictive than they once were; they limit physician choice and eligibility, provide lower benefits, and use managed care for cost containment (D'Andrea & Meyer, 2004).

Private Insurance

Most private insurances pay for at least some rehabilitative services. There is generally a deductible and often a co-pay, which may be higher if the provider is not within the network of providers supplied by the insurance company. In the case where the person has private insurance and Medicare as a secondary payer, much of the therapy services may be covered, provided there is sufficient and ongoing documentation of medical necessity and progress toward goals. Private insurance may also provide disability income insurance, accidental death and dismemberment insurance, or other benefits.

Social Security Disability Income

Social Security Disability Income (SSDI) was established in 1956 as part of the Social Security Disability Act of 1954. This is a federally administered disability insurance program for those who meet the strict definition of disability under Social Security. The criteria for disability is threefold: 1) the person cannot do the same work he or she did before; 2) it is determined that the person cannot adapt to other work because of the existing medical condition; and 3) the disability has lasted for at least 1 year, or is expected to result in death (Social Security Online, 2007). The person must also have worked and paid into the Social Security

program before the disability. SSDI is paid as a monthly benefit.

Supplemental Security Income (SSI) may provide disability benefits for persons who have not worked long enough to receive SSDI. The SSI program pays benefits to disabled adults and children with limited income and resources, or certain older persons with severely limited income. Persons may receive a monthly check, and the SSI program also helps individuals to access Medicare benefits and take advantage of other possible assistance through the federal government. Qualifying for the program is based on income and resources (Social Security Online, 2007).

Disability Benefits for Veterans

The Department of Veterans Affairs, often called the VA, provides a number of benefits for veterans: "Disability compensation is a benefit paid to a veteran because of injuries or diseases that happened while on active duty, or were made worse by active military service. It is also paid to certain veterans disabled from VA health care" (VA, 2011). These benefits are tax free and may include a monthly stipend (ranging from $123 to $2673), priority medical care through the VA, clothing and housing allowances (to make accommodations), adaptive equipment, and various grants as needed (VA, 2010). The VA also provides vocational rehabilitation by maintaining working relationships with many businesses to employ veterans with physical and mental or emotional disabilities. Consultation is available in many areas including employment, assistive technology, case management, work site and job analysis, and help in addressing Americans with Disabilities Act (ADA) compliance issues (VA, 2010).

Vocational Rehabilitation

Vocational rehabilitation is an important part of the rehabilitation process, carrying heavier weight for those of working age and certain racial–ethnic groups for whom work is part of personal identify and reputation. In 1918, Congress passed the Smith-Sears Act to assist with national vocational rehabilitation services to veterans who served in World War I. In 1920, The Smith-Fess Act made vocational rehabilitation services available for all persons with disabilities, not just those with war-related injuries (Buchanan, 1996). More significant legislation was enacted when The Rehabilitation Act of 1973 provided funds to support state vocational rehabilitation programs. The Rehabilitation Services Administration (RSA) of the U.S. Department of Education (2005) coordinates vocational rehabilitation services. The RSA (2007) states that it "oversees grant programs that help individuals with physical or mental disabilities to obtain employment and live more independently through the provision of such supports as counseling, medical and psychological services, job training and other individualized services" (p. 1). This is accomplished through dispensing funds to state grant programs to assist them with finding work-related services or programs for persons with disabilities, particularly the severely disabled. The RSA is the Congressionally appointed federal agency charged with implementing the various titles associated with The Rehabilitation Act of 1973. This agency acts as a resource for information and a leader in advocating at all levels for national programs that help to remove barriers for persons with disabilities (RSA, 2007).

The services provided in vocational rehabilitation are many, but generally include personal counseling, mental and physical health services, and assistance with vocational placement and job training (Kielhofner et al., 2004; Lysaght, 2004; O'Neill et al., 2004; Targett et al., 2004). In addition, the RSA helps administer projects with specific groups of persons such as migrant and seasonal farm workers, American Indians, older adults, and the visually impaired. One principle of vocational rehabilitation is that informed consumer choice promotes enhanced employment outcomes. For vocational rehabilitation to be effective and enhance quality of life for the person with mental disabilities, the agency and counselors must work closely with the employer and the client to find the working environment suited to that individual (Inman, McGurk, & Chadwick, 2007; Morgan, 2007). Employment outcomes are most frequently used as the measure of the success of vocational rehabilitation for those with disabilities (Kosciulek, 2007). More research is needed to explore the factors related to positive outcomes of vocational rehabilitation.

Vocational rehabilitation may not be a goal for all rehabilitation clients. Many older adults requiring rehabilitation services are retired, and employment is not a goal. However, for those younger persons with functional limitations or mental health impairments, work may be directly related to their sense of self and identify within their culture. For these persons, vocational rehabilitation plays an important part in the comprehensive rehabilitation process, and the vocational rehabilitation counselor will be an essential team member.

Americans with Disabilities Act

The ADA enacted in 1990 guarantees individuals with physical disabilities equal access to

Table 24-4 Americans with Disabilities Act	
Title 1: Employment	Employers cannot discriminate against a qualified disabled job applicant or employee in any manner related to employment and benefits.
	Employers must make their existing facilities accessible and usable by individuals with disabilities.
	Accommodations in all aspects of job attainment and performance are required in order to place individuals on an equal plane with the nondisabled.
Title 2: Public Services	Qualified disabled individuals must have access to all services and programs provided by state or local governments. Public rail transportation must be made accessible to disabled individuals and supplemented with paratransit.
Title 3: Public Accommodations Services Operated by Private Entities	Virtually every entity open to the public must now be made accessible to the disabled. A study is to be conducted concerning accessibility of the over-the-road transportation.
Title 4: Telecommunications Relay	Telephone companies are required to furnish telecommunication devices to enable hearing- and speech-impaired individuals to communicate by wire or radio.

Source: Reprinted from Watson, P. (1990). The Americans with Disabilities Act: More rights for people with disabilities. *Rehabilitation Nursing, 15*, 326. Published by the Association of Rehabilitation Nurses, 4700 W. Lake Avenue, Glenview, IL 60025-1485. Copyright © 1990 by the Association of Rehabilitation Nurses. Used with permission.

public accommodations related to transportation, education, and employment. Employment discrimination of qualified applicants because of disabilities is prohibited by this law (U.S. Equal Employment Opportunity Commission, 2008). Although the Rehabilitation Act of 1973 and its amendments covered accessibility to buildings of organizations that received federal financial assistance, the ADA also requires private organizations to comply with accessibility and employment laws. The concept of reasonable accommodation was introduced, requiring employers to make those accommodations within reason that may be necessary for a person with disability. **Table 24-4** provides a summary of the ADA related to the

four major areas it addresses: employment, public services, public accommodations services by practice entities, and telecommunications relay.

REHABILITATION ISSUES AND CHALLENGES

Rehabilitation services provided by an interdisciplinary team within a variety of settings suggest several possible challenges for providers. These include the rising costs of care, caregiver burden, inequities among those with disabilities, the negative image of disability, the changing composition of the disabled population, ethical issues, providing culturally competent care, and professional and informal caregiver issues.

Rising Care Costs

It is estimated that 133 million Americans have at least one chronic illness, with 25% of those individuals having one or more daily activity limitation (Centers for Disease Control and Prevention [CDC], 2009). Forty-two million persons (17% of the U.S. population) were uninsured and 32 million (13%) received Medicaid assistance. Of those uninsured, the major reason cited was cost. About 10.7 million (5%) adults were unable to work because of health-related problems. Persons with less education and who were poor were less likely to be able to work because of health problems (Adams, Dey, & Vickerie, 2007). The American government spends about $200 billion per year on assistance for persons with disabilities (Council of State Administrators of Vocational Rehabilitation, 2004–2005). Given these statistics, major challenges for rehabilitation professionals are to assist persons to attain and regain their health and become productive, working members of society, and to explore other means of providing access to health care.

Caregiver Burden

Because an event requiring rehabilitation happens to the entire family and community, not just the client, it is important to address the needs of caregivers throughout the rehabilitation process and/or chronic illness trajectory. Family members comprise the vast majority (72%) of paid and unpaid caregivers of older persons with functional limitations from chronic disease, with adult children caregivers (42%) and spouses (25%) bearing the largest burden of care (Shirey & Summer, 2000). The caregiver's ability to cope with the care demands is influenced by a variety of factors including the type and severity of illness, the length of quality of recovery, social support, inherent caregiver factors, and coping ability. This may hold true for both formal and informal caregivers (Bushnik, Wright, & Brudsall, 2007). For example, the caregiver spouse of a person with uncomplicated coronary bypass surgery may be able to meet care demands over a limited period of rehabilitation, whereas the older spouse caregiver of a stroke survivor with severe aphasia and functional deficits may be facing years of caregiving—a burden that is often overwhelming.

Caregiver burden, the effects of caregiving-related stress on family members or other care providers, has been associated with a number of health problems in the caregiver. Emotional distress, anxiety, depression, decreased quality of life, hypertension, lowered immune function, and increased mortality are among the concerns noted by researchers of caregivers (Anderson, Linto, & Stewart-Wynne, 1995; Brouwer et al., 2004; Canam & Acorn, 1999; das Chagas Medeiros, Ferraz, & Quaresma, 2000; Grunfeld et al., 2004; Hughes et al., 1999; King, Hartke, & Denby, 2007; Kolanowski, Fick, Waller, & Shea, 2004; Lieberman & Fisher, 1995; Mills, Yu, Ziegler, Patterson, & Grant, 1999; Schulz & Beach, 1999; Shaw et al., 1999; Ski & O'Connell, 2007; Weitzenkamp, Gerhart, Charlifue, Whiteneck, & Savic, 1997; Wu et al., 1999). There is sufficient research since 1995 to demonstrate that the burden of caregiving over time can have a deleterious effect on the health of the family caregiver.

The caregiver burden is thought to be greater when more care is required. Research suggests that although education and training programs have some effect on caregiver stress levels, the benefit is short term and caregivers are likely to need ongoing involvement from care professionals to help maintain their own health (Draper et al., 2007; Halm, Treat-Jacobson, Lindquist, & Savik, 2007; King et al., 2007). Assessment of caregiver burden should be included in the rehabilitation plan of care (see Chapter 10). Early identification and interventions related to managing caregiver stress may result in better outcomes for the entire family, and appropriate discharge planning and follow up are an important part of the process.

Inequities Among Disabled Americans

According to the CDC (CDC, 2007b):

> Despite great improvements in the overall health of the nation, Americans who are members of racial and ethnic minority groups, including blacks or African Americans, Hispanics or Latinos, and other Pacific Islanders, are more likely than whites to have poor health and die prematurely. (paragraph 2)

The groups experiencing the most disparity are the ones predicted to grow at a faster rate than the general population. This is especially true of the Hispanic group, with minorities accounting for about 90% of the predicted population growth by 2050 (Minority Business Development Agency, 1999).

The National Health Interview Survey (NHIS) of 2005

> is a household, multistage probability sample survey conducted annually by interviewers of the U.S. Census Bureau for the CDC's National Center for Health Statistics. In 2005, household interviews were completed

> for 98,649 persons living in 38,509 households, reflecting a household response rate of 86.5%. (Adams et al., 2007, p. 8)

The survey looked at multiple factors including respondent-assessed health status, functional ability, healthcare access, and healthcare insurance coverage. The data revealed several inequities among disabled Americans, similar to the results of the National Organization on Disability (NOD) survey (2004).

The NHIS showed that 3.8 (2% of the U.S. population) million adults need help with ADLs and 7.8 million adults (4%) need assistance with (instrumental activities of daily living [IADLs] such as shopping or household chores). The need for assistance dramatically increases with age, with 10% of those older than 75 years requiring assistance with ADLs and 19% needing help with IADLs (Adams et al., 2007; Fried, Bradley, Williams, & Tinetti, 2001). It is estimated that in 2004, 34% of the noninstitutionalized American population older than age 65 had activity limitations caused by chronic health conditions (Adams et al., 2007). Add to that those older adults who reside in long-term care facilities, and there is a significant number of older adults whose daily lives are affected by chronic illness.

Many persons in minority groups experience a double jeopardy or double minority status when they acquire disability. Caucasians and Asians were more likely to report excellent health than African Americans. Hispanic persons younger than age 65 (34%) were more than 2.5 times as likely as non-Hispanics (14%) in the same age cohort to be uninsured. Both older age and poverty are factors that are associated with poorer health status and increased disability. The poor elderly were three to four times more likely to need assistance with ADLs and IADLs than those who were not poor (Adams et al., 2007).

The survey from the NOD revealed significant differences among groups within the United States related to the factors of employment, income, education, socialization, religious involvement, access to health care, and transportation (NOD, 2004). This survey examined participation gaps between able-bodied and disabled Americans in 10 life areas. Only 35% of disabled Americans reported working full- or part-time compared with 78% of non-disabled Americans. Three times as many disabled Americans live in households with a total income of less than $15,000. Twenty-two percent of disabled Americans reported experiencing job discrimination. Persons with disabilities were less likely to attend church services, dine out, and socialize than nondisabled persons.

In the United States, the groups considered vulnerable populations (in which disparities in access to health care and transportation are often most prominent) include some minority groups, children, the elderly, the poor, those living in rural areas, and those with mental illness (Havercamp, Scandlin, & Roth, 2004; Reichard, Sacco, & Turnbull, 2004; U.S. Department of Health and Human Services & the Agency for Health Quality and Research, 2003). Prisoners are also a vulnerable group. The National Health and Nutrition Examination Survey indicated that non-Hispanic blacks and Mexican Americans generally report more disability than nonminorities, with minority women reporting more disability than men (Ostchega et al., 2000). American Indians have the highest disability rate (25%) of any other ethnic group. The most common types of self-reported disabilities include spinal cord injury, complications from diabetes, blindness, difficulty with ambulation, traumatic brain injury, deafness or hardness of hearing, orthopedic conditions, and mental health problems (Lomay & Hinkebein, 2006). Additional research is needed with these high-risk minority groups to understand these health-care disparities in order to develop strategies to address them.

Stigma of Disability

Although much progress has been made on a national policy level toward dispelling the negative image and stigma associated with disability through modifying rehabilitation models (Brandt & Pope, 1997; WHO, 2002), many persons with disabilities still report feelings of negative reactions from others regarding their differences. The disability could be something as relatively invisible as a hearing aid worn by an adolescent (Kent & Smith, 2006) to obvious employment discrimination for a person with mental illness (Stuart, 2006; Lloyd & Waghorn, 2007). One study found that a positive factor such as exercise done by a person with a physical disability may undermine the negative impressions that some persons have and fight the stigma of disability (Arbour, Latimer, Ginis, & Jung, 2007).

Changes made in today's rehabilitation models portray disability on a continuum, with a prominent factor being the environment. In a classic work by Zola (1982), the author toured a 65-acre utopia in The Netherlands as a professional visitor. The village was designed for those with disabilities who did not fit well into other existing societies, with complete and full accessibility, environmental adaptation, and removal of barriers. Each of the 400 members of the village had to contribute to their self-crafted society. However, in such an environment, persons functioned well and without stigma, because their situation was the new norm. Zola found himself feeling out of place, although able-bodied, suggesting that the environment is a key factor in perception of disability (see Chapter 3).

Persons with disabilities who have helped to change the perception of the public include role models in the arts, science, politics, and sports. Marla Runyon (Olympic runner), the late actor/director Christopher Reeve, actor Michael J. Fox, scientist Stephen Hawking, and Senator Max Cleland are just a few examples of such role models. Runyon is legally blind, yet participated as an Olympic runner in the 2000 games in Sydney, Australia. Christopher Reeve, the actor best known for his role as Superman, was a high-level, ventilator-dependent quadriplegic. Reeve continued to act and direct movies throughout his life and, along with his late wife, Dana, helped establish services for those with spinal cord injuries.

The actor Michael J. Fox experienced early-onset Parkinson's disease and has been a crusader for research in that area. Stephen Hawking, noted physicist and prolific author, was diagnosed with motor neuron disease (amyotrophic lateral sclerosis) at a relatively young age and yet has continued to work. Even after he was completely paralyzed by his disease, he continued to write with the use of technology and his blink reflex. Cleland, a triple amputee, was a United States senator and director of the VA. These individuals may seem remarkable because of their accomplishments; however, there are thousands of other "everyday" citizens with disabilities who are productive members and make significant contributions to society. Their stories are the untold ones.

Ethical and Legal Issues

Rehabilitation professionals are often in positions that require difficult decision making. Masters-Farrell (2006) states that the "conflict occurs when a choice must be made between two equal possibilities" (p. 590) and that an ethical dilemma is present when a situation forces one to evaluate and choose between two equally unattractive choices. For example, take the situation of a nonterminal rehabilitation client who had just told the nurse that he did not wish to be resuscitated if he should "code," but the paperwork for advance directives had not yet been completed, signed, or placed on the chart, and the nurse found him minutes later without a pulse or respirations. Although she must call the code team in this situation, the nurse is in conflict because she has intimate knowledge that this was action was contrary to the client's wishes.

Beauchamp and Childress (2001), in their classic text on principles of biomedical ethics, emphasize four cornerstone principles: respect for person, nonmaleficence, beneficence, and justice. These principles play into many aspects of rehabilitation practice and programming. Common ethical (and often legal) issues that pertain particularly to rehabilitation clients may include the following (Ellis & Hartley, 2004; Kirschner, Stocking, Wagner, Foye, & Siegler, 2001; Masters-Farrell, 2007):

- Withholding or withdrawing treatment
- Determining competence in decision making
- Do not resuscitate (DNR) orders
- Use of physical or chemical restraints
- Genetic screening
- Organ donation

- Guardianship
- Research on human subjects
- Disagreement between family members about treatment options
- Use of complementary and alternative medical treatments
- Advance directives (life-prolonging declarations, living wills, durable power of attorney)
- Informed consent
- Estate planning
- Determining legal death or brain death
- Substance abuse
- Confidentiality
- Defining quality of life
- Self-termination or assisted suicide
- Abuse of the vulnerable
- Allocation of resources and insurance coverage
- End-of-life decisions
- Long-term care placement

Ethics committees are becoming more popular in acute care hospitals and even retirement communities to assist in difficult decision making (Hogstel, Curry, Walker, & Burns, 2004; Hughes, 2004; Johnson, 2004; Nelson, 2004). Ellis and Hartley (2004) view the ethics committee as an interdisciplinary group of healthcare professionals that is established specifically to address ethical dilemmas that occur in a particular setting. Persons serving on an ethics committee may include physicians, nurses, advanced practice nurses, social workers, therapists, pastoral care personnel, members of the community, and an ethicist. The benefits of an ethics committee include allowing many perspectives to be discussed, providing a forum for communication,

fostering development of related policies, promoting awareness of existing and potential issues, and focusing on the patient (Masters-Farrell, 2007). Some disadvantages include the potential for inefficiency and political influence, and lack of time for participation.

Cultural Competency

Cultural sensitivity involves an awareness and consideration of a group's beliefs, values, communication styles, language, and behavior. Providing culturally sensitive rehabilitation care will be an even greater challenge in the future, with the changing demographics and increasing minority elderly population (Niemeier, Burnett, & Whitaker, 2003). How clients and families perceive disability and participate in rehabilitation is heavily influenced by cultural norms and expectations (Campinha-Bacote, 2001). The first step in becoming culturally sensitive is to know one's own self. Although some generalizations will be discussed here related to the major ethnic–racial groups, professionals should avoid stereotyping and seek individual information from each client. If needed, the services of a translator (not a family member) should be used. Because of the vast differences between and within the many cultural groups that rehabilitation professionals serve, it is wise to ask clients about their particular beliefs and practices. Even if one is familiar, for example, with the Lakota Indian health practices, this does not mean that the Navajo will practice precisely the same rituals and observances, although both will value Native American tradition.

African Americans are a group at high risk for many disabilities and chronic illnesses that warrant rehabilitative care, including hypertension, stroke, diabetes, and heart disease. African Americans typically have a close family structure, deep religious affiliations, and share a strong belief against placing older parents in long-term care facilities. They are generally open to rehabilitation programs and tend to experience disabling conditions at a younger age than do Caucasians. Career counseling for African Americans with disabilities should take into account the effects of double minority status: disability and racial. Rehabilitation professionals should realize that prejudice, oppression, and stigma are often attached to both of these factors, and a multidimensional, multicultural approach to care should be used (Mpofu & Harley, 2006).

Hispanic or Latino Americans enjoy strong family bonds. There is generally good family involvement for clients experiencing rehabilitation. However, severe disability may be seen as a punishment from God for some evil or wrongdoing and thus may stigmatize a person or family. Latinos tend to continue to work with a disability, but in some instances may show poorer outcomes, such as difficulty adjusting to life after stroke (Cook, Stickley, Ramey, & Knotts, 2005).

Among Asian cultures, there is a diversity of beliefs. However, a respect for healthcare professionals as well as Eastern healers often means that Asians will seek treatment for rehabilitative conditions. In Chinese and Japanese cultures, there is belief in the need for balance between positive and negative forces, between the hot and cold, between the male and female. These opposing and related forces are referred to as the yin and the yang. When the body is out of harmony, or lacks balance, illness may occur; emotional problems are believed to be linked to a weak character. There may be feelings of guilt and shame in having a disability, because it could indicate punishment for wrongdoing. Work is seen as fundamental to a successful and honorable life, but in Hong Kong, only 2.5% of male Chinese with psychiatric disabilities are permitted to seek employment (Yip & Ng, 2002). Asian Americans often seek alternative or complementary medicine, including herbal remedies, in addition to Western medicine and rehabilitation care.

As of the 2000 Census, there were 4.1 million American Indians living in the United States. These groups in general embrace the interrelatedness of the earth with the body and spirit, but tribes often have their own culturally distinct practices. They rely on a relatively private extended community and kinship ties. Most traditional American Indians value folk medicine over Westernized medical treatments and facilities. There is an innate distrust of those outside their community, given their history of oppression. Mortality has been drastically higher for American Indians when compared to the general U.S. population related to the following: alcoholism, 627%; tuberculosis, 533%; diabetes mellitus, 249%; accidents, 204%; suicide, 72%; pneumonia and influenza, 71%; and homicide, 63% (Indian Health Services [IHS], 2001). Rehabilitation professionals must be aware that today's American Indians may come from a mixed background of tribal customs, and that many will still believe in folk healers.

Several excellent resources are readily available to help develop cultural awareness and sensitivity. A helpful series of monographs online—and updated regularly—and in booklet form are available to assist rehabilitation professionals with cultural information (Center for International Rehabilitation Research Information and Exchange [CIRRIE], 2007). These informative papers provide information on 11 countries of origin for foreign-born groups in the United States including China, Cuba, Dominican Republic, El Salvador, India, Jamaica, Korea, Mexico, Philippines, Vietnam, and Haiti. More than 100 training programs for rehabilitation providers on a variety of issues related to various ethnic groups and disabilities are also available from The National Clearinghouse of Rehabilitation Training Materials (www.ncrtm.org).

Formal and Informal Caregiver Issues

As the population increases and the oldest of the elderly become the fastest growing age group, there will be a lack of physicians and nurses prepared to meet the care demand for the number of persons with chronic illness and disability. Currently, there is a lack of qualified physiatrists and nurses in the United States (Currie, Atchison, & Fiedler, 2002; Dean-Baar, 2003; Verville & DeLisa, 2001). The ARN (Secrest, 2007) has strongly advocated for certification in rehabilitation; there are nearly 10,000 nurses who hold the Certified Rehabilitation Registered Nurse (CRRN) credential. However, few nursing programs provide rehabilitation education as a separate course or have dedicated content to this specialty area. Getting healthcare professionals such as physicians and nurses interested in the specialty has been difficult because of its limited visibility in traditional educational programs (Neal, 2001; Thompson, Emrich, & Moore, 2003). The European Union has addressed concerns regarding a shortage of physicians trained in physical medicine and rehabilitation through the Union of European Medical Specialist (UEMS) by beginning to standardize training and education throughout its 28 member countries. Within these countries there are

13,000 specialists and more than 2800 trainees in physical and rehabilitation medicine (PRM) (Ward & Gutenbrunner, 2006), and the specialty is felt to be robust. Still, there is a concerted effort to recruit and educate physicians in PRM in Europe.

With more than 35 million people in America older than 65 years of age, there is an increased need for professionals trained to provide quality care to older adults. Older adults account for almost one fourth of ambulatory care visits, nearly one half of all hospital stays, and represent 83% of nursing facility residents (Kovner, Mezey, & Harrington, 2002; Mezey & Fulmer, 2002). Most nursing schools in this country have no full-time faculty certified in geriatric nursing; only a few of the nation's medical schools have a geriatric department, and less than 10% require a course in geriatrics (Remsburg & Carson, 2006). As of 2002, there were 63 master's programs that prepared nurses in geriatrics, but only 4,200 certified specialists (Mezey & Fulmer, 2002).

Despite concerted efforts to change it, there continues to be a negative stigma around care of older adults among nursing students. Without education in gerontology, healthcare professionals may not realize the rehabilitation potential of many of these older adults. The common rehabilitative disorders often are seen in the older age group, and even small improvements in function and independence can allow older adults to age in place and remain at home. Even those making long-term care or retirement communities their home can improve their strength and function with small lifestyle changes and exercise.

There is also a growing number of persons whose caregiving needs go unmet (Kennedy, 2001; LaPlante, Kaye, Kang, & Harrington,

2004). More than 34 million persons are limited in some way from usual activities because of chronic illness. It is estimated that there are 3.8 million adults with disabilities who require assistance with ADLs and 7.8 million who need help with IADLs (Adams et al., 2007). Persons who need assistance were more likely to be poor, older, and less educated. Persons whose needs are not met are more likely to experience discomfort, weight loss, dehydration, falls, and burns (LaPlante et al., 2004). Further research is needed to help identify consequences from unmet caregiving needs as well as strategies to address this growing problem.

INTERVENTIONS

The Rehabilitation Process

Rehabilitation is both a philosophy and a discipline (Secrest, 2007). Rehabilitation is based on the premise that all individuals have self-worth and are deserving of dignity, respect, and quality health care regardless of their limitations. Many concepts are imbedded in the field of rehabilitation and are reflected through such common sayings as:

- Rehabilitation begins day one
- What you do not use, you lose
- Progress is measured in small gains
- Independence is better than dependence
- Motivation is a key to success
- All care should include rehabilitation principles
- Activity strengthens and inactivity wastes
- If it can be corrected, it probably could have been prevented

Rehabilitation should begin from the first day the person is in the hospital. When healthcare professionals forget the basic principles of rehabilitation, complications such as contractures, pressure sores, and incontinence ensue. Rehabilitation includes nursing, medical therapies, and social services. It is an interdisciplinary team process focused on maintaining or restoring function, preventing complications, promoting independence and self-care, and enhancing quality of life.

Team Approach

The team approach is most effective when working with clients with complex needs such as those requiring rehabilitative services. Although there are several models used in this approach, the common threads are that the team members work toward goals that are mutually established with the client.

Prevailing models are either multidisciplinary, interdisciplinary, or transdisciplinary. Multidisciplinary teams involve professionals from different disciplines, each treating the client within their various areas; however, they may not coordinate their efforts in the care of a client (Secrest, 2007). The advantage of this type of model is that all professionals bring their education and expertise to promote the best outcomes for the client. However, the major weakness is that communication between and across the disciplines may be lacking.

In the transdisciplinary model, each client has a primary therapist from the team, who may be a nurse, physical therapist, or occupational therapist. One therapist is cross-trained to provide comprehensive care to the client (Secrest,

2007). Although this model may provide for continuity of care, issues surrounding licensure, scope of practice, and accountability abound. In addition, team members are often out of their comfort zone in providing services that they were not specifically trained for. Turf issues often complicate this type of care. Lastly, some organizations that have tried this model have given it up for a different approach because the team was not motivated to embrace it.

The most preferred rehabilitation team model is the interdisciplinary team (see **Table 24-5**). The interdisciplinary team approach involves each team member communicating on a regular basis with each other and establishing common goals for clients (Secrest, 2007). This is often accomplished through weekly team meetings in which the entire team reviews the progress of each client and mutual goals are discussed and updated. The client and family are an important part of the team as well. Nontraditional team members may be added to the team based on the client's needs. Table 24-5 lists other potential team members in addition to the client and family members.

Evaluation of the Client

An important element in considering rehabilitation as an option for any client is proper evaluation of rehabilitation potential. There are many factors that comprise such an evaluation, but several forces seem to play a major role. These include the severity of the illness, injury, or defect; functional level and cognitive status; willingness to participate; internal or external motivation (Kemp, 1986); social support (Fairfax, 2002); and available resources.

Rehabilitation Potential

For purposes of insurance coverage (i.e., the healthcare payers), clients receiving inpatient rehabilitation need to meet the minimum requirements of being able to tolerate at least 3 hours of therapy per day. Generally, a professional is assigned to do an evaluation of rehabilitation potential before the client is admitted to a program. This professional may be a social worker, nurse, case manager, clinical nurse specialist, or other clinician with appropriate education and evaluation skills. No one type of client provides a perfect profile of the usual

Table 24-5   Members of the Rehabilitation Team
Physiatrist
Certified rehabilitation registered nurse (CRRN)
Certified nursing assistant
Physical therapist
Physical therapist assistant
Occupational therapist
Certified occupational therapy assistant
Speech therapist/speech–language pathologist
Audiologist
Dietitian/nutritionist
Social worker
Psychologist
Therapeutic recreation specialist
Pastoral counselor
Prosthetist/orthotist
Case manager

patient. Rather, the evaluator uses his or her assessment skills to consider all the aspects of the person's life that could contribute to success in an intensive therapeutic program such as the likelihood of functional improvement given the person's illness or injury, internal motivation, and available support.

Although general criteria are followed for admission to a rehabilitation program, the uniqueness of each individual is considered by the evaluator. Over time, healthcare professionals develop an intuition that aids them in the selection of clients who are appropriate rehabilitation candidates. There may be occasions when, for example, a person with a low functioning level as a result of traumatic brain injury but who is highly motivated and has strong family support has better rehabilitation outcomes than the stroke patient with minimal functional deficits, but whose negative attitude is a deterrent to readiness for intensive therapy. Sometimes clients will be referred to a transitional care unit or post-acute care prior to rehabilitation admission, and then days or weeks later they may feel the motivation to enter acute rehabilitation.

For each specific disease or condition there are some factors that are associated with either more positive or negative outcomes. For example, history of previous stroke, advanced age, incontinence, and visual–spatial deficits are all associated with poorer outcomes after stroke (Brandstater, 2005). Easton (2001) found that stroke survivors who were older, had more life experience, knew the cause of their stroke, had realistic expectations, good social support, and expressed faith in God seemed to adapt better to their condition after stroke. Outcomes for older stroke survivors have been shown to improve with intensive inpatient rehabilitation (Jett, Warren, & Wirtalla, 2005).

Strengths of the Client, Family, and Environment

Another important factor in the evaluation process is the identification of the client's and family's strengths. Questions to ask during this assessment should include: What can the client do for him- or herself? What does the client see as his or her own strengths and weaknesses? What are the family's strengths and weaknesses? What coping mechanisms does the client typically use, and will they be sufficient for the current crisis? What community resources are available to the family and client? What are the client's personal goals? A highly motivated client and supportive family are important to the success of the rehabilitation process.

Functional Assessment

Although functional assessment is important, the evaluator should not forget that a true evaluation of rehabilitation potential must consider all factors, not just physical or function related. Functional assessment includes an evaluation that identifies one's ability to perform self-care and physical activities. The two approaches generally used are asking questions and observation (Guse, 2006).

A number of tools are available to assess function, although these are mainly aimed at screening for disability. Functional assessment tools include: 1) the development of a client problem list, 2) goal setting based on identified strengths and weaknesses of the client, 3) evaluation of the client's progress and outcomes, 4) measurement of treatment interventions, 5) cost–benefit effectiveness of care, 6) assistance in the rehabilitation program's evaluation and audit, and 7) research (Remsburg & Carson, 2006, p. 601).

CASE STUDY

Adjustment to Life-Altering Condition

Dr. Janes, a community dentist, was diagnosed with MS at age 54. His clinical patterns proved to be the relapsing-remitting type with slowly progressive disability and loss of function over time. By the age of 60, Dr. Janes retired because complications of his MS such as fatigue, visual problems, and poor balance made it difficult to continue his busy pediatric dentistry practice. His wife was frustrated with his decline in health and early retirement. Dr. Janes consulted a clinical nurse specialist during the last hospitalization for a severe exacerbation to help better manage his condition after retirement, now that he was "able to focus on his own health more." A new medication in the group of immunomodifiers proved effective in reducing the number and severity of exacerbations per year and working with the rehabilitation team on an outpatient basis helped to improve Dr. Janes's quality of life.

Discussion Questions

1. What team members would have been involved in Dr. Janes's rehabilitation in the inpatient rehabilitation unit after an acute exacerbation of his MS?
2. What goals would be appropriate for Dr. Janes in the long term? Short term?
3. Name two tools or classification systems that would be appropriate in evaluating Dr. Janes's functional ability.
4. If you developed a long-term plan of care for Dr. Janes, what outcomes would be appropriate over a 10-year period?

Evaluators may use a variety of methods to complete a functional assessment. Generally, a combination of self-report, whether in the form of a questionnaire completed by the person or the interviewer, and observation are used. An example of an easy tool to assess general geriatric health is the Timed Up and Go (TUG) test. The person is asked to rise up from a chair, walk 10 feet, turn around, and sit back down. Increased TUG times have been associated with falls in the elderly (Podsiadlo & Richardson, 1991).

The FIM (Uniform Data System for Medical Rehabilitation, 1997) is the most widely accepted and most used performance-based measure of ADLs (see **Figure 24-1**). A revised version of the FIM (called the Wee-FIM) is available for pediatric patients. The FIM is an instrument that is completed by a trained evaluator to assess 18 performance items on a 7-level scale. The tool is completed upon admission, at discharge, and often several times in between to monitor progress. The total score of all categories can help to show improvement over time. The evaluator may

L E V E L S	7 Complete Independence (Timely, Safely) 6 Modified Independence (Device)	**NO HELPER**	
	Modified Dependence 5 Supervision (Subject = 100%+) 4 Minimal Assist (Subject = 75%+) 3 Moderate Assist (Subject = 50%+) **Complete Dependence** 2 Maximal Assist (Subject = 25%+) 1 Total Assist (Subject = less than 25%)	**HELPER**	

	ADMISSION	DISCHARGE	FOLLOW-UP
Self-Care A. Eating B. Grooming C. Bathing D. Dressing - Upper Body E. Dressing - Lower Body F. Toileting	☐☐☐☐☐☐	☐☐☐☐☐☐	☐☐☐☐☐☐
Sphincter Control G. Bladder Management H. Bowel Management	☐☐	☐☐	☐☐
Transfers I. Bed, Chair, Wheelchair J. Toilet K. Tub, shower	☐☐☐	☐☐☐	☐☐☐
Locomotion L. Walk/Wheelchair M. Stairs	☐☐ W Walk / C Wheelchair / B Both	☐☐ W Walk / C Wheelchair / B Both	☐☐ W Walk / C Wheelchair / B Both
Motor Subtotal Score	☐	☐	☐
Communication N. Comprehension O. Expression	☐☐ A Auditory / V Visual / B Both / V Vocal / N Nonvocal / B Both	☐☐ A Auditory / V Visual / B Both / V Vocal / N Nonvocal / B Both	☐☐ A Auditory / V Visual / B Both / V Vocal / N Nonvocal / B Both
Social Cognition P. Social Interaction Q. Problem Solving R. Memory	☐☐☐	☐☐☐	☐☐☐
Cognitive Subtotal Score	☐	☐	☐
TOTAL FIM Score	☐	☐	☐

NOTE: Leave no blanks. Enter 1 if patient not testable due to risk.

FIGURE 24-1   FIM Instrument.

Source: Copyright © 1997 Uniform Data System for Medical Rehabilitation (UDSmr), a division of UB Foundation Activities, Inc. (UBFA). Reprinted with the permission of UDSmr, University at Buffalo, 232 Parker Hall, 3435 Main Street, Buffalo, NY 14214. All marks associated with IFM and UDSmr are owned by UBFA.

be one person, or different team members may complete various parts of the FIM tool based on their expertise. For example, the nurse may complete the sphincter control item and the speech therapist may complete the communication section. Team members base their evaluation on direct observation of the subject. The items assessed include self-care, sphincter control, transfers, locomotion, communication, and social cognition. The evaluator quantifies each category by determining how much assistance is required in each category. A score of 1 means total assistance was needed and the subject provided less than 25% of the effort. A score of 7 signifies complete independence in a timely and safe manner (i.e., the subject was completely independent in that activity).

The usefulness or accuracy of some of these tools has been called into question by some. It is wise to investigate the development of the instrument and which patient groups were used during its development. In addition, the outcomes of a tool are generally somewhat dependent upon the person using it, so it is essential that evaluators are properly educated in the use of the instrument. Many tools have questionable generalizability to older adults and may not take into consideration the normal effects of aging.

Pain Management

Both acute and chronic pain may be present in rehabilitation clients. Acute pain is thought to be of shorter duration and associated with the insult. Chronic pain, more often seen in those clients with chronic illness and disability, is of longer duration and can result in diminished health, disability, and reduction in quality of life (American Pain Society, 2006; Hertzberg, 2007). Chronic pain has been associated with depression, disability, decreased function, and increased time off of work (Harris, 2000; Lipton, Hamelsky, Kolodner, Steiner, & Stewart, 2000; Walsh, Dumitru, Schoenfeld, & Ramaurthy, 2005). The popularity of pain clinics, whose major purpose is to address chronic, intractable pain, is growing, and referrals are often made to these programs when other interventions fail.

Pain, whether acute and/or chronic, can interfere with rehabilitation goals. Therefore, pain management is a part of most rehabilitation programs. The ARN, in fact, provides specific goals for pain management in clients, stating that rehabilitation nurses should seek to assist clients with acute or chronic pain to improve their physical functioning and thus improve their quality of life (ARN, 1996). Pain is a complex problem that requires a comprehensive approach from an interdisciplinary team using a variety of pharmacologic and nonpharmacologic interventions.

Rehabilitation Nursing

Rehabilitation is a growing specialty, and nursing is an emerging leader in this field. Specialties such as rehabilitation nursing are often impacted by the wars that create larger numbers of veterans with multiple traumatic injuries that require rehabilitation. Rehabilitation nurses are finding themselves working in a wider variety of settings and subspecialties to meet the growing demand for their services. Several of the settings in which rehabilitation nurses may work are discussed in the following sections.

In 1984, the ARN offered the first certification for registered nurses (RNs) working with rehabilitation clients. This credential, the CRRN, is the basic designation for this nursing specialty. There are more than 10,000 CRRNs today (ARN, 2010). In 1997 an advanced practice certification, the certified rehabilitation registered nurse-advanced (CRRN-A) was offered, but because of the smaller number of nurses sitting for the exam and changes in certification methods, it was phased out in 2009. The ARN (2010) also supports a variety of specialized practice roles for rehabilitation nurses. Role descriptions that have been developed by the ARN for rehabilitation nurses include the subspecialties of gerontologic rehabilitation, home care, pain management, pediatric rehabilitation, rehabilitation nurse manager, rehabilitation admissions liaison, advanced practice, case manager, staff nurse, nurse educator, and nurse researcher (see **Table 24-6**).

Table 24-6   Rehabilitation Nursing Role Descriptions
Gerontologic Rehabilitation Nurse
Homecare Rehabilitation Nurse
Pain Management Rehabilitation Nurse
Pediatric Rehabilitation Nurse
Rehabilitation Nurse Manager
Rehabilitation Admissions Liaison Nurse
Advanced Practice Rehabilitation Nurse
Rehabilitation Nurse Case Manager
Rehabilitation Nurse Educator
Rehabilitation Staff Nurse
Rehabilitation Nurse Researcher
Source: Association of Rehabilitation Nurses. (2010). Role description brochures. Retrieved September 21, 2011, from http://www.rehabnurse.org/pubs/role/index.html

Rehabilitation Settings

Rehabilitation services are offered in a wide variety of settings. These may include freestanding rehabilitation facilities, acute rehabilitation within hospitals, long-term care facilities, or the home. Regardless of the setting for care, services should be provided by an interdisciplinary team of trained professionals. In the past, rehabilitation units, especially those within hospitals, served patients with diverse diagnoses. However, as the specialty has grown and the body of research and evidence-based practice expands, it is becoming more common for larger rehabilitation facilities to target services for specific diagnostic groups of clients such as multiple trauma, traumatic brain injury, stroke syndromes, spinal cord injuries, cancer, burns, or human immunodeficiency virus (HIV), or at least to provide dedicated units for persons with similar diagnoses.

Subacute Care Units

Subacute care units are for patients who require more intensive nursing care than the traditional long-term care facility or nursing home can provide, but less than that provided by the acute care hospital or skilled care unit (Mauk, 2006). These units are sometimes referred to as transitional care units. Clients seen in subacute care are typically those who need:

> assistance as a result of non-healing wounds, chronic ventilator dependence, renal problems, intravenous therapy, and coma management and those with complex medical and/or rehabilitation needs, including pediatrics, orthopedics, and neurologic. These units are designed to promote optimum outcomes in the least expensive cost setting. (Easton, 1999, p. 15)

Clients may stay from days to several weeks. Persons who need rehabilitation services but would be unable to tolerate the intensive therapy of acute rehabilitation may be candidates for this level of care.

Skilled Nursing Facilities

Skilled nursing facilities may also provide rehabilitation and can be housed in acute care hospitals, and on independent specialty units, or within long-term care facilities. Remsburg and colleagues caution that not all skilled nursing facilities provide the same level of rehabilitation services, with services ranging from those who are Commission on Accreditation of Rehabilitation Facilities (CARF)–accredited programs and others that offer some restorative care, so consumers should carefully evaluate options when choosing a facility (Remsburg, Armacost, Radu, & Bennett, 1999; Remsburg, Armacost, Radu, & Bennett, 2001; Resnick & Fleishell, 2002).

Several benefits are seen with skilled nursing facilities. The pace is generally slower. Often patients will have more continuity of care with nursing staff than in an acute care hospital. Length of stay is generally longer, perhaps weeks or months instead of days. The focus of treatment is on individual outcomes with less regard to speed of progress (Osterweil, 1990).

Hospitals and Freestanding Facilities

Acute rehabilitation is often provided in acute care hospitals or freestanding rehabilitation facilities. A person requiring inpatient rehabilitation is not just in need of therapy, for if that was the only service required, it could be done on an outpatient basis, as often occurs with such conditions as joint replacement surgery. The person needing intensive inpatient rehabilitation is one who also requires 24-hour nursing care to address such problems as medication management, complex comorbidities, nutrition, swallowing disorders, behavior issues, skin care, and bowel and bladder retraining. Clients in acute rehabilitation may be admitted for a specific diagnosis such as stroke but also have pre- or coexisting conditions that complicate recovery such as hypertension, cancer, diabetes, and renal disease. In addition, the majority of clients treated in acute rehabilitation are older adults. Older adults as a population have unique needs with or without undergoing acute rehabilitation. Generally, to qualify for acute intensive rehabilitation services offered in these facilities, clients must be able to tolerate at least 3 hours of therapy per day, have a goal of discharge to home, and be able to demonstrate progress toward mutually established goals (Mauk & Hanson, 2010). They should also have private insurance or Medicare coverage to cover the high cost of the interdisciplinary services provided by multiple therapies and nursing.

Long-Term Care Facilities or Retirement Communities

Although long-term care facilities often carry a negative stigma with the general public, rehabilitative services offered in these facilities may be quite appropriate for assisting adults in regaining independence and function. Long-term care facilities, especially those offering multiple levels of care, may have accredited rehabilitation units housed within them. Persons making a retirement community their home may also avail themselves of therapeutic services offered within the facility. An increasing number of continuous care retirement communities (CCRCs) have physical or other therapists available to assist with rehabilitation after an accident, surgery, or illness in order to help older adults "age in place." In addition, many CCRCs have begun to offer health promotion activities that include state-of-the-art fitness centers with personal trainers to foster primary prevention as well as rehabilitation.

Community-Based Rehabilitation

Community-based rehabilitation may involve a rehabilitation team or involve only nursing. Community-based nurses may work in outpatient rehabilitation clinics, senior centers, assisted living, home health care, public schools, churches, or function as case managers. According to Parker and Neal-Boylan (2007), community-based rehabilitation is used in a variety of settings including home health care, subacute care, long-term care, and independent living.

Home health care provides services to clients of all ages and emphasizes primary care and case management. It allows individuals and families to remain in the home and still receive services that focus on health restoration and maximizing function. Home care is considered a cost-effective service for those recuperating from an injury or illness who are not able to completely care for themselves (National Association for Home Care and Hospice, 2007). Unique models may even allow CCRCs to provide homecare services covered by Medicare (L. Mullet, personal communication, November 26, 2007).

Subacute care in the community-based model generally provides services to adults

through a team-nursing delivery system, with most of the daily care being provided by nursing assistants, with supervision by licensed practical nurses and case management by RNs. In the long-term care setting, services are offered mainly to geriatric residents using a team approach, with the RN in the role of case manager. In independent living settings, older adults may receive care from personal care attendants. Here again the RN serves as a care manager and client advocate (Parker & Neal-Boylan, 2007).

Rehabilitation Specialties

Within the discipline of rehabilitation, there are many subspecialties. Although most traditional rehabilitation programs provide care to a mixed case of clients, there are both population- and diagnosis-specific units that cater to the needs of smaller, select groups of patients. These types of specialty programs may be inpatient or outpatient and may include geriatrics, pediatrics, cardiac, pulmonary, cancer, HIV, and Alzheimer's disease.

Geriatric Rehabilitation

By 2030, it is estimated that there will be more than 71 million Americans older than age 65, comprising about 20% of the population (CDC, 2007a). The top chronic illnesses that are considered the greatest health burden to society include arthritis, heart disease and stroke, diabetes, and cancer, and more recently obesity and tobacco-related disease (National Center for Chronic Disease Prevention and Health Promotion, 2007). Of the six leading causes of death in older Americans, five are from chronic illnesses, indicating that rehabilitation in geriatric clients should be a priority.

Geriatric rehabilitation focuses on restoring and maintaining optimal function while considering holistically the unique effects of aging on the person (Clark & Siebens, 2005). Programs specifically designed for older adults may have adjusted expectations such as requiring less intensive rehabilitation and preventing potential complications such as falls, dehydration, pressure sores, immobility, delirium, and polypharmacy that occur more frequently in older adults (Beers & Berkow, 2004; Lin & Armour, 2004; Routasalo, Arve, & Lauri, 2004; Worsowicz, Stewart, Phillips, & Cifu, 2004). Geriatric rehabilitation also focuses on enhancing quality of life through the strengthening of social support systems, family involvement, client education, and connection with community resources.

Mauk and Lehman (2007) suggest that there are two ways in which disability affects older adults: acquiring disability at an advanced age, and aging with an earlier onset disability. Factors that may affect an older adult's rehabilitation potential include: age, frailty, the normal aging process, effects of chronic disease, functional and cognitive status, the use of multiple medications, and the presence of social support (Bagg, Pombo, & Hopman, 2002; Bandeen-Roche et al., 2006; Beaupre et al., 2005; Charles & Lehman, 2006; Yu, 2005). The more common acquired disabilities in older adults include stroke, head injury, and fractures from falls. In addition, the various syndromes (such as delirium, dizziness, incontinence, dehydration, and functional loss) that are seen more often in older adults can negatively impact the rehabilitation process (Mauk & Lehman, 2007). Persons aging with a disability tend to experience a greater degree of complications over time. For example,

a man with a lower extremity amputation that occurred in his 20s is much more likely to have arthritis and range-of-motion problems in his shoulders from overuse of a non–weight-bearing joint than the person who has lost this limb later in life. However, the person with lower extremity amputation later in life as a result of peripheral vascular disease secondary to diabetes is at an increased risk for complications because of advanced age and disease process. Therefore, both the disability and the aging process contribute to one's overall rehabilitation potential. Rehabilitation can positively impact older adults by providing services to strengthen both physical and psychosocial functioning.

Pediatric Rehabilitation

Children with functional limitations have different needs and development concerns than adults do. Pediatric rehabilitation involves the collaboration of an interdisciplinary team of professionals to provide a continuum of care for children from the onset of injury or illness until adulthood. The focus of treatment is on adaptation and maximum function to promote independence within the family and society. The ARN (2007) defines pediatric rehabilitation nursing as "the specialty practice committed to improving the quality of life for children and adolescents with disabilities and their families" (p. 1). Professionals working with children practice family-centered care, must be knowledgeable about normal growth and development, and be able to work with an interdisciplinary team to address interventions that include physical, emotional, cultural, educational, socioeconomic, and spiritual dimensions (Edwards, Hertzberg, & Sapp, 2007).

CASE STUDY

Technologic Advances

Ted is a 24-year-old veteran of the Iraq war. He received polytrauma injuries after an improvised explosive device exploded near his tank in the field. He sustained multiple burn injuries, mild brain injury, and an eventual amputation of the left lower leg. After extensive time in rehabilitation at a polytrauma center, he was fitted for a prosthetic C-Leg to allow him to return to his prior love of running. Ted's long-term goal is to compete in the Paralympics, because he had been an athlete prior to his injuries. He has the support of a loving family and young wife of 2 years, as well as his large home church.

Discussion Questions

1. What are some other nonpharmacologic strategies that could be applied to help improve Ted's quality of life?
2. How would the interdisciplinary team assist Ted with developing a long-term plan to cope with the effects of polytrauma?
3. What rehabilitation issues and concerns would be involved in Ted's situation? What psychosocial and emotional factors should be addressed?
4. How should the family and church friends be involved in the plan of care for Ted?
5. Is Ted's goal of competing in the Paralympics realistic? What factors would have to be considered for this to occur?

Some of the common disorders associated with the need for pediatric rehabilitation include: traumatic brain injury, spinal cord injury, burns, cancer, congenital diseases and birth defects, and chronic illness. For example, whether a child sustains a brain injury from an accident or is born with cerebral palsy, the interventions from the interdisciplinary rehabilitation team will be designed to maximize function and help the child attain adulthood as a well-adjusted member of society.

Cardiac Rehabilitation

According to the American Heart Association (AHA, 2011), 1 in 6 deaths in the United States are caused by coronary heart disease. Cardiac rehabilitation "enhances recovery, and secondary prevention measures prevent further complications from disease" (Carbone, 2007). Cardiac rehabilitation is appropriate for persons with congenital or acquired heart disease such as those with myocardial infarction, chronic angina, cardiomyopathy, or postsurgical patients. The aims are to improve functional capacity and to reduce related morbidity and mortality (Singh, Schocken, Williams, & Stamey, 2004). Cardiac rehabilitation following a myocardial infarction has four phases: phase I: acute phase—during the inpatient stay; phase II: convalescent phase—early post-discharge;

phase III: training phase—structured and supervised exercise program; and phase IV: maintenance phase—post-training and lifestyle changes (Shah, 2005; Singh et al., 2004). Measures employed in cardiac rehabilitation include risk factor modification along with medication management and medical interventions. Risk-factor management focuses on smoking cessation, controlling hypertension, decreasing cholesterol, management of diabetes, increasing physical activity, and decreasing stress (AHA, 2011). Client participation in cardiac rehabilitation is an ongoing problem, with recent research suggesting that the strength of physician recommendation, gender (men participated more than women), and disease severity may be the best predictors of whether clients initiate cardiac rehabilitation (Ades, Waldmann, McCann, & Weaver, 1992; Shanks, Moore, & Zeller, 2007).

Pulmonary Rehabilitation

COPD, which includes chronic bronchitis and emphysema, is the third leading cause of death in America (American Lung Association [ALA], 2011). When asthma and other pulmonary problems are factored in, chronic respiratory problems are a leading cause of functional disability in the United States. The primary risk factor for COPD is smoking, and 80–90% of deaths from COPD are attributed to this cause (ALA, 2011). Because of the large numbers of Americans experiencing pulmonary problems, specific programs have been developed to address these needs. The American Association for Respiratory Care (2002) state that essential components of a pulmonary rehabilitation program include: assessment, patient education, exercise, psychosocial interventions, and follow up. Smoking cessation programs are a major

focus in both the prevention and rehabilitative treatment of respiratory problems.

Cancer Rehabilitation

According to the CDC's 2007 data, the top cancer deaths for males across all races include prostate, lung, liver, and colorectal (CDC, 2011a). For women, the leading causes of cancer deaths include lung, breast, and colorectal (CDC, 2011a). Given these statistics, many cancers detected early are highly treatable and need not be viewed as a terminal diagnosis. These data suggest that persons with cancer will not only survive but may require rehabilitation to enhance quality of life and return to optimal functioning after their diagnosis and as part of their treatment. "Cancer rehabilitation is the process that assists the person with cancer in obtaining maximum physical, social, psychological, and work-related functioning during and after cancer treatment" (People Living with Cancer, 2006, p. 1). The goals of cancer rehabilitation include maximizing independence in mobility and ADLs, preserving dignity, and promoting quality of life (Beck, 2003; Gillis, Cheville, & Worsowicz, 2001; Vargo & Gerber, 2005), and are individualized to each person, given the stage of their disease. The cancer rehabilitation team includes all of the usual team members of rehabilitation as well as the oncologist. Quality of life is enhanced through cancer rehabilitation by assistance with ADLs, pain management, improving nutrition, smoking cessation, stress reduction, and improved coping strategies. In one study of women with breast cancer, exercise therapy was found to significantly enhance quality of life (Dale et al., 2007). Rehabilitation can also assist individuals with terminal cancer to live a better quality of life until end of life.

Dementia or Alzheimer's Programs

Alzheimer's disease is a progressive and fatal brain disease that currently affects more than 5 million Americans (National Institute on Aging, 2010). New research from the National Institutes of Health suggests that one in seven Americans older than the age of 71 has some type of dementia (Plassman et al., 2007). Generally occurring in older adults, there are still believed to be between 220,000 and more than half a million cases of early-onset Alzheimer's that affect persons in their 30s, 40s, and 50s (Alzheimer's Association, 2007). It is the most common type of dementia and has no cure. Although Alzheimer's disease is not generally considered a rehabilitation diagnosis, it certainly fits the profile of chronic illness. Those with early-onset Alzheimer's disease would certainly avail themselves of all treatment possible to postpone the inevitable effects of this progressive illness. This would include interventions from the rehabilitation team.

Rehabilitation nurses are often found working in long-term care facilities that serve residents with dementia, and the need is likely to grow. Although the focus of care for older persons with Alzheimer's disease includes rehabilitation goals, realistic outcome planning as the disease progresses will not likely include discharge to home. Persons with Alzheimer's disease may receive services from assisted living, nursing homes, and/or special care units (Alzheimer's Association, 2007). The Alzheimer's unit within the nursing home often becomes the last home that a person with dementia will know. The number of Alzheimer's units within long-term care facilities is increasing owing to the demand for services as the disease progresses, and family caregivers are no longer able to manage persons at home. As their condition deteriorates with advancing dementia, the fundamental principles of rehabilitation still apply to these residents: to assist individuals to remain as independent as possible for as long as possible, to maintain function, and to prevent complications.

HIV/AIDS

An estimated 1,178,350 persons aged 13 and older were living with HIV or acquired immune deficiency syndrome (AIDS) in the United States in 2009 (CDC, 2011b). It is estimated that between 34.6 and 42.3 million people in the world have HIV or AIDS (Monahan, Sands, Neighbors, Marek, & Green, 2007) and about 25 million people worldwide have died from AIDS, including about a half million Americans (CDC, 2006). Although current treatments have dramatically increased the life expectancy for many persons with HIV, those developing AIDS experience many associated neurologic, pulmonary, cardiac, and rheumatologic problems. Rehabilitation programs designed to address all levels of prevention along with the associated health problems inherent with HIV/AIDS are becoming more common. Rehabilitation nurses may work with infected patients from before diagnosis through end of life (Manning & Haldi, 2007). Rehabilitation goals depend on the stage of illness, whether symptomatic, asymptomatic, or terminal, but include interventions such as monitoring client status, careful assessment, addressing psychological needs and responses, balancing energy with rest, medication management, education regarding prevention of transmission, emotional support, and counseling for the person and family.

Ensuring Quality in Rehabilitation Facilities

There are two primary accrediting bodies for rehabilitation providers: the Joint Commission and CARF. Although the Joint Commission accreditation is expected for inpatient rehabilitation providers, CARF accreditation is viewed as a mark of distinction that signifies meeting higher standards for rehabilitation.

The Joint Commission

The oldest and best known accrediting body is the Joint Commission, previously known as the Joint Commission on the Accreditation of Healthcare Organizations. The mission of the Joint Commission is "to continuously improve the safety and quality of care provided to the public through the provision of health care accreditation and related services that support performance improvement in health care organizations" (Joint Commission, 2007, p. 1). The Joint Commission has developed current, professionally based standards for hospitals, long-term care, home health care, and other organizations and uses a survey process to evaluate the compliance of healthcare organizations with these standards. The Joint Commission has a cooperative agreement with CARF regarding the evaluation of rehabilitation facilities. In 1997, the ORYX initiative allowed the integration of outcomes and standard performance measures into the accreditation process and helped organizations identify care issues that required attention (Black, 2007). The Joint Commission holds organizations responsible for providing safe care that meets the standards of the industry and protects public safety. Some

benefits of Joint Commission accreditation and certification include strengthening the trust of the public in the organization, improving risk management, promoting patient safety and comfort, and enhancing staff recruitment into the organization (Black, 2007).

Commission on Accreditation of Rehabilitation Facilities (CARF)

CARF is an independent, not-for-profit organization that accredits rehabilitation programs and services. "CARF reviews and grants accreditation services nationally and internationally on request of a facility or program. Our standards are rigorous, so those services that meet them are among the best available," and CARF accreditation procedures "ensure the highest industry standards possible, providing risk reduction and accountability" (CARF, 2007, p. 1). There are six divisions in CARF's organizational structure: medical rehabilitation, behavioral health, employment and community services, aging services, child and youth services, and opioid treatment (Black, 2007). The most recent publications for CARF include the *Child and Youth Standards Manual* and *Aging Services Standards Manual* (CARF, 2011a, b).

OUTCOME MEASUREMENT AND PERFORMANCE IMPROVEMENT

According to Black (2007), outcomes of care are being emphasized as never before. She lists the following benefits of monitoring outcomes (Black, 2007, p. 395):

- Track efficiency and effectiveness
- Identify trends

- Facilitate communication between the patient, family, treatment team, payers, referral source, and other stakeholders
- Assess follow up measures to determine whether progress is continuing after discharge
- Identify areas for improvement
- Measure access to programs

In rehabilitation, outcomes are key to ensuring that goals are being met. Goal setting in rehabilitation should be mutual between the client and the healthcare team. Individual goals for clients are reviewed systematically at team conferences. Outcome measurement can be used to look at trends within an organization, be benchmarked against industry standards, and compared with best practices.

There are many ways that outcomes can be measured. Accreditation provides one way to ensure that facilities are meeting the industry standards. A variety of tools can also be used to monitor individual and collective rehabilitation outcomes. One of the most commonly used is the FIM instrument (see Figure 24-1). The FIM (Uniform Data System for Medical Rehabilitation, 1997) instrument provides a quantitative measure of function on admission, discharge, and follow up so that data may be compared across time and with other cohorts. This information often proves useful in justifying insurance coverage by demonstrating continued improvement by the client.

There are also many tools and models for performance improvement in health care. Most of these focus on devices to assist team members to improve the quality of care for clients. Diagrams, flow sheets, checklists, charts, and other visuals can enhance performance. Standard setting by national organizations provides an additional means of quality improvement as organizations strive to meet industry

aims. Outcomes measurement and documentation of performance improvement are critical because reimbursement under present payment systems require rehabilitation providers to provide evidence of the effectiveness of their programs and services (Johnston, Eastwood, Wilkerson, Anderson, & Alves, 2005).

Evidence-Based Practice Box

This qualitative study explored and compared the hopes of caregivers and nurses dealing with adolescent patients with acquired brain injury. Four themes of hope were revealed by 21 caregivers (mean age of 45 years). Fourteen nurses' perceptions of hope for recovery of the adolescent patients were also examined. Nurses were found to have different perceptions of recovery than the caregivers, who felt they knew the patient better than the staff. The four themes of hope suggested by the caregivers included: 1) family as important, 2) taking one day at a time, 3) knowing the patient better, and 4) spiritual strength as a major social support. Rehabilitation nurses can learn from this limited study that caregivers believe they can provide good insight into the patient with brain injury and that social supports in the form of family and spirituality were seen as important to this group.

Source: Gebhardt, M. C., Mcgehee, L. A., Grindl, C. G., & Dufour, L. T. (2011). Caregiver and nurse hopes for recovery of persons with acquired brain injury. *Rehabilitation Nursing, 36*(1), 3–12.

Rehabilitation is both a philosophy and an approach to treatment. Describe the philosophy of rehabilitation and how it relates to treatment from an interdisciplinary team of professionals.

Define the following rehabilitation terms in relationship to chronic illness: *impairment, functional limitation, disability,* and *community reintegration.*

Identify three problems in the provision of rehabilitation services to the chronically ill.

Describe the different settings where rehabilitation services can be provided.

What specific issues in rehabilitation make doing research difficult?

Discuss the advantages and disadvantages of the major functional assessment tools mentioned in this chapter.

INTERNET RESOURCES

Alzheimer's Association: www.alz.org
American Heart Association: www.aha.org
American Stroke Association: www.strokeassociation.org
Association of Rehabilitation Nurses: www.rehabnurse.org
Centers for Medicare & Medicaid Services: www.cms.hhs.gov/medicare/
National Institute of Neurological Disorders and Stroke: www.ninds.nih.gov
National Rehabilitation Information Center: www.naric.com
National Rehabilitation Association: www.nationalrehab.org
National Stroke Association: www.stroke.org
The State of Aging and Health in America: www.cdc.gov/aging/data/stateofaging.htm

For a full suite of assignments and additional learning activities, use the access code located in the front of your book and visit this exclusive website: **http://go.jblearning.com/larsen**. If you do not have an access code, you can obtain one at the site.

REFERENCES

Adams, P. F., Dey, A. N., & Vickerie, J. L. (2007). Summary health statistics for the U.S. population: National Health Interview Survey, 2005. National Center for Health Statistics. *Vital Health Statistics, 10*(233). Hyattsville, MD: U.S. Department of Health and Human Services.

Ades, P. A., Waldmann, M. L., McCann, W., & Weaver, S. O. (1992). Predictors of cardiac rehabilitation participation in older coronary patients. *Archives of Internal Medicine, 152*, 1033–1035.

Alzheimer's Association. (2007). Alzheimer's disease. Retrieved September 16, 2011, from: http://www.alz.org/alzheimers_disease_alzheimers_disease.asp

American Association for Respiratory Care. (2002). AARC clinical practice guideline: Pulmonary rehabilitation. *Respiratory Care, 47*(5), 617–625.

American Heart Association. (2011). Heart disease and stroke statistics: 2011 update. Retrieved September 29, 2011, from http://cire.ahajournals.org/content/123/4/el8.full.pdf

American Lung Association. (2011). COPD. Retrieved September 29, 2011, from http://www.lungusa.org/lung-disease/copd/

American Pain Society. (APS). (2006). Pain: Current understanding of assessment, management, and treatments. Retrieved September 29, 2011, from www.ampainsoc.org/education/enduring/

Anderson, C., Linto, J., & Stewart-Wynne, E. (1995). A population-based assessment of the impact and burden of caregiving for long-term stroke survivors. *Stroke, 26*, 843–849.

Arbour, K. P., Latimer, A. E., Ginis, K. A., & Jung, M. E. (2007). Moving beyond the stigma: The impression formation benefits of exercise for individuals with a physical disability. *Adapted Physical Activity Quarterly, 24*(2), 144–159.

Association of Rehabilitation Nurses. (1996). *Scope and standards of advanced clinical practice in rehabilitation nursing.* Glenview, IL: Author.

Association of Rehabilitation Nurses. (2007). ARN positional statement on the role of the nurse in the rehabilitation team. Retrieved September 16, 2011, from: http://www.rehabnurse.org/pdf/PS-Role.pdf

Association of Rehabilitation Nurses. (2008). *Standards and scope of rehabilitation nursing practice.* Glenview, IL: Author.

Association of Rehabilitation Nurses. (2010). Role description brochures. Retrieved September 16, 2011, from: www.rehabnurse.org/pubs/role/index.html

Bagg, S., Pombo, A. P., & Hopman, W. (2002). Effect of age on functional outcomes after stroke rehabilitation. *Stroke, 33,* 179–185.

Bandeen-Roche, K., Xue, Q-L., Ferrucci, L., Walston, J., Guralnik, J. M., Chaves, P. et al. (2006). Phenotype of frailty: Characterization in the women's health and aging studies. *The Journals of Gerontology series A: Biological Sciences and Medical Sciences, 61,* 262–266.

Beauchamp, T. L., & Childress, J. F. (2001). *Principles of biomedical ethics.* New York: Oxford University Press.

Beaupre, L. A., Cinats, J. G., Senthilselvan, A., Scharfenberger, A., Johnston, D. W., & Saunders, L. D. (2005). Does standardized rehabilitation and discharge planning improve functional recovery in elderly patients with hip fracture? *Archives of Physical Medicine and Rehabilitation, 86,* 2231–2239.

Beck, L. A. (2003). Cancer rehabilitation: Does it make a difference? *Rehabilitation Nursing, 28*(2), 32–37.

Beers, M. H., & Berkow, R. (2004). Rehabilitation. The Merck manual of geriatrics. Merck & Co., Medical Services, USMEDA, USHH. Retrieved September 16, 2011, from: www.merck.com/mrkshared/mm_geriatrics/home.jsp

Black, T. (2007). Outcomes measurement and performance improvement. In K. L. Mauk (Ed.), *The specialty practice of rehabilitation nursing: A core curriculum* (pp. 395–411). Glenview, IL: Association of Rehabilitation Nurses.

Blake, D., & Scott, D. (1996). Employment of persons with disabilities. *Physical Medicine and Rehabilitation* (p. 182). Philadelphia: W.B. Saunders.

Brandstater, M. E. (2005). Stroke rehabilitation. In J. DeLisa & B. Gans (Eds.), *Rehabilitation medicine: Principles and practice* (4th ed., pp. 1655–1676). Philadelphia: Lippincott-Raven.

Brandt, E., & Pope, A. (1997). *Enabling America: Assessing the Role of Rehabilitation Science and Engineering.* Committee on Assessing Rehabilitation Science and Engineering. Division of Health Policy. Institute of Medicine. Washington, DC: National Academies Press.

Brouwer, W. B. F., van Exel, N. J. A., van de Berg, B., Dinant, H. J., Koopmanschap, M. A., & van den Bos, G. A. (2004). Burden of caregiving: Evidence of objective burden, subjective burden, and quality of life impacts on informal caregivers of patients with rheumatoid arthritis. *Arthritis and Rheumatism, 51*(4), 570–577.

Buchanan, L. (1996). Community-based rehabilitation nursing. In S. Hoeman (Ed.), *Rehabilitation nursing: Process and application* (2nd ed., pp. 114–129). St. Louis: Mosby.

Bushnik, T., Wright, J., & Burdsall, D. (2007). Personal attendant turnover: Association with level of injury, burden of care, and psychosocial outcome. *Topics in Spinal Cord Injury Rehabilitation, 12*(3), 66–76.

Campinha-Bacote, J. (2001). A model of practice to address cultural competence. *Rehabilitation Nursing, 26*(1), 8–11.

Canam, C., & Acorn, S. (1999). Quality of life for family caregivers of people with chronic health problems. *Rehabilitation Nursing, 24*(5), 192–196.

Carbone, L. (2007). Cardiovascular and pulmonary rehabilitation: Acute and long-term management. In K. L. Mauk (Ed.), *The specialty practice of rehabilitation nursing: A core curriculum* (pp. 238–259). Glenview, IL: Association of Rehabilitation Nurses.

Center for International Rehabilitation Research Information and Exchange, & the National Institute on Disability and Rehabilitation Research. (2007a). The rehabilitation provider's guide to cultures of the foreign-born. Retrieved September 21, 2011, from: cirrie.buffalo.edu/mseries.html

Centers for Disease Control and Prevention. (2006). Overview. Retrieved December 2, 2006, from: www.cdc.gov/hiv/topics/testing/index.htm

Centers for Disease Control and Prevention. (2007a). About minority health. Retrieved December 8, 2007, from: www.cdc.gov/omhd/AMH/AMH.htm

Centers for Disease Control and Prevention (2007b). Disease burden and risk factors. Retrieved November 1, 2011 from: http://www.cdc.gov/omhd/AMH/dbrf.htm

Centers for Disease Control and Prevention. (2007b). The state of aging and health in America report. Retrieved December 1, 2007, from: www.cdc.gov/aging/saha.htm

Centers for Disease Control and Prevention. (2009). Chronic disease and health promotion. Retrieved September 29, 2011, from http://www.cdc.gov/chronicdisease/overview/index/htm

Centers for Disease Control and Prevention. (2011a). United States cancer statistics. Retrieved September 29, 2011, from: http://www.cdc.gov/Features/CancerStatistics/

Centers for Disease Control and Prevention. (2011b). Basic statistics. Retrieved September 29, 2011, from http://www.cdc.gov/hiv/topics/surveillance/basic.htm#hivest

Centers for Medicare & Medicaid Services. (2005). Medicaid at-a-glance 2005. Retrieved September 29, 2011, from: www.cms.hhs.gov/MedicaidDataSourcesGenInfo/02_MAAG2005.asp

Centers for Medicare & Medicaid Services. (2011a). Overview of Inpatient Rehabilitation Facility PPS. Retrieved September 29, 2011, from: www.cms.gov/InPatientRehabFacPPS/

Centers for Medicare & Medicaid Services. (2011b). Medicare and you 2012. Retrieved from http://www.medicare.gov/publications/pubs/pdf/10050.pdf

Charles, C. V., & Lehman, C. (2006). Medications and laboratory values. In K. L. Mauk (Ed.), *Gerontological nursing: Competencies for care* (pp. 293–320). Sudbury, MA: Jones and Bartlett.

Clark, G. S., & Siebens, H. (2005). Geriatric rehabilitation. In J. DeLisa & B. Gans (Eds.), *Physical medicine and rehabilitation: Principles and practice* (4th ed., pp. 1531–1560). Philadelphia: Lippincott Williams & Wilkins.

Commission on Accreditation of Rehabilitation Facilities International (CARF). (2011a). 2011 Aging services program descriptions. Retrieved September 29, 2011, from: http://www.carf.org/ASprogramDescriptions/

Commission on Accreditation of Rehabilitation Facilities International (CARF). (2011b). 2011 Child and youth services program descriptions. Retrieved September 29, 2011, from: http://www.carf.org/WorkArea/DownloadAsset.aspx?

Committee on Accreditation of Rehabilitation Facilities (2007). Payers. Retrieved on November 21, 2007 from: www.carf.org/

Cook, C., Stickley, L, Ramey, K., & Knotts, V. J. (2005). Variables associated with occupational and physical therapy stroke rehabilitation utilization and outcomes. *Journal of Allied Health, 34*(1), 3–10.

Council of State Administrators of Vocational Rehabilitation (2004–2005). Investing in America: The gateway to independence public vocational rehabilitation—A program that works. Retrieved September 21, 2011, from: www.rehabnetwork.org/investing_in_america.htm

Currie, D. M., Atchison, J. W., & Fiedler, I. G. (2002). The challenge of teaching rehabilitative care in medical school. *Academic Medicine, 77*(7), 701–708.

Dale, A. J., Crank, H., Saxton, J. M., Mutrie, N., Coleman, R., & Roalfe, A. (2007). Randomized trial of exercise therapy in women treated for breast cancer. *Journal of Clinical Oncology, 25*(13), 1713–1721.

D'Andrea, D. C., & Meyer, J. D. (2004). Workers' compensation reform. *Clinics in Occupational & Environmental Medicine, 4*, 259–271.

das Chagas Medeiros, M., Ferraz, M., & Quaresma, M. (2000). The effect of rheumatoid arthritis on the quality of life of primary caregivers. *Journal of Rheumatology, 27*(1), 76–83.

Dean-Baar, S. (2003). Nursing shortages affect all levels of the profession. *Rehabilitation Nursing, 28*(4), 102.

Department of Veterans Affairs. (2000). Facts about the Department of Veterans Affairs. Retrieved from: http://www.va.gov/vetdata/Quick_Facts.asp

Department of Veterans Affairs. (2010). Federal benefits for veterans, survivors, and dependents. Retrieved September 21, 2011, from: http://www1.va.gov/opa/publications/benefits_book/federal_benefits.pdf

Department of Veterans Affairs. (2011). Vocational rehabilitation and employment services. Retrieved September 21, 2011, from: http://www.vba.va.gov/bln/vre/

Deutsch, A., & Dean-Baar, S. (2007). Economics and health policy in rehabilitation. In K. L. Mauk (Ed.), *The specialty practice of rehabilitation nursing: A core curriculum* (pp. 35–53). Glenview, IL: Association of Rehabilitation Nurses.

Doherty, R. B. (2004). Assessing the new Medicare prescription drug law. *Annals of Internal Medicine, 141*(5), 391–395.

Draper, B., Bowring, G., Thompson, C., Van Heyst, J., Conroy, P., & Thompson, J. (2007). Stress in caregivers of aphasic stroke patients: A randomized controlled trial. *Clinical Rehabilitation, 21*(2), 122–130.

Easton, K. L. (1999). *Gerontological rehabilitation nursing.* Philadelphia: Saunders.

Easton, K. L. (2001). *The post-stroke journey: From agonizing to owning.* Doctoral dissertation. Wayne State University, Detroit, MI.

Edwards, P. (1992). The evolution of rehabilitation facilities for children. *Rehabilitation Nursing, 17,* 191–192.

Edwards, P. (2007). Rehabilitation nursing: Past, present and future. In K. Mauk (Ed.), *The specialty practice of rehabilitation nursing: A core curriculum* (5th ed., pp. 455–466). Glenview, IL: Association of Rehabilitation Nurses.

Edwards, P., Hertzberg, D., & Sapp, L. (2007). Pediatric rehabilitation nursing. In K. L. Mauk (Ed.), *The specialty practice of rehabilitation nursing: A core curriculum* (pp. 336–358). Glenview, IL: Association of Rehabilitation Nurses.

Ellis, J. R., & Hartley, C. L. (2004). *Nursing in today's world: Trends, issues, and management* (8th ed.). Philadelphia: Lippincott, Williams & Wilkins.

Emmer, S., & Allendorf, L. (2004). The Medicare Prescription Drug, Improvement, and Modernization Act of 2003. *Journal of the American Geriatrics Society, 52*(6), 1013–1015.

Fairfax, J. (2002). *Theory of quality of life of stroke survivors.* Doctoral dissertation. Wayne State University, Detroit, MI.

Federal Register. (2007). Inpatient Rehabilitation Facility Prospective Payment System for Federal Fiscal Year 2008; Proposed Rule. Department of Health and Human Services, *CMS, 72*(88), 26230–26479.

Fried, T. R., Bradley, E. H., Williams, C. S., & Tinetti, M. E. (2001). Functional disability and health care expenditures for older persons. *Archives of Internal Medicine, 161*(21), 2602–2607.

Gillis, T. A., Cheville, A. L., & Worsowicz, G. M. (2001). Cardiopulmonary rehabilitation and cancer rehabilitation: Oncologic rehabilitation. *Archives of Physical Medicine and Rehabilitation, 83*(Suppl. 1), S47–51.

Grunfeld, E., Coyle, D., Whelan, T., Clinch, J., et al. (2004). Family caregiver burden: results of a longitudinal study of breast cancer patients and their principal caregivers. *Canadian Medical Association Journal, 170*(12), 1795–1801.

Guse, L. W. (2006). Assessment of the older adult. In K. L. Mauk (Ed.), *Gerontological nursing: Competencies for care* (pp. 265–292). Sudbury, MA: Jones and Bartlett.

Halm, M. A., Treat-Jacobson, D., Lindquist, R., & Savik, K. (2007). Caregiver burden and outcomes of caregiving of spouses of patient who undergo coronary artery bypass graft surgery. *Heart & Lung, 36*(3), 170–187.

Harris, J. A. (2000). Understanding acute and chronic pain. In P. Edwards (Ed.), *The specialty practice of rehabilitation nursing* (4th ed.). Glenview, IL: Association of Rehabilitation Nurses.

Hartke, R. J., & King, R. B. (2002). Analysis of problem types and difficulty among older stroke caregivers. *Topics in Stroke Rehabilitation, 9*(1), 16–33.

Havercamp, S. M., Scandlin, D., & Roth, M. (2004). Health disparities among adults with developmental disabilities, adults with other disabilities, and adults not reporting disability in North Carolina. *Public Health Reports, 119*(4), 418–426.

Hertzberg, D. (2007). Understanding acute and chronic pain. In K. L. Mauk (Ed.), *The specialty practice of rehabilitation nursing: A core curriculum* (pp. 260–274). Glenview, IL: Association of Rehabilitation Nurses.

Hogstel, M. O., Curry, L. C., Walker, C. A., & Burns, P. G. (2004). Ethics committees in long-term care facilities. *Geriatric Nursing, 25*(6), 364–369.

Hughes, J. A. (2004). Ethics in the emergency department. *Academy of Emergency Medicine, 11*(9), 995–996.

Hughes, S., Giobbie-Hurder, A., Weaver, F., Kubal, J., et al. (1999). Relationship between caregiver burden and health-related quality of life. *The Gerontologist, 39*(5), 534–545.

Indian Health Services. (2001). *Trends in Indian health.* Retrieved September 21, 2011, from: www.ihs.gov/PublicInfo/Publications/trends98/trends98.asp

Inman, J., McGurk, E., & Chadwick, J. (2007). Is vocational rehabilitation a transition to recovery? *British Journal of Occupational Therapy, 70*(2), 60–66.

Jett, D. U., Warren, R. L., & Wirtalla, C. (2005). The relation between therapy intensity and outcomes of rehabilitation in skilled nursing facilities. *Archives of Physical Medicine and Rehabilitation, 86*(3), 373–379.

Johnson, J. A. (2004). Withdrawal of medically administered nutrition and hydration: The role benefits and burdens, and of parents and ethics committees. *Journal of Clinical Ethics, 15*(3), 307–311.

Johnston, M. V., Eastwood, E., Wilkerson, D. L., Anderson, L., & Alves, A. (2005). Systematically assessing and improving the quality and outcomes of medical rehabilitation programs. In J. DeLisa & B. M. Gans (Eds.), *Rehabilitation medicine: Principles and practice* (3rd ed., pp. 1163–1192). Philadelphia: Lippincott-Raven.

Joint Commission. (2007). About the Joint Commission. Retrieved November 21, 2007, from: http://www.jointcommission.org/AboutUs/

Kaiser Commission. (2007). Medicaid and the uninsured. Retrieved December 14, 2007, from: http://www.kff.org/medicaid/upload/7682.pdf

Kelly, P. (1999). Reimbursement mechanisms. In A. S. Luggen & S. Meiner (Eds.), *NGNA core curriculum for gerontological nursing* (pp. 185–186). St. Louis: Mosby.

Kemp, B. (1986). Psychosocial and mental health issues in rehabilitation of older persons. In S. Brody & G. Ruff (Eds.), *Aging and rehabilitation* (pp. 122–158). New York: Springer.

Kennedy, J. (2001). Unmet and undermet need for activities of daily living and instrumental activities of daily living assistance among adults and disabilities: Estimates from the 1994 and 1005 disability followback surveys. *Medical Care, 39*(12), 1305–1312.

Kent, B., & Smith, S. (2006). They only see it when the sun shines in my ears: Exploring perceptions of adolescent hearing aid users. *Journal of Deaf Studies & Deaf Education, 11*(4), 461–476.

Kielhofner, G., Braveman, B., Finlayson, M., Paul-Ward, A., Goldbaum, L., & Goldstein, K. (2004). Outcomes of a vocational program for persons with AIDS.

American Journal of Occupational Therapy, 58(1), 64–72.

King, R. B., Hartke, R. J., & Denby, F. (2007). Problem-solving early intervention: A pilot study of stroke caregivers. *Rehabilitation Nursing, 32*(2), 68–76.

Kirschner, K. L., Stocking, C., Wagner, L. B., Foye, S. J., & Siegler, M. (2001). Ethical issues identified by rehabilitation clinicians. *Archives of Physical Medicine and Rehabilitation, 82* (12 Suppl. 2), S2–8.

Kiselica, D., Sibson, B., & McKenzie-Green, J. (2004). Workers' compensation: A historical review and description of a legal and social insurance system. *Clinics in Occupational and Environmental Medicine, 4*, 237–247.

Kolanowski, A. M., Fick, D., Waller, J. L., & Shea, D. (2004). Spouses of persons with dementia: Their healthcare problems, utilization, and costs. *Research in Nursing & Health, 27*, 296–306.

Kosciulek, J. F. (2007). A test of the theory of informed consumer choice in vocational rehabilitation. *Journal of Rehabilitation, 73*(2), 41–49.

Kottke, F., Stillwell, G., & Lehmann, J. (Eds.). (1982). *Krusen's handbook of physical medicine and rehabilitation* (3rd ed.). Philadelphia: Saunders.

Kovner, C. T., Mezey, M., & Harrington, C. (2002). Who cares for older adults? Workforce implications of an aging society. *Health Affairs (Millwood), 21*(5), 78–89.

LaPlante, M., Kaye, H. S., Kang, T., & Harrington, C. (2004). Unmet need for personal assistance services: estimating the shortfall in hours of help and adverse consequences. *The Journal of Gerontology, Series B, Psychological Science and Social Science, 59*(2), S98–S108.

Larsen, P. (1998). "Rehabilitation." In I. Lubkin & P. Larsen (Eds.), *Chronic illness: Impact and interventions* (4th ed., p. 534).

Lieberman, M., & Fisher, L. (1995). The impact of chronic illness on the health and well-being of family members. *Gerontologist, 35*(1), 94–102.

Lin, J. L., & Armour, D. (2004). Selected medical management of the older adult rehabilitative patient. *Archives of Physical Medicine and Rehabilitation, 85*(Suppl. 3), S76–82.

Lipton, R., Hamelsky, S., Kolodner, K., Steiner, T., & Stewart, W. F. (2000). Migraine, quality of life, and depression: A population-based case-control study. *Neurology, 55*(5), 629–635.

Lloyd, C., & Waghorn, G. (2007). The importance of vocation in recovery for young people with psychiatric disabilities. *British Journal of Occupational Therapy, 70*(2), 50–59.

Lomay, V. T., & Hinkebein, J. H. (2006). Cultural considerations when providing rehabilitation services to American Indians. *Rehabilitation Psychology, 51*(1), 36–42.

Lutz, B. J., & Bowers, B. J. (2003). Understanding how disability is defined and conceptualized in the literature. *Rehabilitation Nursing, 28*(3), 74–78.

Lysaght, R. M. (2004). Approaches to worker rehabilitation by occupational and physical therapists in the United States: Factors impacting practice. *Work, 23*(2), 139–146.

Manning, K., & Haldi, P. (2007). Specific disease processes requiring rehabilitation interventions. In K. L. Mauk (Ed.), *The specialty practice of rehabilitation nursing: A core curriculum* (pp. 275–322). Glenview, IL: Association of Rehabilitation Nurses.

Masters-Farrell, P. A. (2006). Ethical/legal principles and issues. In K. L. Mauk (Ed.), *Gerontological nursing: Competencies for care* (pp. 589–616). Sudbury, MA: Jones and Bartlett.

Masters-Farrell, P. A. (2007). Ethical, moral, and legal considerations. In K. L. Mauk (Ed.), *The specialty practice of rehabilitation nursing: A core curriculum* (pp. 27–34). Glenview, IL: Association of Rehabilitation Nurses.

Mauk, K. L. (2006). Nursing interventions within the Mauk Model of Poststroke Recovery. *Rehabilitation Nursing, 31*(6), 267–263.

Mauk, K. L., & Hanson, P. (2010). Management of common illnesses, diseases, and health conditions. In K. L. Mauk (Ed.), *Gerontological nursing: Competencies for care* (pp. 382–453). Sudbury, MA: Jones & Bartlett .

Mauk, K. L., & Lehman, C. (2007). Geriatric rehabilitation. In K. L. Mauk (Ed.), *The specialty practice of rehabilitation nursing: A core curriculum,* (pp. 359–383). Glenview, IL: Association of Rehabilitation Nurses.

Mezey, M., & Fulmer, T. (2002). The future history of gerontological nursing. *Journal of Gerontology A Biological Sciences Medical Sciences, 57*(7), M438–441.

Mills, P., Yu, H., Ziegler, M., Patterson, T., & Grant, I. (1999). Vulnerable caregivers of patients with Alzheimer's disease have a deficit in circulating CD62L-T lymphocytes. *Psychosomatic Medicine, 61*(2), 168–174.

Minority Business Development Agency. (1999). *Dynamic diversity: Projected changes in U.S. race and ethnic composition 1995 to 2050.* Retrieved September 21, 2011, from: http://www.mbda.gov/sites/default/files/DynamicDiversityProjectedChanges_0.pdf

Monahan, F. D., Sands, J. K., Neighbors, M., Marek, J. F., & Green, C. J. (2007). *Phipps' medical-surgical nursing: Health and illness perspectives* (8th ed.). St. Louis: Mosby Elsevier.

Morgan, J. E. (2007). *Successful outcomes in vocational rehabilitation: The effects of stage of change and relational development.* Doctoral dissertation: Brandeis University.

Mpofu, E., & Harley, D. A. (2006). Racial and disability identity: Implications for the career counseling of African Americans with disabilities. *Rehabilitation Counseling Bulletin, 50*(1), 14–23.

Nadash, P., & Feldman, P. H. (2003). The effectiveness of a "restorative" model of care for home care patients. *Home Healthcare Nurse, 21*(6), 421–423.

National Association for Home Care and Hospice. (2007). Basic statistics about home care. Retrieved September 21, 2011, from: www.nahc.org/facts/07HC_stats.pdf

National Center for Chronic Disease Prevention and Health Promotion, Centers for Disease Control and Prevention. (2007). Quick facts: Economic and health burden of chronic disease. Retrieved September 21, 2011, from: www.cdc.gov/nccdphp/press/#4

National Institute on Aging. (2010). Alzheimer's disease fact sheet. Retrieved September 21, 2011, from: http://www.nia.nih.gov/Alzheimers/Publications/adfact.htm

National Organization on Disability. (2004). Executive summary of the 2000 N.O.D./Harris survey of Americans with disabilities. Retrieved September 21, 2011, from: http://www.nod.org/research_publications/nod_harris_survey/2000_survey_of_americans_with_disabilities/

Neal, L. J. (2001). Using rehabilitation theory to teach medical-surgical nursing to undergraduate students. *Rehabilitation Nursing, 26*(2), 72–75, 77.

Nelson, W. (2004). Addressing rural ethics issues. The characteristics of rural healthcare settings pose unique ethical challenges. *Healthcare Executive, 19*(4), 36–37.

Niemeier, J. P., Burnett, D. M., & Whitaker, D. A. (2003). Cultural competence in the multidisciplinary rehabilitation setting: Are we falling short of meeting needs? *Archives of Physical Medicine and Rehabilitation, 84*(8), 1240–1245.

O'Neill, J. H., Zuger, R. R., Fields, A., Fraser, R., & Pruce, T. (2004). The program without walls: Innovative approach to state agency vocational rehabilitation of persons with traumatic brain injury. *Archives of Physical Medicine and Rehabilitation, 85*(4), S68–72.

Ostchega, Y., Harris, T., Hirsch, R., Parsons, V., Kingston, R., & Katzoff, M. (2000). The prevalence of functional limitations and disability in older persons in the U.S.: Data from the National Health and Nutrition Examination Survey III. *Journal of the American Geriatrics Society, 48*, 1132–1135.

Osterweil, D. (1990). Geriatric rehabilitation in the long-term care institutional setting. In B. Kemp, K. Brummel-Smith, & J. Ramsdell (Eds.), *Geriatric rehabilitation* (pp. 347–456). Boston: Little, Brown.

Parker, B. J., & Neal-Boylan, L. (2007). Community and family-centered rehabilitation nursing. In K. L. Mauk (Ed.), *The specialty practice of rehabilitation nursing: A core curriculum* (pp. 13–26). Glenview, IL: Association of Rehabilitation Nurses.

People Living with Cancer. (2006). Rehabilitation. Retrieved December 1, 2007, from: http://www.cancer.net/patient/Survivorship/Rehabilitation/#mainContent.idmainContent

Pierce, L., Steiner, V., Govoni, A., Hicks, B., Thompson, T., & Friedemann, M. (2004). Caring-Web Internet-based support for rural caregivers of persons with stroke show promise. *Rehabilitation Nursing, 29*(3), 95–99, 103.

Pierce, L. L., Steiner, V., Hicks, B., & Holzaepfel, A. L. (2006). Problems of new caregivers of persons with stroke. *Rehabilitation Nursing, 31*(4), 166–172.

Plassman, B. L., Langa, K. M., Fisher, G. G., Heeringa, S. G., Weir, D. R., Ofstedal, M. B., et al. (2007). Prevalence of dementia in the United States: The aging, demographics, and memory study. *Neuroepidemiology, 29,* 125–132.

Podsiadlo, D., & Richardson S. (1991). The timed "up & go": A test of basic functional mobility for frail elderly persons. *Journal of the American Geriatric Society, 39,* 142–148.

Pope, A. M., & Tarlov, A. R. (1991). *Disability in America: Toward a national agenda for prevention.* Washington, DC: National Academy Press.

Pryor, J. (2002). Rehabilitative nursing: A core nursing function across all settings. *Collegian, 9*(2), 11–15.

Rehabilitation Services Administration. (2007). About RSA. Retrieved December 9, 2007, from: www.ed.gov/about/offices/list/osers/rsa/about.html

Reichard, A., Sacco, T. M., & Turnbull, H. R., III. (2004). Access to health care for individuals with developmental disabilities from minority backgrounds. *Mental Retardation, 42*(6), 459–470.

Remsburg, R. (2004). Restorative care activities. In B. Resnick (Ed.), *Restorative care nursing for older adults: A guide for all care settings* (pp. 74–95). New York: Springer.

Remsburg, R., Armacost, K., Radu, C., & Bennett, R. (1999). Comparison of two models of restorative care in the nursing home. *Geriatric Nursing, 20*(6), 321–326.

Remsburg, R., Armacost, K., Radu, C., & Bennett, R. (2001). Impact of a restorative care program in the nursing home. *Educational Gerontology: An International Journal, 27,* 261–280.

Remsburg, R., & Carson, B. (2006). Rehabilitation. In I. Lubkin & P. Larsen (Eds.). *Chronic illness: Impact and interventions* (pp. 579–616). Sudbury, MA: Jones and Bartlett.

Resnick, B., & Fleishell, A. (2002). Developing a restorative care program: A five-step approach that involves the resident. *American Journal of Nursing, 102*(7), 91–95.

Resnick, B., & Remsburg, R. (2004). Overview of restorative care. In B. Resnick (Ed.), *Restorative care nursing for older adults: A guide for all care settings,* (pp. 1–12). New York: Springer.

Routasalo, P., Arve, S., & Lauri, S. (2004). Geriatric rehabilitation nursing: Developing a model. *International Journal of Nursing Practice, 10*(5), 207–215.

Rusk, H. (1965). Preventive Medicine, curative medicine—The rehabilitation. *New Physician, 59*(4), 156–160.

Santerre, R. E. (2002). The inequity of Medicaid reimbursement in the United States. *Applied Health Economics and Health Policy, 1*(1), 25–32.

Schulz, R., & Beach, S. (1999). Caregiving as a risk factor for mortality: The caregiver health effects study. *Journal of the American Medical Association, 282*(23), 2215–2219.

Secrest, J. A. (2007). Rehabilitation and rehabilitation nursing. In K. Mauk (Ed.), *The specialty practice of rehabilitation nursing: A core curriculum* (5th ed., pp. 2–12). Glenview, IL: Association of Rehabilitation Nurses.

Secrest, J. A., & Thomas, S. P. (1999). Continuity and discontinuity: The quality of life following stroke. *Rehabilitation Nursing, 24*(6), 240–246.

Secrest, J. A., & Zeller, R. (2003). Measuring continuity and discontinuity following stroke. *Journal of Nursing Scholarship, 35*(3), 243–249.

Secrest, J. A., & Zeller, R. (2007). The relationship of continuity and discontinuity, functional ability, depression, and quality of life over time in stroke survivors. *Rehabilitation Nursing, 32*(4), 158–164.

Shah, S. K. (2005). Cardiac rehabilitation. In J. DeLisa & B. M. Gans (Eds.), *Rehabilitation medicine: Principles and practice* (3rd ed., pp. 1811–1842). Philadelphia: Lippincott-Raven.

Shanks, L. C., Moore, S. M., & Zeller, R. A. (2007). Predictors of cardiac rehabilitation initiation. *Rehabilitation Nursing, 32*(4), 152–157.

Shaw, W., Patterson, T., Ziegler, M., Dimsdale, J., et al. (1999). Accelerated risk of hypertensive blood pressure recordings among Alzheimer caregivers. *Journal of Psychosomatic Medicine, 43*(3), 215–227.

Shirey, L., & Summer, L. (2000). *Caregiving: Helping the elderly with activity limitations. Challenges for the 21st century: Chronic and disabling conditions.* Washington, DC: National Academy on an Aging Society.

Singh, V. N., Schocken, D. D., Williams, K., & Stamey, R. (2004). Cardiac rehabilitation. *EMedicine.* Retrieved September 21, 2011, from: www.emedicine.com/pmr/topic180.htm

Ski, C., & O'Connell, B. (2007). Stroke: The increasing complexity of carer needs. *Journal of Neuroscience Nursing, 39*(3), 172–179.

Social Security Online. (2007). Supplemental security income. Retrieved September 21, 2011, from: www.ssa.gov/pubs/11000.html#part3

Stuart, H. (2006, September). Mental illness and employment discrimination. *Current Opinion in Psychiatry, 5*, 522–526.

Targett, P., Wehman, P., & Young, C. (2004). Return to work for persons with spinal cord injury: Designing work supports. *Neurorehabilitation. 19*(2), 131–139.

Thompson, T. L., Emrich, K., & Moore, G. (2003). The effect of curriculum on the attitudes of nursing students toward disability. *Rehabilitation Nursing, 28*(1), 27–30.

Uniform Data System for Medical Rehabilitation. (1997). FIM™ Instrument. University at Buffalo, Buffalo, NY, 14214.

U.S. Department of Education. (2005). Office of Special Education and Rehabilitation Services. Rehabilitation Services Administration. Retrieved September 21, 2011, from: http://www.ed.gov/about/offices/list/osers/index.html

U.S. Department of Health and Human Services, & The Agency for Health Quality and Research. (2003). The national health disparities report, 2003. Retrieved September 21, 2011, from: http://www.ahrq.gov/qual/nhdr03/nhdrsum03.htm

U.S. Equal Opportunity Employment Commission. (2008). Americans with Disabilities Act. Retrieved September 29, 2011 from www.eeoc.gov/facts/fs-ada.html

Vargo, M. M., & Gerber, L. H. (2005). Rehabilitation for patients with cancer diagnoses. In J. DeLisa & B. Gans (Eds.), *Physical medicine and rehabilitation: Principles and practice* (4th ed., pp. 1771–1794). Philadelphia: Lippincott Williams & Wilkins.

Verville, R., & DeLisa, J. A. (2001). The evolution of Medicare financing policy for graduate medical education and implications for PM&R: A commentary. *Archives of Physical Medicine and Rehabilitation, 82*(4), 558–562.

Walsh, N. E., Dumitru, D., Schoenfeld, L. S., & Ramaurthy, S. (2005). Treatment of the patient with chronic pain. In J. DeLisa & B. Gans (Eds.), *Physical medicine and rehabilitation: Principles and practice* (4th ed., pp. 493–530). Philadelphia: Lippincott Williams & Wilkins.

Ward, A. B., & Gutenbrunner, C. (2006). Physical and rehabilitation medicine in Europe. *Journal of Rehabilitation Medicine, 38*, 81–86.

Watson, P. (1990). The Americans with Disabilities Act: More rights for people with disabilities. *Rehabilitation Nursing*, 15, 326. Published by the Association of Rehabilitation Nurses, 4700 W. Lake Avenue, Glenview, IL 60025-1485.

Weitzenkamp, D., Gerhart, K., Charlifue, S., Whiteneck, G., & Savic, G. (1997). Spouses of spinal cord injury survivors: The added impact of caregiving. *Archives of Physical Medicine and Rehabilitation, 78*(8), 822–827.

Whyte, J. (1998). Enabling America: A report from the Institute of Medicine on rehabilitation science and engineering. *Archives of Physical Medicine and Rehabilitation, 79*(11), 1477–1480.

World Health Organization. (1980). International classification of impairments, disabilities and handicaps. Geneva, Switzerland: Author.

World Health Organization. (2002). *Towards a common language for functioning, disability and health ICF.* Retrieved September 21, 2011, from: www.who.int/classifications/icf/training/icfbeginnersguide.pdf

World Health Organization. (2007). International classification of functioning, disability, and health. Retrieved December 5, 2007, from: http://www.who.int/classifications/icf/en

Worsowicz, G. M., Stewart, D. G., Phillips, E. M., & Cifu, D. X. (2004). Geriatric rehabilitation: Social and economic implications of aging. *Archives of Physical Medicine and Rehabilitation, 85*(Suppl. 3), S3–6.

Wu, H., Wang, J., Cacioppo, J., Glaser, R., Kiecolt-Glaser, J. K., & Malarkey, W. B. (1999). Chronic stress associated with spousal caregiving of patients with Alzheimer's dementia is associated with down regulation of B-lymphocyte GH mRNA. *Journal of Gerontology A Biologic Science/Medical Science, 54*(4), M212–215.

Yip, K., & Ng, Y. (2002). Chinese cultural dynamics of unemployability of male adults with psychiatric disabilities in Hong Kong. *Psychiatric Rehabilitation Journal, 26*(2), 197–202.

Yu, F. (2005). Factors affecting outpatient rehabilitation outcomes in elders. *Journal of Nursing Scholarship, 37*(3), 229–236.

Zola, I. K. (1982). *Disincentives to independent living.* Lawrence, KS: Research and Training Center on Independent Living, University of Kansas.

INDEX

Page numbers followed by a *t* or *f* indicate tables or figures, respectively.